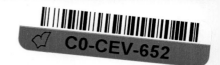
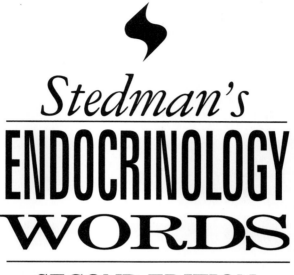

Stedman's
ENDOCRINOLOGY
WORDS

SECOND EDITION

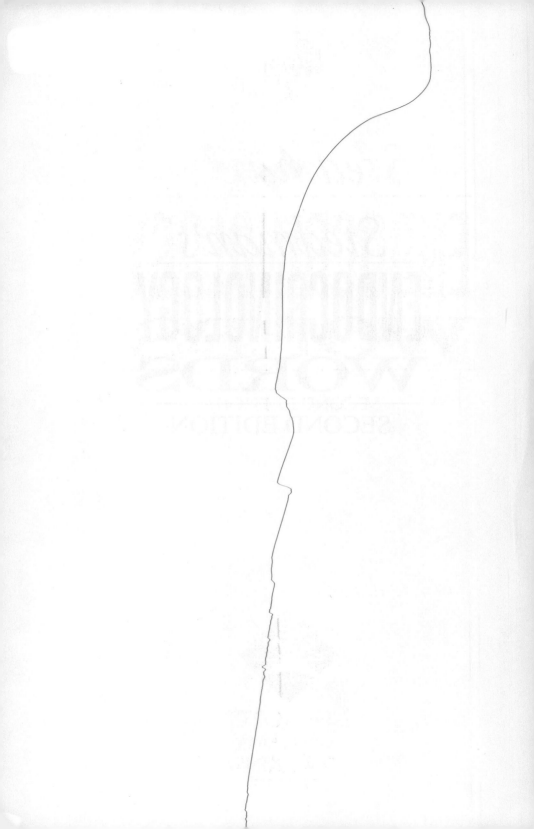

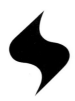

Stedman's
ENDOCRINOLOGY
WORDS

SECOND EDITION

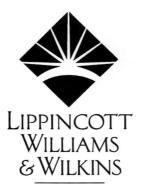

LIPPINCOTT
WILLIAMS
& WILKINS

Publisher: Julie K. Stegman
Senior Product Manager: Eric Branger
Managing Editor: Amy Millholen
Typesetter: Josephine Bergin
Printer & Binder: Malloy Litho, Inc.

Second Edition, 2006

Library of Congress Cataloging-in-Publication Data

Stedman's endocrinology words.— 2nd ed.
　　p. ; cm.— (Stedman's word books)
Includes bibliographical references.
ISBN 0-7817-6173-5 (alk. paper)
　1. Endocrinology—Terminology. I. Stedman, Thomas Lathrop, 1853-1938. II. Title: Endocrinology words. III. Series.
　[DNLM: 1. Endocrine Glands—Terminology—English. 2. Endocrine System Diseases—Terminology—English. WK 15 S812 2006]
RC649.S74 2006
616.4'001'4--dc22

2005019443

06
1 2 3 4 5 6 7 8 9 10

Contents

Acknowledgements

An important part of our editorial process is the involvement of medical transcriptionists—as advisors, reviewers, and editors.

We extend special thanks to Sandy Kovacs and Patty White for editing the manuscript and helping to resolve many difficult questions. Our appreciation also goes to Janet West for revising and developing the appendices. We are grateful to advisory board members Ann Hall, Angela Kelly, Andrea Linderman, Beth Pessetto, and Janet West, who shared their valuable judgment, insight, and perspective.

Our appreciation goes to the following contributors who helped to enhance the A-to-Z content for this edition: Sue Bartolucci, Marty Cantu, Trista DiPaula, Ann Hall, Robin Koza, Helen Littrell, Andrea Linderman, Beth Pessetto, Lauri Rebar, and Janet West. We also extend thanks to Jeanne Bock and Andrea Linderman for their assistance with the Sample Reports appendix. Thanks to Helen Littrell for performing the final prepublication review.

We thank Barb Ferretti, who played an integral role in the process by reviewing the content files for format and updating the manuscript.

As with all our Stedman's word references, this resource incorporates the suggestions and expertise of our many contacts in the medical transcriptionist community. Thanks to all of our advisory board participants, reviewers, and editors; AAMT meeting attendees; and others who have written us with requests and comments—keep talking, and we'll keep listening.

Editors' Preface

How would you define a partner? The Merriam-Webster on-line dictionary says a partner is "one associated with another especially in an action." Synonyms are "associate," "colleague," and "spouse." How boring life would be if we did not have partners, people to share the work and also the fun?

My partner in editing this second edition of *Stedman's Endocrinology Words* was Patty White, CMT, FAAMT. We live many, many miles apart, yet through advances in technology, we can work closely together to create an updated reference book to put on your bookshelf. This book would not be as comprehensive and complete if I did not have Patty as my partner. She brings a different perspective to the table because she has worked as an editor for a national MT service for many years.

I like to think of my reference books as my partners in the quest for excellent quality reports. Without them, I would not feel confident in the accuracy of many new terms that come across my headsets every day. It is our hope that this book will be one of your partners.

Endocrinology can be a challenging specialty to transcribe because of the unusual syndromes, multiple hormones and genes, and medications that are discussed in detail in consultations and office notes. There are many terms related to diabetes and the symptoms/conditions that can develop as a sequela of diabetes such as renal insufficiency or failure, retinopathy, and neuropathy. Exciting advances have been made in diabetes care over the past few years, and we have included many new terms related to diabetes, such as new devices for insulin administration and drugs that have been recently approved for use by the FDA. There is a new section in the appendix that shows a list of diseases that can affect each gland in the endocrine system. Review the sample reports. There are many excellent examples of clinic notes, H&Ps, discharge summaries, consultations, and operation reports. We have added some interesting illustrations related to hemodialysis and peritoneal dialysis. These certainly help me to understand that complicated process more fully.

I would like to thank Amy Millholen for giving Patty and I the opportunity to "partner" with her. Once again, LWW has stepped up and filled the need for updated reference materials for medical transcriptionists, and for this we thank you very much!

Enjoy this book, use it to help you produce the highest quality reports you possibly can, and put that partner on its shelf to rest after a day of intense transcription.

As a final note, here are comments from Patty: To answer the question that my partner, Sandy Kovacs, CMT, FAAMT, posed in the preface of the first edition of *Endocrinology Words*, "Yes, I love reference books." My office bookshelf is filled with a rainbow of books, many of which I've had the pleasure to work on. Sandy and I were privileged to edit the first edition of *Stedman's Endocrinology Words* a few years ago and have teamed again in hopes of making this second edition even more useful. Every time I think that there can't be enough new terms to warrant a new edition of any title, I'm totally amazed at what needs to be added during the review process. Today's ongoing research into the causes and cures of such common problems as thyroid disorders and the ever-increasing incidence of diabetes, as well as many other endocrine conditions, produces a continuous supply of new terms, so much so that we as MTs cannot stop learning even if we wanted to. I hope you enjoy learning these new words as much as we do.

Sandy Kovacs, CMT, FAAMT
Patricia White, CMT, FAAMT

Publisher's Preface

Stedman's Endocrinology Words, Second Edition, offers an authoritative assurance of quality and exactness to the wordsmiths of the healthcare professions—medical transcriptionists, medical editors and copyeditors, health information management personnel, court reporters, and the many other users and producers of medical documentation.

In *Stedman's Endocrinology Words, Second Edition*, users will find thousands of words as they relate to the thyroid, diabetes, and hormones. Users will also find terms for protocols, diagnostic and therapeutic procedures, new techniques, and lab tests, as well as equipment names, and abbreviations with their expansions. The appendix sections provide anatomical illustrations with useful captions and labels, sample reports, and common terms by procedure, as well as normal lab values, endocrine gland locations and functions, endocrine glands and associated products, common disorders by gland, diabetes classifications, complications of diabetes, wound care products, and drugs by indication.

This compilation of more than 37,600 terms, fully cross-indexed for quick access, includes over 1,500 more terms than the first edition. The extensive A-Z list was developed from manufacturers' literature, scientific reports, books, journals, CDs, and web sites (please see list of References on page xvii).

We at Lippincott Williams & Wilkins strive to provide you with the most up-to-date and accurate word references available. Your use of this Word Book will prompt new editions, which we will publish as often as updates and revisions justify. We welcome your suggestions for improvements, changes, corrections, and additions—whatever will make this Stedman's product more useful to you. Please complete the postage-paid card in this book for future suggestions and recommendations, or visit us online at www.stedmans.com.

Explanatory Notes

Medical transcription is an art as well as a science. Both approaches are needed to correctly interpret the dictation of a physician, whose language is a product of education, training, and experience. This variety in medical language means that there are several acceptable ways to express certain terms, including jargon. *Stedman's Endocrinology Words, Second Edition*, provides variant spellings and phrasings for many terms. These elements, in addition to complete cross-indexing, make *Stedman's Endocrinology Words, Second Edition*, a valuable resource for determining the validity of terms as they are encountered.

Alphabetical Organization

Alphabetization of main entries is letter by letter as spelled, ignoring punctuation, spaces, prefixed numbers, or other characters. For example:

Potter facies
pouch
POU1F1 gene

Terms beginning or ending with Greek letters show the Greek letters spelled out and listed alphabetically. For example:

gamma
interferon g.
neuropeptide g.
g. unit

In subentry alphabetization, the abbreviated singular form or the spelled-out plural form of the noun main entry word is ignored.

Format and Style

All main entries are in boldface to expedite locating a sought-after term, to enhance distinction between main entries and subentries, and to relieve the textual density of the pages.

Irregular plurals and variant spellings are shown on the same line as the singular or preferred form of the word. For example:

locus, pl. loci
disk, disc

Hyphenation

As a rule of style, multiple eponyms (e.g., Prader-Willi syndrome) are hyphenated. Also, hyphens have been added between a manufacturer and one or more eponyms (e.g., Vital-Metzenbaum dissecting scissors). Please note that in many cases, hyphenation is a question of style, not of accuracy, and thus is a matter of choice.

Possessives

Possessive forms have been dropped in this reference for the sake of consistency and conformance with the guidelines of the American Association for Medical Transcription (AAMT) and other groups. Please note, however, that in many cases, retaining the possessive, like hyphenating, is a question of style, not of accuracy, and thus is a matter of choice. To form the possessive of a word, simply add the apostrophe or apostrophe "s" to the end of the word.

Cross-indexing

The word list is in an index-like main entry-subentry format that contains two combined alphabetical listings:

(1) A noun main entry-subentry organization, which is typical of the A-Z section of medical dictionaries like *Stedman's*:

cancer
   liver c.
   medullary thyroid c.

puberty
   pseudoprecocious p.
   stalled p.

(2) An *adjective* main entry-subentry organization, which lists words and phrases as you hear them. The main entries are the adjectives or modifiers in a multiword term. The subentries are the nouns around which the terms are constructed and to which the adjectives or modifiers pertain:

hereditary
    h. angioneurotic edema
    h. ataxia

partial
    p. hypopituitarism
    p. insulin resistance

This format provides the user with more than one way to locate and identify a multiword term. For example:

peripheral
    p. blood lymphocyte

lymphocyte
    peripheral blood l.

thyroid
    t. radioiodine uptake

uptake
    thyroid radioiodine u.

QuickLance
    Q. lancing device

device
    QuickLance lancing d.

It also allows the user to see together all terms that contain a particular descriptor, as well as all types, kinds, or variations of a noun entity. For example:

calcitonin
    c. monomer
    c. receptor
    salmon c.

primary
    p. infertility
    intrathyroidal p.
    p. macronodular hyperplasia

Wherever possible, abbreviations are separately defined and cross-referenced. For example:

TBS
total body scan

total
t. body scan (TBS)

scan
total body s. (TBS)

References

In addition to the manufacturers' literature we gather at various medical meetings, scientific reports from hospitals, and the lists of our MT Editorial Advisory Board members (from their daily transcription work), we used the following sources for new terms in *Stedman's Endocrinology Words, Second Edition.*

Books

Becker KL, Bilezikian JP, Bremner WJ, et al. Principles and Practice of Endocrinology and Metabolism, 3rd ed. Baltimore: Lippincott Williams & Wilkins, 2000.

Braverman LE, Utiger RD (eds.). Werner & Ingbar's The Thyroid: A Fundamental and Clinical Text, 9th ed. Philadelphia: Lippincott Williams Wilkins, 2005.

Burch WM. Endocrinology, 3rd ed. Baltimore: Lippincott Williams & Wilkins, 1994.

Bushinsky DA. Renal Osteodystrophy. Philadelphia: Lippincott-Raven Publishers, 1998.

Camacho PM, Gharib H, Sizemore GW (eds.). Evidence-Based Endocrinology. Philadelphia: Lippincott Williams Wilkins, 2003.

Copeland EM, Bland KI, Deitch EA, et al. Year Book of Surgery 2000. St. Louis: Mosby, 2000.

Falk SA. Thyroid Disease, 2nd ed. Philadelphia: Lippincott-Raven Publishers, 1997.

Gass GH, Kaplan HM, eds. Handbook of Endocrinology, 2nd ed, Volumes 1 & 2. Boca Raton: CRC Press, 1996.

Greenspan FS, Strewler GJ. Basic & Clinical Endocrinology, 5th ed. New York: McGraw-Hill, 1997.

Guyton AC, Hall JE. Human Physiology and Mechanisms of Disease, 6th ed. Philadelphia: Saunders, 1996.

Guyton AC, Hall JE. Textbook of Medical Physiology, 9th ed. Philadelphia: Saunders, 1995.

Henderson KE, Baranski TJ, Bickel PE (eds.). The Washington Manual: Endocrinology Subspecialty Consult. Philadelphia: Lippincott Williams Wilkins, 2005.

Kacsoh B. Endocrine Physiology. New York: McGraw-Hill, 2000.

Kahn CR, Weir GC, King GL, Jacobson AM, Moses AC, Smith RJ (eds.). Joslin's Diabetes Mellitus, 14th ed. Philadelphia: Lippincott Williams Wilkins, 2005.

Kettyle WM, Arky RA. Lippincott's Pathophysiology Series: Endocrine Pathophysiology. Philadelphia: Lippincott-Raven Publishers, 1998.

Krisht A, Tindall G. Pituitary Disorders. Baltimore: Lippincott Williams & Wilkins, 1998.

Lance LL. 2005 Quick Look Drug Book. Baltimore: Lippincott Williams & Wilkins, 2005.

Lavin N (ed.). Manual of Endocrinology and Metabolism, 3rd ed. Philadelphia: Lippincott Williams Wilkins, 2002.

LeRoith D, Taylor SI, Olefsky JM (eds.). Diabetes Mellitus: A Fundamental and Clinical Text, 3rd ed. Philadelphia: Lippincott Williams Wilkins, 2004.

Martin CR. Dictionary of Endocrinology and Related Biomedical Sciences. Oxford: Oxford University Press, 1995.

McDermott MT. Endocrine Secrets, 2nd ed. Philadelphia: Hanley & Belfus, Inc., 1998.

Pescovitz OH, Eugster EA (eds.). Pediatric Endocrinology: Mechanisms, Manifestations, and Management. Philadelphia: Lippincott Williams Wilkins, 2004.

Pyle V. Current Medical Terminology, 8th ed. Modesto: Health Professions Institute, 2000.

Reece EA, Coustan DR, Gabbe SG. Diabetes in Women: Adolescence, Pregnancy, and Menopause, 3rd ed. Philadelphia: Lippincott Williams Wilkins, 2004.

Skyler JS (ed.). Atlas of Diabetes, 2nd ed. Philadelphia: Lippincott Williams Wilkins, 2002.

Speroff L, Fritz MA. Clinical Gynecologic Endocrinology and Infertility, 7th ed. Philadelphia: Lippincott Williams Wilkins, 2005.

Stedman's Medical Dictionary, 27th ed. Baltimore: Lippincott Williams & Wilkins, 2000.

Styne DM. Pediatric Endocrinology. Philadelphia: Lippincott Williams Wilkins, 2004.

Tessier C. The American Association of Medical Transcriptionists Book of Style. Modesto: AAMT, 1995.

Weintraub BD. Molecular Endocrinology. New York: Raven Press, Ltd., 1994.

Wilson JD, Foster DW, Kronenberg HM, Larsen PR. Williams Textbook of Endocrinology, 9th ed. Philadelphia: Saunders, 1998.

Journals

Current Opinion in Endocrinology & Diabetes. Philadelphia: Lippincott Williams Wilkins, 2004.

The Endocrinologist. Philadelphia: Lippincott Williams Wilkins, 2004-2005.

Endocrinology. Bethesda: The Endocrine Society, 2000.

Internal Medicine. Montvale, NJ: Medical Economics, 1996-1997.

Menopause. Philadelphia: Lippincott Williams Wilkins, 2004-2005.

Molecular Endocrinology. Bethesda: The Endocrine Society, 2000.

Images

Agur AMR, Lee MJ. Grant's Atlas of Anatomy, 10th ed. Baltimore: Lippincott Williams & Wilkins, 1999.

Barratt-Dimes MA. Parkton, MD. Stedman's Medical Dictionary, 27th ed. Baltimore: Lippincott Williams & Wilkins, 2000.

Caldwell S. Pikesville, MD. Stedman's Medical Dictionary, 27th ed. Baltimore: Lippincott Williams & Wilkins, 2000.

Hardy NO. Westport, CT. Stedman's Medical Dictionary, 27th ed. Baltimore: Lippincott Williams & Wilkins, 2000.

LifeART Nursing 2, CD-ROM. Baltimore: Lippincott Williams & Wilkins.

LifeART Nursing 3, CD-ROM. Baltimore: Lippincott Williams & Wilkins.

LifeART Pediatrics 1, CD-ROM. Baltimore: Lippincott Williams & Wilkins.

LifeART Super Anatomy Collection 4, CD-ROM. Baltimore: Lippincott Williams & Wilkins.

LifeART Super Anatomy Collection 9, CD-ROM. Baltimore: Lippincott Williams & Wilkins.

MediClip Clinical OB/GYN Images, CD-ROM. Baltimore: Lippincott Williams & Wilkins.

From Pillitteri A. Maternal and Child Nursing, 4th Ed. Philadelphia: Lippincott, Williams & Wilkins, 2003.

Sauerland, EK. Grant's Dissector, 12th ed. Baltimore: Lippincott Williams & Wilkins, 1999.

Senkarik M. San Antonio, TX. Stedman's Medical Dictionary, 27th ed. Baltimore: Lippincott Williams & Wilkins, 2000.

From Smeltzer SC, Bare BG. Textbook of Medical-Surgical Nursing, 9th ed. Philadelphia: Lippincott Williams & Wilkins, 2000.

Ward L. Salt Lake City, UT. Stedman's Medical Dictionary, 27th ed. Baltimore: Lippincott Williams & Wilkins, 2000.

Websites

http://diabetes.about.com

http://www.aace.com

http://www.diabetesnet.com

http://www.diabetes.org/professionalpublications

http://www.endo.edoc.com

http://www.endocrine.medscape.com/Medscape/features/JournalScan/public/index_JournalScan.html

http://www.eurothyroid.org

http://hpisum.com

http://www.jdf.org

http://www.mtdesk.com/newterms.shtml

http://www.niddk.nih.gov

http://www.thyroid.org

CD

UpToDate Clinical Reference Library on CD, Version 8:2. Wellesley, MA: UpToDate, 2000.

A

alpha-preprotachykinin A
aminopeptidase A
bafilomycin A
beta-hydroxy-beta-methylglutaryl-
coenzyme A (HMG-CoA)
beta-preprotachykinin A
biochanin A
botulinum toxin type A
bovine chromogranin A (bCgA)
A cell
coenzyme A (CoA)
cyclosporin A
A element insulin gene promoter
gamma-preprotachykinin A
hemoglobin A
hemophilia A
hepatitis A
hypervitaminosis A
immunoglobulin A (IgA)
inhibin A
Orexin A
platelet-derived growth factor A
(PDGF-A)
proenkephalin A
A proliferation-inducing ligand
(APRIL)
protein kinase A (PKA)

a

phosphorylase *a*

A_0

hemoglobin A_0

A_1

A_1 cell
vitamin A_1

A-1

apoprotein A-1

A2

thromboxane A2 (TXA2, TxA2)

A_2

A_2 cell
phospholipase A_2 (PLA_2)
vitamin A_2

3A

A_4

leukotriene A_4 (LTA_4)

A9

coxsackievirus A9

A23187

Ca^{2+} ionophore A23187

AA

arachidonic acid
platelet-derived growth factor AA

A_1a

hemoglobin A_1a

AA-NAT

arylalkylamine *N*-acetyltransferase

AASH

adrenal androgen-stimulating hormone

AAV

adeno-associated virus

Ab

antibody
TPO Ab
thyroperoxidase antibody

A_1b

hemoglobin A_1b

AB amyloidosis

abarelix

Abbott AxSYM assay

ABC

adenosine triphosphate binding cassette

abdominal

a. obesity
a. paracentesis
a. stria

abdominoperineal resection

abducent nerve

aberrant

a. behavior
a. expression
a. mediastinal thyroid tissue
a. motility
a. ribonucleic acid

abetalipoproteinemia

recessive a.

abiotic environmental factor

ablation

alcohol a.
cell-specific a.
ovarian a.
thyroidal a.
thyroid gland a.

abluminal compartment

abnormal

a. fetal growth
a. ocular movement
a. parathyroid gland
a. regulation of calcium-dependent
parathyroid hormone secretion
a. set point

abnormality

congenital a.
endocrine a.
gastric motor a.
gastric myoelectric a.
lipid a.
multiple endocrine a.'s (MEA)
primary immunoregulatory a.
pupillary a.

abnormality *(continued)*
    receptor-binding a.
    set point a.
    thyroid-stimulating hormone a.
ABP
  androgen-binding protein
abscess
    amebic brain a.
    gas-containing a.
    parathyroidal a.
    pituitary a.
abscissa
absent septum pellucidum
Absidia
absolute
    a. leptin deficiency
    a. leptin resistance
    a. thyroidal uptake rate
absorbable gelatin film roll
absorptiometry
    dual-energy x-ray a. (DEXA, DXA)
    dual-photon a.
    dual-x-ray a.
    single-photon a. (SPA)
absorption
    calcium a.
    enhanced proximal tubular salt a.
    enteral aluminum a.
    fluid a.
    gastrointestinal calcium a.
    insulin a.
    intestinal a.
    net calcium a.
    salt a.
absorptive
    a. endocytosis
    a. hypercalciuria
abzyme
A/C
  albumin creatinine
    A/C ratio
A_{1c}, $A1_c$
    glycated hemoglobin A_{1c}
    hemoglobin A_{1c} (HbA_1c)
    spuriously elevated hemoglobin A_{1c}
acarbose
    a. cardiovascular risk reduction
    a. coagulation activation
    a. combination therapy
    a. hypoglycemia
    a. insulin sensitivity
    a. lipid metabolism
    a. plasma insulin
    a. type 2 diabetes mellitus risk reduction
    a. with insulin
    a. with metformin

ACAT
  acyl-coenzyme A cholesterol acyltransferase
ACC
  aplasia cutis congenita
accelerated
    a. catabolism
    a. thyrotoxicosis
Accelerator
    Triax Metabolic A.
accessory
    a. adrenocortical rest
    a. molecule
Access Ostase blood test
acclimation
acclimatization
accommodative target
accretion
    bone mass a.
    bone mineral a.
Accu-Chek
    A.-C. Active glucose meter
    A.-C. Advantage glucose meter
    A.-C. Advantage non-wipe blood glucose monitoring system
    A.-C. Comfort Curve test strip
    A.-C. Compact glucose meter
    A.-C. Complete blood glucose monitoring system
    A.-C. Complete glucose meter system
    A.-C. II Freedom
    A.-C. III
    A.-C. Instant glucose meter
    A.-C. InstantPlus
    A.-C. Simplicity blood glucose monitoring system
    A.-C. SoftClix lancet device
    A.-C. Soft Touch lancing device
    A.-C. Voicemate glucose meter
accuDEXA bone mineral assessment device
Acculink Modem
accumulation
    aluminum a.
    intrahepatocellular triglyceride a.
    osteoid a.
    visceral fat a.
Accutility Software
acebutolol
acellular desquamated keratin
Acephen
acervulus, pl. **acervuli**
    acervuli cerebri
acesulfame-K
acesulfame potassium
acetate
    buserelin a.
    calcium a.

cortisone a.
Cortone A.
cyproterone a.
depot medroxyprogesterone a.
(DMPA)
desmopressin a.
estradiol/norethindrone a.
Florinef A.
fludrocortisone a.
leuprolide a.
medroxyprogesterone a. (MPA)
megestrol a. (MA)
nomegestrole a.
norethindrone a.
paramethasone a.
pexiganan a.
pramlintide a.
sermorelin a.
sodium a.
[13C]-acetate test
acetazolamide
Acetest
acetic acid
acetoacetate
acetoacetic acid
acetoacetyl-CoA thiolase
acetohexamide
acetone
acetylate
acetylation
histone a.
acetylcholine (ACh)
acetyl-CoA deficiency
acetyl-coenzyme A
acetylcysteine
acetylglucosamine
acetyl-L-carnitine
acetylsalicylic acid
acetyltransferase
bacterial chloramphenicol a.
choline a. (ChAT)
histone a. (HAT)
_N_-acetyltransferase
arylalkylamine _N_-a. (AA-NAT)
ACh
acetylcholine
ACh receptor-inducing activity
(ARIA)
**achalasia-addisonianism-alacrima
syndrome**
achlorhydria
gastric a.

syndrome of watery diarrhea,
hypokalemia, and a.
watery diarrhea, hypokalemia, a.
(WDHA)
achondrogenesis type II
acid
aberrant ribonucleic a.
acetic a.
acetoacetic a.
acetylsalicylic a.
3′,5′ adenylic a.
alanine amino a.
alpha-amino-3-hydroxy-5methyl-4-
isoxazole propionic a.
amino a.
aminoisobutyric a. (AIBA)
antidouble-stranded
deoxyribonucleic a.
arachidonic a. (AA)
ascorbic a.
a. ash diet
aspartic a.
azaprostanoic a.
B9-B23 amino a.'s
benzoic a.
beta-cell nonesterified fatty a.
bile a.
branched-chain amino a.
calcitroic a.
carbonic a.
a. cholesteryl ester hydrolase
deficiency
9-_cis_ retinoic a. (RXR)
13-_cis_ retinoic a.
citric a.
complementary deoxyribonucleic a.
(cDNA)
deoxyribonucleic a. (DNA)
dicarboxylic a.
diethylamine triamine pentaacetic a.
(DTPA)
dihomo-gamma-linoleic a.
2′4-dihydroxybenzoic a.
dihydroxymandelic a. (DOMA)
dihydroxyphenylacetic a. (DOPAC)
4,4′-di-isothiocyanatostilbene-2,2′-
disulfonic a. (DIDS)
dimercaptosuccinic a. (DMSA,
DMSA-V-Tc99-m)
docosahexaenoic a. (DHA)
edetic a.
eicosapentaenoic a. (EPA)

NOTES

3

acid *(continued)*
  ergogenic a.
  essential fatty a. (EFA)
  ethacrynic a.
  ethylenediaminetetraacetic a.
    (EDTA)
  excitatory amino a.
  fatty a.
  ferrous salt and ascorbic a.
  ferrous sulfate, ascorbic acid,
    vitamin B complex, and folic a.
  fibric a.
  flufenemic a.
  folic a.
  free fatty a. (FFA)
  gamma-aminobutyric a. (GABA)
  gamma-carboxyglutamic a.
  gamma-carboxylated glutamic a.
  gamma-linolenic a. (GLA)
  glucaneogenic amino a.'s
  glucuronic a.
  glutamic a.
  glycyrrhetinic a.
  glycyrrhizinic a.
  homogentisic a.
  homovanillic a. (HVA)
  hyaluronic a.
  5-hydroperoxyeicosatetraenoic a. (5-
    HPETE)
  12-hydroperoxyeicosatetraenoic a.
    (12-HPETE)
  hydrophobic amino a.
  hydroxyeicosatetraenoic a. (HETE)
  5-hydroxyeicosatetraenoic a. (5-
    HETE)
  12-hydroxyeicosatetraenoic a. (12-
    HETE)
  15-hydroxyeicosatetraenoic a. (15-
    HETE)
  2-hydroxyglutaric a.
  5-hydroxyindoleacetic a. (5-HIAA)
  hydroxyisovaleric a.
  13-hydroxyoctadecadienoic a. (13-
    HODE)
  iodoamino a.
  iopanoic a.
  isobutyric a.
  isovaleric a.
  lactic a.
  linoleic a.
  mefenamic a.
  messenger ribonucleic a. (mRNA)
  5-methoxyindoleacetic a.
  2-methylbutyric a.
  methylmalonic a.
  mitochondrial deoxyribonucleic a.
    (mDNA, mtDNA)
  monosaturated fatty a.
  nalidixic a.

  nicotinic a.
  N-methyl D-aspartic a.
  nondissociated a.
  nonessential fatty a.'s
  nonesterified fatty a. (NEFA)
  okadaic a.
  oleic a.
  omega-3 polyunsaturated fatty a.
  orotic a.
  palmitic a.
  palmitoleic a.
  pantothenic a.
  paraaminobenzoic a.
  paraaminosalicylic a.
  peracetic a.
  a. phosphatase deficiency
  phosphatidic a.
  plasma free fatty a.
  polyunsaturated fatty a. (PUFA)
  potassium citrate and citric a.
  preproinsulin messenger
    ribonucleic a.
  pyroglutamic a.
  pyrophosphoric a.
  a. resistant/coated preparation
  resorcylic a.
  retinoic a.
  ribonucleic a. (RNA)
  sialic a.
  small nuclear ribonucleic a.
    (snRNA)
  a. solochrome azurin
  stearic a.
  sulfhydryl amino a.
  technetium-99m
    dimercaptosuccinic a. (^{99m}Tc-
    DMSA)
  tetraiodoacetic a.
  tetraiodothyroacetic a.
  thyroacetic a.
  tiglic a.
  tranexamic a.
  tranexamine a.
  transfer ribonucleic a. (tRNA)
  trans-retinoic a. (RAR)
  tricarboxylic a. (TCA)
  triiodoacetic a.
  triiodothyroacetic a.
  3,5,3'-triiodothyroacetic a. (TRIAC)
  unesterified arachidonic a.
  unsaturated fatty a.
  uric a.
  ursodeoxycholic a. (UDCA)
  valproic a.
  vanillylmandelic a. (VMA)
  vitamin B complex with vitamin C
    and folic a.
  zoledronic a.
acid-base balance

acidemia
 arginosuccinic a.
 glutaric a. type II
 isovaleric a.
 methylmalonic a.
 propionic a.
acidification
acid-labile subunit (ALS)
acidophil, acidophile
 somatotroph a.
acidophilic
 a. adenoma
 a. cell
 a. tumor
acidophilus
 lactobacillus a.
acidosis
 aldosterone-deficient hyperkalemic a.
 anion-gap a.
 chronic metabolic a.
 diabetic a. (DA)
 hyperchloremic metabolic a.
  (HCMA)
 lactic a.
 metabolic a.
 nonketotic hypoglycemic a.
 renal tubular a. (RTA)
 respiratory a.
 uncompensated metabolic a.
 uremic metabolic a.
acidotic coma
acid-Schiff
acid-Schiff-positive
 periodic a.-S.-p.
acid-stable protein
acid-tyrosine
 asparticacid/glutamic a.-t. (Asp/Glu-
  Tyr)
aciduria
 argininosuccinic a.
 glutaric a. type II
 methylmalonic a.
 propionic a.
 pyroglutamic a.
acinar
 a. differentiation
 a. gland
acinus, pl. **acini**
 glandular acini
Aciphex
acipimox

ACL
 acromegaly, cutis verticis, leukoma
  ACL syndrome
acne
 cystic a.
 steroid a.
acneiform eruption
ACPR30
 adipocyte complement related protein of
 30 kd
acquired
 a. end-organ resistance
 a. hypogonadotropic hypogonadism
 a. hypothyroidism
 a. immune deficiency
 a. immune deficiency syndrome
  (AIDS)
 a. immunity
 a. immunodeficiency syndrome
  (AIDS)
 a. immunodeficiency syndrome-
  related complex
 a. nephrogenic diabetes insipidus
 a. organification defect
 a. perforating dermatosis (APD)
 a. von Willebrand disease (AvWD)
acral
 a. enlargement
 a. overgrowth
acrodermatitis
acrodynia
acrodysostosis
acromegalic
 a. feature
 a. patient
 a. rosary
 a. symptom
acromegaloidism
acromegaly
 a., cutis verticis, leukoma (ACL)
 a., cutis verticis, leukoma
  syndrome
 ectopic a.
 hypothalamic a.
 pituitary tumor-related a.
acromelic shortening
acroosteolysis
acropachy
 thyroid a.
acrophase
acrosin

NOTES

acrosomal
- a. cap
- a. enzyme
- a. reaction
- a. vesicle

acrosome
- a. phase
- a. reaction

Actagen-C

ACTH
adrenocorticotrophin hormone
adrenocorticotropic hormone
- ACTH hypersecretion
- ACTH resistance

Acthar

ACTH-dependent Cushing syndrome

ACTH-independent
- A.-i. bilateral macronodular hyperplasia (AIBH)
- A.-i. Cushing syndrome

ACTH-producing thymoma

Acthrel

actin
- a. fibril
- a. filament
- a. scavenger system

actin-binding protein

actin-myosin complex

Actinobacillus actinomycetemcomitans

Actinomyces naeslundii

actinomycetemcomitans
- *Actinobacillus a.*

actinomycin

actinomycin-D

actinomycosis

action
- altered androgen a.
- antigonadotropic a.
- antinociceptive a.
- antipsoriatic a.
- autocrine a.
- extracellular cathepsin a.
- glucocorticoid a.
- hemocrine a.
- hypotriglyceridemic a.
- insulin a.
- intracrine a.
- neonatal diabetes mellitus insulin a.
- nongenomic a.
- paracrine a.
- peak a.
- phosphaturic a.
- pituitary resistance to thyroid hormone a.
- a. potential
- thyroid hormone a.
- thyromimetic a.

Actiq Oral Transmucosal

activated
- a. charcoal
- a. Hageman factor
- a. protein C resistance

activating
- a. cytokine
- a. factor

activation
acarbose coagulation a.
- adrenergic receptor a.
- Akt a.
- atypical protein kinase C a.
- B-cell a.
- ectopic intrapancreatic protease a.
- a. energy
- gonadotropin-releasing hormone a.
- G protein a.
- insulin-stimulated sympathetic a.
- neutrophil a.
- purinergic a.
- steroid hormone receptor a.
- TC-10 cell a.
- transcriptional a.

activational hormone

activator
allosteric a.
- kallikrein a.
- plasminogen a.
- a. protein-1 (AP-1)
- a. protein-1 element
- a. protein-1 transcription factor
- tissue-type plasminogen a.
- urokinase plasminogen a.
- urokinase-type plasminogen a.

active
- a. immunity
- a. renin
- a. salt transport
- a. variceal hemorrhage
- a. vitamin D_3

Activella

activin
- a. A receptor
- a. cell-surface receptor type I, II
- a. receptor (ActR)
- a. receptor I (ActRI)
- a. receptor IB (ActRIB)
- a. receptor II (ActRII)
- a. receptor IIB (ActRIIB)
- a. signaling

activinlike receptor kinase

activin-nonresponsive pituitary tumor

activity
ACh receptor-inducing a. (ARIA)
- adenylate cyclase a.
- adenylyl cyclase a.
- adrenomedullary a.
- 1-alpha-hydroxylase a.
- 5-alpha-reductase a. (5-alpha-RA)

anticonvulsive a.
antidiuretic a.
antirachitic a.
bactericidal a.
baroreflex a.
calorigenic a.
carbonic anhydrase a.
cholinergic a.
differentiation-inhibiting a.
fibrinolytic a.
gastric motor a.
hCG-modulated thyroid a.
hepatic fibrogenic a.
hepatic lipase a.
high impact a.
histone deacetylase a.
human chorionic gonadotropin-modulated thyroid a.
increased adenyl cyclase a.
insulinlike a. (ILA)
melanoma growth stimulatory a. (MGSA)
monodeiodinase a.
5'-monodeiodinase a.
monodeiodination a.
neutrophil respiratory burst a. (NRBA)
nonsuppressible insulinlike a. (NSILA)
osteoclast a.
osteoclastic a.
phagocytic a.
phosphatase a.
physical a.
plasma aldosterone concentration/plasma renin a. (PAC/PRA)
plasma renin a. (PRA)
plasmin renin a. (PRA)
platelet a.
postreceptor pyruvate dehydrogenase a.
protein-dimerizing a.
proteolytic a.
receptor tyrosine kinase a.
a. rhythm
serum vasopressinase a.
stromal osteoclast-forming a. (SOFA)
suppressed plasma renin a.
thyroid peroxidase a.
thyroid trapping a.

tyrosine kinase a.
uterine contractile a.
Actonel
Actos
ActR
    activin receptor
ActRI
    activin receptor I
ActRIB
    activin receptor IB
ActRII
    activin receptor II
ActRIIB
    activin receptor IIB
acuity
    visual a.
acustimulation
Acusyst-Xcell monoclonal antibody culturing system
acute
    a. addisonian crisis
    a. adrenal crisis
    a. adrenal insufficiency
    a. arterial occlusion
    a. fatty liver of pregnancy
    a. hemorrhagic pancreatitis (AHP)
    a. hypoglycemia
    a. infectious hepatitis
    a. insulin response (AIR)
    a. insulin response testing
    a. lymphoblastic leukemia
    a. lymphocytic leukemia (ALL)
    a. lymphocytic thyroiditis
    a. myelogenous leukemia
    a. necrotizing pancreatitis (ANP)
    a. painful neuropathy
    a. phase reactant
    a. phase response (APR)
    a. phase response syndrome
    A. Physiology and Chronic Health Evaluation (APACHE II)
    a. primary hyperparathyroidism
    a. recurrent pancreatitis
    a. streptococcal gangrene
    a. suppurative thyroiditis
    a. uric acid nephropathy
    a. water intoxication
    a. Wolff-Chaikoff effect
Acutrim
    A. 16 Hour
    A. Late Day
    A. II, Maximum Strength

NOTES

acylated ghrelin
acylation
    protein a.
acylation-stimulating protein
acylcarnitine
    fatty a.
acyl-CoA
    long chain fatty a.-C. (LCFA-CoA)
acyl-coenzyme A cholesterol
  acyltransferase (ACAT)
acyltransferase
    acyl-coenzyme A cholesterol a.
    (ACAT)
    alpha-glycerophosphate a.
    glycerol-3-PO4 a. (G3PAT)
    lecithin-cholesterol a. (LCAT)
AD
    androstenedione
AD-36 adenovirus
ADA
    adenosine deaminase
    American Diabetes Association
ADAM
    androgen deficiency in aging males
adamantinomatous craniopharyngioma
adaptation
    hypothermic cold a.
adaptational response
adaptor protein
ADCC
    antibody-dependent cell cytotoxicity
    antibody-dependent cellular cytotoxicity
ADD1
    adipocyte determination and
    differentiation factor-1
add-back regimen
Addison disease
addisonian crisis
adduct
    ketamine a.
ADEKs pediatric drops
adenine
    a. nucleotide sulfonylurea receptor
    a. nucleotide translocase
    a. phosphoribosyltransferase
    a. phosphoribosyltransferase
    deficiency
adeno-associated
    a.-a. virus (AAV)
    a.-a. virus vector
adenocarcinoma
    mucin-producing a.
    pancreatic a. (PAC)
adenocyst
adenohypophysial
    a. capillary
    a. corticotroph cell
    a. gangliocytoma
    a. hormone

    a. neuronal choristoma
    a. system
adenohypophysial-thyroid axis
adenohypophysis
adenoid
    a. appearance
    a. facies
adenoma
    acidophilic a.
    adrenal a.
    adrenocortical a.
    adrenocorticotropic hormone cell a.
    aldosterone-producing a. (APA)
    aldosterone-secreting a.
    alpha subunit-secreting pituitary a.
    basophilic a.
    beta-cell a.
    C-cell a.
    a. charcoal
    chromophobe a.
    chromophobic a.
    clinically nonfunctioning pituitary a.
    colloid a.
    corticotroph a.
    corticotropin-secreting a.
    cortisol-producing cortical a.
    cortisol-secreting a.
    dense staining of a.
    ectopic adrenal a.
    ectopic pituitary a.
    embryonal a.
    endocrine-inactive pituitary a.
    fetal a.
    follicular a.
    gangliocytoma-pituitary a.
    GH cell a.
    GH-secreting pituitary a.
    giant invasive pituitary a.
    glycoprotein-producing a.
    gonadotrope a.
    gonadotroph cell a.
    gonadotroph pituitary a.
    gonadotropic a.
    gonadotropin-producing pituitary a.
    gonadotropin-secreting a.
    growth hormone cell a.
    growth hormone-producing giant
    invasive a.
    growth hormone-prolactin cell a.
    growth hormone-secreting
    pituitary a.
    Hürthle cell a.
    hyalinizing trabecular a.
    intraductal pancreatic a.
    intrapituitary a.
    intrasellar a.
    invasive hormonally active
    pituitary a.

invasive hormonally inactive
pituitary a.
islet cell a.
lactotroph a.
left anterior mediastinal a.
macrofollicular a.
mammosomatotroph cell a.
mediastinal parathyroid a.
mixed GH cell-prolactin cell a.
mixed GH-PRL cell a.
mixed GH-secreting and prolactin-
secreting a.
mixed growth hormone cell-
prolactin cell a.
mixed growth hormone-prolactin
cell a.
mixed growth hormone-secreting
and prolactin-secreting a.
multicentric islet cell a.
nonfamilial parathyroid a.
nonfunctional pituitary a.
nonfunctioning pituitary a. (NFPA)
nonsecreting pituitary a.
nonsecretory adrenal a.
nontoxic thyroid a.
null-cell a.
oncocytic a.
oxyphilic a.
papillary a.
parathyroid a.
pituitary a.
plurihormonal a.
PRL-cell a.
PRL-secreting a.
prolactin cell a.
prolactin-producing pituitary a.
prolactin-secreting a.
recurrent a.
residual a.
secreting pituitary a.
silent ACTH a.
silent corticotrope a. subtype I, II,
III
silent corticotroph cell a.
silent gonadotroph cell a.
silent somatotroph a.
solitary a.
somatotroph cell a.
thyroid gland a.
thyrotrope a.
thyrotroph cell a.
thyrotroph-derived a.

thyrotropin-secreting pituitary a.
toxic a.
trabecular a.
TSH-secreting pituitary a. (TSH-
oma)
unilateral aldosterone-producing a.
adenoma-carcinoma sequence
adenoma-gangliocytoma
mixed pituitary a.-g.
adenomatosis
islet cell a.
multiple endocrine a.
adenomatous
a. adrenal gland
a. goiter
a. hyperplasia
a. polyposis
a. tumor
adenomectomy
surgical a.
transsphenoidal microsurgical a.
transsphenoidal pituitary a.
transsphenoidal selective a.
adenomyomatosis
adenopathy
multiple endocrine a.'s (MEA)
adenosine
a. cyclic monophosphate
a. deaminase (ADA)
a. deaminase deaminate
a. deaminase locus
a. 5′ diphosphate (ADP)
a. diphosphate ribosylation
a. 5′ monophosphate (AMP)
a. monophosphate-activated protein
kinase (AMPK)
a. monophosphate deaminase 1
(AMPD1)
a. monophosphate deaminase
deficiency
a. triphosphatase (ATPase)
a. 5′ triphosphate (ATP)
a. triphosphate binding cassette
(ABC)
a. triphosphate binding cassette
superfamily
a. triphosphate potassium channel
a. triphosphate potassium channel
hyperpolarized resting membrane
potential
a. triphosphate potassium opener

NOTES

adenosine *(continued)*
 a. triphosphate-sensitive
  potassium$_{ATP}$ channel
 a. triphosphate-sensitive potassium
  channel beta-cell
adenosis
 sclerosing a.
adenosyltransferase
 methionine a.
adenovirus
 AD-36 a.
 a. E1A protein
 recombinant a.
 a. vector
adenylate
 a. cyclase
 a. cyclase activity
 a. cyclase desensitization
 a. cyclase moiety
 a. cyclase stimulator
 a. cyclase system
adenylation
adenyl cyclase
3′,5′ adenylic acid
adenylosuccinate lyase deficiency
adenylyl
 a. cyclase
 a. cyclase activity
 a. cyclase agonist forskolin
 a. cyclase cascade
 a. cyclase pathway
ADH
 antidiuretic hormone
adherens
 cumulus a.
 a. junction
 zonula a.
adhesion
 endothelial-leukocyte a.
 a. molecule
 a. molecule-like from the X-
  chromosome (ADMLX)
 periovarian a.
adhesiveness
 platelet a.
ADICOL
 advanced insulin infusion with a control
  loop
 ADICOL system
Adipex-P
adipocyte
 a. complement related protein of
  30 kd (ACPR30)
 deficiency of a.
 a. determination and differentiation
  factor-1 (ADD1)
 a. differentiation-related protein
  (ADRP)
 a. lipolysis mechanism

 a. lipolysis regulation
 a. phosphodiesterase 3B
adipocyte-derived peptide
adipocytokines
adipogenesis
adipo-hypothalamic axis
adipokine
adipokinetic hormone
adipoleptin growth hormone axis
adiponectin
adipose
 a. tissue
 a. tissue regulation
 a. tissue-uncoupling protein
adiposity
 aging a.
 intraabdominal a.
 truncal a.
adiposogenital
 a. dystrophy
 a. syndrome
adipostat
adiposus
 panniculus a.
adipsia, type A, B, C
adipsic disorder
adipsin
adjuvant
 a. chemotherapy
 complete Freund a. (CFA)
ad libitum
Adlone Injection
ADM
 atypical diabetes mellitus
administration
 glycerol a.
 intensive insulin a.
 mannitol a.
 pharmacologic estrogen a.
 pulsed a.
ADMLX
 adhesion molecule-like from the X-
  chromosome
adnexa
 cutaneous a.
adolescence
 constitutional delay in growth
  and a. (CDGA)
adolescent
 a. metformin monotherapy
 a. type 2 diabetes mellitus
ADP
 adenosine 5′ diphosphate
adrenal
 a. adenoma
 a. androgen
 a. androgen deficiency
 a. androgenesis
 a. androgen excess

a. androgen-stimulating hormone (AASH)
a. cancer
a. capsular distention
a. carcinoma
a. cortex
a. cortex cell
a. corticosteroid (mineralocorticoid)
a. cortisol
a. crisis
a. diabetes
a. dysfunction
a. gland
a. gland limb
a. gland margin
a. hemorrhage
a. hypoplasia congenita (AHC)
hypothalamopituitary a. (HPA)
a. incidentaloma
a. insufficiency
a. medulla
a. medullary disease
a. medullary hormone
a. medullary hyperplasia
a. medullary paraganglioma
a. necrosis
a. pheochromocytoma
a. pseudotumor
a. remodeling
a. reserve
a. rest
a. rest tissue
a. scintigraphy
a. screening
a. steroidogenesis
a. steroidogenic cascade
a. steroid precursor
a. tuberculosis
a. vein
a. vein aldosterone ratio
a. vein sampling
a. vein thrombosis
a. venous sampling (AVS)
a. zona fasciculata
a. zona glomerulosa
a. zona reticularis
adrenalectomize
adrenalectomy (ADX)
laparoscopic a. (LA)
open a. (OA)
unilateral a.

adrenalectomy/oophorectomy
Adrenalin Chloride
adrenaline
adrenalitis
autoimmune a.
infectious a.
adrenarche
precocious a.
premature a.
adrenergic
a. agent
a. antagonist
a. blockade
a. nervous system
a. receptor
a. receptor activation
adrenocortical
a. adenoma
a. atrophy
a. carcinoma
a. cell
a. function
a. hormone
a. regeneration
a. thyroid interaction
a. tumorigenesis
adrenocorticotrophic hormone hypersecretion
adrenocorticotrophin
a. hormone (ACTH)
a. stimulation test
adrenocorticotropic
a. hormone (ACTH)
a. hormone cell adenoma
a. hormone-dependent Cushing syndrome
a. hormone hypersecretion
adrenocorticotropic-adrenal axis
adrenocorticotropin
human chorionic a.
adrenodoxin reductase
adrenogenital syndrome
adrenoleukodystrophy
familial a.
neonatal a.
recessive a.
sex-linked a.
X-linked recessive a.
adrenomedullary
a. activity
a. cell

NOTES

adrenomedullary *(continued)*
    a. hormonal system
    a. hyperplasia
adrenomedullin (AM)
    a. hormone
adrenomyeloneuropathy
adrenopause
ADRP
    adipocyte differentiation-related protein
adult
    a. adrenal cortex
    a. cystinosis
    growth hormone-deficient a.
    hypopituitary a.
    latent autoimmune diabetes of a.'s
      (LADA)
    a. Leydig cell failure
    a. polycystic kidney disease
    a. respiratory distress syndrome
    a. rickets
    a. T-cell leukemia (ATL)
    a. zone
adult-onset
    a.-o. diabetes
    a.-o. diabetes mellitus
advanced
    a. glycation end-product (AGE)
    a. glycation end-product formation
    a. glycosylation end-product (AGE,
      AGEP)
    a. insulin infusion with a control
      loop (ADICOL)
adventitia
    perithyroidal a.
Advicor Versus Other Cholesterol-
  Modulating Agents Trial
  (ADVOCATE)
ADVOCATE
    Advicor Versus Other Cholesterol-
    Modulating Agents Trial
ADX
    adrenalectomy
adynamia
adynamic
    a. bone disease
    a. bone disorder
    a. bone lesion
AEIOU TIPS
    alcohol, epilepsy, insulin, overdose,
    uremia, trauma, infection, psychiatric,
    stroke
Aerobacter
aerodigestive tract
Aerodiol
aeruginosa
    Pseudomonas a.
AERx diabetes management system
AF-1
    antifertility factor-1

AFC
    antral follicle count
affected sibling pair (ASP)
affective illness
afferent
    a. arteriole
    a. arteriole hyalinization
    a. axon
    beta-endorphinergic a.
    histaminergic a.
    noradrenergic a.
    a. pathway
    a. signal
    a. system
    vagal a.
affinity
    a. attenuated total reflectance
      spectroscopy
    a. chromatography
    a. evanescent wave spectroscopy
    a. fluorescence spectroscopy
    insulin binding a.
    a. surface plasmon spectroscopy
Affymetrix GeneChip technology
AFP
    alpha-fetoprotein
African trypanosomiasis
AFTN
    autonomously functioning thyroid nodule
agammaglobulinemia
agarose gel electrophoresis
AGD
    antigonadotropic decapeptide
AGE
    advanced glycation end-product
    advanced glycosylation end-product
age
    bone a.
    bone age/chronologic a. (BA/CA)
    delayed bone a.
    large for gestational a. (LGA)
    a., metastases, extent and size
      (AMES)
    A., Metastases, Extent and Size
      risk criteria
    a. pigment
    small for gestational a. (SGA)
agenesis
    gonadal a.
    Leydig cell a.
    müllerian a.
    pituitary a.
    renal a.
    sacral a.
    thyroid a.
    unilateral renal a.
agent
    adrenergic a.
    alkylating a.

alpha-adrenergic a.
anticholinergic a.
antidiabetic a.
antifungal a.
antihyperglycemic a.
antimycotic a.
antiresorptive a.
antiserotonergic a.
beta-adrenergic a.
biguanide oral antihyperglycemic a.
bipyridine inotropic a.
bone formation-stimulating a.
bone-resorbing a.
bone resorption-inhibiting a.
calcimimetic a.
dopamine a.
erectogenic a.
first-generation a.
formation-stimulating a.
formation-stimulation a.
gastric prokinetic a.
goitrogenic a.
hypoglycemic a.
hypolipidemic a.
inactive a.
lipid-lowering a.
nonsteroidal antiinflammatory a.
oral antidiabetic a.
oral hypoglycemic a.
orexigenic a.
paracrine a.
phosphate-binding a.
rheologic a.
second-generation a.
serotonergic a.
sulfonylurea a.
thiazide diuretic a.
tocolytic a.
uricosuric a.

AGEP
advanced glycosylation end-product
age-related osteoporosis
agglutination
labial fusion a.
agglutinin
fluorescein-labeled pea a.
fluorescein-labeled peanut a.
aggregated human IgG (AHuG)
aggregation
arachidonate-induced platelet a.
platelet a.

aggressive
a. hypothalamic lymphoma
a. insulin-dependent diabetes (AID)
a. insulin-dependent diabetes loci
a. xanthomatosis
aging
a. adiposity
programmed theory of a.
stochastic theory of a.
agoiterous autoimmune thyroiditis
agonist
beta a.
beta-adrenergic a.
beta-receptor a.
calcium receptor a.
cholinergic M-receptor a.
D_2 a.
dopamine receptor a.
dopaminergic a.
E_2 a.
GnRH a.
gonadotropin-releasing hormone a. (GnRHa)
mineralocorticoid a.
partial a.
PPAR-gamma partial a.
purinergic a. (PIA)
serotogenic a.
agonist-antagonist
mixed a.-a.
agonist-receptor interaction
agouti protein
agouti-related protein
agouti-related
a.-r. peptide
a.-r. transcript
AGP
alpha$_1$-acid glycoprotein
agranulocytosis
infantile a.
AHA
autoimmune hemolytic anemia
AHC
adrenal hypoplasia congenita
AHG
antihemophilic globulin
AHO
Albright hereditary osteodystrophy
AHP
acute hemorrhagic pancreatitis

NOTES

AhR
    arylhydrocarbon receptor
      AhR nuclear translocator (ARNT)
Ah receptor
AHuG
    aggregated human IgG
A-hydroCort Injection
AI
    apolipoprotein deficiency AI
AIBA
    aminoisobutyric acid
AIB1 coactivator
AIBH
    ACTH-independent bilateral
    macronodular hyperplasia
AICAR
    5-amino-4-imidazolecarboxamide
    riboside
    aminoimidazole carboximide riboside
AID
    aggressive insulin-dependent diabetes
AIDS
    acquired immune deficiency syndrome
    acquired immunodeficiency syndrome
AIDS-related complex (ARC)
AIGF
    androgen-induced growth factor
AILD
    angioimmunoblastic lymphadenopathy
    with dysproteinemia
AIP
    autoimmune pancreatitis
AIR
    acute insulin response
AIRE
    autoimmune regulator
      AIRE gene
      AIRE gene mutation
airway
    a. hyperactivity
    a. obstruction
    a. resistance
AIS
    androgen insensitivity syndrome
AITD
    autoimmune thyroid disease
    autoimmune thyroid disorder
AKA
    alcoholic ketoacidosis
AKAP
    A-Kinase anchoring protein
    protein kinase A pathway
A-Kinase anchoring protein (AKAP)
AKR gene
Akt
    protein kinase B
      Akt activation
      Akt oncogenic serine-threonine
      kinase

Ala-Ala
    HOKT3-gamma1 nonmitogenic anti-CD3
    antibody
    Ala-Ala preventing diabetes mellitus
alacrima
Alagille syndrome
alanine
    a. amino acid
    a. aminotransferase
    a. cycle
    a. transaminase
alarlike extension
alar plate
ALB
    albumin
Albers-Schönberg disease
Albert Glyburide
albicans
    Candida a.
    corpus a.
albinism
    ocular a.
    oculocutaneous a. (OCA)
Albright
    A. hereditary osteodystrophy (AHO)
    A. hereditary osteodystrophy
    syndrome
albumin (ALB)
    bovine serum a. (BSA)
    a. creatinine (A/C)
    serum a.
    a. solution
albumin-bound
    a.-b. calcium
    a.-b. testosterone level
albumin:creatinine ratio
albuminoid protein
albuminuria
albuterol
    ipratropium and a.
Alcian blue
alcohol
    a. ablation
    a. dehydrogenase
    a., epilepsy, insulin, overdose,
    uremia, trauma, infection,
    psychiatric, stroke (AEIOU TIPS,
    AEIOU TIPS)
    a. intolerance
    sugar a.
alcoholic ketoacidosis (AKA)
alcohol-induced
    a.-i. birth defect
    a.-i. hypoglycemia
alcoholism
    pseudo-Cushing syndrome of a.
alcohol-related chronic pancreatitis
aldehyde
    a. dehydrogenase

a. fuchsin
a. thionin
a. thionin staining technique
aldehyde-thionin-positive vesicle
Aldo
aldosterone
aldohexose
aldo-keto
a.-k. reductase
a.-k. reductase gene
aldolase level
aldose
a. reductase
a. reductase inhibitor (ARI)
a. reductase polyol pathway
aldosterone (Aldo)
a. baroreceptor
a. cardiomyocyte
a. diabetic vasculopathy
a. escape
a. escape phenomenon
a. excretion
plasma a.
a. receptor
recumbent a.
a. resistance
a. secretory rate
serum a.
a. synthase deficiency
a. synthesis
urine a.
aldosterone-deficient hyperkalemic acidosis
aldosterone-18-glucuronide
aldosterone-producing adenoma (APA)
aldosterone/renin ratio (ARR)
aldosterone-secreting adenoma
aldosterone-stimulating hormone (ASH)
aldosterone-to-renin ratio
aldosteronism
glucocorticoid-remediable a. (GRA)
glucocorticoid-suppressible a.
idiopathic a.
primary a. (PAL)
aldosteronoma
Aldurazyme
alendronate (ALN)
a. sodium
Alesse
alfa
dornase a.

epoetin a.
thyrotropin a.
alfacalcidol
alglucerase
algodystrophy
algogenic
alimentary
a. form
a. hypoglycemia
aliquot
alizapride
alkali
alkaline
a. phosphatase antialkaline phosphatase (APAAP)
a. phosphatase antialkaline phosphatase antibody test
alkaloid
ergot a.
opium a.
semisynthetic ergot a.
alkalosis
hypokalemic metabolic a.
metabolic a.
respiratory a.
Alka-Mints
alkaptonuria
Alkphase-B serum bone turnover assay
alkylated androgenic steroid
alkylating agent
ALL
acute lymphocytic leukemia
allele
DQ a.
DR a.
DR4 a.
HLA a.
human leukocyte antigen a.
mutant a.
5T a.
allele-specific
a.-s. oligonucleotide (ASO)
a.-s. oligonucleotide hybridization
Allen test
Allerfrin w/Codeine
allergic
a. salute
a. shiner
allergy
insulin a.
AllerMax Oral
Allescheria boydii

NOTES

Allgrove syndrome
alloantigen
allocation
    pancreas transplantation organ a.
allograft
    fetal a.
    freeze-dried a.
    human a.
    islet a.
alloimmune disorder
alloimmunity
allopregnanolone
allopurinol
allosteric
    a. activator
    a. effect
    a. effector
    a. inhibitor
    a. stimulator
allotypes
    Gm a.
alloxan
ALN
    alendronate
alone
    bladder-drained pancreaticoduodenal transplant a.
    islet transplantation a. (ITA)
    pancreas transplant a. (PTA)
    pancreas transplantation a. (PTA)
    pancreaticoduodenal transplant a.
alopecia
    a. androgenica
    a. areata
    total a.
Alora transdermal
alpha
    a. antagonist
    ER a.
    estrogen receptor a.
    follitropin a.
    hepatocyte nuclear factor 1 a.
    hepatocyte nuclear factor 4 a.
    HNF-1 a.
    HNF-4 a.
    a. subunit-secreting pituitary adenoma
    a. subunit-secreting tumor
    a. TC-1/9 cell
    thyrotropin a.
    transforming growth factor a. (TGF-A)
    a. v beta 3 vitronectin receptor integrin
alpha₁
    a.₁ antitrypsin deficiency
    thymosin a.₁ (T alpha₁)

alpha₂
    a.₂ antagonist
    a.₂ receptor
alpha₁-acid glycoprotein (AGP)
alpha-adrenergic
    a.-a. agent
    a.-a. blocker
    a.-a. effect
    a.-a. receptor
alpha₂-adrenergic
    a.-a. catecholamine
    a.-a. receptor
alpha₁-adrenergic receptor
alpha-amidation
alpha-amino-3-hydroxy-5methyl-4-isoxazole propionic acid
5-alpha-androstane-3-alpha,17-beta-diol
    5-alpha-a.-d. glucuronide
alpha-antitrypsin deficiency
Alphabetic multivitamin supplement
alpha-cell
    islet a.-c.
5-alpha-dihydrotestosterone
3-alpha-diol
3-alpha-diol-G
alpha-fetoprotein (AFP)
9alpha-fludrocortisone
9alpha-fluorocortisol
alpha-galactosidase deficiency
alpha-glucosidase inhibitor
alpha-glutamyl
alpha-glycerol phosphate
alpha-glycerophosphate
    a.-g. acyltransferase
    a.-g. dehydrogenase
alpha-hCG
    alpha-human chorionic gonadotropin
3-alpha-HSD
    3-alpha-hydroxysteroid dehydrogenase
alpha₂-HS-glycoprotein
alpha-human chorionic gonadotropin (alpha-hCG)
16-alpha-hydroxyestrone
1-alpha-hydroxylase
    1-a.-h. activity
    25-hydroxy-vitamin D 1-a.-h. (1-alpha-OHase)
20-alpha-hydroxylase
17-alpha-hydroxylase/17,20-lyase (p450c17) deficiency
1-alpha-hydroxylation
3-alpha-hydroxysteroid dehydrogenase (3-alpha-HSD)
6-alpha-hydroxytetrahydro-11-deoxycortisol
1-alpha-hydroxyvitamin D₃
alpha-lactalbumin
alpha₂-macroglobulin

alpha-mannosidosis
alpha-melanocyte-stimulating hormone
    (alpha-MSH)
alpha-methyldopa
alpha-methyldopamine
alpha-methylnorepinephrine
7-alpha-methyl-19-nortestosterone
    (MENT)
alpha-methyl-tyrosine
alpha-MSH
    alpha-melanocyte-stimulating hormone
    alpha-MSH hormone
1-alpha-OHase
    25-hydroxy-vitamin D 1-alpha-
    hydroxylase
1-alpha-OH-cholecalciferol
alpha-preprotachykinin A
5-alpha-RA
    5-alpha-reductase activity
5-alpha-reductase
    5-a.-r. activity (5-alpha-RA)
    5-a.-r. enzyme
    5-a.-r. type II
alpha-thalassemia
alpha-thyroid stimulating hormone
    subunit
alpha-TSH subunit
alprenolol
Alredase
alrestatin
ALS
    acid-labile subunit
    amyotrophic lateral sclerosis
    antilymphocytic serum
Alstrom syndrome
Altea
    A. MicroPor
    A. MicroPor laser
alteration
    gain-of-function a.
    lipoprotein a.
altered
    a. androgen action
    a. degradation of parathyroid
    hormone
    a. set point
alternate cover test
alternative sweetener
aluminum
    a. accumulation
    a. bone disease
    a. bone level

a. burden
a. deposit
a. effect
a. gel
a. hydroxide
a. hydroxide and magnesium
    carbonate
a. hydroxide, magnesium hydroxide,
    and simethicone
a. hydroxide and magnesium
    trisilicate
a. intoxication
a. loading
Maloney stain for a.
a. overload
a. retention
a. salt
tissue a.
a. toxicity
aluminum-associated osteomalacia
aluminum-containing
    a.-c. medication
    a.-c. phosphate binder
aluminum-contaminated
    a.-c. casein hydrolysate
    a.-c. dialysate
aluminum-induced osteomalacia
aluminum-related
    a.-r. bone disease
    a.-r. osteomalacia
alveolar
    a. bone
    a. type II cell
Alzheimer disease
AM
    adrenomedullin
Amadori product
Amadori-type rearrangement
Amaryl glimepiride tablet
amastia
ambient temperature
ambiguous genitalia
ambisexual development
Amcort Injection
AME
    apparent mineralocorticoid excess
amebic brain abscess
ameloblast
amelogenesis imperfecta
Amen Oral
amenorrhea
    athletic a.

NOTES

amenorrhea *(continued)*
    exercise-related a.
    functional hypothalamic a. (FHA)
    hypothalamic a.
    lactational a.
    postpill a.
    primary a.
    psychogenic a.
    secondary a.
amenorrhea-galactorrhea syndrome
American
    A. Association of Clinical
      Endocrinologists
    A. Diabetes Association (ADA)
    A. Diabetes Association
      classification system
    A. Diabetes Association guidelines
    A. Joint Commission on Cancer
    A. Thyroid Association
    A. Urologic Association (AUA)
    A. Urologic Association symptom
      score
Amerlite MAB free T4 assay
AMES
    age, metastases, extent and size
    AMES risk criteria
A-methaPred Injection
AMF
    autocrine motility factor
AMH
    anti-müllerian hormone
amidating enzyme
amidation
amide
    tripeptide a.
amikacin
amiloride-sensitive proton exchange
amine
    a. precursor uptake and
      decarboxylation (APUD)
    a. precursor uptake and
      decarboxylation cell
    a. precursor uptake and
      decarboxylation series
    sympathomimetic a.
amino
    a. acid
    a. acid delivery
    a. acid-peptide hormone
    a. acid sequence analysis
    a. acid substitution
    a. terminal domain
    a. terminus
5-amino-4-imidazolecarboxamide riboside
   (AICAR)
aminoaciduria
    dibasic a.
aminoacyl-tRNA complex

Amino-Cerv Vaginal Cream
aminoglutethimide therapy
aminoglycoside
5-amino group
aminoguanide
aminoguanidine
aminoimidazole carboximide riboside
   (AICAR)
aminoisobutyric acid (AIBA)
aminopeptidase
    a. A
    a. B
    cysteine a.
    insulin-responsive a. (IRAP)
aminophylline
aminoterminal leader
aminotransferase
    alanine a.
    aspartate a.
    serum alanine a.
    tyrosine a.
aminotriazole (ATA)
amiodarone-associated thyrotoxicosis
amiodarone-induced
    a.-i. destructive thyrotoxicosis
    a.-i. hypothyroidism
amiodarone thyrotoxicosis
Amipaque
ammonium chloride
amnioblast
amniocentesis
amnionic cavity
amniotic fluid
amorphous
    a. calcium
    a. calcium phosphate
    a. urate
amoxicillin
Amoxil
AMP
    adenosine 5′ monophosphate
    cyclic AMP (cAMP)
AMP-activated protein kinase (AMPK)
AMPD1
    adenosine monophosphate deaminase 1
amperometric
    a. glucosensor
    a. glucose oxidase electrode
    a. meter
amperometry
amphenone
amphetamine
    dextroamphetamine and a.
amphetamine-related transcript system
amphiregulin
amphotericin B
amphoteric molecule
ampicillin

AMPK
    adenosine monophosphate-activated
      protein kinase
    AMP-activated protein kinase
amplification
    a. factor
    germline a.
    a. refractory mutation system
      (ARMS)
    somatic a.
amplitude
    cycle a.
    prolactin pulse a.
    pulse a.
ampullary stone
ampulla of the vas deferens
AMV
    avian myeloblastosis virus
amygdala
amylacea
    corpora a.
amylase
amylin
amyloid
    beta-cell islet a.
    a. deposit
    a. fibril
    a. goiter
    immune a.
    islet a.
    a. peptide
    pituitary a.
amyloidic disease
amyloidogenesis
    beta-cell islet a.
amyloidogenicity
amyloidosis
    AB a.
    beta$_2$-microglobulin a.
    cutaneous lichen a.
    dialysis-associated a.
    dialysis-related a. (DRA)
    familial oculoleptomeningea a.
    senile systemic a.
amyotrophic lateral sclerosis (ALS)
amyotrophy
    diabetic a.
ANA
    antinuclear antibody
anabolic
    a. steroid
    a. therapy

anabolic-androgenic
    a.-a. steroid
    a.-a. steroid binding
Anabolin
anabolism
Anadrol
anaerobic glycolysis
anagen
analbuminemia
analog, analogue
    bromoaurone a.
    gastrin a.
    GnRH a.
    gonadotropin-releasing hormone a.
    insulin a.
    narcotine a.
    noncalcemic a.
    radiolabeled somatostatin a.
    somatostatin a.
    steroid a.
    thromboxane a.
    vitamin D a.
analysis, pl. analyses
    amino acid sequence a.
    computer-aided sperm a. (CASA)
    computer-assisted semen a. (CASA)
    crystallographic stone a.
    energy-dispersive x-ray a. (EDXA)
    flow cytometric a.
    immunocytochemical a.
    immunohistochemical a.
    isobologram a.
    Kyte-Doolittle hydropathy a.
    mass isotopomer distribution a.
    (MIDA)
    Northern blot a.
    pedigree a.
    phenotype-genotype a.
    Pulsar a.
    semen a.
    single-stranded conformation
      polymorphism a.
    Southern blot a.
    Western blot a.
analyte
analytical sensitivity
analyzer
    pulse-height a.
anamnestic
    a. antibody response
    a. element
anandamide

NOTES

anaphylaxis
anaplastic
    a. astrocytoma
    a. thyroid cancer
    a. thyroid carcinoma
anastomosis
    jejunocolic a.
anastomotic blood supply
anastrozole
Anavar
Andractim
Andro
androblastoma
Androcur Depot
Androderm
    A. testosterone transdermal patch
    A. Transdermal System
Andro/Fem
Androgel
androgen
    adrenal a.
    a. antagonist
    a. deficiency in aging males (ADAM)
    a. deficient
    a. excess
    a. insensitivity syndrome (AIS)
    a. milieu
    a. receptor (AR)
    a. receptor gene
    a. receptor gene mutation
    a. replacement therapy (ART)
    a. resistance
    a. resistance syndrome
    a. sensitivity
androgen-binding protein (ABP)
androgenesis
    adrenal a.
androgenica
    alopecia a.
androgenic follicle
androgen-induced growth factor (AIGF)
androgen-lowering therapy
androgen-producing tumor
androgen-secreting neoplasm
androgen-type hirsutism
androgynous
android
    a. fat distribution
    a. obesity
Andro-L.A. Injection
Androlone-D
Andropatch
andropause
    surgical a.
Andropository Injection
Androsorb
androstane derivative

androstanediol glucuronide
androstenedione (AD, D4-A)
androsterone glucuronide (AoG)
anechoic focus
anemia
    autoimmune hemolytic a. (AHA)
    Cooley a.
    a. of end-stage renal disease
    Fanconi a.
    hemolytic a.
    hypoproliferative a.
    leukoerythroblastic a.
    megaloblastic a.
    microcytic a.
    myelophthisic a.
    normocytic normochromic a.
    pernicious a.
    sickle cell a.
    sideroblastic a.
    unexplained microcytic a.
AnemiaPro Self-Screening Kit
anencephaly
anephric
anergy
    clonal a.
anestrous condition
aneuploid
aneuploidia
aneuploidy
    sex chromosome a.
aneurysm
    carotid a.
    dot a.
    giant carotid a.
    pituitary a.
ANF
    atrial natriuretic factor
ANG
    angiogenin
Angel Hypoglycemic capsule
Angelman syndrome
angiitis
angioedema
angiofibroma
angiogenesis
angiogenic growth factor
angiogenin (ANG)
angioimmunoblastic lymphadenopathy with dysproteinemia (AILD)
angioinvasion
angioma
    retinal capillary a.
angiomyelolipoma
angiopathy
    diabetic a.
angiopoietin
angiosarcoma
    thyroid a.
angiostatin

angiotensin
a. I, II, III
a. II antidiuretic hormone
a. I and II assay
angiotensin-converting
a.-c. enzyme
a.-c. enzyme inhibitor
angiotensinergic fiber
angular cheilitis
ANH
atrial natriuretic hormone
anhedonia
anhidrosis
distal a.
anhydrase
carbonic a. II (CA II)
anicteric cholestasis
animal protein diet
Animas
A. R-1000 insulin pump
A. R-1000 sensor
anion
bicarbonate a.
a. gap
a. of the Hofmeister series
peroxynitrite a.
anion-gap acidosis
anisocoria with ipsilateral mydriasis
anisotropine
ankle
a. pressure
a. reflex time
ankylosing hyperostosis of spine
ankyrin deficiency
anlage
cartilaginous a.
lateral thyroid a.
medial a.
median a.
thyroid a.
anlagen
annexin I, II, IV
annular
a. array
a. pancreas
annulare
granuloma a.
annulus
Zinn a.
Anodynos-DHC
anomalous pancreaticobiliary union

anomaly
congenital forebrain a.
conotruncal a.
diethylstilbestrol-associated a.
Ebstein a.
ectodermal a.
endocrine a.
müllerian a.
anophthalmos
anorchia
bilateral a.
congenital a.
anorchism
anorectal
a. atresia
a. function
anorectic
anorectin
anorexia nervosa
anorexigenic
anosmia
anosmin
anosmin-1
anovulation
chronic hyperandrogenic a.
chronic hypoandrogenic a.
clomiphene-resistant a.
eugonadotrophic a.
hyperandrogenic a.
hypothalamic a.
WHO class 1, 2, 3 a.
anovulatory
a. cycle
a. infertility
Anovulin
ANP
acute necrotizing pancreatitis
atrial natriuretic peptide
ansa
a. cervicalis nerve
a. hypoglossal nerve
Antagon
antagonism
insulin a.
antagonist
adrenergic a.
alpha a.
alpha$_2$ a.
androgen a.
dihydropyridine a.
histamine (H$_2$) a.
5HT$_2$ receptor a.

NOTES

antagonist *(continued)*

 5-hydroxytryptamine subtype 2 receptor a.
 inotropic glutamate receptor a.
 insulin a.
 interleukin-1 receptor a. (IL-1RA)
 JMV1155 gastrin receptor a.
 nonpeptide a.
 partial agonist-partial a.
 selective aldosterone a.
 selective 5HT$_2$ receptor a.

antegrade instrumentation
antenatal Bartter syndrome
antenatal-hypercalciuric variant
anterior

 a. choroidal artery
 a. clinoid process
 a. commissure
 a. communicating artery
 a. incisural space
 a. pituitary function
 a. pituitary gland
 a. pituitary lobe
 a. pole
 a. scalene muscle

anterograde flow
anteroventral 3rd ventricle (AV3V)
anthracycline
anthropometrics
anthropometry
anthropozoonosis
anti-37K antibody
antiadrenal antibody
antiandrogen
antiapoptotic factor
antiarrhythmic
antibiotic

 oral a.
 a. resistance gene

antibody (Ab)

 antiadrenal a.
 antibovine serum albumin a.
 anti-BrDU a.
 antibromodeoxyuridine a.
 anti-BSA a.
 anticarcinoembryonic antigen monoclonal a.
 anticardiolipin immunoglobulin M a.
 anti-CD3 monoclonal a.
 anti-CEA monoclonal a.
 antiidiotype a.
 antiidiotypic a.
 anti-IL-2R a. (anti-IL-2R Ab) antiinterleukin-2 antibody
 antiinsulin receptor a.
 antiinterleukin-2 a. (anti-IL-2R antibody)
 antiislet cell a.

anti-37K a.
anti-La a.
antimicrosomal a.
antineutrophil cytoplasmic a.
antinuclear a. (ANA)
antipituitary a.
anti-Ro a.
antisomatostatin a.
anti-Tg a.
antithyroid peroxidase a.
antithyroid-stimulating hormone a.
anti-TPO a.
anti-TSH a.
complement-fixing thyroid a.
cytoplasmic islet-cell a.
DuPan-2 a.
a. epitope
GAD65 a.
growth-blocking a.
growth-stimulating a.
heterophilic a.
HOKT3-gamma1 nonmitogenic anti-CD3 a. (Ala-Ala)
insulin receptor a.
islet cell cytoplasmic a.
islet cell surface a. (ICSA)
a. Ki
maternal blocking a.
MIB-1 a.
microsomal a.
monoclonal a. (MAb, Mab)
nonmitogenic anti-CD3 a.
ovarian a.
pituitary cell-surface a.
polyclonal anti-T-cell a.
primary a.
radiolabeled monoclonal a.
a. response
secondary a.
sensitive transcription factor 1 a.
serum antiinsulin a.
serum microsomal a.
thyroglobulin a. (TgAb)
thyroid microsomal a.
thyroid peroxidase a.
thyroid-stimulating a. (TSAb)
thyroid-stimulating-blocking a. (TSBAb)
thyroid-stimulating hormone-binding inhibitor a.
thyroid-stimulating hormone receptor a. (TSH-RAb)
thyroid stimulation-blocking a. (TSBAb)
thyroperoxidase a. (TPO Ab)
thyrotropin receptor a.
thyrotropin receptor-stimulating a. (TSH-RAb)
a. titer

transplacental a.
TSH-binding inhibitory a.
TSH-R a.
TSH receptor-blocking a.
TSH receptor-stimulating a.
TSH stimulation blocking a.
  (TSBAb)
uteroglobin a.
antibody-dependent
  a.-d. cell cytotoxicity (ADCC)
  a.-d. cell-mediated cytotoxicity
  a.-d. cellular cytotoxicity (ADCC)
  a.-d. cytotoxicity test
antibovine serum albumin antibody
anti-BrDU antibody
antibromodeoxyuridine antibody
anti-BSA antibody
anticarcinoembryonic
  a. antigen
  a. antigen monoclonal antibody
anticardiolipin immunoglobulin M
  antibody
anti-CD3 monoclonal antibody
anti-CEA monoclonal antibody
anticholinergic
  a. agent
  a. side effect
anticipatory control
anticonvulsant-associated hypocalcemia
anticonvulsive activity
anticus
  scalenus a.
antidiabetic
  a. agent
  a. medication
antidiuresis
antidiuretic
  a. activity
  a. hormone (ADH)
antidouble-stranded
  a.-s. deoxyribonucleic acid
  a.-s. DNA
antiendomysial
antiestrogen drug
antifertility factor-1 (AF-1)
antifungal agent
anti-GAD autoantibody
antigalactic
antigen
  anticarcinoembryonic a.
  autoimmune thyroid-related a.-1
    (ATRA1)

B8 a.
B-cell a.
beta-cell a.
breast cancer a. (BRCA)
carcinoembryonic a. (CEA)
CD1 a.
cell-surface a.
cognate a.
colloid a.
coxsackievirus B a.
cryptococcal a.
factor VIII-related a.
factor VIII ristocetin cofactor a.
histocompatibility locus a. (HLA)
HLA-A a.
HLA-B a.
HLA-B8 a.
HLA-C a.
HLA-D a.
HLA-DP a.
HLA-DQ a.
HLA-DR a.
HLA-DR3 a.
HLA-DR4 a.
HLA-DR5 a.
HLA-Dw3 a.
HNK-1 a.
homologous thyroid a.
human leukocyte a. (HLA)
H-Y a.
immune response a.
islet cell a. (ICA)
leu-7 a.
leukocyte common a.
microsomal a.
a. presentation autoantibodies
proliferating cell nuclear a.
  (PCNA)
prostate-specific membrane a.
  (PSMA)
Rh blood group a.
Rhesus factor blood group a.
SV40 large T a.
T-cell a.
testis-determining a. (TDA)
thyroglobulin a.
thyroid peroxidase a.
tumor-specific a. (TSA)
antigen-1
  fertilization a.-1 (FA-1)
  lymphocyte function-associated a.-1
    (LFA-1)

NOTES

antigen-2
>cytotoxic lymphocyte a.-2 (CTLA-4)

antigen-125
>cancer a.-125 (CA125)

antigenic property

antigen-presenting cell (APC)

antigen-specific
>a.-s. preventive therapy
>a.-s. suppressor T cell

antigliadin

antiglucocorticoid

antiglutamic acid decarboxylase autoantibody

antigonadotropic
>a. action
>a. decapeptide (AGD)

antigonadotropin
>pineal a. (PAG)

antihemophilic globulin (AHG)

antihormone
>estrogen receptor a.
>steroid hormone receptor a.

antihyperglycemic agent

antihypertensive therapy

antiidiotype antibody

antiidiotypic antibody

anti-IL-2R Ab
>anti-IL-2R antibody

anti-IL-2R antibody (anti-IL-2R Ab)

antiinsulin
>a. autoantibody
>B-cell a.
>a. receptor antibody

antiinterleukin-2 antibody (anti-IL-2R antibody)

antiislet cell antibody

antiknock mix

anti-La antibody

antilipolytic effect

antilymphocytic serum (ALS)

antimetabolite

antimicrobial
>a. therapy
>topical a.

antimicrosomal antibody

antimitotic effect

antimongoloid

anti-müllerian
>a.-m. hormone (AMH)
>a.-m. hormone deficiency

antimycotic agent

antineutrophil cytoplasmic antibody

antinociceptive action

antinuclear antibody (ANA)

antiobesity hormone

antiovulatory

antioxidant
>a. defense
>probucol a.

antiperistaltic

antiphospholipid (APL)
>a. syndrome

antipituitary antibody

antiport
>sodium a.

antiporter

antiprogestin

antipsoriatic action

antipyretics

antipyrine

antirachitic
>a. activity
>a. effect
>a. property

antirachitogenic effect

antiresorptive
>a. agent
>a. therapy

antireticulin

antiretroviral therapy

anti-Ro antibody

antisense nucleotide

antisera (*pl. of* antiserum)

antiserotonergic agent

antiserotoninergic effect

antiserum, pl. **antisera**

antisomatostatin antibody

antisteatotic hormone

antistress effect

anti-Tg antibody

antithrombin III level

antithrombotic factor

antithymocyte globulin

antithyroglobulin autoantibody

antithyroid
>a. antibody titer
>a. drug (ATD)
>a. medication
>a. peroxidase
>a. peroxidase antibody

antithyroid-stimulating
>a.-s. hormone
>a.-s. hormone antibody

antithyroperoxidase (anti-TPO)
>a. level

anti-TPO
>antithyroperoxidase
>anti-TPO antibody

anti-TSH antibody

antral
>a. follicle
>a. follicle count (AFC)

Anxanil Oral

AoG
>androsterone glucuronide

aortic
- a. allograft conduit
- a. arch
- a. arch interruption
- a. root dilatation

AP
- area postrema

AP-1
- activator protein-1
- AP-1 element
- AP-1 transcription factor

APA
- aldosterone-producing adenoma
- unilateral APA

APAAP
- alkaline phosphatase antialkaline phosphatase

APACHE II
- Acute Physiology and Chronic Health Evaluation
- APACHE II score

apathetic
- a. hyperthyroidism
- a. thyrotoxicosis

apatite crystal

APC
- antigen-presenting cell

APD
- acquired perforating dermatosis

APECED
- autoimmune polyendocrinopathy-candidiasis-ectodermal dystrophy

ApEn
- approximate entropy

Apert syndrome

aperture
- palpebral a.

aphrodisiac drug

apical
- a. iodide channel
- a. membrane
- a. membrane of proximal convoluted tubule cell

apituitarism

APL
- antiphospholipid

aplasia
- congenital bilateral a.
- congenital thymic a.
- a. cutis
- a. cutis congenita (ACC)
- germinal cell a.

- Leydig cell a.
- pituitary a.
- renal a.

aplastic
- a. bone disease
- a. bone disorder
- a. bone lesion
- a. uremic osteodystrophy

apo
- apolipoprotein
- apo A-I concentration
- apo B mRNA-editing catalytic polypeptide-1 (apobec-1)
- Apo Bromocriptine
- apo E genotype

apo-AI level

apo B
- apolipoprotein B

apobec-1
- apo B mRNA-editing catalytic polypeptide-1

Apo-Chlorpropamide

apocrine
- a. body odor
- a. secretion
- a. sweat gland

apoD
- apoprotein D

Apo-Gain

Apo-Glyburide

apolipoprotein (apo)
- a. B (apo B)
- a. B gene
- C a.
- a. C
- a. deficiency AI
- a. deficiency B
- a. deficiency E
- a. type 3

apomorphine

apophyseal joint

apoplectic hemorrhage

apoplexy
- pituitary tumor a.

Apo-Prednisone

apoprotein
- a. A-1
- a. D (apoD)

apoptosis
- cardiomyocyte a.
- osteoblast a.

NOTES

apoptosis *(continued)*
    osteoclast a.
    a. pathway
aporeceptor
apoT3R-mediated repression
Apo-Tolbutamide
apparatus
    distal Golgi a.
    Golgi a.
    juxtaglomerular a. (JGA)
    proximal Golgi a.
    Warburg a.
apparent mineralocorticoid excess (AME)
appearance
    adenoid a.
    cotton-wool a.
    "dewdrop on a rose petal" a.
    dripping-candle-wax a.
    signet-ring a.
    sucked-candy a.
appendiceal carcinoid
appendicular skeleton
appetite
    salt a.
    a. suppressant
apple-green birefringence
appositional
    a. crystal proliferation
    a. growth
Appraise diabetes monitoring system
approach
    bayesian a.
    candidate gene a.
    endonasal endoscopic
      transsphenoidal a.
    endonasal transseptal a.
    meal-planning a.
    pterional a.
    sublabial transseptal a.
    transcallosal-transforaminal a.
    translateral retroperitoneal a.
    transnasal-transseptal a.
    transsphenoidal a.
approximate entropy (ApEn)
APR
    acute phase response
APRIL
    A proliferation-inducing ligand
a priori
Aprodine w/C
aprotinin
    high-dose intraperitoneal a.
APS
    autoimmune polyendocrine syndrome
APS-1
    autoimmune polyendocrine syndrome 1
APS-2
    autoimmune polyendocrine syndrome 2

APS-3
    autoimmune polyendocrine syndrome 3
aptamer
APUD
    amine precursor uptake and
      decarboxylation
      APUD cell
      APUD series
apudoma
AQ2
    aquaporin-2
      AQ2 water channel
AQP
    aquaporin
Aquacare Topical
AquaMEPHYTON Injection
aquaporin (AQP)
aquaporin-2 (AQ2)
    a.-2 water channel
aquaresis
Aquasol A, E
aqueduct
    nonsyndromic familial enlarged
      vestibular a.
    a. of Sylvius
aqueous
    a. humor
    a. solution
Aquest
AR
    androgen receptor
    Axid AR
arabinoside
    cytosine a.
arachidonate
arachidonate-induced platelet aggregation
arachidonic
    a. acid (AA)
    a. acid cascade
arachnoid
    a. cyst
    a. membrane
arachnoidal sheet
arachnoiditis
    chiasmal a.
arbor
    dendritic a.
arborization
arbovirus
ARC
    AIDS-related complex
    arcuate nucleus of the hypothalamus
arch
    aortic a.
    branchial a.
arci *(pl. of arcus)*
arcuata
    pars a.

arcuate
    a. nucleus
    a. nucleus of the hypothalamus (ARC)
arcus, pl. **arci**
    corneal a.
    a. senilis
area
    extrasplanchnic a.
    hypophysiotropic a. (HTA)
    lateral retrochiasmatic a.
    osteoid a. (OA)
    parapituitary a.
    periaqueductal gray a.
    posterior hypothalamic a. (PHA)
    a. postrema (AP)
    retrochiasmatic a.
    rostral a.
    sacral autonomic a.
areata
    alopecia a.
Aredia
areflexia
arenacea
    corpora a.
argentaffin
    a. cell
    a. reaction
argentaffinoma
Argesic-SA
arginase
arginine
    a. infusion test
    a. tolerance test (ATT)
    a. vasopressin (AVP)
    a. vasopressor precursor
    a. vasotocin (AVT)
argininosuccinate lyase
argininosuccinic aciduria
arginosuccinic acidemia
Arg mutation
argon laser
argyrophil cell
ARI
    aldose reductase inhibitor
ARIA
    ACh receptor-inducing activity
ariboflavinosis
A-ring
    aromatic A-r.
Aristocort
    A. Forte Injection

    A. Intralesional Injection
    A. Oral
Aristospan
    A. Intraarticular Injection
    A. Intralesional Injection
Arm-a-Med
    A.-a-M. isoetharine
    A.-a-M. isoproterenol
    A.-a-M. metaproterenol
Armour Thyroid
ARMS
    amplification refractory mutation system
Arnold-Healy-Gordon syndrome
ARNT
    AhR nuclear translocator
arom
    P450 a.
Aromasin
aromatase
    cytochrome P450 a.
    a. deficiency
    a. enzyme complex
    a. gene
    a. inhibition
    a. inhibitor
    a. inhibitor testolactone
    a. P450
aromatic
    a. ammonia spirit
    a. A-ring
    a. L-amino acid decarboxylase
aromatization
aromatize
ARR
    aldosterone/renin ratio
array
    annular a.
arrest
    follicular a.
    germinal a.
arrested follicular cyst
arrhenoblastoma
arsenite
ART
    androgen replacement therapy
arterial
    a. bruit
    A. Disease Multiple Intervention Trial
    a. embolization
    a. reconstruction

NOTES

arterial *(continued)*
a. stimulation and venous sampling (ASVS)
arteriole
afferent a.
efferent a.
juxtaglomerular afferent a.
arteriosum
ligamentum a.
arteriovenous
a. difference
a. malformation (AVM)
arteritis
giant-cell a.
secondary a.
artery
anterior choroidal a.
anterior communicating a.
carotid a.
celiac a.
cerebral a.
choroid a.
common hepatic a. (CHA)
communicating a.
coronary a.
dorsal pancreatic a.
feeding a.
gastroduodenal a. (GDA)
helicine a.
hepatic a.
hypophysial a.
iliac a.
inferior pancreaticoduodenal a.
inferior parathyroid a.
inferior phrenic a.
inferior thyroid a.
mesenteric a.
ophthalmic a.
posterior cerebral a.
posterior communicating a.
profunda penis a.
renal a.
splenic a.
superior hypophyseal a.
superior mesenteric a. (SMA)
superior pancreaticoduodenal a.
superior parathyroid a.
thyroid ima a.
uterine arcuate a.
Artha-G
arthropathy
Charcot a.
destructive a.
diabetic neuropathic a.
neuropathic a.
pyrophosphate a.
Arthus phenomenon

articular
a. cartilage
a. overgrowth
articulation
vomerosphenoidal a.
artifact
starburst a.
artifactual hypoglycemia
artificial
a. endocrine pancreas
a. insemination with donor sperm
ARVDD-1
type 1 autosomal recessive vitamin D dependency
arylalkylamine *N*-acetyltransferase (AA-NAT)
arylhydrocarbon receptor (AhR)
arylmethyl group
arylsulfatase C
arytenoid
oblique a.
transverse a.
ascending pyelonephritis
Ascensia
A. Autodisc test strip
A. Breeze blood glucose monitoring system
A. Breeze glucometer
A. Breeze testing kit
A. DEX2 diabetes care system
A. Elite test strip
A. Elite XL diabetes care system
A. Microlet Adjustable lancing device
A. Microlet Vaculance lancing device
Aschoff body
ascitic fluid test
ascorbate
sodium a.
ascorbic acid
aseptate hypha
ASH
aldosterone-stimulating hormone
Asherman syndrome
Ashkenazi Jew
asialoglycoprotein receptor
asialo-human chorionic gonadotropin
asialyloglycoprotein
Askanazy cell
ASO
allele-specific oligonucleotide
ASP
affected sibling pair
Asp57
asparaginase
asparagine
thyroglobulin a.
asparagine-linked glycosylation moiety

aspart
> insulin a.
> a. insulin

aspartame

aspartamine

aspartate aminotransferase

aspartic
> a. acid
> a. endopeptidase cathepsin D

asparticacid/glutamic acid-tyrosine (Asp/Glu-Tyr)

aspartyl endoprotease

aspartylglycosaminuria

A-Spas S/L

aspergilloma
> renal a.

aspergillosis

Aspergillus
> *A. flavus*
> *A. fumigatus*
> A. infection
> A. thyroiditis

Aspergum

aspermia

Asp/Glu-Tyr
> asparticacid/glutamic acid-tyrosine

aspiration
> CT-guided fine-needle a.
> cyst a.
> fine-needle a. (FNA)
> gastric a.
> pulmonary a.

assay
> Abbott AxSYM a.
> Alkphase-B serum bone turnover a.
> Amerlite MAB free T4 a.
> angiotensin I and II a.
> avidin-biotin complex a.
> binding a.
> bioavailable testosterone a.
> blood spot a.
> chemiluminescence a.
> chemiluminescent a.
> Chiron ACS:180 a.
> chromatin immunoprecipitation a.
> colorimetric a.
> combination a.
> competitive zona binding a.
> cortisol a.
> electrophoretic gel mobility shift a. (EMSA)
> enzyme-linked immunosorbent a. (ELISA)
> free androgen index a.
> glycohemoglobin a.
> hemizona a.
> human zona binding a.
> immunochemiluminescence a. (ICMA)
> immunochemiluminescent a. (ICMA)
> immunochemiluminometric a. (ICMA)
> immunometric a. (IMA)
> immunoprecipitation a.
> immunoradiometric a. (IRMA)
> lithostathine a.
> mutation-enriched restriction fragment length polymorphism a.
> nuclear runoff a.
> OptiQuant a.
> parathyroid hormone a.
> pigeon crop sac-stimulation a.
> proliferation a.
> Pyrilinks-D deoxypyridinoline crosslinks urine a.
> radioreceptor a. (RRA)
> reverse dot blot a.
> reverse hemolytic plaque a.
> TBII a.
> third-generation a.
> thyroglobulin a.
> ThyroTest rapid a.
> thyroxine radioisotope a. (T_4RIA)
> total testosterone a.
> TSI a.
> type 1 diabetes mellitus combination autoantibody a.'s
> in vitro collagen invasion a.
> Xenopus oocyte expression a.

assessment
> histomorphometric a.
> visual field a.
> in vivo a.
> volume a.

assignment
> gender a.

assisted
> a. reproduction technique
> a. reproductive technology

association
> American Diabetes A. (ADA)
> American Thyroid A.
> American Urologic A. (AUA)

NOTES

association *(continued)*
    British Diabetes A.
    cell a.
    HLA DR antigen a.
    human leukocyte antigen DR
      antigen a.
Assure blood glucose monitoring system
asteroides
    Nocardia a.
asthenia
asthenospermia
asthma
    bronchial a.
Astramorph PF Injection
astressin
astrocyte
astrocytoma
    anaplastic a.
    hypothalamic a.
    juvenile pilocytic a.
    low-grade a.
ASVS
    arterial stimulation and venous sampling
asymmetric neuropathy
asymptomatic
    a. hyponatremia
    a. pheochromocytoma
    a. synechia
ATA
    aminotriazole
Atarax Oral
ataxia
    cerebellar a.
    familial cerebral a.
    Friedreich a.
    gait a.
    hereditary a.
    limb a.
    myxedema a.
    spinocerebellar a. types I, II, III,
      VI, VII
    a. telangiectasia
    a. telangiectasia mutated (ATM)
    a. telangiectasia mutated gene
ATD
    antithyroid drug
athelia
atherogenesis
atherogenic dyslipidemia
atherogenicity
atherosclerosis
    PPAR-gamma a.
atherothrombosis
athetoid movement
athletic amenorrhea
athymia
athyreosis
athyreotic cretin
athyrotic

ATL
    adult T-cell leukemia
AtLast blood glucose monitoring system
ATM
    ataxia telangiectasia mutated
    ATM gene
atmospheric pressure
Atolone Oral
atom
    phenolic orthohydrogen a.
atomic absorption spectrophotometry
atomization
atorvastatin calcium
Atozine Oral
ATP
    adenosine 5′ triphosphate
ATPase
    adenosine triphosphatase
    ouabain-sensitive Na^+-K^+ ATPase
    sarcoplasmic/endoplasmic reticulum
      calcium ATPase (SERCA)
ATRA1
    autoimmune thyroid-related antigen-1
atresia
    anorectal a.
    biliary a.
    duodenal a.
    follicular a.
atretic follicular cyst
atrial
    a. fibrillation
    a. flutter
    a. myxoma
    a. natriuretic factor (ANF)
    a. natriuretic hormone (ANH)
    a. natriuretic peptide (ANP)
    a. tachyarrhythmia
atriopeptin
atrophic
    a. autoimmune hypothyroidism
    a. chronic autoimmune thyroiditis
    a. gastritis
    a. Hashimoto thyroiditis
    a. vaginitis
atrophy
    adrenocortical a.
    band a.
    bow-tie a.
    bull's eye-type macular a.
    cortical a.
    dentatorubral-pallidoluysian a.
    (DRPLA)
    disuse a.
    exhaustion a.
    fiber a.
    fibrous a.
    genital a.
    gyrate a.
    interosseous a.

multiple system a.
neurogenic a.
olivopontocerebellar a.
postinflammatory testicular a.
postpubertal testicular a.
spinal muscular a. types I, II, III
spinobulbar muscular a.
Sudeck a.
testicular a.
type II muscle fiber a.
atropine plus diphenoxylate
ATT
arginine tolerance test
AtT20 pituitary cell line
Attache food scale
attention-deficit hyperactivity disorder
attenuate
attenuation
attractin
atypia
cytologic a.
nuclear a.
atypical
a. antipsychotic medication
a. charcoal
a. diabetes
a. diabetes mellitus (ADM)
a. mycobacterium
a. protein kinase C
a. protein kinase C activation
a. protein kinase C and insulin
a. teratoma
AUA
American Urologic Association
AUA symptom score
AUG codon
Aurbach pseudohypoparathyroidism
aureus
Staphylococcus a.
aurone
autacoid
autoantibodies
a. against insulin
antigen presentation a.
glucose transporter 2 a.
phogrin a.
autoantibody
anti-GAD a.
antiglutamic acid decarboxylase a.
antiinsulin a.
antithyroglobulin a.
competitive insulin a.

GAD65 a.
heat shock protein a.
HLA a.
insulin a. (IAA)
insulin-receptor a.
islet antigen a. (IAA)
islet antigen 2 a.
islet cell a.
plasmic islet cell a.
a. production
receptor a.
sperm a.
thyroglobulin a.
thyroid hormone a.
thyroid peroxidase a.
thyroid-stimulating hormone
  receptor a. (TSH-RAb)
thyrotropin receptor a. (TRAb)
TSH receptor a.
autoantigen
extrathyroid a.
islet a.
type 1 diabetes mellitus a.
Autoclix fingerstick device
autocrine
a. action
a. cell
a. communication
a. effect
a. motility factor (AMF)
a. secretion
a. suppressor
a. system
autograft
a. bone
islet a.
autoimmune
a. adrenalitis
a. diabetes
a. diabetes mellitus
a. diathesis
a. endocrine disease
a. hemolytic anemia (AHA)
a. hepatitis
a. hyperthyroidism
a. hypoglycemia
a. hypoparathyroidism
a. hypophysitis
a. nervous system screening
a. neuromuscular junction disorder
a. oophoritis
a. pancreatitis (AIP)

NOTES

autoimmune *(continued)*
   a. polyendocrine syndrome (APS)
   a. polyendocrine syndrome 1 (APS-1)
   a. polyendocrine syndrome 2 (APS-2)
   a. polyendocrine syndrome 3 (APS-3)
   a. polyendocrinopathy-candidiasis-ectodermal dystrophy (APECED)
   a. polyglandular endocrinopathy
   a. polyglandular failure
   a. polyglandular hypofunction
   a. regulator (AIRE)
   a. regulator gene
   a. signal
   a. thrombocytopenia purpura
   a. thyroid disease (AITD)
   a. thyroid disorder (AITD)
   a. thyroid hyperfunction
   a. thyroiditis
   a. thyroid-related antigen-1 (ATRA1)
   a. thyrotoxicosis
autoimmunity
   iodide-induced a.
   islet a.
   maternal a.
   polyglandular a.
   transgenic models for a.
   type 1A diabetes mellitus a.
   type 2 diabetes mellitus a.
autoinfarction
   complete a.
Autolance
auto-Lancet Mini lancing device
Autolet
   A. Clinisafe lancing device
   A. fingerstick device
   A. Lite lancing device
   A. Mini lancing device
autonomic
   a. cooling mechanism
   a. dysfunction
   a. function
   a. nervous system
   a. neuropathy
   a. polyneuropathy
   a. postganglionic nerve terminal
autonomous
   a. adrenal hyperplasia
   a. hyperfunction
   a. nodular hyperplastic gland
   a. nodule
   a. parathyroid chief cell proliferation
   a. toxic nodule
autonomously functioning thyroid nodule (AFTN)

autonomy
   masked thyroid a.
   nodular a.
   thyroid gland a.
autophosphorylation
   insulin-stimulated a.
autoproteolysis
autoradiography
   receptor a.
   thyamidine a.
   thymidine a.
autoregulation
   glucose a.
autosomal
   DAZ-like a. (DAZLA)
   deleted in azoospermia-like a. (DAZLA)
   a. dominant condition
   a. dominant diabetes mellitus
   a. dominant disorder
   a. dominant hypocalcemia
   a. dominant hypoparathyroidism
   a. dominant osteosclerosis
   a. dominant toxic thyroid hyperplasia
   a. karyotypic disorder
   a. recessive disease
   a. recessive disorder
   a. recessive hypophosphatemic rickets
autosome
   X chromosome to a. (X:A)
autosympathectomy
autotransplantation
   parathyroid a.
Avandia
avian-intracellulare
   Mycobacterium a.-i.
avian myeloblastosis virus (AMV)
avidin
avidin-biotin complex assay
avidity
avium-intracellulare
   Mycobacterium a.-i.
AVM
   arteriovenous malformation
Avon Longitudinal Study of Pregnancy and Childhood
AVP
   arginine vasopressin
AVS
   adrenal venous sampling
AVT
   arginine vasotocin
AV3V
   anteroventral 3rd ventricle
AvWD
   acquired von Willebrand disease
axes *(pl. of axis)*

axial
   a. osteomalacia
   a. QCT
   a. skeleton
Axid AR
axillary hair
axis, pl. **axes**
   adenohypophysial-thyroid a.
   adipo-hypothalamic a.
   adipoleptin growth hormone a.
   adrenocorticotropic-adrenal a.
   brain-gut a.
   endocrine a.
   enteroinsular a. (EIA)
   fetal-hypothalamic-pituitary-adrenal a.
   GHRH-GH-IGF a.
   gonadal a.
   growth hormone/insulin-like growth
      factor a.
   growth hormone-releasing hormone-
      growth hormone-insulin-like
      growth hormone a.
   HPA a.
   HPG a.
   HPT a.
   hyperparathyroidism a.
   hypothalamic-pituitary a.
   hypothalamic-pituitary-adrenal a.
   hypothalamic-pituitary-gonadal a.
   hypothalamic-pituitary-ovarian a.
   hypothalamic-pituitary-thyroid a.
   hypothalamopituitary-
      adrenocortical a.
   pituitary-gonadal a.
   pituitary-hypothalamic a.
   pituitary-thyroid a.
   pituitary-thyroidal a.
   putative neural a.
   renin-aldosterone a.
   renin-angiotensin-aldosterone a.
   serotonergic a.
   somatotropic a.
   thyroid a.
axon
   afferent a.
   a. response of Lewis
   sympathetic preganglionic a.
axonemal
   a. complex
   a. structure
axoneme
Ayala disease
Aygestin
azaprostanoic acid
azathioprine
AZF
   azoospermia factor
azide
   sodium a.
azidothymidine (AZT)
azithromycin
azoospermia
   deleted in a. (DAZ)
   a. factor (AZF)
azoospermia-homologue
   deleted in a.-h. (DAZH)
azotemia
   prerenal a.
AZT
   azidothymidine
azurin
   acid solochrome a.

NOTES

B

aminopeptidase B
amphotericin B
apolipoprotein B (apo B)
apolipoprotein deficiency B
cathepsin B
B cell
compound B
coxsackievirus B
hepatitis B
inhibin B
liposomal amphotericin B
B lymphocyte
B oncogene
Orexin B
pocket P9 insulin B
procarboxypeptidase B (PCPB)
proenkephalin B
protein kinase B (Akt, PKB)
B vitamin therapy

b

phosphorylase *b*

1B

protein-tyrosine phosphatase 1B
(PTP1B)

B2

thromboxane B2 (TXB2, TxB2)

2B

protein phosphatase 2B

B₂

prostaglandin B₂

3B

adipocyte phosphodiesterase 3B
hepatocyte phosphodiesterase 3B

B₄

leukotriene B₄ (LTB₄)

B₆

vitamin B₆

17B

17B estradiol
Vagifem 17B

B100

familial defective apolipoprotein
B100

BA/CA

bone age/chronologic age

bacillus, pl. **bacilli**

b. Calmette-Guérin (BCG)
b. Calmette-Guérin vaccine
Döderlein b.
tubercle b.

background retinopathy
bacteremia
bacterial

b. chloramphenicol acetyltransferase

b. infection
b. overgrowth (BO)
b. thyroiditis
b. translocation

bactericidal

b. activity
b. killing

bacteriophage lambda repressor
bacteriuria
Bacteroides

B. dermatitidis
B. fragilis

baculovirus vector
bafilomycin A
BAH

bilateral adrenal hyperplasia

Bailey-Pinneau table
B/Akt

protein kinase B/Akt

balance

acid-base b.
calcium b.
carbon b.
energy b.
glomerulotubular b.
metabolic b.
nitrogen b.
phosphate b.
phosphorus b.
potassium b.
redox b.
water b.

balanced electrolyte solution (BES)
balding

frontotemporal b.
temporal b.

baldness

male pattern b.

Bamforth-Lazarus syndrome
B9-B23 amino acids
Bancap HC
band

b. atrophy
Broca diagonal b.
C b.
floating beta b.
G b.
hypoechoic b. (halo)
b. keratopathy
Q b.

Bannayan-Ruvalcaba-Riley syndrome
Bannayan-Zonana syndrome
Banophen Oral
Banthine
B8 antigen

bar
  Greenberg b.
  ZNP B.
Bardet-Biedl syndrome
bare lymphocyte syndrome
barium
  b. contrast esophagography
  b. swallow
beta-ARK
  beta-adrenergic receptor kinase
Barker hypothesis
baroreceptor
  aldosterone b.
  carotid sinus b.
  high-pressure b.
  low-pressure b.
baroreflex activity
baroregulation
barostat
  electronic b.
Barr body
barrier
  blood-brain b. (BBB)
  blood-cerebrospinal fluid b.
  blood-testis b.
  perivitelline b.
Bartholin gland
Bartter syndrome
basal
  b. aluminum level
  b. body temperature (BBT)
  b. catecholamine secretion
  b. cell nevus syndrome
  b. compartment
  b. encephalocele
  b. ganglia
  b. ganglion calcification
  b. glycemia
  b. 24-hour UFC excretion
  b. 24-hour urine free cortisol
    excretion
  b. insulin
  b. insulin secretion
  b. insulin therapy
  b. lamina
  b. metabolic rate (BMR)
  b. metabolism
  b. plasma cortisol
  b. plasma GH level
  b. plasma growth hormone level
  b. plate
  b. promoter element (BPE)
  b. rate
  b. repression
  b. serum prolactin level
  b. sphincter pressure
  b. surface
  b. telencephalon

  b. thermogenesis
  b. thyroxine
basale
  stratum b.
basalis
  decidua b.
Basaljel
base
  Schiff b.
  skull b.
Basedow
  B. disease
  B. paraplegia
baseline
  b. aldosterone/plasma renin activity
    ratio
  b. BMI
  b. body mass index
basement membrane
base-substitution effect
basic
  b. fibroblast growth factor (bFGF)
  b. helix-loop-helix (bHLH)
  b. helix-loop-helix transcription
    factor
  b. multicellular unit (BMU)
  OneTouch B.
  B. Rest-Activity Cycle (BRAC)
basilar
  b. cistern
  b. meningitis
  b. sinus
basis pedunculi
basisphenoid
basolateral plasma membrane
basophil
basophilic
  b. adenoma
  b. cell
  b. cell invasion
B25-Asp-insulin
Bassen-Kornzweig syndrome
BAT
  brown adipose tissue
Bayer glucometer
bayesian approach
Bayes rule
BB
  platelet-derived growth factor BB
BBB
  blood-brain barrier
4-1BBL
  4-1BB ligand
4-1BB ligand (4-1BBL)
BBM
  brush-border membrane
BBS
  BES buffered saline

BBT
  basal body temperature
B$_c$
  vitamin B$_c$
B-cell
  B.-c. activation
  B.-c. adenosine triphosphate-sensitive potassium$_{ATP}$ channel
  B.-c. antigen
  B.-c. antigen receptor (BCR)
  B.-c. antiinsulin
  B.-c. autoimmune thyroid disease
  B.-c. function
  B.-c. growth factor (BCGF)
  B.-c. intrathyroid
  B.-c. lymphoma
  B.-c. ontogeny
  B.-c. preservation
  B.-c. rejuvenation
  B.-c. repertoire
  B.-c. second signal
BCG
  bacillus Calmette-Guérin
  BCG vaccine
bCgA
  bovine chromogranin A
  synthetic bCgA
BCGF
  B-cell growth factor
bcl-2
BCR
  B-cell antigen receptor
BDGF
  bone-derived growth factor
B-D Glucose
BD Lancet device
BDNF
  brain-derived neurotropic factor
BDS
  botanical dietary supplement
beading
  venous b.
becaplermin
Becker muscular dystrophy gene
Beckwith-Wiedemann syndrome
bedtime
  b. insulin
  b. insulin, daytime sulfonylurea (BIDS)
bedwetting
beef insulin
beer potomania

behavior
  aberrant b.
  hyperoral b.
  b. modification
  oscillatory b.
behavioral
  b. research
  b. rhythm
  B. Risk Factor Surveillance System (BRFSS)
  b. therapy
Belix Oral
belladonna
  b. and opium
  b., phenobarbital, and ergotamine tartrate
Bel-Phen-Ergot S
Benadryl Oral
Ben-Allergin-50 Injection
bendroflumethiazide
Benedict test
benfluorex
benign
  b. charcoal
  b. cystic lesion
  b. cystic teratoma
  b. cystinosis
  b. familial hypercalciuria
  b. hypocalciuric hypercalcemia
  b. intracranial hypertension
  b. nodular disease
  b. nodular goiter
  b. optic glioma
  b. pituitary cyst
  b. prostatic fibroadenoma
  b. prostatic hypertrophy
  b. sporadic adrenal pheochromocytoma
benzene
benzoate
benzodiazepine (BZD)
  gamma-aminobutyric acid/b. (GABA/BZD)
benzoic acid
benzonatate
benzophenone
benzothiophene
benzoyl peroxide
benzphetamine
beraprost
Berardinelli-Seip syndrome

NOTES

37

Bercu
  B. patient
  B. patient of Kindred S
beriberi
Berry ligament
Berubigen
berylliosis
beryllium
BES
  balanced electrolyte solution
  BES buffered saline (BBS)
Besnier prurigo
Beta-2
beta
  b. agonist
  b. blocker
  b. cell destruction
  b. cell dysmaturation syndrome
  b. cell hyperplasia
  b. cell polypeptide
  b. cell replacement
  b. cell secretory granule
  b. cell transplant
  ER b.
  estrogen receptor b.
  follitropin b.
  b. granin
  hepatocyte nuclear factor 1 b.
  HNF-1 b.
  integrin alpha v b. 3
  nuclear factor b.
  retinoic acid X receptor b.
  b. Tc-6 cell
  thymosin $b_{.4}$ (Tb_4)
  transforming growth factor b.
    (TGF-B)
beta-adrenergic
  b.-a. agent
  b.-a. agonist
  b.-a. blocker
  b.-a. effect
  b.-a. receptor
  b.-a. receptor kinase (beta-ARK)
  b.-a. vasodilation
beta$_2$-adrenergic
  b.$_2$-a. catecholamine
  b.$_2$-a. receptor
beta$_1$-adrenergic receptor
beta-agonist
beta-alanine transaminase
beta-aminobutyrate
beta-aminoisobutyrate
beta-antagonist
beta-arrestin protein
beta-carotene
beta-catenin
beta-cell
  b.-c. adenoma

  b.-c. adenosine triphosphate
    potassium channel
  adenosine triphosphate-sensitive
    potassium channel b.-c.
  b.-c. antigen
  b.-c. CA2+-activated K+ channel
  b.-c. calcium channel
  chronic hyperglycemia
    pancreatic b.-c.
  b.-c. cytokine
  b.-c. cytokine transgenic expression
  b.-c. cytotoxic T-lymphocyte
  cytotoxic T-lymphocyte b.-c.
  b.-c. delayed rectifier voltage-gated
    K channel
  b.-c. expansion
  b.-c. function
  b.-c. gap junction
  b.-c. glucose-mediated depolarization
    K_{ATP} channel
  b.-c. glucose-mediated depolarization
    potassium$_{ATP}$ channel
  b.-c. glucose sensitivity
  b.-c. granule pool
  b.-c. hyperglycemia
  b.-c. hypothesis
  b.-c. impairment
  interferon gamma b.-c.
  b.-c. intracellular channel
  b.-c. ion channel
  islet b.-c.
  b.-c. islet amyloid
  b.-c. islet amyloidogenesis
  b.-c. K_v and CA_v channel
  b.-c. lmx1.1 protein
  b.-c. mass
  b.-c. melanin concentrating hormone
  MHC b.-c.
  b.-c. nonesterified fatty acid
  b.-c. nonselection cation channel
  pancreatic islet b.-c.
  pancreatic transcription factor 1 b.-
    c.
  b.-c. phenotype
  b.-c. potassium$_{ATP}$ channel
  b.-c. potassium$_{ATP}$ channel
    reconstruction
  potassium$_{ATP}$ whole-cell b.-c.
  b.-c. rest
  b.-c. reversible immortalization
  b.-c. secretory granule channel
  b.-c. secretory pathway
  b.-c. set point
  b.-c. transgene
  b.-c. tumor necrosis factor-alpha
  b.-c. voltage-gated calcium channel
  whole-cell K_{ATP} b.-c.
beta-cellulin

beta-END
    beta-endorphin
beta-endorphin (beta-END)
    plasma b.-e.
beta-endorphinergic afferent
beta-estradiol
17-beta-estradiol valerate
beta-galactosidase
beta-gamma complex
beta-glucuronidase
17-beta-glucuronide
betaglycan
beta-granule
    b.-g. plasma membrane transport
    b.-g. storage pool
beta-hCG
    beta-human chorionic gonadotropin
3-beta-HSD
    3-beta-hydroxysteroid dehydrogenase
11-beta-HSD
    11-beta-hydroxysteroid dehydrogenase
11-beta-HSD1
    11-beta-hydroxysteroid dehydrogenase
    type 1
11-beta-HSD2
    11-beta-hydroxysteroid dehydrogenase
    type 2
17-beta-HSD
    17-beta-hydroxysteroid dehydrogenase
17-beta-HSD1
    17-beta-hydroxysteroid dehydrogenase
    type 1
17-beta-HSD2
    17-beta-hydroxysteroid dehydrogenase
    type 2
17-beta-HSD3
    17-beta-hydroxysteroid dehydrogenase
    type 3
17-beta-HSD4
    17-beta-hydroxysteroid dehydrogenase
    type 4
17-beta-HSD5
    17-beta-hydroxysteroid dehydrogenase
    type 5
beta-human chorionic gonadotropin
  (beta-hCG)
17-beta-hydroxyandrogen
beta-hydroxy-beta-methylglutaryl-
  coenzyme A (HMG-CoA)
beta-hydroxybutyrate
beta-hydroxylase
    dopamine b.-h. (DBH)

21-beta-hydroxylase
11-beta-hydroxylase deficiency (11-beta-
  OHD)
3-beta-hydroxysteroid
    3-b.-h. dehydrogenase (3-beta-HSD)
    3-b.-h. dehydrogenase deficiency
    3-b.-h. dehydrogenase insufficiency
11-beta-hydroxysteroid
    11-b.-h. dehydrogenase (11-beta-
    HSD)
    11-b.-h. dehydrogenase type 1 (11-
    beta-HSD1)
    11-b.-h. dehydrogenase type 2 (11-
    beta-HSD2)
17-beta-hydroxysteroid
    17-b.-h. dehydrogenase (17-beta-
    HSD)
    17-b.-h. dehydrogenase type 1 (17-
    beta-HSD1)
    17-b.-h. dehydrogenase type 2 (17-
    beta-HSD2)
    17-b.-h. dehydrogenase type 3 (17-
    beta-HSD3)
    17-b.-h. dehydrogenase type 4 (17-
    beta-HSD4)
    17-b.-h. dehydrogenase type 5 (17-
    beta-HSD5)
betaine
beta-lactamase
Betalin S
beta-lipoprotein (beta-LPH)
beta-lipotropin
beta-LPH
    beta-lipoprotein
beta-mannosidosis
beta-melanocyte-stimulating hormone
  (beta-MSH)
betamethasone
beta$_2$-microglobulin
    b.$_2$-m. amyloid deposition
    b.$_2$-m. amyloidosis
beta$_2$-microglobulinemia
beta-MSH
    beta-melanocyte-stimulating hormone
beta-nerve growth factor
11-beta-OHD
    11-beta-hydroxylase deficiency
beta-ol-dehydrogenase deficiency
beta-oxidation
beta-preprotachykinin A

B

NOTES

beta-receptor
    b.-r. agonist
    pinealocyte b.-r.
beta-secretase
beta-sitosterol
beta-thalassemia
beta-thyroid-stimulating
    b.-t.-s. hormone (beta-TSH)
    b.-t.-s. hormone gene
beta-TSH
    beta-thyroid-stimulating hormone
    beta-TSH gene
bethanechol
bexarotene
Bexophene
bFGF
    basic fibroblast growth factor
BFR
    bone formation rate
bG
    blood glucose
    Chemstrip bG
BGP
    bone G1a protein
    BGP protein
bHLH
    basic helix-loop-helix
    bHLH transcription factor
biallelic expression
biantennary
Biatain
bicalutamide
bicarbonate
    b. anion
    diabetic ketoacidosis b.
    serum b.
    sodium b.
    b. therapy
Bicitra
BIDS
    bedtime insulin, daytime sulfonylurea
    BIDS therapy
bifid scrotum
bifidus
    lactobacillus b.
biglycan bone sialoprotein
biguanide
    hypoglycemia b.
    b. oral antihyperglycemic agent
bihormonal effector
bilateral
    b. adrenal disease
    b. adrenal hyperplasia (BAH)
    b. adrenal vein catheterization
    b. anorchia
    b. hemianopsia
    b. idiopathic hyperaldosteronism
    b. IHA
    b. macronodular hyperplasia

    b. pes cavus deformity
    b. salpingo-oophorectomy (BSO)
bile
    b. acid
    b. acid resin
    b. acid sequestrant
    b. composition
    b. duct
    b. flow
bile-binding resin
bile-salt malabsorption
biliary
    b. atresia
    b. cirrhosis
    b. colic
    b. fistula
    b. sludge
    b. worm
biliointestinal bypass
biliopancreatic
    b. bypass
    b. diversion
bilirubin
    conjugated b.
bilirubinemia
biliverdin
bimanual synkinesis
bimodal pattern
binder
    aluminum-containing phosphate b.
    phosphate b.
binder-1
    Grb2-associated b.-1 (Gab-1)
binding
    anabolic-androgenic steroid b.
    b. assay
    calcium b.
    b. capacity
    fragment antigen b. (Fab)
    ^{3}H-imipramine b.
    insulin b.
    nonspecific b. (NSB)
    phosphate b.
    phosphorus b.
    phosphotyrosine b. (PTB)
    PPAR DNA b.
    protein b.
    protein-tyrosine b. (PTB)
    receptor ligand b.
    thyroglobulin b.
    total androgen b.
bioactivation
bioactive
    b. mediator
    b. parathyroid hormone
bioamine neurotransmitter
bioartificial pancreas
bioassay
    cytochemical b. (CBA)

endogenous estrogen b.
in vitro b.
in vivo b.
bioavailable
    b. fluoride
    b. testosterone assay
    b. testosterone level
Biocef
biochanin A
biochemical
    b. gate
    b. hypothyroidism
    b. marker
    b. remission
biochemically euthyroid
bioeffect
bioelectrical impedance
bioengineered living-skin equivalent
bioequivalence
biofeedback training
bioflavanoid
biographer
    GlucoWatch B.
bioidentical hormone
bioinactive
bioinactivity
    gonadotropin b.
bioincompatibility
    hemodialysis membrane b.
bioineffective
biologic
    b. catalyst
    b. half-life
biology
    molecular b.
    vascular cell b.
bioluminescence detection
biometric assessment of fetal growth
biopsy
    fine-needle aspiration b. (FNAB)
    FNA b.
    large-needle aspiration b. (LNAB)
    percutaneous b.
    thyroid b.
biorhythm
    pseudoperiodic b.
    true periodic b.
biorhythmicity
biosensor
    implantable b.
Biostator

biosynthesis
    catecholamine b.
    cortisol b.
    hormone b.
    prolactin b.
    steroid b.
    thyroglobulin b.
biosynthetic
    b. growth hormone
    b. hexosamine
    b. human insulin
biotechnology
biotic
biotin cofactor deficiency
biotinylated-nucleotide protocol
Biozyme-C
biphasic
    b. insulin
    b. insulin secretion
biphenyl
    polybrominated b. (PBB)
    polychlorinated b. (PCB)
biphosphonate
bipotential gonad
bipyridine
    inotropic b.
    b. inotropic agent
Birbeck granule
bird-like facies
birefringence
    apple-green b.
birefringent
    b. collagen fibril
    b. pattern
bisalbuminemia
bis-mannose photolabel
Bismatrol
bismuth subsalicylate
bisoprolol
4,5-bisphosphate
    phosphatidylinositol 4,5-b. (PIP_2)
bisphosphonate
    osteoporosis b.
bitemporal
    b. defect
    b. hemianopia
    b. hemianopsia
bitolterol
black
    b. cohosh
    b. pus
    b. thyroid

NOTES

Blackfan-Diamond syndrome
bladder
    b. drainage
    b. exstrophy
bladder-drained pancreaticoduodenal transplant alone
blade-of-grass lesion
blastocoele
blastocyst
blastogenesis
blastolemmase
blastomere
Blastomyces dermatitidis
blastomycetica
    erosio interdigitalis b.
blastomycosis
    North America b.
    South American b.
blepharitis
blepharophimosis, ptosis, epicanthus inversus syndrome
blind hemihypophysectomy
blind-loop syndrome
blockade
    adrenergic b.
    Evaluation of PTCA to Improve Long-Term Outcome by C7E3 GpIIb/IIIa Receptor B. (EPILOG)
    potassium$_{ATP}$ b.
blocker
    alpha-adrenergic b.
    beta b.
    beta-adrenergic b.
    calcium channel b. (CCB)
    dopaminergic b.
    glycoprotein IIb and IIIb b.
    noradrenergic b.
    potassium$_{ATP}$ channel b.
block-replace regimen
Blomstrand lethal chondrodysplasia
blood
    circulating b.
    citrated b.
    b. clotting cascade
    b. free thyroxine
    b. glucose (bG)
    b. glucose buffer system
    b. glucose concentration
    b. glucose meter
    b. glucose monitoring
    b. glucose testing
    b. pressure
    b. pressure dysregulation
    b. purification therapy
    b. sampling
    b. spot assay
    b. sugar
    b. urea nitrogen (BUN)

    b. volume
    b. volume change
blood-borne pathogen
blood-brain barrier (BBB)
blood-cerebrospinal fluid barrier
blood-testis barrier
Bloom syndrome
blot
    Northern b.
    Southern b.
    Western b.
Blount disease
blue
    Alcian b.
    methylene b.
    b. patch
    b. tinge sclera
    Urolen b.
blueberry lesion
blue-diaper syndrome
blue-toe syndrome
blunt estrogenic stimulation
blunting
    b. of nocturnal thyroid-stimulating hormone surge
    b. of nocturnal TSH surge
BMAL1
    brain/muscle ARNT-like protein 1
    BMAL1 protein
BMD
    bone mineral density
BMI
    body mass index
    baseline BMI
BMP
    bone morphogenetic protein
    bone morphogenic protein
BMR
    basal metabolic rate
BMU
    basic multicellular unit
BNP
    brain natriuretic peptide
BO
    bacterial overgrowth
body
    Aschoff b.
    Barr b.
    Call-Exner b.
    carotid b.
    b. cell mass
    b. composition
    b. densitometry
    Doehle b.
    F b.
    b. fluid osmolality
    b. habitus
    Herring b.
    hyaline b.

ketone b.
lysosomal dense b.
mammillary b.
b. mass index (BMI)
oxytocinergic cell b.
polar b.
psammoma b.
Schumann b.
ultimobranchial b. (UB)
b. water
b. water osmolality
b. weight
X b.
Y b.
yellow b.
BodyGem metabolism monitor
bolus therapy
bombesin
b. infusion
mammalian b.
bombesin-like peptide
bond
noncovalent b.
selenosulfide b.
bone
b. age
b. age/chronologic age (BA/CA)
b. alkaline phosphatase
alveolar b.
autograft b.
cancellous b.
b. carbonate
b. cell
b. cell receptor
compact b.
b. consolidation
cortical b.
b. crisis
b. deficiency
b. densitometry
b. effect
b. embedding
fibrous dysplasia of b.
b. fluid
b. formation rate (BFR)
b. formation-stimulating agent
b. G1a protein (BGP)
b. growth
b. histology
b. hunger
hungry b.
hyoid b.

intramembranous b.
lamellar b.
long b.
b. loss
b. marrow
b. marrow-derived myogenic
  progenitor
b. marrow-derived stromal cell
b. marrow element
b. marrow function
b. marrow stroma
b. marrow transplantation
b. mass
b. mass accretion
b. mass density
membranous b.
b. mineral
b. mineral accretion
b. mineral density (BMD)
b. mineral metabolism
b. morphogenetic factor 7 signaling
b. morphogenetic protein (BMP)
b. morphogenetic protein-2
b. morphogenetic protein-4
b. morphogenetic protein-7
b. morphogenic protein (BMP)
b. mucormycosis
osteoclastic b.
Paget disease of b.
pagetic b.
b. pain
b. quantum
rachitic b.
b. reconstruction
b. remodeling
b. resorption
b. resorption-inhibiting agent
sarcomatous b.
b. scan
b. sialoprotein (BSP)
sphenoid b.
spongy b.
spotted b.
b. structural unit
trabecular b.
b. turnover
undercalcified b.
von Recklinghausen disease of b.
wormian b.
woven b.
bone-age radiography
bone-derived growth factor (BDGF)

NOTES

bone-forming
    b.-f. cell
    b.-f. cell transplantation
bone-related protein
bone-resorbing
    b.-r. agent
    b.-r. cytokine
    b.-r. osteoclast
bone-specific
    b.-s. alkaline phosphatase
    b.-s. cathepsin
    b.-s. protein
bone-within-bone
Bontril
    B. PDM
    B. Slow-Release
bony
    b. exostosis
    b. reservoir
border
    ruffled b.
borderline diabetes
Borjeson-Forssman-Lehman syndrome
Borrelia
bossing
    frontal b.
B&O Supprettes
botanical dietary supplement (BDS)
botulinum
    b. A toxin
    b. injection
    b. toxin type A
bound
    b. hormone
    total b. (TB)
bovine
    b. chromogranin A (bCgA)
    b. insulin
    b. parathyroid hormone (bPTH)
    pegademase b.
    b. serum albumin (BSA)
    b. viral diarrhea mucosal disease (BVD-MD)
    b. viral diarrhea mucosal disease virus
bow
    Cupid b.
    b. leg
bowel-associated dermatosis-arthritis syndrome
Bowman
    B. capsule
    B. gland
bow-tie atrophy
box
    CAAT b.
    consensus TATA b.
    Goldberg-Hogness b.
    high mobility group b.

    HMG b.
    TATA b.
    toe b.
boydii
    Allescheria b.
BPE
    basal promoter element
B2036-PEG
bPTH
    bovine parathyroid hormone
BRAC
    Basic Rest-Activity Cycle
brachial
    b. plexus
    b. pressure
brachial-to-penile Doppler blood pressure ratio
bradycardia
bradykinin
    desArg b.
BRAF
Bragg peak proton irradiation therapy
brain
    b. development
    gliotic b.
    b. hormone
    b. isoenzyme
    b. $K_{IR}6.2/SUR1$ potassium$_{ATP}$ channel
    b. masculinization
    b. monoamine
    b. natriuretic peptide (BNP)
    b. necrosis
    b. tumor
brain-derived neurotropic factor (BDNF)
brain-gut
    b.-g. axis
    b.-g. peptide
brain/muscle
    b./m. AhR nuclear translocator-like protein 1
    b./m. ARNT-like protein 1 (BMAL1)
brainstem reticular formation
2-Br-alpha-ergocryptine mesylate
branch
    b. chain 2-ketoacid decarboxylase
    b. chain ketoaciduria
    choroidal b.
    b. retinal vein occlusion
    thymic b.
branched-chain amino acid
branchial
    b. arch
    b. pouch
    b. pouch dysembryogenesis
branching enzyme
brandenberg
    Salmonella b.

Bra Pocket pump holder
BRCA
>breast cancer antigen
>BRCA gene

BRCA1
>BRCA1 gene
>BRCA1 mutation

BRCA2
>BRCA2 gene
>BRCA2 mutation

BrDU
>bromodeoxyuridine

breast
>b. arterial calcification
>b. cancer
>b. cancer antigen (BRCA)
>b. cancer antigen 1, 2 mutation
>b. cancer cell
>b. cancer gene
>b. development
>fibroadenomatous hyperplasia of b.
>b. lobule
>b. milk
>b. parenchyma
>pigeon b.
>b. silicone implant
>b. stimulation
>b. tumor

breast/ovarian cancer syndrome
breath
>fruity b.

Brenner tumor
Brevicon
BRFSS
>Behavioral Risk Factor Surveillance System

Bricanyl
bridge
>cytoplasmic b.
>disulfide b.
>intermolecular dityrosine b.

bridged sella turcica
Brief Index of Sexual Functioning for Women
British Diabetes Association
brittle-bone disease
brittle diabetes
broad
>b. beta disease
>b. ligament

Broca diagonal band
Bromanate DC

bromergocryptine
bromide
>butylscopolamine b.
>cyanogen b.

bromoaurone analog
bromocriptine
>Apo B.
>b. therapy

bromodeoxyuridine (BrDU)
>b. uptake

bromodiphenhydramine and codeine
bromoflavone
bromophenolic ring
brompheniramine, phenylpropanolamine, and codeine
Bromsulphalein (BSP)
bronchial
>b. asthma
>b. carcinoid variant syndrome
>b. lavage
>b. microcarcinoid

bronchocentric granulomatosis
bronze
>b. diabetes
>b. disease

brown
>b. adipose tissue (BAT)
>b. fat
>b. tumor

Brown-Schilder disease
Brown-Séquard organotherapy
BRR syndrome
brucei
>*Trypanosoma b.*

Brucella melitensis
brucellosis
Bruchner reflex
bruit
>arterial b.

Brunner gland
brush-border
>b.-b. alpha-glucosidase enzyme
>b.-b. membrane (BBM)

brush cytology
brushite
Bruton
>B. disease
>B. tyrosine kinase
>B. tyrosine kinase gene

BSA
>bovine serum albumin

NOTES

BSO
  bilateral salpingo-oophorectomy
BSP
  bone sialoprotein
  Bromsulphalein
BTK gene
bubble boy disease
BUBRI
buccal
  b. smear
  b. testosterone
buciclate
  testosterone b.
bud
  thyroid b.
buffalo hump
buffer
  b. nerve
  proton b.
buffered citrate
buffering
  hydrogen ion b.
buildup
  callus b.
bulb
  jugular b.
  olfactory b.
bulbi (*pl. of* bulbus)
bulbospongiosus muscle
bulbourethral
  b. gland
  b. gland of Cowper
bulbus, pl. **bulbi**
  b. penis
  b. vestibuli
bulging
  chondrocostal junction b.
bulimia nervosa
bulla, pl. **bullae**
  diabetic b.
bullosa
  epidermolysis b.
bullosis diabeticorum
bullous
  b. diabeticorum
  b. pemphigoid
bull's eye-type macular atrophy
bulsulfan
bumetanide
bumetanide-sensitive sodium-postassium-2 chloride cotransporter

bumpy lips
BUN
  blood urea nitrogen
bundle
  medial forebrain b.
  myelinated fiber b.
  nigrostriatal b.
  ventral adrenergic b.
Buprenex
buprenorphine
bupropion
burden
  aluminum b.
Burin variant
Burkitt lymphoma
burnout
  diabetes b.
bursting pattern
Buschke-Ollendorff syndrome
buserelin acetate
busulfan
butalbital compound and codeine
butanol-extractable iodine
butanone
butorphanol
button infuser
butylscopolamine bromide
B-variant
  estrogen receptor B-v.
BVD-MD
  bovine viral diarrhea mucosal disease
  BVD-MD virus
B_x
  vitamin B_x
bypass
  biliointestinal b.
  biliopancreatic b.
  dorsalis pedis arterial b.
  gastric b.
  intestinal b.
  jejunoileal b.
  Roux-en-Y gastric b.
bystander
  b. effect
  b. stimulation
  b. T-cell proliferation hypothesis
BZD
  benzodiazepine

C

C apolipoprotein
apolipoprotein C
arylsulfatase C
atypical protein kinase C
C band
C cell
C cell hyperplasia
hemoglobin C
hepatitis C
high-density lipoprotein C (HDL-C)
mitomycin C
C peptide
phospholipase C (PLC)
protein kinase C (PKC)
very low density lipoprotein C
(VLDL-C)

C1 element insulin gene promoter
C2 element insulin gene promoter
C$_4$
leukotriene C$_4$ (LTC$_4$)
C-19
C-19 progestin
C-19 steroid
C-21
C-21 progestin
C-21 steroid
CA
CA II deficiency
CA II gene
CA125
cancer antigen-125
Ca^{2+}
cytoplasmic Ca^{2+}
free Ca^{2+}
Ca^{2+} ionophore A23187
Ca^{2+} ionophore drug
Ca^{2+} pump
total Ca^{2+}
CAAT box
Ca^{2+}-ATPase
calmodulin-dependent C.-A.
cabergoline
cachectin
cachexia
cancer c.
diencephalic c.
exophthalmic c.
neuropathic c.
CACS
coronary artery calcium score
cadaveric pancreas transplantation
cadaver pancreas
cadherin
cadmium telluride detector

café
c. au lait lesion
c. au lait macule
c. au lait pigmentation
c. au lait spot
cafeteria diet
caffeine
orphenadrine, aspirin, and c.
Caffey syndrome
CAH
congenital adrenal hyperplasia
CA II
carbonic anhydrase II
CA II deficiency
CA II gene
CAIS
complete androgen insensitivity
syndrome
calbindin
c. D$_{9K}$
c. D$_{28K}$
c. 9-kDA
CALCA gene
Cal Carb-HD
calcemic
c. effect
c. response
Calci-Chew
Calciday-667
calcifediol
calciferol metabolite
calcification
basal ganglion c.
breast arterial c.
dystrophic c.
ectopic c.
extracellular c.
extraskeletal c.
laminated c.
metastatic extraosseal c.
ocular c.
pathologic c.
popcorn c.
provisional c.
soft-tissue c.
tumor-like c.
vascular c.
visceral c.
zone of provisional c.
calcified
c. desquamated debris
c. malignant insulinoma
Calcijex
Calcimar

calcimimetic
    c. agent
    c. compound
    c. drug
Calci-Mix
calcineurin inhibitor
calcinosis
    c. circumscripta
    toxic c.
    tumoral c.
    c. universalis
calciopenic rickets
calciotropic peptide hormone
calcipenia
calciphylaxis
calcipotriol
calcitonin (CT)
    c. gene
    c. gene expression
    c. gene-related hormone (CGRH)
    c. gene-related peptide (CGRP)
    human c.
    c. monomer
    c. receptor
    salmon c.
calcitonin-induced phosphaturia
calcitriol
    c. deficiency
    c. therapy
calcitriol-mediated hypercalcemia
calcitroic acid
calcitrol
calcitropic hormone
calcium
    c. absorption
    c. acetate
    albumin-bound c.
    amorphous c.
    atorvastatin c.
    c. balance
    c. bilirubinate granule
    c. binding
    c. carbonate and magnesium
      carbonate
    c. carbonate oxyphil cell
    c. carbonate and simethicone
    c. channel blocker (CCB)
    circulating c.
    c. citrate
    c. complex
    complexed c.
    cytoplasmic c.
    cytosolic free c.
    c. deficiency
    c. degradation
    c. deposition
    c. efflux
    endogenous fecal c.
    c. flux

    c. glubionate
    c. glucoheptonate
    c. gluconate
    c. gradient
    c. homeostasis
    c. homeostatic factor
    c. hydrogen phosphate
    immunoradiometric assay of
      circulating c.
    intracellular c.
    c. iodide
    c. ion
    c. ion concentration
    ionic c.
    c. ionophore
    c. ionophore challenge
    c. lactate
    c. loading
    c. malabsorption
    c. oxalate
    c. oxalate dihydrate crystal
    c. oxalate monohydrate crystal
    c. oxalate renal stone
    c. phosphate compound
    c. phosphate crystal
    c. phosphorus metabolism
    physiologically active c.
    c. pump
    c. pyrophosphate
    c. receptor agonist
    c. release
    c. release-activated cation channel
    c. resorption
    c. salt
    c. sensor
    serum ionized c.
    c. stimulation test
    c. times phosphorus product
    total intestinal c.
    c. transport
    c. uptake
    urinary c.
calcium-binding
    c.-b. protein
    c.-b. protein synthesis
calcium/creatinine ratio
calcium-dependent protein kinase
calcium-induced calcium release (CICR)
calcium-lowering hormone
calcium-regulating hormone
calcium-sensing receptor (CaR)
calcium-to-creatinine ratio
calculation
    Friedewald c.
calculus, pl. **calculi**
    intrapancreatic c.
    renal c.
Calderol
caldesmon

calendar
    PRISM c.
California Diabetes and Pregnancy Sweet Success Guidelines
californica
    Torpedo c.
calipers
    Prader c.
Call-Exner body
callosum
    corpus c.
    dysgenesis of corpus c.
callus buildup
Calmette-Guérin
    bacillus C.-G. (BCG)
calmodulin-dependent
    c.-d. Ca^{2+}-ATPase
    c.-d. protein kinase (CaM-kinase)
calmodulin protein
Calm-X Oral
calnexin
caloric intake
calorigenic activity
calorimetry
calpactin
calpain-10 gene
Cal-Plus
Caltrate
calvarial
    c. osteomalacia
    c. thickening
CAM
    cell-cell adhesion molecule
camera
    Planar gamma c.
CaM-kinase
    calmodulin-dependent protein kinase
cAMP
    cyclic adenosine monophosphate
    cyclic 3′,5′-adenosine monophosphate
    cyclic AMP
    cyclic arginine monophosphate
    dibutyryl cAMP
    nephrogenous cAMP
    cAMP response element-binding (CREB)
cAMP-response
    c.-r. element (CRE)
    c.-r. element modulator (CREM)
camptomelic
    c. dwarfism
    c. dysplasia

camsylate
    trimethaphan c.
Camurati-Engelmann disease
Canadian Diabetes Association Clinical Practice Guidelines
Canadian-Dutch Mennonite kindreds
Canadian/European Cyclosporine Study
canal
    craniopharyngeal c.
    Dorello c.
    haversian c.
    optic c.
    Volkmann c.
canalicular testis
canaliculus, pl. **canaliculi**
Canavan disease
cancellous bone
cancer
    adrenal c.
    American Joint Commission on C.
    anaplastic thyroid c.
    c. antigen-125 (CA125)
    breast c.
    c. cachexia
    differential thyroid c. (DTC)
    differentiated thyroid c. (DTC)
    endometrial c.
    estrogen receptor-positive breast c.
    European Organization for Research and Treatment of C. (EORTC)
    European Prospective Investigation of C. (EPIC)
    familial colorectal c.
    familial gastric c.
    familial medullary thyroid c. (FMTC)
    familial nonmedullary thyroid c.
    familial ovarian c.
    follicular thyroid c.
    hereditary nonpolyposis colon c. (HNPCC)
    hormone-resistant breast c.
    liver c.
    medullary thyroid c. (MTC)
    pancreas c.
    papillary thyroid c.
    thyroid c.
    Union Internationale Contre le C. (UICC)
Candida albicans

NOTES

candidal
  c. vaginitis
  c. vulvitis
candidate
  c. gene
  c. gene approach
candidiasis
  c. endocrinopathy syndrome
  hypoparathyroidism, adrenal
    insufficiency, mucocutaneous c.
    (HAM)
  mucocutaneous c.
  vaginal c.
  vulvovaginal c.
candiduria
canine distemper virus
cantharides
canthomeatal line
Cantil
Cantrell
  pentalogy of C.
CAP
  catabolite activator protein
  Cbl/Cbl-associated protein
  chronic alcoholic pancreatitis
  contraction-associated protein
cap
  acrosomal c.
  c. phase
capacitance measurement
capacitation of the spermatozoa
capacity
  binding c.
  reduced exercise c.
  reserve c.
  vital c.
cap-binding complex
CAPD
  chronic ambulatory peritoneal dialysis
  continuous ambulatory peritoneal dialysis
capillary
  adenohypophysial c.
  c. basement membrane width
    (CBMW)
  c. blood glucose monitoring
  c. blood sugar (CBS)
  c. endothelium
  c. filtrate collector
  c. leak syndrome
capita (*pl. of* caput)
Capital and codeine
capitalis
  plexus pancreaticus c.
Capoten
CAPP
  Captopril Prevention Project
caproate
  hydroxyprogesterone c.
capsaicin

Capsin
capsularis
  decidua c.
capsulatum
  Histoplasma c.
capsule
  Angel Hypoglycemic c.
  Bowman c.
  Diabetes Hypoglucose c.
  internal c.
  c. of islet
  Pearl Hypoglycemic c.
  pregabalin c.
  tense tumor c.
  thyroid c.
  Tongyi Tang Diabetes c.
  Zhen Qi c.
captopril
  C. Prevention Project (CAPP)
  c. test
caput, pl. **capita**
  c. epididymis
Capzasin-P
CaR
  calcium-sensing receptor
Carafate
carbamazepine
carbamide drug
carbamoyl
  c. phosphate synthase
  c. phosphate synthetase I
    deficiency
carbamoyltransferase
  ornithine c.
carbamylcholine
  muscarinic agonist c.
carbenoxolone
carbetapentane
Carb-HD
  Cal C.-H.
carbidopa
  levodopa and c.
carbimazole
carbodiimide modified heteroduplex
  screening method
carbohydrate
  complex c.
  c. counting
  c. intolerance
  c. malabsorption
  c. meal
  c. metabolism
  c. metabolism change
  c. moiety
  c. nutrient
  refined c.
  c. response
  simple c.

carbohydrate-deficient
    c.-d. glycoprotein (CDG)
    c.-d. glycoprotein syndrome
carbohydrate-induced
  hypertriglyceridemia
carbon
    c. balance
    c. disulfide
carbonate (CO_3^{2-})
    aluminum hydroxide and
      magnesium c.
    bone c.
    calcium carbonate and
      magnesium c.
    dihydroxyaluminum sodium c.
    c. ion
    lithium c.
    magnesium c.
carbonic
    c. acid
    c. anhydrase activity
    c. anhydrase enzyme
    c. anhydrase II (CA II)
    c. anhydrase II deficiency
    c. anhydrase II gene
    c. anhydrase II isoenzyme
    c. anhydrase inhibitor
carboplatin
carboxamide-Dome
    dimethyl triazeno imidazole c.-D.
      (DTIC-Dome)
carboxyesterase
carboxykinase
carboxylase
    hydroxymethylglutaryl-coenzyme
      A c.
    3-methylcrotonyl c.
    propionyl-coenzyme A c.
    pyruvate c.
carboxyl kinase
carboxyl-terminal region
carboxyl-terminus domain
carboxymethylation
carboxypeptidase
    dipeptidyl c.
    c. E
    c. H (CPH)
carboxyterminal cross-linked telopeptide
  of type I collagen (ICTP)
carboxytermini
carbuncle
carcinoembryonic antigen (CEA)

carcinogenesis
    radioactive iodine-induced c.
    RAI-induced c.
carcinogenic
carcinoid
    appendiceal c.
    c. crisis
    primary ovarian c.
    sporadic c.
    c. syndrome
    thymic c.
    c. tumor
    type 1, 2, 3 gastric c.
carcinoidlike tumor
carcinoma
    adrenal c.
    adrenocortical c.
    anaplastic thyroid c.
    differentiated thyroid c.
    embryonal c.
    encapsulated angioinvasive c.
    epithelial thyroid c.
    familial medullary thyroid c.
      (FMTC)
    familial thyroid c.
    follicular epithelial c.
    follicular thyroid c.
    giant cell c.
    infantile embryonic c.
    infiltrating ductal c.
    infiltrating lobular c.
    insular c.
    invasive ductal c. (IDC)
    islet cell c.
    lipid-laden homogeneous
      adrenocortical c.
    medullary thyroid c. (MTC)
    Merkel cell c.
    mucoepidermoid c.
    nevoid basal cell c.
    nonpapillary thyrogenic c.
    nonsmall cell c.
    occult c.
    pancreatic duct cell c. (PDC)
    papillary renal c.
    papillary thyroid c. (PTC)
    parathyroid c.
    pituitary c.
    pleomorphic c.
    radiation-associated papillary
      thyroid c.
    c. of Sakamoto

C

NOTES

carcinoma *(continued)*
    sclerosing mucoepidermoid c.
    c. showing thymuslike
      differentiation (CASTLE)
    small cell c.
    spindle cell c.
    thyrogenic c.
    thyroglossal duct c.
    thyroid gland c.
    thyroid mucoepidermoid c.
    thyroid papillary c.
    thyroid squamous cell c.
    thyrotroph c.
    Warthin-like papillary c.
    c. with thymus-like differentiation
      tumor
carcinomatosa
    peritonitis c.
carcinosarcoma
    thyroid c.
cardiac
    c. abnormality, abnormal facies,
      thymic hypoplasia, cleft palate,
      hypocalcemia (CATCH)
    c. endocrine aldosterone system
    c. fibrosis
    c. gene expression
    c. index
    c. looping
    c. mucormycosis
    c. output
    c. steroidogenic system
cardiofaciocutaneous syndrome
cardiogenic shock
cardiometabolic syndrome
cardiomyocyte
    aldosterone c.
    c. apoptosis
cardiomyopathy
    diabetic c.
    hypertensive c.
    hypertrophic c.
cardioprotective effect
cardiotropin-1 (CT-1)
cardiovascular
    c. autonomic neuropathy
    c. disorder
    c. dysmetabolic syndrome
    c. effect
Cardura
CARE
    Cholesterol and Recurrent Events
    CARE study
carinatum
carinii
    Pneumocystis c.
carmoisin
Carmol Topical

Carney
    C. complex
    C. syndrome
    triad of C.
    C. triad
carnitine
    c. acylcarnitine translocase
      deficiency
    c. palmitoyltransferase I (CPTI)
    c. palmitoyltransferase I deficiency
    c. palmitoyltransferase II (CPTII)
    c. palmitoyltransferase II deficiency
    c. shuttle
Carnitor
carnosinase
carnosine
carotenoderma
carotid
    c. aneurysm
    c. artery
    c. body
    c. body tumor
    c. sinus
    c. sinus baroreceptor
Carpenter syndrome
carpopedal spasm
carpotarsal osteolysis
carrier
    c. detection
    dolichol phosphate c.
    c. protein
CART
    cocaine and amphetamine regulated
      transcript
cartilage
    articular c.
    c. calcification failure
    cricoid c.
    hyaline c.
    Meckel c.
    c. oligomeric matrix protein
    preosseous c.
    thyroid c.
cartilaginous anlage
cartridge
    Genotropin two-chamber c.
    Novolin 85/15 PenFill c.
    sorbent dialysis c.
CASA
    computer-aided sperm analysis
    computer-assisted semen analysis
cascade
    adenylyl cyclase c.
    adrenal steroidogenic c.
    arachidonic acid c.
    blood clotting c.
    insulin phosphorylation c.
    MAPK c.

microtubule-associated protein
kinase c.
mitogen-activated protein kinase c.
protein kinase C c.
protein kinase/phosphatase c.

caseating granuloma

casein
c. hydrolysate
c. kinase I, II

CASH
cortical androgen-stimulating hormone

Casodex

cassava

cassette
adenosine triphosphate binding c.
(ABC)

CASTLE
carcinoma showing thymuslike
differentiation
CASTLE tumor

Castleman disease

castration
c. cell
chemical c.

CAT
chloramphenicol acetyl transferase
coital alignment technique

catabolic stress

catabolism
accelerated c.
fat c.
muscle c.
statin c.

catabolite
c. activator protein (CAP)
c. regulatory protein

Cataflam Oral

catagen

catalysis

catalyst
biologic c.

catalytic homodimer

catamenial
c. epilepsy
c. seizure

cataplexy

Catapres

CATCH
cardiac abnormality, abnormal facies,
thymic hypoplasia, cleft palate,
hypocalcemia
CATCH 22 syndrome

catch trial

catecholamine
alpha$_2$-adrenergic c.
beta$_2$-adrenergic c.
c. biosynthesis
fetal c.
fractionated urinary c.
c. receptor gene
c. response
c. surge

catecholaminergic system

catecholamine-secreting cell

catechol compound

catecholestrogen

catechol-*O*-methyltransferase (COMT)

cathepsin
c. B
c. B enzyme
bone-specific c.
c. D
c. H
c. K
c. K gene
c. L
c. O
c. S

catheterization
bilateral adrenal vein c.

cationic trypsinogen gene

caucus
Congressional Diabetes C.

caudal regression syndrome

caveola, pl. **caveolae**

caveolin

cavernosum
corpus c.

cavernous
c. hemangioma
c. sinus
c. sinus sampling (CSS)
c. sinus syndrome
c. sinus thrombophlebitis

cavity
amnionic c.
endometrial c.
intrasellar c.
medullary c.
nasal c.

Cayler cardiofacial syndrome

CBA
cytochemical bioassay

NOTES

53

CBAVD
    congenital bilateral absence of the vas
      deferens
CBD
    common bile duct
CBF
    cerebral blood flow
CBG
    corticosteroid-binding globulin
    cortisol-binding globulin
Cbl/Cbl-associated protein (CAP)
CBMW
    capillary basement membrane width
CBP
    CREB-binding protein
CBS
    capillary blood sugar
c/c
    Snp5 c/c
CCAAT element insulin gene promoter
CCAAT/enhancer binding protein (C/EBP)
CCB
    calcium channel blocker
CCCT
    clomiphene citrate challenge test
CCD
    cortical collecting duct
C-cell
      C-c. adenoma
      C-c. complex
CC-EPT
    continuous-combined estrogen-
      progestogen therapy
ccHRT
    continuous-combined hormone
      replacement therapy
CCK
    cholecystokinin
CCK-A and CCK-B
    cholecystokinin A and cholecystokinin B
      CCK-A and CCK-B receptor
CCK-C
    cholecystokinin-C
CCK-8-S
    cholecystokinin-8-S
CCPT
    chronic calcific pancreatitis of the tropics
C-Crystals
CD
      CD 27 ligand (CD 27L)
      CD 30 ligand (CD 30L)
      CD 40 ligand
CD4+
      C. T cell
      C. T-cell receptor transgene
CD8+
      C. phenotype

      C. T cell
      C. T-cell receptor transgene
CD154
CD38
CD1 antigen
CD4 helper lymphocyte
CD8 suppressor lymphocyte
Cdc42
CDE
    Certified Diabetes Educator
CDG
    carbohydrate-deficient glycoprotein
CDGA
    constitutional delay in growth and
      adolescence
CDI
    central diabetes insipidus
    controlled diabetes insipidus
CDK, Cdk
    cyclin-dependent kinase
CD 27L
    CD 27 ligand
CD 30L
    CD 30 ligand
cDNA
    complementary deoxyribonucleic acid
    complementary DNA
CDR3
    third complementarity determining region
CDU
    color Doppler ultrasonography
CEA
    carcinoembryonic antigen
Cebid
C/EBP
    CCAAT/enhancer binding protein
      C/EBP transcription factor
cecocentral
      c. defect
      c. scotoma
Cecon
cecum
      foramen c.
CEE
    conjugated equine estrogen
CEEP
    conjugated equine estrogen plus
      norgestrel
cefadroxil
Cefanex
cefdinir
Cefol Filmtabs
ceftazidime
Celestone
      C. Oral
      C. Phosphate Injection
      C. Soluspan
celiac
      c. artery

c. disease
c. plexus
c. sprue

cell

A c.
A$_1$ c.
A$_2$ c.
acidophilic c.
adenohypophysial corticotroph c.
adrenal cortex c.
adrenocortical c.
adrenomedullary c.
alpha TC-1/9 c.
alveolar type II c.
amine precursor uptake and
  decarboxylation c.
antigen-presenting c. (APC)
antigen-specific suppressor T c.
apical membrane of proximal
  convoluted tubule c.
APUD c.
argentaffin c.
argyrophil c.
Askanazy c.
c. association
autocrine c.
B c.
c. basement membrane
basophilic c.
beta Tc-6 c.
bone c.
bone-forming c.
bone marrow-derived stromal c.
breast cancer c.
C c.
calcium carbonate oxyphil c.
castration c.
catecholamine-secreting c.
CD4+ T c.
CD8+ T c.
CFU-E c.
chemoreceptive c.
chief c.
Chinese hamster ovary c.
CHO c.
chromaffin c.
chromophilic c.
chromophobic c.
ciliated c.
clear c.
clonal c.
colony-forming unit erythroid c.

compact c.
corticotropic c.
Crooke c.
cuboidal epithelioid c.
c. culture study
cumulus granulosa c.
cycling c.
D c.
delta c.
determined osteoprogenitor c.
ECL c.
electrically excitable c.
endocrine effector c.
endothelial c. (EC)
enterochromaffin c. (EC)
enterochromaffin-like c.
epithelioid giant c.
eukaryotic c.
exocrine c.
F c.
Fischer rat thyroid line-5 c.
foam c.
foamy c.
follicular c.
folliculostellate c.
FRTL-5 c.
G c.
ghost c.
glial c.
glucagonlike peptide-1 pancreatic
  endocrine c.
goblet c.
gonadectomy c.
gonadotroph c.
granular chromophil c.
granulated c.
granulosa lutein c.
growth hormone c.
growth hormone-expressing c.
growth hormone-prolactin c.
helper T c.
HI-K$_{IR}$6.2 beta c.
hilar c.
hilus c.
HIT-T15 c.
Hofbauer c.
homeobox gene expressed in
  ES c.'s (HESX1)
hormone-secreting c.
horny c.
host c.
human pluripotent stem c.

NOTES

55

cell *(continued)*
    Hürthle c.
    hybridoma c.
    hypochromic microcytic red blood c.
    inflammatory c.
    insulinoma c.
    insulin-producing c.
    intercalated c.
    islet c.
    JG c.
    Jurkat c.
    juxtaglomerular c.
    Kornchenzellen c.
    Kulchitsky c.
    Kupffer c.
    L c.
    LAK c.
    Langerhans c.
    Leydig c.
    lipid-laden clear c.
    lipoid c.
    lutein c.
    lymphoid c.
    lymphokine-activated killer c.
    macula densa c.
    mammosomatotroph c.
    marrow hematopoietic stem c.
    mast c.
    medullary c.
    melanotropic c.
    membrana granulosa c.
    mesangial c.
    mesenchymal stem c.
    mesodermal c.
    murine L c.
    myelomonocytic c.
    myoepithelial c.
    myoid c.
    natural killer c.
    neoplastic adenohypophysial c.
    neuroendocrine c.
    neuroglia c.
    neurohormonal c.
    neurosecretory c.
    NK c.
    NKT c.
    noncontractile c.
    noncornified c.
    nongranular clear chromophobe c.
    null c.
    osteoblastlike osteosarcoma c.
    osteoprogenitor c.
    ovarian granulosa c.
    oxyphil c.
    pancreatic acinar c.
    pancreatic islet beta c.
    parabasal c.
    paracrine c.
    parafollicular calcitonin-producing c.
    parathyroid hormone-related protein-transfected RIN-141 c.
    pathognomonic Askanazy c.
    peripheral cytotrophoblast c.
    peritubular endothelial c.
    pituitary lactotroph c.
    pluripotent hematopoietic c.
    pluripotential precursor c.
    pluripotential stromal c.
    pluripotent stem c.
    PMN c.
    polarized c.
    polyclonal B, T c.
    polygonal c.
    polyhedral c.
    polymorphonuclear c.
    polypeptide-producing c.
    polyploidic c.
    precursor c.
    pregnancy c.
    primordial germ c. (PGC)
    progenitor c.
    prokaryotic c.
    prolactin hormone-expressing c.
    pseudogiant c.
    PTHrP-transfected RIN-141 c.
    Purkinje c.
    red blood c. (RBC)
    renal carcinoma c.
    resting c.
    Schwann c.
    secondary interstitial c.
    c. senescence
    Sertoli c.
    Sertoli-Leydig c.
    sickle c. (SC)
    c. signaling
    somatostatin-producing delta c.
    somatotroph c.
    somatotropic c.
    spindle c.
    stem c.
    stromal c.
    suppressor T c.
    supraopticohypophysial c.
    surrogate beta c.
    sympathetic c.
    syncytiotrophoblast c.
    T c.
    tall c.
    target c.
    TC-6-10 c.
    Th1 c.
    Th2 c.
    theca externa c.
    theca interna c.
    theca interstitial c.
    theca lutein c.

T helper 1, 2 c.
thyroidal C c.
thyroid C c.
thyroid deficiency c.
thyroidectomy c.
thyroid epithelial c.
thyroid follicular c.
thyroid parafollicular c.
thyrotroph c.
thyrotropic c.
thyrotropin-stimulating hormone-
  expressing c.
transient amplifying c.
trophoblast c.
tumor c.
vascular smooth muscle c. (VSMC)
white blood c. (WBC)
zona fasciculata c.
zona glomerulosa c.
cell-bone matrix interaction
cell-cell adhesion molecule (CAM)
CellCept
cell-cycle regulation
cell-mediated
  c.-m. immunity
  c.-m. toxicity
cell-signaling mechanism
cell-specific ablation
cell-surface antigen
cell-to-cell communication
cellular
  c. dehydration
  c. immunity
cellulitis
  necrotizing c.
  nonclostridial anaerobic c.
  orbital c.
  synergistic necrotizing c.
cellulose
  c. sodium phosphate
  c. sulfate
cellulose-derived matrix
Cel-U-Jec Injection
cement line
cementum
Cenestin
Cenolate
center
  central thermoregulatory c.
  germinal c.
  C. for Human Islet Transplantation
  hypothalamic c.

Joslin Diabetes C.
New England Diabetes and
  Endocrinology C.
X inactivation c. (Xic)
centigray (cGy)
centiMorgan (cM)
central
  c. adrenocortical insufficiency
  c. diabetes insipidus (CDI)
  c. hyperhidrosis
  c. hyperthyroidism
  c. hypoadrenalism
  c. hypogonadism
  c. hypogonadism type IA, IB, IIA,
    III
  c. hypothyroidism
  c. necrosis
  c. nervous system (CNS)
  c. obesity
  c. pontine myelinolysis
  c. precocious puberty (CPP)
  c. scotoma
  c. serous chorioretinopathy (CSCP)
  c. thermoregulatory center
centrifugation
  isopycnic c.
centriole
centripetal obesity
cephalexin
cephalic
  c. parenchymography
  c. phase
cephalosporin
c-erbA
  protooncogene c-e.
c-erbA-beta
  c-e.-b. receptor
  c-e.-b. thyroid hormone receptor
    gene
c-erbA-beta-1 defect
c-erbA-beta-2 defect
cerebellar
  c. ataxia
  c. cortex
  c. vermis
cerebelloretinal hemangioblastomatosis
cerebellum
cerebral
  c. artery
  c. blood flow (CBF)
  c. cortex
  c. edema

C

NOTES

cerebral (*continued*)
    c. gigantism
    c. palsy
    c. peduncle
    c. salt wasting
    c. tetany
    c. vein thrombosis
cerebri
    acervuli c.
    epiphysis c.
    pseudomotor c.
    pseudotumor c.
cerebrospinal
    c. fluid (CSF)
    c. fluid ACE level
    c. fluid angiotensin-converting
      enzyme level
    c. fluid fistula
    c. fluid rhinorrhea
cerebrotendinous xanthomatosis
Ceredase
Cerezyme
cerivastatin
Cerose-DM
Certified Diabetes Educator (CDE)
cerulein
ceruleus
    locus c.
ceruloplasmin
cervical
    c. factor infertility
    c. goiter
    c. lymph node (CLN)
    c. mucosa
    c. mucous plug
    c. sensory nerve
cervicodorsal fat pad
cervix uterus
Cesamet
cetrorelix
cetylmyristoleate (CMO)
    c. II
Cevalin
Cevi-bid
Ce-Vi-Sol
CFA
    complete Freund adjuvant
CFC BioScanner System
C-fiber pain
c-*fms* oncogene
c-*fos*
    c. gene
    c. mapping
    c. promoter
    protooncogene c.
cFos-cJun heterodimer
CFRD
    cystic fibrosis-related diabetes

CFTR
    cystic fibrosis transmembrane regulator
      CFTR gene
CFU-E
    colony-forming unit erythroid
      CFU-E cell
CG
    chorionic gonadotropin
CGI
    glycoprotein crystal growth inhibitor
      CGI protein
CGL
    chronic granulocytic leukemia
    congenital generalized lipodystrophy
cGMP
    cyclic guanosine monophosphate
    cyclic 3′,5′-guanosine monophosphate
    5′-cyclic guanosine monophosphate
      cGMP phosphodiesterase
cGMP-dependent protein kinase
CGMS
    continuous glucose monitoring system
CGRH
    calcitonin gene-related hormone
CGRP
    calcitonin gene-related peptide
cGy
    centigray
CHA
    common hepatic artery
ChAgly
chain
    jugular c.
    mitochondrial electron transport c.
    myosin heavy c. (MHC)
    myosin light c. (MLC)
    nascent protein c.
    oligosaccharide c.
    sympathetic c.
challenge
    calcium ionophore c.
    deferoxamine c.
    DFO c.
change
    blood volume c.
    carbohydrate metabolism c.
    Crooke hyaline c.
    fluorotic c.
    intracytoplasmic oncocytic c.
    oxyphilic c.
    peripheral circulatory c.
    polyneuropathy, organomegaly,
      endocrinopathy, monoclonal
      component, skin c.'s (POEMS)
    polyneuropathy, organomegaly,
      endocrinopathy, M proteins,
      skin c.'s (POEMS)
    rachitic c.
    sexual dimorphic physical c.

channel
adenosine triphosphate potassium c.
adenosine triphosphate-sensitive potassium$_{ATP}$ c.
apical iodide c.
aquaporin-2 water c.
AQ2 water c.
B-cell adenosine triphosphate-sensitive potassium$_{ATP}$ c.
beta-cell adenosine triphosphate potassium c.
beta-cell CA2+-activated K+ c.
beta-cell calcium c.
beta-cell delayed rectifier voltage-gated K c.
beta-cell glucose-mediated depolarization K$_{ATP}$ c.
beta-cell glucose-mediated depolarization potassium$_{ATP}$ c.
beta-cell intracellular c.
beta-cell ion c.
beta-cell K$_v$ and CA$_v$ c.
beta-cell nonselection cation c.
beta-cell potassium$_{ATP}$ c.
beta-cell secretory granule c.
beta-cell voltage-gated calcium c.
brain K$_{IR}$6.2/SUR1 potassium$_{ATP}$ c.
calcium release-activated cation c.
collecting tubule sodium c.
cystic fibrosis transmembrane conductance regulator chloride c.
epithelial sodium c. (ENaC)
inward-directed voltage-gated Ca^{2+} c.
inward-rectifying K$^+$-c. 6.2 (K$_{ir}$6.2)
iodide c.
ion c.
kainate receptor c.
ligand-gated c.
L-type calcium c.
potassium$_{ATP}$ c.
potassium leak c.
potassium $_{IR}$6.2 sulfonylurea receptor 1 potassium$_{ATP}$ c.
T-type calcium c.
voltage-dependent anion c. (VDAC)
voltage-dependent calcium c. (VDCC)
voltage-gated Ca^{2+} c.
voltage-gated K$^+$ c.
voltage-gated Na$^+$ c.
channel-forming integral protein (CHIP)

CHAOS
coronary artery disease, hypertension, adult-onset diabetes, obesity, and stroke
chaperone
molecular c.
characteristic
chronobiologic c.
charcoal
activated c.
adenoma c.
atypical c.
benign c.
c. hemoperfusion
Charcot
C. arthropathy
C. foot
C. foot phenomenon
C. fracture
C. joint
C. joint disease
C. neuroarthropathy
Charcot-Marie disease
Charcot-Marie-Tooth disease
charge
energy c.
chart
growth-velocity c.
intrauterine growth c.
National Center for Health Statistics c.
chase incubation
ChAT
choline acetyltransferase
checklist
thyroid symptom c.
Chediak-Higashi syndrome
cheilitis
angular c.
cheiropathy
chelation
chelator
fura-2 fluorescent Ca^{2+} c.
quin-2 fluorescent Ca^{2+} c.
cheloni
Mycobacterium c.
chemical
c. castration
endocrine disrupting c. (EDC)
c. gradient
c. messenger
xenobiotic c.

NOTES

chemiluminescence
> c. assay
> c. detection

chemiluminescent
> c. assay
> c. immunoassay (CLIA)
> c. reagent

Chemistrip
> Micral C.

chemodectoma
> thyroid c.

chemoembolization
> transcatheter arterial c. (TACE)

chemokine
> growth factor-inducible c. (FIC)
> c. receptor

chemoreceptive cell
chemoreceptor
> macula densa c.

chemosis
> conjunctival c.

chemosurgery
chemotactic factor
chemotaxis
> neutrophil c.

chemotherapy
> adjuvant c.
> cytotoxic c.

Chemstrip
> C. bG
> C. MatchMaker blood glucose meter

Chiari-Frommel syndrome
chiasm
> optic c.

chiasmal
> c. arachnoiditis
> c. compression
> c. glioma
> c. neuritis
> c. syndrome

chiasmapexy
chiasmatic
> c. cistern
> c. sulcus
> c. syndrome

chiasmatis
> cisterna c.

chiasmopathy
Chicago
> insulin C. (Phe-B25-Leu)

chief cell
child
> growth hormone-deficient c.
> rachitic c.
> vitamin D-replete c.

childhood
> Avon Longitudinal Study of Pregnancy and C.

> c. Cushing syndrome
> c. Graves disease
> c. head and neck irradiation
> c. hypothyroidism
> c. obesity

Child-Pugh
> C.-P. class
> C.-P. disease

chimeric
> c. protein
> c. pseudogene
> c. receptor

chimerism
chimerization
Chinese
> C. hamster ovary (CHO)
> C. hamster ovary cell

CHIP
> channel-forming integral protein

Chiron ACS:180 assay
chiropody
Chlamydia trachomatis
chloasma gravidarum
chlorambucil
chloramphenicol acetyl transferase (CAT)
chlorbutanol
chlordiazepoxide
> clidinium and c.

chloride
> Adrenalin C.
> ammonium c.
> c. channel gene CLCNKB
> methyl c.
> potassium c.
> thallium c. (TI-201)
> ^{201}Tl-thallous c.
> zinc c.

chlorodeoxyadenosine
chloroquine
chlorothiazide
chlorotrianisene
chlorpromazine
chlorpropamide
chlorpyrifos
chlorthalidone
CHO
> Chinese hamster ovary
> CHO cell

choice
> Medi-Jector C.

cholangitis
> primary sclerosing c. (PSC)
> sclerosing c. (SC)

cholecalciferol
cholecystography
cholecystokinin (CCK)
> c. A and cholecystokinin B (CCK-A and CCK-B)

c. A and cholecystokinin B
  receptor
c. glycemic index
cholecystokinin-C (CCK-C)
cholecystokinin-8-S (CCK-8-S)
choledochal cyst
choledochocele
cholera
pancreatic c.
c. toxin
cholerae
Vibrio c.
CholestaGel
cholestane
cholestanol
cholestasis
anicteric c.
intrahepatic c.
cholestatic
c. hepatitis
c. jaundice
c. liver disease
cholesteatoma
cholesterol
c. desmolase
c. desmolase deficiency
c. embolus
high-density lipoprotein c. (HDL-C)
lipid c.
low-density lipoprotein c. (LDL-C)
c. monohydrate crystal
C. and Recurrent Events (CARE)
C. and Recurrent Events study
c. spike
total c. (TC)
c. transport
cholesteryl
c. ester
c. ester storage disease
c. ester transfer protein
cholestyramine resin
choline
c. acetyltransferase (ChAT)
c. magnesium trisalicylate
c. salicylate
cholinergic
c. activity
c. effect
c. M-receptor agonist
c. neuron
c. nicotinic receptor
c. pathway

chondrocalcinosis
chondrocostal junction bulging
chondrocyte
c. proliferation
c. terminal differentiation
chondrocytic
c. growth
c. lineage
chondrodysplasia
Blomstrand lethal c.
Jansen metaphyseal c. (JMC)
c. punctata
Schmid-type metaphyseal c.
chondrodystrophia punctata
chondroitin sulfate
chondroma
pulmonary c.
chondroprotective effect
chondrosarcoma
Chooz
chordoma
sacrococcygeal c.
chorea
Huntington c.
choreiform movement
choreoathetosis
Chorex
choriocarcinoma
primary ovarian c.
testicular c.
chorion
c. frondosum
c. laeve
leafy c.
chorionepithelioma
chorionic
c. gonadotropin (CG)
c. gonadotropin-secreting tumor
c. gonadotropin stimulation test
c. plate
c. sac
c. somatomammotropin (CS)
c. thyrotropin
c. villus
c. villus sampling (CVS)
chorioretinopathy
central serous c. (CSCP)
choristoma
adenohypophysial neuronal c.
intrasellar adenohypophyseal
  neuronal c.

C

NOTES

choristoma *(continued)*
    pituitary adenoma-adenohypophyseal
      neuronal c. (PANCH)
    pituitary adenoma-neuronal c.
choroid
    c. artery
    c. plexus
choroidal
    c. branch
    c. fissure
Choron
chromaffin
    c. cell
    c. granule
    c. tissue
    c. vesicle
Chromagen OB
chromalum-hematoxylin
    Gomori c.-h.
Chroma-Pak
chromatid
    sister c.
chromatin
    c. derepression
    c. immunoprecipitation assay
    sex c.
    supercoiled c.
    X, Y c.
chromatin-positive seminiferous tubule
  dysgenesis
chromatofocusing
chromatography
    affinity c.
    denaturing high-pressure liquid c.
      (dHPLC)
    exclusion c.
    gas c.
    gel filtration c.
    high-performance liquid c. (HPLC)
    ion exchange c.
chromogen
chromogranin
    c. A
    c. A, B, C protein
chromogranin-secretogranin protein
chromophil
chromophilic
    c. cell
    c. hypophysis
chromophobe
    c. adenoma
    c. tumor
chromophobic
    c. adenoma
    c. cell
    c. pattern
chromosomal
    c. damage
    c. disorder

    c. instability
    c. mosaicism
chromosome
    c. 20
    c. deletion
    c. 7, 12, 20 disorder
    c. duplication
    heterodisomic c.
    c. 6 HLA
    c. 11 insulin gene
    isodisomic c.
    c. 6p21.3
    c. 17p12-13
    c. 18p11
    phosphatase and tensin homologue
      deleted on c. (PTEN)
    phosphate-regulating gene with
      homologies to endopeptidases
      found at the HYP locus on the
      X c. (PEX)
    c. 11p15 insulin gene region
    c. 3q27
    c. 5q31
    c. 5q35.3
    c. 10q
    c. 12q
    c. 12q15
    c. 1q21-q23
    c. 6q22-q23
    c. 11q23-q25
    c. ring
    sex-determining region of the Y c.
      (SRY)
    SRY c.
    c. 7 T-cell receptor beta chain
      locus
    c. translocation
chronic
    c. active hepatitis
    c. alcoholic pancreatitis (CAP)
    c. ambulatory peritoneal dialysis
      (CAPD)
    c. autoimmune theory
    c. autoimmune thyroiditis
    c. calcific pancreatitis of the
      tropics (CCPT)
    c. cystic mastitis
    c. dehydration
    c. dialysis patient
    c. fatigue syndrome
    c. fibrous thyroiditis
    c. glucocorticoid deficiency
    c. granulocytic leukemia (CGL)
    c. granulomatous disease
    c. hemodialysis
    c. hyperandrogenic anovulation
    c. hypercortisolism
    c. hyperglycemia impaired insulin
      secretion

c. hyperglycemia pancreatic beta-cell
c. hypoandrogenic anovulation
c. hypoglycemia
c. inflammatory demyelinating polyneuropathy (CIDP)
c. interstitial nephritis
c. lobular hyperplasia
c. lymphocytic hypophysitis
c. lymphocytic thyroiditis
c. metabolic acidosis
c. myelogenous leukemia (CML)
c. renal failure (CRF)
c. renal insufficiency (CRI)
c. water intoxication
chronobiologic characteristic
chronopharmacologic
chronopharmacology
chronopharmacotherapy
chronotherapy
chronotropic
CHUK
conserved helix-loop-helix ubiquitous kinase
chupatti flour
Chvostek
C. sign
C. test
11-C-hydroxyephedrine scintigraphy
chylomicronemia syndrome
chylomicron retention disease
chymotrypsin
chymotrypsinogen-related 30-kd protein/chymotrypsin
Cialis
ciamexone
Cibacalcin
ciclopirox
CICR
calcium-induced calcium release
CIDP
chronic inflammatory demyelinating polyneuropathy
ciglitazone
ciliary neurotrophic factor (CNTF)
ciliated cell
cilostazol
cimetidine
cinereum
hamartoma of tuber c.
tuber c.

cingulate
c. cortex
c. gyrus
cingulum
circadian
c. clock
c. gating
c. hormonal rhythm
c. locomotor output cycles kaput (CLOCK)
c. oscillator
c. pattern
c. rhythm of hormone secretion
c. variation
circadian/diurnal hormonal rhythm
circannual
c. rhythm
c. rhythmicity of steroid
circulating
c. blood
c. calcium
c. estrogen level
c. lipolytic enzyme
c. proinsulin-like peptide
circulation
enterohepatic c.
fetomaternal c.
hypophysial-portal c.
hypophysial stalk c.
portal c.
vitelline c.
circulatory shock
circumferential lamella
circumoral numbness
circumscripta
calcinosis c.
osteoporosis c.
circumventricular organ (CVO)
CIRP
cold-inducible ribonucleic acid-binding protein
cold-inducible RNA-binding protein
cirrhosis
biliary c.
hepatic c.
primary biliary c.
cis
c. element
c. Golgi network
c. mechanism

NOTES

cis-acting
>> c.-a. DNA element
>> c.-a. factor

cisapride
cis-**clomiphene citrate**
cisplatin
Cis-platinum
13-*cis* retinoic acid
9-*cis* retinoic acid (RXR)
cistern
>> basilar c.
>> chiasmatic c.
>> interpeduncular chiasmatic c.
>> suprasellar c.

cisterna, pl. **cisternae**
>> c. chiasmatis
>> endoplasmic reticulum cisternae

cisternography
>> contrast c.

citalopram
Citracal
citrate
>> buffered c.
>> calcium c.
>> *cis*-clomiphene c.
>> clomiphene c.
>> fentanyl c.
>> gallium c. (Ga-67)
>> c. ion
>> potassium c.
>> ranitidine bismuth c.
>> sildenafil c.
>> c. synthase
>> trans clomiphene c.
>> Zuclomiphene c.

citrated blood
citric
>> c. acid
>> c. acid cycle

Citrobacter diversus
citrullinemia
CJD
>> Creutzfeldt-Jakob disease

cJun
>> c. gene
>> c. molecule

cJunN-terminal
>> c.-t. kinase (JNK)
>> c.-t. kinase serine phosphorylation

c-jun **promoter**
CK
>> creatine kinase

clamp
>> euglycemic insulin c.
>> hyperglycemic glucose c.
>> hypoglycemic c.
>> insulin c.
>> Kelly c.

>> Ochsner c.
>> patch c.

clarithromycin
class
>> Child-Pugh c.
>> c. II HLA locus
>> c. II human leukocyte antigen locus
>> c. III major histocompatibility complex molecule
>> c. I, II MHC molecule
>> c. III MHC molecule
>> c. II major histocompatibility complex molecule
>> c. I major histocompatibility complex molecule

classical
>> c. hydroxylase deficiency
>> c. XO karyotype

classic homocystinuria
classification
>> clinicopathologic c.
>> DeGroot c.
>> diabetes mellitus c.
>> McMaster c.
>> TNM c.
>> tumor/node/metastases c.
>> White c.

clathrin
clathrin-coated
>> c.-c. pit
>> c.-c. vesicle

claudication
>> intensive intermittent c.

clavicular fat pad
claw-toe deformity
CLCNKB
>> chloride channel gene C.

clean-catch urine
clear
>> c. cell
>> c. cell metaplasia
>> c. cytoplasm
>> c. zone

clearance
>> cortisol c.
>> creatinine c.
>> free water c.
>> glucose c.
>> insulin c.
>> iron c.
>> osmolar c.

cleavage
>> collagenase c.
>> ether-link c.
>> posttranslational c.
>> c. product
>> proteolytic c.

P450 side chain c. (P450SCC)
side chain c. (SCC)

cleft
hypophysial c.
c. of the Rathke pouch
synaptic c.

clefting
facial c.

cleidocranial dysplasia

Cleocin
C. HCl Oral
C. Pediatric Oral
C. Phosphate Injection
C. Vaginal

CLI
corpus luteum insufficiency

CLIA
chemiluminescent immunoassay

clidinium and chlordiazepoxide

climacteric
male c.

Climara transdermal

climax
female c.

clindamycin

Clindex

clinical
c. hypoglycemia
c. hypothyroidism
c. insulin sensitivity
c. obesity
c. trial

clinically
c. euthyroid
c. hyperthyroid
c. nonfunctioning pituitary adenoma
c. significant macular edema
(CSME)
c. silent tumor

clinicopathologic classification

clinodactyly

clinoid process

Clinoril

CLIP
corticotropin-like intermediate lobe
peptide

clitoridis
frenulum c.
glans c.

clitoris

clitoromegaly

clitoroplasty

clival
c. indentation
c. portion

clivus
upper c.

CLN
cervical lymph node

cloacal exstrophy

CLOCK
circadian locomotor output cycles kaput
CLOCK gene
CLOCK protein

clock
circadian c.

clodronate

clofibrate

Clomid

clomiphene
c. citrate
c. citrate challenge test (CCCT)

clomiphene-resistant anovulation

clonal
c. anergy
c. cell
c. deletion
c. expansion
c. neoplasm
c. rejection

clonality

cloned steroid acute respiratory protein

clonidine
c. diabetic neuropathy
c. gel
c. hydrochloride
c. suppression test

cloning
expression c.

Clonorchis sinensis

Clopra

clorgyline

closed-loop insulin delivery system

clostridia

Clostridium septicum

closure
epiphyseal c.

clotrimazole

clotting
c. factor II, V, VII, X

clouded sensorium

clozapine

cluster
consanguineous c.

NOTES

C

65

clustering
    risk factor c.
Clyde mood scale
cM
    centiMorgan
CML
    chronic myelogenous leukemia
CMO
    cetylmyristoleate
    corticosterone methyl oxidase
        CMO I
        CMO I, II deficiency
CMP
    comprehensive metabolic panel
    cow's milk protein
c-*mpl* ligand
CMV
    cytomegalovirus
c-myc
    c-m. oncogene
    c-m. protein
    c-m. protooncogene
CNP
    C-type natriuretic peptide
CNS
    central nervous system
CNTF
    ciliary neurotrophic factor
CO_3^{2-}
    carbonate
CoA
    coenzyme A
coactivator
    AIB1 c.
    GRIP 1 c.
    NCoA-1, -2 c.
    p/CIP c.
    p160 family of c.'s
    c. protein
    receptor-associated c. 3 (RAC3)
    SRC-1 c.
    TIF2 c.
    TRAM-1 c.
coagulability
    red cell c.
coagulation
    c. defect
    disseminated intravascular c. (DIC)
    red cell c.
coalesce
    tubuli recti c.
coarsened facial feature
CoAs
    long chain acyl C. (LCAcoA, LC-CoAs)
coast
    c. of California smooth margin
    c. of Maine irregular margin
coated pit

cobalamin metabolism
cobalt-knife radiosurgery
COBE 2991 computerized centrifuge system
Cobex
COC
    combined oral contraceptive
cocaine
    c. and amphetamine regulated transcript (CART)
    c. and amphetamine-responsive transcript
Coccidioides
    C. immitis
    C. immitis thyroiditis
coccidioidomycosis
coccidioidomycosis-induced thyroiditis
Cockayne syndrome
Codamine
codeine
    bromodiphenhydramine and c.
    brompheniramine, phenylpropanolamine, and c.
    butalbital compound and c.
    Capital and c.
    Empirin with c.
    Fiorinal with C.
    Phenergan VC with c.
    terpin hydrate and c.
codfish vertebra
codon
    c. 12, 13, 61
    AUG c.
    glutamic acid c. (GAA)
    premature top c. (TAA)
Codoxy
coelomic
    c. epithelium
    c. metaplasia
coenzyme
    c. A (CoA)
    c. Q10
cofactor
    mahogany c.
    plasma ristocetin c.
Coffin-Lowry syndrome
Co-Gesic
cognate antigen
Cohen syndrome
coherence therapy
cohosh
    black c.
coital alignment technique (CAT)
colchicine
cold
    C. GLUT-4
    c. intolerance
    c. mass

c. naïve
c. nodule
cold-inducible
c.-i. ribonucleic acid-binding protein (CIRP)
c.-i. RNA-binding protein (CIRP)
cold-shock protein
colestipol
colestyramine
coli
Escherichia c.
familial polyposis c.
colic
biliary c.
renal c.
collagen
carboxyterminal cross-linked telopeptide of type I c. (ICTP)
c. cross-link
C-telopeptide of c.
C-terminal telopeptide of type I c.
c. fiber
c. fibril
c. gene
c. molecule
c. monomer
N-telopeptide c.
N-terminal telopeptide of type I c.
c. synthesis
c. type I
type I, II, IX, X c.
collagenase
c. cleavage
C. Santyl ointment
collagenoma
collagenosis
Collagraft
collecting
c. tubule
c. tubule sodium channel
collection
24-hour urine c.
urine c.
collector
capillary filtrate c.
colli
pterygium c.
colliculus
c. seminalis
superior c.
Collier sign

collimation
converging hole c.
parallel hole c.
pinhole c.
collimator
flat-field c.
pinhole c.
colloid
c. adenoma
c. antigen
c. cyst
c. droplet
eosinophilic c.
c. goiter
c. osmotic pressure
c. stage
sticky c.
thyroid c.
viscous c.
colloidal
c. gold-198
c. yttrium-91
Colo-205 colorectal cancer cell line
coloboma, pl. **colobomata**
c. dysplasia
retinal c.
uveal c.
colobomatous dysplasia
colocalize
colony-forming
c.-f. unit erythroid (CFU-E)
c.-f. unit erythroid cell
colony morphology
colony-stimulating
c.-s. factor
c.-s. factor-1
color
c. Doppler scan
c. Doppler ultrasonography (CDU)
c. duplex ultrasonography
c. vision
colorectal
c. cancer cell line
c. tumorigenesis
colorimetric
c. assay
c. method
column
intermediolateral cell c.
intermediolateral gray c.
trophoblastic cell c.

NOTES

coma
>acidotic c.
>diabetic ketoacidosis-related c.
>hyperammonemic c.
>hyperglycemic c.
>hyperosmolar nonketotic c.
>hypoglycemic c.
>myxedema c.
>nonketotic hyperosmolar c.

Combantrin
Combid
combination
>c. assay
>c. therapy

combined
>c. hyperlipidemia
>c. immunodeficiency
>c. oral contraceptive (COC)
>c. PET/CT
>c. pituitary hormone deficiency (CPHD)
>c. therapy

CombiPatch
combretastatin
comedone
commissure
>anterior c.
>habenular c.

common
>c. bile duct (CBD)
>c. hepatic artery (CHA)

communicating artery
communication
>autocrine c.
>cell-to-cell c.

comorbid
comorbidity
compact
>c. bone
>c. cell

Companion 2 self blood glucose monitoring device
comparator element
compartment
>abluminal c.
>basal c.
>early endosomal c.
>extramitochondrial c.
>hematopoietic c.
>interstitial fluid c.
>intramitochondrial c.
>intravascular c.
>lateral sellar c.
>luminal c.
>suprasellar c.
>transcellular fluid c.

compartmentalization
compartmentation
Compazine

compensated
>c. euthyroidism
>c. iodine deficiency

compensation
>respiratory c.

compensatory
>c. feedback
>c. hyperinsulinemia
>c. hyperinsulinemia insulin-resistance syndrome
>c. hyperparathyroidism
>c. hypertrophy
>c. ligand-induced upregulation of tissue receptor

competitive
>c. insulin autoantibody
>c. zona binding assay

complement
>c. defect
>c. level

complementary
>c. and alternative therapy
>c. deoxyribonucleic acid (cDNA)
>c. DNA (cDNA)

complement-fixing thyroid antibody
complete
>c. androgen insensitivity syndrome (CAIS)
>c. androgen sensitivity
>c. autoinfarction
>c. Freund adjuvant (CFA)
>c. hydatidiform mole
>c. hypopituitarism
>c. precocious puberty
>c. testicular feminization

complex
>acquired immunodeficiency syndrome-related c.
>actin-myosin c.
>AIDS-related c. (ARC)
>aminoacyl-tRNA c.
>aromatase enzyme c.
>axonemal c.
>beta-gamma c.
>calcium c.
>cap-binding c.
>c. carbohydrate
>Carney c.
>C-cell c.
>corepressor c.
>Dandy-Walker c.
>ferrous sulfate, ascorbic acid, and vitamin B c.
>c. genetic disorder
>glycine cleavage c.
>Golgi c.
>G-protein trimeric c.
>GTP-dependent regulatory protein c.

guanosine triphosphate-dependent
  regulatory protein c.
hormone receptor-ligand c.
c. hyperthyroxinemia
hypothalamohypophyseal c.
immune c.
iron dextran c.
150-kDa ternary c.
ligand-receptor c.
major histocompatibility c. (MHC)
NeoVadrin B C.
nuclear pore c.
polysaccharide-iron c.
preinitiation c. (PIC)
receptor-ligand c.
19S cap c.
ternary c.
thyroperoxidase-iodide c.
transthyretin-ligand c.
transthyretin thyroid hormone
  analogue c.
TTR-ligand c.
TTR-thyroid hormone analogue c.
tubular bulbo c.
vitamin B c.

complexed calcium
compliance
insulin c.
vascular c.
complication
diabetes-specific c.
Epidemiology of Diabetes
  Interventions and C.'s (EDIC)
long-term c.
microvascular c.
sinonasal c.
component
group-specific c. (Gc)
intrathoracic goitrous c.
RI regulatory c.
RII regulatory c.
Composite Cultured Skin
composition
bile c.
body c.
side-chain c.
water c.
compound
c. B
calcimimetic c.
calcium phosphate c.
catechol c.

dihydrocodeine c.
gadolinium-chelated c.
glutahione c.
c. heterozygosity
iodolipid c.
lanthanum-containing c.
pentazocine c.
c. S
SH c.
sulfhydryl c.
thiourea c.
thyromimetic c.
zirconium-containing c.
comprehensive metabolic panel (CMP)
compression
chiasmal c.
c. neuropathy
spinal cord c.
compressive
c. mononeuropathy
c. neuropathy
comprised glucose counterregulation
computed
c. tomography (CT)
c. tomography under endoscopic
  retrograde pancreatography (ERP-
  CT)
computer
c. tomographic methods of axial
  skeleton (axial QCT)
c. tomographic methods of
  peripheral skeleton (pQCT)
computer-aided sperm analysis (CASA)
**computer-assisted semen analysis
(CASA)**
**computerized continuous subcutaneous
insulin infusion pump**
COMT
catechol-*O*-methyltransferase
concanavalin-A
concentration
apo A-I c.
blood glucose c.
calcium ion c.
dialysate calcium c.
glucose c.
glycogen c.
inactive renin c.
insulin c.
intrathyroid iodide c.
ionized calcium c.
leptin c.

NOTES

concentration *(continued)*
    midnight plasma cortisol c.
    minimal detectable c. (MDC)
    plasma aldosterone c. (PAC)
    plasma glucose c.
    platelet lipid peroxide c.
    postprandial glucose c.
    postprandial insulin c.
    salivary cortisol c.
    serum albumin c.
    serum cholesterol c.
    serum 18-hydroxycorticosterone c.
    serum IGF-1 c.
    serum IGFBP-3 c.
    serum insulinlike growth factor-1 c.
    serum insulinlike growth factor
      binding protein-3 c.
    serum ionized calcium c.
    serum leptin c.
    tissue c.
    total serum calcium c.
    urine c.
conchal-type sphenoid sinus
concretion
    prostatic c.
condition
    anestrous c.
    autosomal dominant c.
    diabetes associated with certain c.'s
    pathophysiological c.
    rheumatic c.
conductivity
    total body electrical c. (TOBEC)
conduit
    aortic allograft c.
confabulation
confluence
    superior mesenteric-portal vein c.
      (SM-PVC)
conformational dependent epitope
congenic mapping
congenita
    adrenal hypoplasia c. (AHC)
    aplasia cutis c. (ACC)
congenital
    c. abnormality
    c. adrenal dysplasia
    c. adrenal hyperplasia (CAH)
    c. androgen insensitivity
    c. anorchia
    c. aplasia of the parathyroid
    c. bilateral absence of the vas
      deferens (CBAVD)
    c. bilateral aplasia
    c. bone defect
    c. bone disorder
    c. cretinism
    c. cytomegalovirus infection

    dosage-sensitive sex reversal-adrenal
      hypoplasia c. (DSS-AHC)
    c. erythropoietic porphyria
    c. facial diplegia
    c. forebrain anomaly
    c. generalized lipoatrophy
    c. generalized lipodystrophy (CGL)
    c. GH resistance syndrome
    c. growth hormone resistance
      syndrome
    c. hereditary lymphedema
    c. hyperinsulinism
    c. hyperthyroidism
    c. hypoaldosteronism
    c. hypophosphatemia
    c. hypothyroidism
    c. ichthyosis
    c. intrathyroidal cyst
    c. leptin resistance
    c. lipoatrophic diabetes
    c. lipoid adrenal hyperplasia
    c. lipoid adrenal hypoplasia
    c. malformation
    c. rubella syndrome (CRS)
    c. thymic aplasia
    c. virilizing adrenal hyperplasia
Congest
Congressional Diabetes Caucus
conical lobe
conjugate
    glucuronide c.
    sulfate c.
conjugated
    c. bilirubin
    c. equine estrogen (CEE)
    c. equine estrogen plus norgestrel
      (CEEP)
conjunctival
    c. chemosis
    c. edema
    c. erythema
connection
    corticohypothalamic c.
    intracavernous venous c.
connective
    c. tissue
    c. tissue disease
    c. tissue growth factor (CTGF)
connexin-37 (Cx37)
connexin-43 (Cx43)
connexin protein
Conn syndrome
conotruncal
    c. anomaly
    c. malformation
consanguineous
    c. cluster
    c. parents
consanguinity

consciousness osmolarity value
consensus
    c. sequence
    c. TATA box
consensus-response element
conserved helix-loop-helix ubiquitous
  kinase (CHUK)
consolidation
    bone c.
constant
    equilibrium association c. (K_a)
    equilibrium dissociation c. (K_d)
    Faraday c.
    universal gas c.
constitutional
    c. delay
    c. delay in growth and
    adolescence (CDGA)
    c. precocious puberty
constitutive
    c. heterochromatin
    c. secretion
constriction
    hourglass c.
consumption
    energy c.
    oxygen c.
    platelet c.
contamination
    endotoxin c.
content
    glycogen c.
    intramyocellular lipid c. (IMLC)
    keratin c.
    phosphorus c.
    sialic acid c.
    total body bone mineral c.
    (TBBMC)
contiguous gene syndrome
continuous
    c. ambulatory peritoneal dialysis
    (CAPD)
    c. ambulatory radiolucent cyst
    c. capillary endothelium
    c. conjugated equine estrogen
    c. glucose monitoring system
    (CGMS)
    c. hormone replacement therapy
    c. positive airway pressure
    c. regional arterial infusion (CRAI)
    c. subcutaneous insulin infusion
    (CSII)

    c. subcutaneous insulin infusion
    pump
continuous-combined
    c.-c. estrogen-progestogen therapy
    (CC-EPT)
    c.-c. hormone replacement therapy
    (ccHRT)
contraception
    postcoital c.
contraceptive
    combined oral c. (COC)
    estrogen-progesterone c.
    oral c.
    postcoital c.
    progesterone-based c.
contractile protein
contraction-associated protein (CAP)
contrainsulin hormone
contralateral lobe
contrasexual
    c. precocity
    c. pubertal development
contrast
    c. cisternography
    c. dynamic study
    nonionic iodinated c.
control
    anticipatory c.
    diet c.
    feedback c.
    glycemic c.
    hypothalamic-pituitary c.
    metabolic c.
    neuroendocrine c.
    preconceptional glycemic c.
    roller coaster glucose c.
    ventilatory c.
controlled diabetes insipidus (CDI)
conventional
    c. radiotherapy
    c. therapy
converging hole collimation
convertase
    prohormone c.
    prohormone c. 1 (PC1)
    prohormone c. 2 (PC2)
    prohormone c. 3 (PC3)
    proprotein c. (PC)
Cooley anemia
cool nodule
Cooper
    suspensory ligaments of C.

C

NOTES

copeptin
Cope syndrome
copolymer
   ethylene-vinyl acetate c.
copper deposition
CoR
   corepressor
cord
   tethered c.
cordocentesis
coregulator molecule
corepressor (CoR)
   c. complex
   nuclear receptor c. (N-CoR)
core promoter
CorFlow
Corgonject
Cori
   C. cycle
   C. disease
corneal
   c. arcus
   c. leukoma
   c. ulceration
Cornelia de Lange syndrome
coronal
   c. plane
   c. postgadolinium study
   c. slice
corona radiata
coronary
   c. artery
   c. artery calcium score (CACS)
   c. artery disease, hypertension,
      adult-onset diabetes, obesity, and
      stroke (CHAOS)
   c. blood flow
corpus, pl. corpora
   c. albicans
   corpora amylacea
   corpora arenacea
   c. callosum
   c. cavernosum
   c. hemorrhagicum
   c. luteum
   c. luteum insufficiency (CLI)
   c. spongiosum
   c. uterus
corpuscle
   Hassall c.
corrodens
   Eikenella c.
Cortef Oral
cortex, pl. cortices
   adrenal c.
   adult adrenal c.
   cerebellar c.
   cerebral c.
   cingulate c.

ovarian c.
c. pancreas
piriform c.
thickening of c.
cortical
   c. amygdaloid nucleus
   c. androgen-stimulating hormone
      (CASH)
   c. atrophy
   c. bone
   c. collecting duct (CCD)
   c. nephron
corticalis
   hyperostosis c.
cortices (pl. of cortex)
corticohypothalamic connection
corticoid-induced osteopenia
corticomedullary osmotic gradient
corticopupillary osmolality gradient
corticorelin ovine triflutate
corticospinal tract dysfunction
corticostatin
corticosteroid
   high-dose c.
   c. receptor
   c. therapy
corticosteroid-binding globulin (CBG)
corticosterone
   c. methyl oxidase (CMO)
   c. methyl oxidase II
   c. methyl oxidase II deficiency
   serum c.
corticotrope
   pituitary c.
corticotroph
   c. adenoma
   c. cell hyperplasia
   c. stimulation test
   c. tumor
corticotropic cell
corticotropin
corticotropin-dependent Cushing
   syndrome
corticotropin-like intermediate lobe
   peptide (CLIP)
corticotropinoma
   pituitary c.
corticotropin-releasing
   c.-r. factor (CRF)
   c.-r. hormone (CRH)
   c.-r. hormone-binding protein
      (CRH-BP)
   c.-r. hormone 1R (CRH1R)
   c.-r. hormone 2R (CRH2R)
   c.-r. hormone test
corticotropin-secreting adenoma
cortisol (F)
   adrenal c.
   c. assay

basal plasma c.
c. biosynthesis
c. clearance
fetal adrenal c.
fetal plasma c.
free c.
24-hour urine free c.
morning c.
c. nadir
plasma c.
postcosyntropin plasma c.
random c.
c. resistance syndrome
salivary c.
c. secretion
urinary free c.
urine free c. (UFC)
cortisol-binding globulin (CBG)
cortisol-producing cortical adenoma
cortisol-secreting
c.-s. adenoma
c.-s. lesion
cortisone acetate
Cortone Acetate
Cortrosyn
C. stimulation test
C. stimulation testing
Corynebacterium
cosecrete
cosmesis
cosmid
cosyntropin stimulation test
Cotazym
Cotazym-S
cotransporter
bumetanide-sensitive sodium-
postassium-2 chloride c.
Na^+-phosphate c.
sodium glucose c. (SGLT)
sodium glucose c.-1 (SGLT1)
sodium glucose c.-2 (SGLT2)
sodium-potassium-2 chloride c.
(NKCC2)
cotton pledget packing
cotton-wool
c.-w. appearance
c.-w. spot
cotyledon
coulometric meter
coulometry
coumestan
coumestrol

counseling
genetic c.
health status c.
preconception c.
count
antral follicle c. (AFC)
counter
Geiger c.
whole-body c.
counterion
counterregulation
comprised glucose c.
defective glucose c.
c. of hypoglycemia
impaired glucose c.
c. mechanism
counterregulatory hormone
countertransport system
counting
carbohydrate c.
^{40}K c.
coupled amplification and sequencing technique
coupling
c. domain
c. factor
iodothyronine c.
iodotyrosine c.
c. phase
receptor-effector c.
stimulus-secretion c.
synthesis-secretion c.
COUP-TF
COUP-TF thyroid hormone receptor auxillary protein
Courtois
coverage
rainbow c.
Cowden
C. disease
C. syndrome
Cowper
bulbourethral gland of C.
C. gland
cow's milk protein (CMP)
COX
cyclooxygenase
COX-1
cyclooxygenase-1
COX-2
cyclooxygenase-2

NOTES

COX-3
cyclooxygenase-3
coxsackievirus
c. A
c. A9
c. B
c. B antigen
c. B-induced diabetes mellitus
group B c.
COZ
cranioorbitozygomatic osteotomy
CozMore insulin technology system
C-peptide
C-p. level
C-p. suppression test
CPH
carboxypeptidase H
CPHD
combined pituitary hormone deficiency
CPP
central precocious puberty
CPTI
carnitine palmitoyltransferase I
CPTI deficiency
CPTII
carnitine palmitoyltransferase II
CPTII deficiency
CRAI
continuous regional arterial infusion
cranial
c. diabetes insipidus
c. irradiation
c. mononeuropathy
c. nerve palsy
c. nerves II through XII
c. neuropathy
c. sclerosis
craniodiaphysial dysplasia
craniomegaly
craniometaphyseal dysplasia
cranioorbitozygomatic osteotomy (COZ)
craniopharyngeal
c. canal
c. duct
craniopharyngioma
adamantinomatous c.
cystic c.
papillary c.
pituitary c.
craniostenosis
craniosynostosis
nonsyndromic coronal c.
primary c.
craniotabes
craving
salt c.
CRE
cAMP-response element

cyclic adenosine monophosphate
regulatory element
C-reactive protein (CRP)
cream
Amino-Cerv Vaginal C.
dehydroepiandrosterone c.
DHEA c.
fluocinolone acetonide c.
Locilex pexiganan acetate c.
Locilex topical c.
Medrol Veriderm C.
Pro-Gest c.
VANIQA c.
creatine kinase (CK)
creatinine
albumin c. (A/C)
c. clearance
urinary c.
creatinuria
CREB
cAMP response element-binding
cyclic adenosine 3′,5′-monophosphate
response element-binding
CREB-binding protein (CBP)
CREM
cAMP-response element modulator
cremasteric fascia
cremaster muscle
Creme
Gormel C.
Creon 10, 20
Creo-Terpin
crest
mammary c.
neural c.
vagal neural c.
cretin
athyreotic c.
cretinism
congenital c.
endemic c.
goitrous c.
myxedematous endemic c.
neurologic endemic c.
Creutzfeldt-Jakob disease (CJD)
CRF
chronic renal failure
corticotropin-releasing factor
CRH
corticotropin-releasing hormone
placental CRH
CRH stimulation test
CRH-binding protein (CRH-BP)
CRH-BP
corticotropin-releasing hormone-binding
protein
CRH-binding protein
CRH-mRNA transcript

CRH1R
corticotropin-releasing hormone 1R
CRH2R
corticotropin-releasing hormone 2R
CRH-R1 receptor
CRI
chronic renal insufficiency
cribriform plate
cricoarytenoid
lateral c.
posterior c.
cricoid cartilage
cricothyroid
c. joint
c. membrane
c. muscle
cri du chat syndrome
Crinone bioadhesive progesterone gel
crinophagy
crisis, pl. **crises**
acute addisonian c.
acute adrenal c.
addisonian c.
adrenal c.
bone c.
carcinoid c.
fetal/neonatal adrenal c.
hyperglycemic c.
hypoglycemia c.
parathyroid c.
salt-losing c.
salt-wasting c.
thyroid c.
thyrotoxic c.
cristae
tubular c.
criterion, pl. **criteria**
Age, Metastases, Extent and Size
risk criteria
AMES risk criteria
National Cholesterol Education
Program criteria
NCEP criteria
Whipple triad criteria
Critic-Aid skin paste
CrkII protein
CrkI protein
CrkL protein
Crk protein
Crohn disease
Crolom
cromolyn sodium

Crooke
C. cell
C. hyaline change
C. hyalinization
crossed test
crossing nasal retinal fiber
Crosslaps immunoassay
cross-link
collagen c.-l.
pyridinium c.-l.
pyridinoline c.-l.
total deoxypyridinoline c.-l.
trifunctional pyridinium c.-l.
urinary N-telopeptide collagen c.-l.
cross-reactive
trophoblast-lymphocyte c.-r. (TLX)
cross-talk
transcriptional c.-t.
Crouzon
C. disease
C. syndrome
CRP
C-reactive protein
CRS
congenital rubella syndrome
crus, gen. **cruris**
diaphragmatic c.
c. penis
ulcus cruris
cryoglobulin level
cryosurgery
hepatic c.
cryptic
c. hydroxylase deficiency
c. hyperandrogenemia
cryptococcal
c. antigen
c. infection
cryptococcosis
Cryptococcus neoformans
cryptomenorrhea
cryptorchidism
cryptorchism
crystal
apatite c.
calcium oxalate dihydrate c.
calcium oxalate monohydrate c.
calcium phosphate c.
cholesterol monohydrate c.
cystine c.
hydroxyapatite c.
Reinke c.

NOTES

crystal *(continued)*
    struvite c.
    uric acid c.
crystalline zinc insulin (CZI)
crystallized HLA-A2 molecule
crystallographic stone analysis
crystallography
    x-ray c.
crystalloid
    Reinke c.
crystalluria
Crystamine
CS
    chorionic somatomammotropin
CSCP
    central serous chorioretinopathy
CSF
    cerebrospinal fluid
        CSF rhinorrhea
CSII
    continuous subcutaneous insulin infusion
CSME
    clinically significant macular edema
c-*src*
    protooncogene c.
CSS
    cavernous sinus sampling
C-18 steroid
CT
    calcitonin
    computed tomography
        dynamic spiral CT
        helical CT
        spiral CT
CT-1
    cardiotropin-1
C-telopeptide of collagen
C-terminal
        C-t. assay for parathyroid hormone
        C-t. assay for PTH
        C-t. propeptide
        C-t. telopeptide of type I collagen
        C-t. type I collagen telopeptide
C-termini
CTGF
    connective tissue growth factor
CT-guided fine-needle aspiration
CTLA-4
    cytotoxic lymphocyte antigen-2
ctor-kB IkK mediated signaling pathway
C-type natriuretic peptide (CNP)
cube
    porous calcium phosphate c.
cubitus valgus
cuboidal epithelioid cell
cue
    nonphotic c.
Cullen sign

culture
    monolayer c.
    semen c.
cumulus, pl. **cumuli**
    c. adherens
    c. granulosa cell
    c. oophorus
Cunninghamella
Cupid bow
cuprophane dialysis membrane
curette, curet
    Hardy ring c.
current
    microscopic c.
Curretab Oral
curve
    dose-response c.
    growth hormone dose-response c.
Cushing
    C. disease
    C. disease of the omentum
    C. forceps
    C. procedure
    C. syndrome
custom-healing orthotic
cutaneous
    c. adnexa
    c. flushing
    c. hamartoma
    c. hyperpigmentation
    c. infection
    c. lichen amyloidosis
    c. lupus
    c. myxoma
    c. photoaging
    c. pigmentation
    c. vasodilation
cutis
    aplasia c.
    c. verticis
    c. verticis gyrata
cuvette
CVO
    circumventricular organ
CVS
    chorionic villus sampling
Cx37
    connexin-37
Cx43
    connexin-43
cyanide-nitroprusside
cyanocobalamin
cyanogen bromide
cyanogenic glucoside
cyanoglucoside
5-cyano group
Cyanoject
cyclase
    adenyl c.

cyclase

adenylate c.
adenylyl c.
guanylate c.
guanylyl c.
thyroid adenylate c.

cycle

alanine c.
c. amplitude
anovulatory c.
Basic Rest-Activity C. (BRAC)
citric acid c.
Cori c.
dark-light c.
endometrial c.
estrous c.
free-running melatonin c.
futile c.
glucose-fatty acid c.
Krebs c.
menstrual c.
ornithine c.
ovarian c.
ovulatory c.
prolactin secretion during
  menstrual c.
Randle c.
remodeling c.
reverse Randle c.
sleep-wake c.
substrate c.
urea c.
Vollman c.

cycler

thermal c.

cyclic

c. adenosine monophosphate
  (cAMP)
c. 3′,5′-adenosine monophosphate
  (cAMP)
c. adenosine monophosphate
  dependent protein kinase
c. adenosine monophosphate
  regulatory element (CRE)
c. adenosine monophosphate
  regulatory element insulin gene
  promoter
c. adenosine 3′,5′-monophosphate
  response element-binding (CREB)
c. AMP (cAMP)
c. AMP response-element binding
  protein
c. arginine monophosphate (cAMP)

c. arginine monophosphate response
  element-binding
c. conjugated estrogen
c. endoperoxide prostaglandin G_2
c. GMP
c. guanosine monophosphate
  (cGMP)
c. 3′,5′-guanosine monophosphate
  (cGMP)
5′-c. guanosine monophosphate
  (cGMP)
c. guanosine 3′,5′-monophosphate-
  dependent protein kinase
c. guanosine monophosphate-
  phosphodiesterase
c. hyperthermia
c. hypothermia
c. nucleotide phosphodiesterase
c. porphyria

cyclical

c. Cushing disease
c. ethinyl estradiol
c. hormone replacement therapy
c. supplementation

**5′-cyclic guanosine monophosphate
  (cGMP)**

cyclicity

endogenous c.

cyclin

c. D3
c. D gene
c. D1 protein

cyclin-dependent kinase (CDK, Cdk)

cycling

c. cell
liver glycogen c.

cyclocephaly

cyclodextrin

testosterone c.

Cyclofem

cycloheximide

Cyclo(His-Pro)

Cyclomen

cyclooxygenase (COX)

c. pathway

cyclooxygenase-1 (COX-1)

cyclooxygenase-2 (COX-2)

cyclooxygenase-3 (COX-3)

cyclophosphamide

cyclopia

cycloplegic refraction

cyclosporin A

NOTES

cyclosporine
> c. A-induced osteopenia
> c. A-induced resorption

cyclotron
Cycrin Oral
Cyomin
CYP
> cytochrome P450 enzyme
> cytochrome pigment
> cytochrome protein

CYP27
> cytochrome P450 enzyme 27

CYP11A gene
CYP17 gene
CYP19 gene
CYP1A1 gene
CYP21B deficiency
cypionate
> testosterone c.

cyproheptadine hydrochloride
cyproterone acetate
cyst
> arachnoid c.
> arrested follicular c.
> c. aspiration
> atretic follicular c.
> benign pituitary c.
> choledochal c.
> colloid c.
> congenital intrathyroidal c.
> continuous ambulatory
>   radiolucent c.
> dermoid c.
> endolymphatic c.
> epidermal c.
> epidermoid c.
> familial thyroglossal duct c.
> follicular c.
> intrasellar hydatid c.
> luteal c.
> microphthalmic c.
> multiple luteinized theca c.
> nabothian c.
> ovarian endometriosis c.
> parathyroid c.
> pars intermedia c.
> pituitary c.
> pleuropericardial c.
> Rathke cleft c.
> Rathke pouch c.
> renal c.
> sellar c.
> subchondral c.
> suprasellar epidermoid c.
> theca-lutein c.
> thin-walled simple c.
> thyroglossal duct c.

cystadenocarcinoma
> ductectatic-type mucinous c.
> mucinous c.

cystadenoma
> epididymal c.
> mucinous c.

cystathionase
cystathionine
> c. synthase
> c. synthase deficiency

cystathioninuria
cysteine
> c. aminopeptidase
> c. endopeptidase

cysteine-penicillamine
cystic
> c. acne
> c. bone lesion
> c. craniopharyngioma
> c. fibrosis
> c. fibrosis-related diabetes (CFRD)
> c. fibrosis transmembrane
>   conductance regulator chloride
>   channel
> c. fibrosis transmembrane regulator
>   (CFTR)
> c. fibrosis transmembrane regulator
>   gene
> c. hygroma
> c. hyperplasia
> c. mastitis
> c. neurilemoma
> c. nodule
> c. ovary

cystica
> osteitis fibrosa c.

cystine
> c. crystal
> c. knot
> c. renal stone

cystinosis
> adult c.
> benign c.
> infantile c.
> juvenile c.
> nephropathic c.

cystinuria
cystinuric
> homozygous c.

cystogastrostomy
cystometrogram
cystopathy
cystosarcoma phylloides
cytoarchitectonically
cytochemical bioassay (CBA)
cytochrome
> c. C oxidase deficiency
> c. oxidase
> c. P450

c. P450 aromatase
c. P450 enzyme (CYP)
c. P450 enzyme 19
c. P450 enzyme 27 (CYP27)
c. P450 enzyme 1A1
c. P450 enzyme 11A
c. P450 enzyme 21B
c. P450 family of enzymes
c. P450 hemoprotein
c. pigment (CYP)
c. protein (CYP)
cytodiagnosis
cytodifferentiation
cytokeratin
cytokine
activating c.
beta-cell c.
bone-resorbing c.
c. deletion
c. gene
inflammatory c.
osteoporotic c.
c. production
proinflammatory c.
c. studies in isolated pancreatic
islets
tumor necrosis factor-related
activation-induced c. (TRANCE)
type 2 helper T-cell c.
cytokine-induced thyroiditis
cytokinin-regulated
c.-r. kinase
c.-r. kinase I, II
c.-r. kinase I, II protein
c.-r. kinase L
c.-r. kinase L protein
Cytolex
cytologic atypia
cytology
brush c.
**cytomegalic-type congenital adrenal
hypoplasia**
cytomegalovirus (CMV)
Cytomel
C. Oral
C. suppression test

cytoplasm
clear c.
dark c.
perikaryal c.
cytoplasmic
c. bridge
c. Ca^{2+}
c. calcium
c. estrogen
c. islet-cell antibody
c. pseudopod
c. receptor
cytoreduction surgery
cytoreductive surgery
cytosine arabinoside
cytosine-guanine dinucleotide
cytoskeleton
cytosol
neuronal c.
cytosolic
c. enzyme
c. free calcium
c. osmolality
cytotoxic
c. chemotherapy
c. lymphocyte antigen-2 (CTLA-4)
c. T lymphocyte
c. T-lymphocyte beta-cell
cytotoxicity
antibody-dependent cell c. (ADCC)
antibody-dependent cell-mediated c.
antibody-dependent cellular c.
(ADCC)
immune cell-mediated c.
T-cell mediated c.
cytotrophoblast
Langhans c.
villous c.
cytsol
CZI
crystalline zinc insulin

NOTES

79

D

apoprotein D (apoD)
aspartic endopeptidase cathepsin D
cathepsin D
D cell
hypervitaminosis D
immunoglobulin D (IgD)
phospholipase D (PLD)

D1

type 1 deiodinase

D$_1$

vitamin D$_1$

D2

T$_4$5'-deiodinase type 2
type 2 deiodinase

D$_2$

D$_2$ agonist
prostaglandin D$_2$ (PGD$_2$)
vitamin D$_2$

D3

type 3 deiodinase
cyclin D3

D$_3$

active vitamin D$_3$
1-alpha-hydroxyvitamin D$_3$
1,25-dihydroxyvitamin D$_3$
labile previtamin D$_3$
previtamin D$_3$
vitamin D$_3$

D$_4$

leukotriene D$_4$ (LTD$_4$)

DA

diabetic acidosis
dopamine

D4-A

androstenedione

dacarbazine (DTIC)
d'accoucheur

main d.

daclizumab
dactinomycin
DAG

diacylglycerol

daidzein
DAIS

Diabetes Atherosclerosis Intervention
Study

DAISY

Diabetes Autoimmunity Study in the
Young

Dakin solution
Dalgan
Dalrymple sign
dalton

damage

chromosomal d.
oxidative d.

Damason-P
Dana Diabecare insulin pump
danazol
Dandy-Walker

D.-W. complex
D.-W. syndrome

Danocrine
dantrolene
DAO

diamine oxidase

Dapa
Dapacin
Da Qing study
Darbid
Darier sign
dark cytoplasm
dark-light cycle
DASP

Diabetes Autoantibody Standardization
Program

database

National Cardiac Surgery D.
(NCSD)
Online Mendelian Inheritance of
Man d. (OMIM)

daunomycin
daunorubicin
dawn phenomenon
DAX-1 gene
day

Acutrim Late D.

Dayto Himbin
DAZ

deleted in azoospermia

DAZH

DAZ-homologue
deleted in azoospermia-homologue

DAZ-homologue (DAZH)
DAZLA

DAZ-like autosomal
deleted in azoospermia-like autosomal

DAZ-like autosomal (DAZLA)
DBD

DNA-binding domain

D$_{beta}$

total body bone mineral density

db gene
DBH

dopamine beta-hydroxylase

DBP

vitamin D-binding protein

D

DCCT
Diabetes Control and Complications Trial
D-chiro-inositol
DCT
distal convoluted tubule
DDAVP
desamino D-arginine vasopressin
DDD
dichlorodiphenyldichloroethane
DDT
dichlorodiphenyltrichloroethane
de
de Lange syndrome
de Morsier syndrome
de novo
de novo hyperinsulinemia
de novo synthesis
de Quervain nonsuppurative
thyroiditis
deacetylase
histone d. (HDAC)
deacetylation
histone d.
deaf mutism
deafness
diabetes insipidus, diabetes mellitus,
optic atrophy, and d.
diabetes insipidus, diabetes mellitus,
progressive bilateral optic atrophy,
and sensorineural d. (DIDMOAD)
maternally inherited diabetes and d.
(MIDD)
sensorineural d.
deaminase
adenosine d. (ADA)
adenosine monophosphate d. 1
(AMPD1)
polyethylene glycol-adenosine d.
(PEG-ADA)
deaminate
adenosine deaminase d.
death
granulosa cell d.
debridement
minor mechanical d.
debris
calcified desquamated d.
Debrisan
debulked
debulking
transsphenoidal d.
d. of tumor
Decadron
D. Injection
D. Oral
Decadron-LA
Deca-Durabolin
Decaject
Decaject-LA

decanoate
Hybolin D.
nandrolone d.
decapacitation factor
decapeptide
antigonadotropic d. (AGD)
decarboxylase
aromatic L-amino acid d.
branch chain 2-ketoacid d.
dihydroxyphenylalanine d.
DOPA d.
glutamic acid d. (GAD)
ornithine d. (ODC)
decarboxylation
amine precursor uptake and d.
(APUD)
decidua
d. basalis
d. capsularis
d. parietalis
deciliter
milligrams per d. (mg/dL)
decline
response curve d.
Declomycin
DECODE
Diabetes Epidemiology Collaborative
Analysis of Diagnostic Criteria in
Europe study
decompensation
metabolic d.
decompression
gastric d.
deconvolution
decorin
decorticate rigidity
decreased
d. flare reaction
d. lean mass
d. libido
d. mineral apposition rate
d. oxygen tension
d. thyroid reserve
dedifferentiation
defect
acquired organification d.
alcohol-induced birth d.
bitemporal d.
cecocentral d.
c-erbA-beta-1 d.
c-erbA-beta-2 d.
coagulation d.
complement d.
congenital bone d.
enzyme d.
granulosa cell d.
hemianopic d.
insulin secretory d.
iodide organification d.

iodide transport d.
iodine organification d.
iodine-trapping d.
iodotyrosine coupling d.
iodotyrosine dehalogenase d.
luteal phase d.
mineralization d.
mitochondrial d.
monocular temporal arcuate d.
neural tube d.
organification d.
osmoregulatory d.
pupillary d.
rachitic-like skeletal d.
rake d.
regulatory gene d.
structural gene d.
superotemporal hemianoptic d.
testicular enzyme d.
thyroglobin synthesis d.
thyroid hormone receptor d.
thyroid hormonogenesis d. IIB
ventricular septal d. (VSD)
visual field d.
defective glucose counterregulation
defense
antioxidant d.
defensin
deferens, pl. **deferentia**
ampulla of the vas d.
congenital bilateral absence of the
vas d. (CBAVD)
ductus d.
vas d.
deferoxamine (DFO)
d. challenge
d. test
d. therapy
deficiency
absolute leptin d.
acetyl-CoA d.
acid cholesteryl ester hydrolase d.
acid phosphatase d.
acquired immune d.
adenine phosphoribosyltransferase d.
adenosine monophosphate
deaminase d.
adenylosuccinate lyase d.
d. of adipocyte
adrenal androgen d.
aldosterone synthase d.
alpha-antitrypsin d.

alpha$_1$ antitrypsin d.
alpha-galactosidase d.
17-alpha-hydroxylase/17,20-lyase
(p450c17) d.
ankyrin d.
anti-müllerian hormone d.
aromatase d.
11-beta-hydroxylase d. (11-beta-
OHD)
3-beta-hydroxysteroid
dehydrogenase d.
beta-ol-dehydrogenase d.
biotin cofactor d.
bone d.
CA II d.
calcitriol d.
calcium d.
carbamoyl phosphate synthetase
I d.
carbonic anhydrase II d.
carnitine acylcarnitine translocase d.
carnitine palmitoyltransferase I d.
carnitine palmitoyltransferase II d.
cholesterol desmolase d.
chronic glucocorticoid d.
classical hydroxylase d.
CMO I, II d.
combined pituitary hormone d.
(CPHD)
compensated iodine d.
corticosterone methyl oxidase II d.
CPTI d.
CPTII d.
cryptic hydroxylase d.
CYP21B d.
cystathionine synthase d.
cytochrome C oxidase d.
20,22-desmolase (P450scc) d.
dihydrobiopterin synthase d.
dihydropteridine reductase d.
enzyme d.
estrogen d.
factor VIII, IX d.
familial glucocorticoid d. (FGD)
familial growth hormone d.
follicle-stimulating hormone d.
FSH d.
galactose-l-phosphate
uridyltransferase d.
glucocerebrosidase d.
glucocorticoid receptor d.
glucose-6-phosphatase d.

D

NOTES

deficiency *(continued)*
glycerol kinase d.
glycoprotein neuraminidase d.
glycosylasparaginase d.
gonadotropin d.
gonadotropin-releasing hormone d.
G6PD d.
growth hormone d.
hepatic lipase d.
heterozygous cystathione beta
  synthase d.
HPRT d.
hydroxylase d.
11-hydroxylase d.
17-hydroxylase d.
21-hydroxylase d.
3-hydroxy-3-methylglutaryl-CoA
  carboxylase d.
hypothalamic gonadotropin-releasing
  hormone d.
hypoxanthine-guanine
  phosphoribosyltransferase d.
idiopathic growth hormone d.
insulin d.
iodide d.
iodine d.
isolated gonadotropin d.
isolated growth hormone d.
  (IGHD)
isolated growth hormone d. type
  IB (IGHD-IB)
isolated growth hormone d. type II
  (IGHD-II)
isolated growth hormone d. type
  III (IGHD-III)
isomerase dehydrogenase d.
17-ketosteroid reductase d.
3-ketothiolase d.
late onset hydroxylase d.
LCAD d.
LCAT d.
LCHAD d.
LDL d.
leptin d.
LHRH d.
lipoprotein lipase d.
long chain acyl-CoA
  dehydrogenase d.
long chain 3-hydroxyacyl-CoA
  dehydrogenase d.
low-density lipoprotein d.
luteal phase d.
luteinizing hormone-releasing
  hormone d.
magnesium d.
MCAD d.
medium chain acyl-CoA
  dehydrogenase d.

3-methylcrotonyl-CoA
  carboxylase d.
mineral d.
multiple anterior pituitary
  hormone d.
multiple sulfatase d.
nonclassical hydroxylase d.
nonclassical 21-hydroxylase d.
nonclassic 21-hydroxylase d.
ornithine transcarbamylase d.
OTC d.
P450 aromatase (placental) d.
partial 21-hydroxylase d.
P450c17 d.
P450c21 d.
peripheral glucocorticoid d.
PGK d.
phosphate d.
phosphoglycerate kinase d.
phosphoglycerate mutase d.
pituitary d.
placental aromatase d.
placental-fetal aromatase d.
placental hormone d.
placental sulfatase d.
pluriglandular endocrine d.
plurihormonal d.
PNP d.
polyglandular endocrine d.
postprandial insulin d.
primary immune d. (PID)
prolactin d.
pseudocholinesterase d.
purine nucleoside phosphorylase d.
red-green d.
reductase d.
5-reductase d.
relative leptin d.
salt-losing d.
short chain acyl-CoA
  dehydrogenase d. (SCAD)
side chain cleavage d.
single hormone d.
somatotropin d.
StAR d.
steroid acute regulatory protein d.
steroid acute respiratory protein d.
steroid 5-alpha-reductase d.
steroidogenic acute regulatory
  protein d.
steroid sulfatase d.
TBG d.
TH beta-receptor d.
thyroid-stimulating hormone d.
thyroxine-binding globulin d.
TSH d.
very long chain acyl-CoA
  dehydrogenase d.
vitamin D receptor d.

xanthine oxidase d.
X-linked severe combined
   immune d. (X-SCID)
deficiency/resistance
   leptin d.
deficient
   androgen d.
deficit
   free water d.
   pancreatic exocrine d.
   pituitary hormone d.
definitive placenta
deformans
   osteitis d.
deformity
   bilateral pes cavus d.
   claw-toe d.
   Erlenmeyer flask d.
   Madelung d.
   rachitic d.
   saddlenose d.
   skeletal d.
Degas
degeneration
   macular d.
   sarcomatous d.
   wallerian d.
degenerative enthesopathy
deglutition
deglycosylated
deglycosylation
degradation
   calcium d.
   hormone d.
   insulin d.
   receptor d.
   T-lymphocyte insulin binding
      and d.
DeGroot classification
DEHAL1 gene mutation
dehalogenase
   iodotyrosine d.
dehiscence
   wound d.
dehydration
   cellular d.
   chronic d.
   extracellular fluid d.
dehydroalanine (DHA)
dehydroandrosterone sulfate rhythm

7-dehydrocholesterol
11-dehydrocorticosterone (DHC)
dehydroepiandrosterone (DHEA)
   d. cream
   d. sulfate (DHEAS, DHEA-S)
   d. supplement
dehydroestrone
dehydrogenase
   alcohol d.
   aldehyde d.
   alpha-glycerophosphate d.
   3-alpha-hydroxysteroid d. (3-alpha-
      HSD)
   3-beta-hydroxysteroid d. (3-beta-
      HSD)
   11-beta-hydroxysteroid d. (11-beta-
      HSD)
   17-beta-hydroxysteroid d. (17-beta-
      HSD)
   17-beta-hydroxysteroid d. type 1
      (17-beta-HSD1)
   17-beta-hydroxysteroid d. type 2
      (17-beta-HSD2)
   17-beta-hydroxysteroid d. type 3
      (17-beta-HSD3)
   17-beta-hydroxysteroid d. type 4
      (17-beta-HSD4)
   17-beta-hydroxysteroid d. type 5
      (17-beta-HSD5)
   glucose-6-phosphate d. (G6PD,
      G6PDH)
   glyceraldehyde-3-phosphate d.
      (GAPDH)
   glycerol-3-phosphate d.
   hydroxysteroid d. (HSD)
   11-hydroxysteroid d.
   isovaleryl-CoA d.
   lactate d. (LDH)
   lactic d.
   long chain acyl-CoA d. (LCAD)
   long chain 3-hydroxyacyl-CoA d.
      (LCHAD)
   lysine d.
   medium chain acyl-CoA d.
      (MCAD)
   pyrroline-5-carboxylate d.
   pyruvate d. (PDH)
   sarcosine d.
   very long chain acyl-CoA d.
      (VLCAD)
deiodinase
   d. enzyme

D

NOTES

deiodinase *(continued)*
    iodothyronine d.
    iodotyrosine-specific d.
    type 1 d. (D1)
    type 2 d. (D2)
    type 3 d. (D3)
deiodinate
deiodination
    sequential d.
Deknatel tape
Deladumone
Delalutin
Delatestryl Injection
delay
    constitutional d.
    neurodevelopmental d.
delayed
    d. bone age
    d. brain radionecrosis
    d. epiphyseal fusion
    d. puberty
    d. rectifier voltage-gated beta-cell adenosine triphosphate potassium
deleted
    d. in azoospermia (DAZ)
    d. in azoospermia-homologue (DAZH)
    d. in azoospermia-like autosomal (DAZLA)
deletion
    chromosome d.
    clonal d.
    cytokine d.
    gene d.
    germline d.
    somatic d.
delipidation
delirium
    toxic d.
delivery
    amino acid d.
    portal insulin d.
    salt d.
Delphian lymph node
delta cell
Delta-Cortef Oral
Delta-D
delta-5-desaturase enzyme
delta-6-desaturase enzyme
deltanoid
Deltasone
Del-Vi-A
demeclocycline
dementia
    dialysis d.
Demerol
demineralization
Demulen
demyelinating disorder

demyelination
    d. injury
    osmotic d.
demyelinative neuropathy
denaturation
denaturing
    d. gradient gel electrophoresis (DGGE)
    d. high-pressure liquid chromatography (dHPLC)
dendrite
    Purkinje cell d.
dendritic arbor
denervation
    pancreatic d.
    portohepatic d.
    sympathetic d.
DENIS
    Deutsch Nicotinamide Diabetes Intervention Study
densa
    macula d.
dense
    d. LDL
    d. staining of adenoma
densitometer
    Hologic QDR 4500 DXA bone d.
densitometry
    body d.
    bone d.
density
    bone mass d.
    bone mineral d. (BMD)
    endothelin receptor d.
    d. of the fat-free mass (d_{FFM})
    d. of the fat mass (d_{FF})
    femoral neck bone d.
    low bone d.
    lumbar spine bone d.
    total body bone mineral d. (D_{beta}, TBBMD)
dental
    d. lamina
    d. papilla
dentatorubral-pallidoluysian atrophy (DRPLA)
Dent disease
dentin
    radicular d.
dentinal tubule
dentine
dentinogenesis imperfecta
Denver shunt
Denys-Drash syndrome
21-deoxidation
21-deoxyaldosterone
deoxycorticosterone (DOC)
11-deoxycorticosterone (DOC)
deoxycorticosterone-producing tumor

deoxycortisol
11-deoxycortisol
21-deoxycortisol
2-deoxyglucose
deoxyinosine triphosphate (dITP)
deoxynucleotide triphosphate (dNTP)
17-deoxy pathway
deoxypyridinoline (DPD)
deoxyribonucleic acid (DNA)
17-deoxysteroid
depAndrogyn
depAndro Injection
dependency
    type 1 autosomal recessive vitamin
      D d. (ARVDD-1)
depGynogen Injection
dephosphorylate
depigmentation
    progressive d.
depletion
    hypertonic volume d.
    magnesium d.
    phosphate d.
    potassium d.
    volume d.
depMedalone Injection
Depo-Estradiol Injection
Depogen Injection
Depoject Injection
depolarization
Depo-Medrol Injection
Depopred Injection
Depo-Provera Injection
deposit
    aluminum d.
    amyloid d.
    metastatic d.
deposition
    beta$_2$-microglobulin amyloid d.
    calcium d.
    copper d.
    glycosaminoglycan d.
    iron d.
    laminin d.
    retroorbital fat d.
deposteroid
depot
    Androcur D.
    Lupron D.
    d. medroxyprogesterone acetate
      (DMPA)
    Nutropin D.

    Sandostatin LAR D.
    Testoviron D. 50, 100
Depo-Testadiol
Depotest Injection
Depotestogen
Depo-Testosterone Injection
Depot-Ped
    Lupron D.-P.
deprenyl
depressive disorder
deprivation
    estrogen d.
    insulin d.
    water d.
depsipeptide
depth
    erosion d. (EDe)
    d. perception
derangement
derepression
    chromatin d.
derivative
    androstane d.
    ergoline d.
    Ergot Alkaloid and D.
    estrane d.
    fibric acid d.
    imidazole d.
    lipid d.
    müllerian d.
    pregnane d.
    proopiomelanocortin d.
dermal/epidermal composite graft
dermal papilla
dermatan sulfate
dermatitidis
    Bacteroides d.
    Blastomyces d.
dermatitis
    eczematoid d.
    d. herpetiformis
    lichenified d.
    perioral d.
dermatofibrosis lenticularis disseminata
dermatomyositis
dermatophyte infection
dermatosis
    acquired perforating d. (APD)
dermoid cyst
dermopathy
    diabetic d.
    d. of Graves disease

D

NOTES

dermopathy *(continued)*
 infiltrative d.
 pretibial d.
 thyroid d.
DES
 diethylstilbestrol
1-desamino-8-d arginine vasopressin
desamino D-arginine vasopressin (DDAVP)
desArg
 d. bradykinin
 d. kallidin
desaturase
 stearoyl acyl-CoA d.
desensitization
 adenylate cyclase d.
 postreceptor d.
 receptor d.
desethylamiodarone
desferrioxamine therapy
desialylation
desiccated thyroid
designer estrogen
desipramine hydrochloride
desirable body weight
desmolase
 cholesterol d.
20,22-desmolase (P450scc) deficiency
desmoplastic stroma
desmopressin
 d. acetate
 intranasal d.
desmosome
desmosterol
Desogen
desogestrel
 ethinyl estradiol and d.
desoxycorticosterone
Desoxyn
destruction
 beta cell d.
 osteoarticular d.
 d. thyroiditis
destruction-induced thyrotoxicosis
destructive
 d. arthropathy
 d. thyrotoxicosis
desynchronization
desynchrony
detection
 bioluminescence d.
 carrier d.
 chemiluminescence d.
 D. of Ischemia in Asymptomatic Diabetes (DIAD)
 D. of Ischemia in Asymptomatic Diabetics (DIAD)
 liquid chromatography with electrochemical d. (LCED)

 sex-determining region Y gene d.
 SRY d.
 Y chromosome d.
detector
 cadmium telluride d.
detemir
 insulin d.
Detensol
deterioration
 microarchitectural d.
determinant
 immunodominant serologic d.
 ligand binding d.
determined osteoprogenitor cell
deuterated water technique
Deutsch Nicotinamide Diabetes Intervention Study (DENIS)
devascularization
development
 ambisexual d.
 brain d.
 breast d.
 contrasexual pubertal d.
 Griffiths Scales of Infant D.
 isosexual pubertal d.
 premature sexual d.
 pubertal d.
 thyroid gland d.
device
 Accu-Chek SoftClix lancet d.
 Accu-Chek Soft Touch lancing d.
 accuDEXA bone mineral assessment d.
 Ascensia Microlet Adjustable lancing d.
 Ascensia Microlet Vaculance lancing d.
 Autoclix fingerstick d.
 auto-Lancet Mini lancing d.
 Autolet Clinisafe lancing d.
 Autolet fingerstick d.
 Autolet Lite lancing d.
 Autolet Mini lancing d.
 BD Lancet d.
 Companion 2 self blood glucose monitoring d.
 E-Z Lets II lancing d.
 Genotropin Pen 5 growth hormone delivery d.
 Gentle-Lance lancet d.
 Glucolet Automatic lancing d.
 GlucoWatch glucose monitoring d.
 Haemolance Plus lancet d.
 intrauterine d. (IUD)
 Lasette laser lancing d.
 Lasette Plus assisted blood sampling d.
 Lite Touch lancing d.
 macroencapsulation d.

Mirena intrauterine d.
Monojector fingerstick d.
O$_2$ disposable boot d.
oxygen disposable boot d.
Penlet II Automatic blood
sampling d.
Prestige Lite Touch lancing d.
Progestasert intrauterine d.
progestin-containing intrauterine d.
QuickLance lancing d.
Select-Lite lancing d.
steroid-releasing intrauterine d.
Tenderlett Jr. lancing d.
Tenderlett Toddler lancing d.
UltraTLC adjustable lancing d.
vacuum constrictive d.
vacuum tumescence d.

"dewdrop on a rose petal" appearance

DEXA
dual-energy x-ray absorptiometry
DEXA scan

Dex-A-Diet
Maximum Strength D.-A.-D.

dexamethasone
d. suppression test
d. suppression therapy

dexamethasone-suppressed
d.-s. bovine corticotropin-releasing
hormone
d.-s. corticotropin-releasing hormone
stimulation
d.-s. CRH stimulation

**dexamethasone-suppressible
hyperaldosteronism**

Dexasone

Dexatrim
Maximum Strength D.
D. Pre-Meal

Dexedrine

dexfenfluramine

DexFerrum

Dexone

Dex series meters

dextran
parenteral iron d.

dextranomer

dextroamphetamine and amphetamine

dextromethorphan

dextrose
dialysate d.

Dextrostix

Dey-Dose
D.-D. isoproterenol
D.-D. metaproterenol

Dey-Lute isoetharine

dezocine

DFEN
D-fenfluramine

D-fenfluramine (DFEN)

d$_{FF}$
density of the fat mass

d$_{FFM}$
density of the fat-free mass

DFO
deferoxamine
DFO challenge
DFO test

DGGE
denaturing gradient gel electrophoresis

DHA
dehydroalanine
docosahexaenoic acid

DHC
11-dehydrocorticosterone
Duradyne DHC
DHC Plus

DHEA
dehydroepiandrosterone
dihydroepiandrosterone sulphate
DHEA cream
DHEA sulfate

DHEAS, DHEA-S
dehydroepiandrosterone sulfate

DHPG
dihydroxyphenylglycol

dHPLC
denaturing high-pressure liquid
chromatography

DHS
diabetic hyperosmolar state

DHT
dihydrotestosterone
DHT gel

Diabenal

diabesity

DiaBeta

diabetes
adrenal d.
adult-onset d.
aggressive insulin-dependent d.
(AID)
d. associated with certain
conditions

NOTES

diabetes *(continued)*
   d. associated with certain syndrome
   D. Atherosclerosis Intervention Study (DAIS)
   atypical d.
   D. Autoantibody Standardization Program (DASP)
   autoimmune d.
   D. Autoimmunity Study in the Young (DAISY)
   borderline d.
   brittle d.
   bronze d.
   d. burnout
   congenital lipoatrophic d.
   D. Control and Complications Trial (DCCT)
   cystic fibrosis-related d. (CFRD)
   Detection of Ischemia in Asymptomatic D. (DIAD)
   Diabetes Prevention Trial of Type 1 D. (DPT-1)
   drug-induced d.
   d. in early pregnancy (DIEP)
   D. in Early Pregnancy Study
   d. education
   d. education program
   D. Epidemiology Collaborative Analysis of Diagnostic Criteria in Europe study (DECODE)
   EURODIAB Controlled Trial of Lisinopril in Insulin Dependent D. (EUCLID)
   European Association for the Study of D.
   familial autoimmunity in d. (FAD)
   fibrocalculous pancreatic d. (FCPD)
   Flatbush d.
   gestational d.
   D. Hypoglucose capsule
   idiopathic d.
   immune-mediated d. (IMD)
   d. insipidus
   d. insipidus, diabetes mellitus, optic atrophy, and deafness
   d. insipidus, diabetes mellitus, progressive bilateral optic atrophy, and sensorineural deafness (DIDMOAD)
   insulin-dependent d. (IDD)
   insulin-resistant d.
   J-type d.
   juvenile d.
   juvenile-onset d. (JOD)
   ketosis-prone d.
   ketosis-resistant d.
   labile d.
   latent autoimmune d.
   lipoatrophic d.

   maturity-onset d. (MOD)
   d. mellitus
   d. mellitus classification
   D. Mellitus Insulin-Glucose Infusion in Acute Myocardial Infarction (DIGAMI)
   D. Mellitus Insulin-Glucose Infusion in Acute Myocardial Infection study
   d. mellitus, pregnancy classification, class A, B, C, D, E, F
   mitochondrial d.
   nephrogenic d.
   occult d.
   ocular complications of d.
   overt d.
   pancreatic d.
   pituitary d.
   postpubertal d.
   D. Prediction and Prevention Project (DIPP)
   pregestational d.
   prepubertal d.
   D. Prevention Program (DPP)
   D. Prevention Study
   D. Prevention Trial
   D. Prevention Trial research study
   D. Prevention Trial of Type 1 Diabetes (DPT-1)
   protein-deficient pancreatic d.
   renal d.
   secondary d.
   d. self-management
   small bowel d.
   steroid-induced d.
   sugar d.
   transient neonatal d.
   Troglitazone in Prevention of D. (TRIPOD)
   type 1, 2 d.
   unstable d.
   virus-induced d.
diabetes-deafness syndrome
diabetes-specific
   d.-s. complication
   d.-s. distress
diabetic
   d. acidosis (DA)
   d. amyotrophy
   d. angiopathy
   d. autonomic neuropathy
   d. bulla
   d. cardiomyopathy
   d. cerebral edema
   d. dermopathy
   Detection of Ischemia in Asymptomatic D.'s (DIAD)
   d. diarrhea
   d. dyslipidemia

d. enteropathy
d. fetopathy
d. foot
d. foot syndrome
d. gastroparesis
d. hand syndrome
d. hyperosmolar state (DHS)
d. ketoacidosis (DKA)
d. ketoacidosis bicarbonate
d. ketoacidosis-related coma
d. lipoatrophy
d. lipohypertrophy
d. male sexual dysfunction
d. mastopathy
d. microangiopathy
d. microvascular disease
d. mononeuropathy
d. muscle infarction
d. myelopathy
d. myocardial infarction
d. nephropathy
d. neuropathic arthropathy
nonobese d.
d. osteopathy
d. papillopathy
d. pregnancy
d. retinopathy
D. Retinopathy Study (DRS)
D. Retinopathy Vitrectomy Study (DRVS)
d. screening
d. thick skin
D. Tussin
D. Tussin Allergy Relief
D. Tussin Children's Formula
D. Tussin DM Maximum Strength Cough Suppressant/Expectorant
d. ulcer
d. vasculopathy
diabeticorum
bullosis d.
bullous d.
gastroparesis d.
necrobiosis lipoidica d. (NLD)
scleredema d.
DiabetiDerm
DiabetiSweet sugar substitute
diabetogenecity
diabetogenesis
diabetogenic
d. effect
d. epistasis

d. haplotype
d. heterodimer
d. locus
d. stimulus
diabetologist
Diab II
Diabinese
diacetate
ethinyl estradiol and ethynodiol d.
ethynodiol d.
progestin ethynodiol d.
diacylglycerol (DAG)
DIAD
Detection of Ischemia in Asymptomatic Diabetes
Detection of Ischemia in Asymptomatic Diabetics
DIAD study
diagnosis, pl. **diagnoses**
prenatal d.
presymptomatic d.
diagnostant
pancreatic functioning d. (PFD)
diagnostic
female sexual function d. (FSFD)
d. imaging
Dialume
dialysate
aluminum-contaminated d.
d. calcium concentration
d. dextrose
high-calcium d.
low-calcium d.
dialysis
chronic ambulatory peritoneal d. (CAPD)
continuous ambulatory peritoneal d. (CAPD)
d. dementia
equilibrium tracer d.
d. membrane
d. modality
peritoneal d. (PD)
dialysis-associated amyloidosis
dialysis-related amyloidosis (DRA)
dialytic therapy
dialyzable factor
diameter
myofiber d.
Diamicron
diamine oxidase (DAO)
Diamyd

D

NOTES

Dianabol
Diane-35
Dianette
diapedesis
diaphoresis
diaphragm
 urogenital d.
diaphragmal opening
diaphragma sella
diaphragmatic crus
diaphyseal, diaphysial
 d. cortical hyperostosis
 d. dysplasia
 d. sclerosis
diaphysis
diarrhea
 diabetic d.
 osmotic d.
 toxin-induced d.
 X-linked polyendocrinopathy
  immune dysfunction and d.
  (XPID)
diary
 diet d.
 food d.
 sugar d.
Diasensor
 D. 2000 glucose monitor
 D. 1000 sensor
diastase
diastrophic
 d. dystrophia (DTD)
 d. dystrophia gene
diathesis
 autoimmune d.
 hemorrhagic d.
diazoxide
dibasic
 d. aminoaciduria
 d. calcium phosphate
dibenzodiazepine
 tricyclic d.
Dibenzyline
dibromochloropropane
dibutyryl
 d. cAMP
 d. cyclic arginine monophosphate
DIC
 disseminated intravascular coagulation
Dicarbosil
dicarboxylic acid
dichlorodiphenyldichloroethane (DDD)
dichlorodiphenyltrichloroethane (DDT)
dicumarol
didanosine
DIDMOAD
 diabetes insipidus, diabetes mellitus,
  progressive bilateral optic atrophy, and
  sensorineural deafness

Didrex
Didronel
DIDS
 4,4′-di-isothiocyanatostilbene-2,2′-
  disulfonic acid
diencephalic
 d. cachexia
 d. epilepsy
 d. syndrome
 d. syndrome of infancy
diencephalon
dienogest
 progestin d.
DIEP
 diabetes in early pregnancy
diet
 acid ash d.
 animal protein d.
 cafeteria d.
 d. control
 d. diary
 d. education
 euglycemic d.
 HCF d.
 high-carbohydrate high-fiber d.
 high glycemic index d.
 high-phosphorus d.
 high-salt d.
 hypocaloric d.
 isocalorically substituted d.
 low glycemic index d.
 low-phosphorus d.
 low-protein d.
 Mediterranean d.
 phenylalanine-restricted d.
 step 2 d.
 very low calorie d.
dietary
 d. calcium intake
 d. fiber
 d. phosphorus
 d. protein
diethylamine triamine pentaacetic acid
 (DTPA)
diethylpropion
diethylstilbestrol (DES)
diethylstilbestrol-associated anomaly
diet-induced
 d.-i. metabolic syndrome
 d.-i. obesity (DIO)
 d.-i. steatosis
dieting
 inappropriate d.
difference
 arteriovenous d.
differential thyroid cancer (DTC)
differentiated
 d. thyroid cancer (DTC)
 d. thyroid carcinoma

d. thyroid carcinoma, intermediate type

differentiation
acinar d.
carcinoma showing thymuslike d. (CASTLE)
chondrocyte terminal d.
morphologic d.
neurogenic d. 1 (neuroD1)
normal sexual d.
prechondrocyte d.
sexual d.
spindled and epithelial tumor with thymus-like d. (SETTLE)

differentiation-inhibiting activity

diffuse
d. endocrine system
d. idiopathic skeletal hyperostosis (DISH)
d. neuroendocrine system (DNES)
d. papillomatosis
d. renal ischemia
d. toxic goiter

diffusion
proton d.

diflunisal

DIGAMI
Diabetes Mellitus Insulin-Glucose Infusion in Acute Myocardial Infarction
DIGAMI study

Di-Gel

DiGeorge
D. sequence
D. syndrome

Digepepsin

Digess 8000

DigiScope

digitalis

digital vasospasm

digitonin

digoxin

dihomo-gamma-linoleic acid

dihydrobiopterin
d. synthase deficiency
d. synthetase

dihydrocodeine compound

dihydroepiandrosterone sulphate (DHEA)

dihydroequilenin

dihydrogen phosphate

dihydropteridine
d. reductase
d. reductase deficiency

dihydropyridine antagonist

dihydrotachysterol

dihydrotestosterone (DHT)
d. gel

dihydroxyacetone

dihydroxyaluminum sodium carbonate

2′4-dihydroxybenzoic acid

1,25-dihydroxycholecalciferol

5,6-dihydroxyindole

dihydroxymandelic acid (DOMA)

dihydroxyphenylacetic acid (DOPAC)

dihydroxyphenylalanine (DOPA)
d. decarboxylase

dihydroxyphenylglycol (DHPG)

dihydroxyvitamin D

24,25-dihydroxyvitamin D (24,25(OH)$_2$D$_3$)

25-dihydroxyvitamin D (25(OH)$_2$D$_3$)

1,25-dihydroxyvitamin D$_3$

Dihyrex Injection

diiodinated tyrosine (DIT)

3,5-diiodotyrosine (DIT)

diketopiperazine

Dilantin

dilatation
aortic root d.
d. of aortic root
fusiform d.

dilated
d. eye examination
d. fundus examination
d. pupil examination

dilation
triventricular d.

Dilaudid
D. Injection
D. Oral
D. suppository

Dilaudid-HP Injection

Dilor

diltiazem

diluent

dilution
isotope d.

dimenhydrinate

dimer
glucocorticoid receptor d.
type II regulatory d. (RII)
type I regulatory d. (RI)

D

NOTES

dimercaptosuccinate
pentavalent d. (DMSA)
^{99m}Tc-pentavalent d.
dimercaptosuccinic acid (DMSA, DMSA-V-Tc99-m)
dimeric form
dimerization
estrogen receptor d.
PPAR d.
Dimetabs Oral
3,5-dimethyl-3′-isopropyl-L-thyronine (DIMIT)
dimethyl triazeno imidazole carboxamide-Dome (DTIC-Dome)
diminished ovarian reserve
DIMIT
3,5-dimethyl-3′-isopropyl-L-thyronine
DIMOAD syndrome
dimorphic
sexually d.
dimorphism
sexual d.
dimorphous
Dinate Injection
2,4-dinitrophenylhydrazine test
dinucleotide
cytosine-guanine d.
nicotinamide-adenine d. (NAD)
DIO
diet-induced obesity
Dioval Injection
dioxin receptor
dioxolone
imidazole d.
dioxygenase
4-hydroxyphenylpyruvate d.
2,3-dioxygenase
indoleamine 2,3-d. (IDO)
dipalmitoylphosphatidylcholine (DPPC)
dipeptidyl
d. carboxypeptidase
d. peptidase
d. peptidase IV (DPIV, DPP-IV)
Diphenhist
diphenoxylate
atropine plus d.
diphenyl
d. ether linkage
d. ether moiety
diphenylhydantoin
diphosphate
adenosine 5′ d. (ADP)
guanosine 5′ d. (GDP)
inositol d.
uridine 5′-d.
diphosphate-binding
guanosine d.-b.
1,3-diphosphoglycerate
diphosphonate

diphtheroid
diplegia
congenital facial d.
Diplococcus pneumoniae
diplopia
diplosome
diplotene
DIPP
Diabetes Prediction and Prevention Project
Type 1 Diabetes Prediction and Prevention Study
DIPP Study
dipsogenic
d. diabetes insipidus
d. stimulus
Dipyridamole Aspirin Microangiopathy of Diabetes Study
Disalcid
disc, disk
morning glory d.
neovascularization of d. (NVD)
d. pallor
discontinuous capillary endothelium
disease
acquired von Willebrand d. (AvWD)
Addison d.
adrenal medullary d.
adult polycystic kidney d.
adynamic bone d.
Albers-Schönberg d.
aluminum bone d.
aluminum-related bone d.
Alzheimer d.
amyloidic d.
anemia of end-stage renal d.
aplastic bone d.
autoimmune endocrine d.
autoimmune thyroid d. (AITD)
autosomal recessive d.
Ayala d.
Basedow d.
B-cell autoimmune thyroid d.
benign nodular d.
bilateral adrenal d.
Blount d.
bovine viral diarrhea mucosal d. (BVD-MD)
brittle-bone d.
broad beta d.
bronze d.
Brown-Schilder d.
Bruton d.
bubble boy d.
Camurati-Engelmann d.
Canavan d.
Castleman d.
celiac d.

Charcot joint d.
Charcot-Marie d.
Charcot-Marie-Tooth d.
childhood Graves d.
Child-Pugh d.
cholestatic liver d.
cholesteryl ester storage d.
chronic granulomatous d.
chylomicron retention d.
connective tissue d.
Cori d.
Cowden d.
Creutzfeldt-Jakob d. (CJD)
Crohn d.
Crouzon d.
Cushing d.
cyclical Cushing d.
Dent d.
dermopathy of Graves d.
diabetic microvascular d.
ductus-dependent congenital heart d.
endocrine d.
end-stage renal d. (ESRD)
Engelmann d.
Erdheim-Chester d.
euthyroid Graves d.
exocrine pancreas d.
extrathyroidal manifestation of
  Graves d.
Fabry d.
Farber d.
fibrocystic breast d.
fibro-inflammatory d.
Forbes d.
fulminant Letterer-Siwe d.
Gagel d.
Gaucher d.
gestational trophoblastic d.
Gierke d.
Glanzmann d.
glomerular d.
glucagon storage d.
glycogen storage d., types I/Ia, 1I,
  III, IV, V, VI, VII, VIII
graft-versus-host d.
granulomatous d.
Graves d. (GD)
Gull d.
GVH d.
Hand-Schüller-Christian d.
Hansen d.
Hashimoto d.

hepatic d.
Hers d.
Hirschsprung d.
Hodgkin d.
Huntington d.
hyaline membrane d.
hyperabsorptive hypercalciuric
  stone d.
hyperparathyroid bone d.
hypophosphatemic bone d.
hypothalamic-pituitary d.
I-cell d.
idiopathic Addison d.
inclusion cell d.
intestinal d.
iron storage d.
Jakob-Creutzfeldt d.
Jamaican vomiting d.
Jod-Basedow d.
Kearns-Sayre d.
Kennedy d.
Krabbe d.
kwashiorkor d.
Kyrle d.
Laron d.
Leigh d.
Lesch-Nyhan d.
Letterer-Siwe d.
Lhermitte-Duclos d.
liver d.
Lowe d.
low-turnover d.
lung d.
Lyme d.
Machado-Joseph d.
macrovascular d.
mad cow d.
maple syrup urine d.
marble bone d.
Meige d.
Menkes d.
metabolic bone d.
micronodular adrenal d.
microvascular d.
Milroy d.
Modification of Diet in Renal D.
  (MDRD)
monostotic d.
National Institute of Diabetes and
  Digestive and Kidney D.'s
  (NIDDK)
neurodegenerative d.

NOTES

disease *(continued)*
    Newcastle bone d.
    Niemann-Pick d.
    node-based malignant
      lymphoproliferative d.
    nonendocrine d.
    nonthyroid d.
    Norrie d.
    obstructive intestinal d.
    ophthalmic Graves d.
    Osler-Rendu-Weber d.
    Paget d.
    Parkinson d.
    Parry d.
    pathologic parathyroid d.
    Pelizaeus-Merzbacher d.
    pelvic inflammatory d.
    peptic ulcer d.
    peripheral arterial d. (PAD)
    peripheral vascular d.
    Peyronie d.
    pigmented nodular adrenocortical d.
      (PNAD)
    pituitary Cushing d.
    pituitary-dependent Cushing d.
    Plummer d.
    plurihormonal Cushing d.
    polycystic kidney d.
    polycystic ovarian d.
    polycystic ovary d. (PCOD)
    polyostotic Paget d.
    Pompe glycogen storage d., type II
    postpartum thyroid d. (PPTD)
    predominant hyperparathyroid
      bone d.
    pregnancy nodular thyroid d.
    pulmonary d.
    Pyle d.
    rachitic d.
    Recklinghausen d.
    renal d.
    renovascular d.
    restrictive lung d.
    Ribbing d.
    Riedel d.
    runt d.
    Salla d.
    Sandhoff d.
    SC d.
    Schindler d.
    sellar d.
    severe combined
      immunodeficiency d. (SCID)
    sialic acid storage d.
    sickle cell d.
    Simmonds d.
    stigmata of Cushing d.
    suprasellar d.
    Swiss cheese d.

    Tangier d.
    Tay-Sachs d.
    thyrocardiac d.
    thyroid eye d.
    thyroid inflammatory d.
    thyrotoxic Graves d.
    trophoblastic d.
    tubulointerstitial renal d.
    type IV glycogen storage d.
    type I von Willebrand d.
    unilateral adrenal d.
    unstable Cushing d.
    van Buchem d.
    venous thromboembolic d.
    VHL d.
    von Basedow d.
    von Gierke d.
    von Hippel-Lindau d.
    von Recklinghausen d.
    von Willebrand d.
    wasting d.
    Whipple d.
    Wilson d.
    Wolman d.
    X-linked lymphoproliferative d.
disease-management program
disequilibrium
    linkage d.
Disetronic
    D. Diaport pump
    D. Dihedi 25 insulin pump
    D. D-Tron insulin pump
    D. Pen
DISH
    diffuse idiopathic skeletal hyperostosis
disk *(var. of* disc)
dismutase
    superoxide d.
disodium
    edetate d.
    etidronate d.
    d. etidronate
    tiludronate d.
disomy
    uniparental d.
disopyramide
disorder
    adipsic d.
    adynamic bone d.
    alloimmune d.
    aplastic bone d.
    attention-deficit hyperactivity d.
    autoimmune neuromuscular
      junction d.
    autoimmune thyroid d. (AITD)
    autosomal dominant d.
    autosomal karyotypic d.
    autosomal recessive d.
    cardiovascular d.

chromosomal d.
chromosome 7, 12, 20 d.
complex genetic d.
congenital bone d.
demyelinating d.
depressive d.
dysbaric d.
eating d.
endocrine d.
familial lipid d.
Fredrickson classification of
  lipid d.'s
glucocorticoid-resistant depressive d.
growth d.
heredofamilial d.
hyperprolactinemic d.
hypoactive sexual desire d.
  (HSDD)
hypodipsic d.
hypoglycemic d.
hypothalamic-pituitary d.
infiltrative d.
International Council for Control of
  Iodine Deficiency D. (ICCIDD)
iodine-deficiency d. (IDD)
IPEX d.
ketoacid d.
late luteal phase d.
lipid d.
lymphoproliferative d.
major depressive d. (MDD)
monogenic d.
multihormonal system d.
neuromuscular junction d.
neuropsychiatric d.
nonsyndromic autosomal
  recessive d.
pancreatic d.
paroxysmal pain d.
peroxisomal d.
pituitary d.
posttransplantation
  lymphoproliferative d. (PTLD)
premenstrual dysphoric d. (PMDD)
Riedel d.
seasonal affective d. (SAD)
sexual differentiation d.
sperm transport d.
vocal cord d.
disordered water metabolism
disruptor
endocrine d.

dissection
en bloc d.
disseminata
dermatofibrosis lenticularis d.
disseminated
d. fat necrosis
d. histiocytosis X
d. intravascular coagulation (DIC)
d. mucormycosis
d. strongyloidosis
disseminatum
xanthoma d.
distal
d. anhidrosis
d. convoluted tubule (DCT)
d. Golgi apparatus
d. motor axonal loss
d. renal tubular acidosis type 4
d. sensory neuropathy
d. sensory polyneuropathy
d. small-fiber neuropathy
d. subtotal pancreatectomy
d. symmetric diabetic neuropathy
d. symmetric sensorimotor
  polyneuropathy
distalis
pars d.
distant metastasis
distention
adrenal capsular d.
distichiasis
distinct nodule
distress
diabetes-specific d.
epidermic d.
distribution
android fat d.
Gaussian d.
glove-and-stocking d.
gynoid fat d.
phosphorus d.
stocking-glove d.
disturbance
visual field d.
disulfide
d. bridge
carbon d.
d. isomerase
d. loop
disuse atrophy

D

NOTES

DIT
diiodinated tyrosine
3,5-diiodotyrosine
Dital
dITP
deoxyinosine triphosphate
Diucardin
diuresed
diuresis
osmotic d.
pressure d.
solute d.
spontaneous d.
water d.
diuretic
loop d.
osmotic d.
potassium-sparing d.
d. therapy
thiazide d.
Diurigen
Diuril
diurnal rhythm
divalent ion
diversion
biliopancreatic d.
diversus
Citrobacter d.
diverticulitis
diverticulum, pl. **diverticula**
epiphrenic d.
Meckel d.
posterior gastric d.
thyroid d.
division
meiotic d.
parvocellular d.
divisum
pancreas d.
D$_{9K}$
calbindin D$_{9K}$
D$_{28K}$
calbindin D$_{28K}$
DKA
diabetic ketoacidosis
DLD-1 colorectal cancer cell line
DLP
dyslipoproteinemia
D-Med Injection
D-methylmalonyl-CoA
DMN
dorsomedial nucleus
D-Modem and insulin pump therapy
DMPA
depot medroxyprogesterone acetate
DMSA
dimercaptosuccinic acid
pentavalent dimercaptosuccinate
rhenium-188 DMSA

DMSA-V-Tc99-m
dimercaptosuccinic acid
DNA
deoxyribonucleic acid
antidouble-stranded DNA
complementary DNA (cDNA)
DNA fingerprints
mitochondrial DNA
DNA ploidy
putative regulatory sequence DNA
DNA sequencing
DNA topoisomerase II (Top2)
DNA-binding domain (DBD)
DNCP
duct-narrowing chronic pancreatitis
DNES
diffuse neuroendocrine system
DN-PHIP
dominant-negative mutant of PHIP
dNTP
deoxynucleotide triphosphate
DOC
deoxycorticosterone
11-deoxycorticosterone
docetaxel
docking protein
docosahexaenoic acid (DHA)
Döderlein bacillus
Doehle body
Dolacet
Dolene
dolichol phosphate carrier
dolichostenomelia
dolichyl phosphate
Dolobid
Dolophine
Dolorac
DOMA
dihydroxymandelic acid
domain
amino terminal d.
carboxyl-terminus d.
coupling d.
DNA-binding d. (DBD)
extracellular d.
hexameric d.
hormone-binding d. (HBD)
insulin receptor transmembrane d.
kringle d.
leucine-zipper d.
ligand-binding d. (LBD)
phosphotyrosine-binding d. (PTB)
pleckstrin homology d.
pleiotropic d.
PPAR functional d.
PPAR-gamma functional d.
recognition d.
Src homology 2 d.

trans-activation d. (TAD)
transmembrane d.
dominant
d. follicle
d. thyroid nodule
dominant-negative mutant of PHIP (DN-PHIP)
domperidone
donation
segmental pancreas d.
Donnamar
Donnan effect
Donnatal
Donnazyme
Donohue leprechaun syndrome
donor
pancreas transplant registry of living segmental d.
DOPA
dihydroxyphenylalanine
DOPA decarboxylase
L-dopa
DOPAC
dihydroxyphenylacetic acid
dopamine (DA)
d. agent
d. agonist therapy
d. beta-hydroxylase (DBH)
d. enzyme
d. receptor
d. receptor agonist
dopaminergic
d. agonist
d. blocker
d. drug
d. neuron
d. receptor
d. system
d. tone
Dopar
Doppler-derived pressure measurement
Doppler velocimetry
Dopram
Dorcol
Dorello canal
Dormarex 2 Oral
Dormin Oral
dornase alfa
dorsal
d. motor nucleus
d. pancreatic artery

dorsalis
d. pedis arterial bypass
tabes d.
dorsocervical fat pad
dorsomedial
d. nucleus (DMN)
d. nucleus of the hypothalamus
dorsum sella
dosage-sensitive
d.-s. sex (DSS)
d.-s. sex reversal
d.-s. sex reversal-adrenal hypoplasia congenital (DSS-AHC)
d.-s. sex reversal gene
dose
growth hormone d.
intravaginal d.
mixed d.
steroid d.
supraphysiologic d.
tapering d.
dose-response curve
dosimetric scheme
dosimetry
dosing
pulse d.
Dospan
Tenuate D.
Dostinex tablet
dot
d. aneurysm
d. and blot hemorrhages
double-duct sign
double-labeling technique
Douglas
rectouterine recess of D.
dowager hump
down
milk let d.
downgaze
impaired d.
downregulate
downregulation
insulin-induced receptor d.
downstream signaling pathway
Down syndrome
doxapram
doxazosin
doxercalciferol
doxorubicin
doxycycline
DPC4 gene

D

NOTES

DPD
deoxypyridinoline
D-penicillamine
DPIV
dipeptidyl peptidase IV
DPP
Diabetes Prevention Program
DPPC
dipalmitoylphosphatidylcholine
DPPHR
duodenum-preserving pancreatic head resection
DPP-IV
dipeptidyl peptidase IV
DPT-1
Diabetes Prevention Trial of Type 1 Diabetes
DPT-1 research study
DQ
DQ allele
DQ alpha sequence
DQ8
HLA D.
DR4 allele
DRA
dialysis-related amyloidosis
drag
solvent d.
drainage
bladder d.
enteric d.
urinary d.
DR allele
Dramamine Oral
Dramilin Injection
Drash syndrome
dripping-candle-wax appearance
Drisdol
drive
ventilatory d.
droepiandrosterone
droloxifene
dronabinol
droperidol and fentanyl
droplet
colloid d.
drops
ADEKs pediatric d.
Fer-In-Sol d.
rose bengal d.
vitamin C d.
drospirenone
DRPLA
dentatorubral-pallidoluysian atrophy
DRS
Diabetic Retinopathy Study
drug
antiestrogen d.
antithyroid d. (ATD)

aphrodisiac d.
Ca^{2+} ionophore d.
calcimimetic d.
carbamide d.
dopaminergic d.
hypothyroid d.
immunosuppressive d.
lipid-lowering d.
lipophilic d.
methylxanthine d.
nitrous oxide-donor d.
NO-donor d.
nonsteroidal antiinflammatory d. (NSAID)
sulfonylurea hypoglycemic d.
sympatholytic d.
sympathomimetic d.
thionamide antithyroid d.
thiourea d.
drug-induced
d.-i. diabetes
d.-i. diabetes mellitus
d.-i. hypercalcemia
d.-i. hypoglycemia
d.-i. lupus
DRVS
Diabetic Retinopathy Vitrectomy Study
DSS
dosage-sensitive sex
DSS gene
DSS reversal
DSS-AHC
dosage-sensitive sex reversal-adrenal hypoplasia congenital
D-stix
DTC
differential thyroid cancer
differentiated thyroid cancer
DTD
diastrophic dystrophia
DTD gene
D-thyroxine
DTIC
dacarbazine
DTIC-Dome
dimethyl triazeno imidazole carboxamide-Dome
DTPA
diethylamine triamine pentaacetic acid
D-Tron insulin pump
dual-energy x-ray absorptiometry (DEXA, DXA)
dual-phase spiral computed tomography
dual-photon absorptiometry
dual-x-ray absorptiometry
Dubovitz syndrome
Duchenne-Becker muscular dystrophy
Duchenne muscular dystrophy

duct
- bile d.
- common bile d. (CBD)
- cortical collecting d. (CCD)
- craniopharyngeal d.
- d. ectasia
- ejaculatory d.
- excretory d.
- extrahepatic bile d.
- intrahepatic bile d.
- intralobular d.
- ipsilateral paramesonephric d.
- lactiferous d.
- main pancreatic d. (MPD)
- medullary collecting d. (MCD)
- müllerian d.
- parafollicular d.
- paramesonephric d.
- prostatic d.
- thyroglossal d.
- wolffian d.

ductectatic-type mucinous cystadenocarcinoma
duct-narrowing chronic pancreatitis (DNCP)
ductule
- efferent d.

ductuli efferentes
ductus
- d. deferens
- d. epididymis

ductus-dependent congenital heart disease
Duet glucose control monitor
dulcitol
Dull-C
duloxetine
dumbbell-shaped tumor
dumping syndrome
Dunnigan syndrome
DuoCet
Duo-Cyp
duodenal
- d. atresia
- d. intubation test

duodenography
- hypotonic d.

duodenum-preserving pancreatic head resection (DPPHR)
DuPan-2 antibody
duplication
- chromosome d.

Dupuytren
dura
- lamina d.

Duradyne DHC
Duragesic transdermal
dural microclip
Duralone Injection
Duramorph Injection
Duratest Injection
Duratestrin
Durathate Injection
Duricef
Durrax Oral
Duvoid
dwarf
- Levi-Lorain d.

dwarfism
- camptomelic d.
- emotional deprivation d.
- Laron d.
- Laron-type d. (LTD)
- osteodysplastic primordial d.
- panhypopituitary d.
- pituitary d.
- psychosocial d.
- Seckel bird-headed d.
- short-limbed d.
- d. of Sindh

DX
DXA
- dual-energy x-ray absorptiometry

dydrogesterone
dye
- fluorescein d.
- iodinated contrast d.
- oral cholecystographic d.
- radiopaque d.

dye-diluting technique
Dymelor
Dymenate Injection
DynA
- dynorphin A

dynamic
- d. computed tomography
- d. equilibrium
- d. histomorphometry
- d. spiral CT

dynamometer
- isokinetic d.

dynein

NOTES

dynorphin
    d. A (DynA)
    d. system
dyphylline
Dyrexan-OD
dysalbuminemia
    familial d.
dysalbuminemic hyperthyroxinemia
dysarthria
dysautonomia
    familial d.
dysbaric disorder
dysbetalipoproteinemia
    familial d.
    gas d.
dyschondrosteosis
    Leri-Weill d. (LWD)
dysembryogenesis
    branchial pouch d.
dysesthesia
dysfunction
    adrenal d.
    autonomic d.
    corticospinal tract d.
    diabetic male sexual d.
    endothelial cell d.
    erectile d. (ED)
    exocrine pancreatic d.
    extraocular muscle d.
    female sexual d. (FSD)
    gonadal d.
    G protein d.
    luteal d.
    maternal postpartum thyroid d.
    menstrual d.
    neonatal thyroid d.
    ovarian steroidogenic d.
    parathyroid gland d.
    pilosebaceous d.
    pituitary d.
    postpartum thyroid d.
    sexual d.
    sphincter of Oddi d.
    thyroid d.
    transient neonatal thyroid d.
dysgammaglobulinemia
dysgenesis
    chromatin-positive seminiferous
     tubule d.
    d. of corpus callosum
    epiphyseal d.
    gonadal d.
    incomplete XY gonadal d.
    mixed gonadal d.
    ovarian d.
    pure gonadal d.
    seminiferous tubule d.
    thyroid d. (TD)
    45,X gonadal d.

    46,XX gonadal d.
    46,XY gonadal d.
dysgenetic gonad
dysgerminoma
    pineal d.
    primary suprasellar d.
dysgeusia
dysglycemic macroangiopathy
dyshomogenesis
dyshormonogenesis
    thyroid d.
dyshormonogenetic goiter
dysinsulinism
dyskinesia
dyslipidemia
    atherogenic d.
    diabetic d.
dyslipidosis
dyslipoproteinemia (DLP)
dysmenorrhea
dysmorphic facies
dysmotility
    esophageal d.
    ocular d.
dysosteosclerosis
dysostosis multiplex
dyspareunia
dysphonia
    spasmodic d.
dysplasia
    camptomelic d.
    cleidocranial d.
    coloboma d.
    colobomatous d.
    congenital adrenal d.
    craniodiaphysial d.
    craniometaphyseal d.
    diaphyseal d.
    fibrous d. (FD)
    Kniest d.
    Kniest-Stickle d.
    Langer mesomelic d.
    mammary d.
    mesometric d.
    metaphyseal d.
    Mondini d.
    oculodentoosseous d.
    polyostotic fibrous d. (PFD)
    primary pigmental nodular
     adrenal d.
    primary pigmented nodular
     adrenal d.
    progressive diaphyseal d.
    Schmid-type metaphyseal d.
    septooptic d.
    spondyloepiphyseal d. (SED)
    spondylometaphyseal d.
    Strudwick-type
     spondyloepimetaphyseal d.

thanatophoric d. type I, II
X-linked hypohidrotic ectodermal d.

dyspnea
recumbent d.

dyspraxia
speech d.

dysproteinemia
angioimmunoblastic
lymphadenopathy with d. (AILD)

dysregulation
blood pressure d.
hypothalamic d.
immune d.
theca interstitial cell d.
thecal d.

dysthyroid orbitopathy
dystonia type 1
dystonic reaction
dystopia
pituitary d.

dystrophia
diastrophic d. (DTD)

dystrophica
myotonia d.

dystrophic calcification
dystrophy
adiposogenital d.
autoimmune polyendocrinopathy-
candidiasis-ectodermal d.
(APECED)
Duchenne-Becker muscular d.
Duchenne muscular d.
fascioscapulohumeral muscular d.
mixed sclerosing bone d.
muscular d.
myotonic d.
oculopharyngeal muscular d.
reflex sympathetic d.

NOTES

D

E

apolipoprotein deficiency E
carboxypeptidase E
hemoglobin E
hepatitis E
immunoglobulin E (IgE)

1/35E

Norethin 1/35E

E₁

estrone
prostaglandin E_1 (PGE_1)

E₂

estradiol
E_2 agonist
prostaglandin E_2 (PGE_2)
E_2 receptor

E₃

estriol
prostaglandin E_3

E₄

leukotriene E_4 (LTE_4)

EAAE

experimental allergic autoimmune
encephalitis

EAAT2 protein

early

e. collecting tubule
e. endosomal compartment
e. hypocalcemia
e. pregnancy factor (EPF)
e. pubertal hyperandrogenism
e. satiety
E. Treatment Diabetic Retinopathy
Study (ETDRS)

early-onset

e.-o. idiopathic chronic pancreatitis
e.-o. uterine leiomyoma

Easprin

easy satiety

EAT

experimental autoimmune thyroiditis

eating disorder

E-box

E-b. element insulin gene promoter
E-b. motif

Ebstein anomaly

EBV

Epstein-Barr virus

EC

endothelial cell
enterochromaffin cell

E-cadherin protein

ecchymosis

eccrine sweat gland

ecdysone receptor

ECF

extracellular fluid

echinococcal thyroiditis

Echinococcus granulosus

echo

fast asymmetric spin e.

echogenicity

echogenic ovarian stroma

echotexture

echovirus 6

ECL

enterochromaffin-like
ECL cell
ECL cell hyperplasia

eclosion hormone

ECM

extracellular matrix

E-Complex-600

***Eco*RI**

ectasia

duct e.

ecthyma gangrenosis

ectoderm

stomodeal e.

ectodermal anomaly

ectoenzyme

thyroid-releasing hormone-
degrading e.
TRH-degrading e. (TRH-DE)

ectohormone

ectopia lentis

ectopic

e. acromegaly
e. ACTH-secreting tumor
e. ACTH secretion
e. ACTH syndrome
e. adrenal adenoma
e. adrenocorticotropic hormone
secretion
e. adrenocorticotropic hormone
syndrome
e. calcification
e. corticotropin-releasing hormone
syndrome
e. CRH syndrome
e. Cushing syndrome
e. endometrium
e. expression
e. growth hormone-releasing
hormone secretion
e. hormone production
e. hormone receptor
e. hormone syndrome
e. intrapancreatic protease activation
e. neoplasm

E

ectopic *(continued)*
    e. neuroendocrine tumor
    e. paraneoplastic ACTH production
    e. pinealoma
    e. pituitary adenoma
    e. pregnancy
    e. thyroid
    e. thyroid tissue
ectoplasmic specialization
eczematoid dermatitis
ED
    erectile dysfunction
EDC
    endocrine disrupting chemical
EDe
    erosion depth
Edecrin
edema
    cerebral e.
    clinically significant macular e.
      (CSME)
    conjunctival e.
    diabetic cerebral e.
    hereditary angioneurotic e.
    interstitial e.
    macular e.
    neurogenic pulmonary e.
    optic disc e.
    periorbital e.
    pulmonary e.
    refeeding e.
    Reinke e.
    type 1, 2 angioneurotic e.
edetate disodium
edetic acid
EDF
    erythroid differentiation factor
EDIC
    Epidemiology of Diabetes Interventions
    and Complications
Edinger-Westphal nucleus
Edmonton Protocol
EDRF
    endothelium-derived relaxing factor
EDTA
    ethylenediaminetetraacetic acid
education
    diabetes e.
    diet e.
educator
    Certified Diabetes E. (CDE)
EDXA
    energy-dispersive x-ray analysis
EFA
    essential fatty acid
effect
    acute Wolff-Chaikoff e.
    allosteric e.
    alpha-adrenergic e.

aluminum e.
anticholinergic side e.
antilipolytic e.
antimitotic e.
antirachitic e.
antirachitogenic e.
antiserotoninergic e.
antistress e.
autocrine e.
base-substitution e.
beta-adrenergic e.
bone e.
bystander e.
calcemic e.
cardioprotective e.
cardiovascular e.
cholinergic e.
chondroprotective e.
diabetogenic e.
Donnan e.
endocrine e.
estrogenic e.
extrahepatic e.
gastrointestinal e.
growth hormone protein-sparing e.
hair e.
hepatic e.
hormone-dependency e.
hydrogen-bonding e.
ileal-brake e.
immunoregulatory e.
incretin e.
insulinomimetic e.
Jod-Basedow e.
K_m e.
lag e.
maternotoxic e.
metabolic e.
multiplier e.
muscle e.
neuropsychiatric e.
nongenomic e.
paracrine e.
peak e.
physiologic e.
piezoelectric e.
ring-substitution e.
Somogyi e.
stalk section e.
Staub-Traugott e.
vitamin D e.
Wolff-Chaikoff e.
effective
    e. circulating volume
    e. half-life
    e. osmolality
effector
    allosteric e.
    bihormonal e.

E. mechanism
e. organ
efferent
e. arteriole
e. ductule
e. system
efferentes
ductuli e.
effluent
thyroid venous e.
effluvium
telogen e.
efflux
calcium e.
hepatic glucose e.
iodide e.
net e.
parathyroid hormone-mediated
calcium e.
PTH-mediated calcium e.
eflornithine hydrochloride
Efudex
EFV
extracellular fluid volume
EGF
endothelial growth factor
epidermal growth factor
heparin-binding EGF
EGF receptor
EGF-like growth factor
EGGCT
extragonadal germ cell tumor
EGP
endogenous glucose production
Ehlers-Danlos syndrome types I, II, III, IV, VII
EIA
enteroinsular axis
enzyme immunoassay
eicosanoid synthesis
eicosapentaenoic acid (EPA)
EIF2AK3 gene mutation
Eikenella corrodens
ejaculation
premature e.
retrograde e.
ejaculatory duct
ejection
milk e.
elastase
plasma polymorphonuclear e.
(PMN-3)

elastase-1 level
elastin
elastography
magnetic resonance e. (MRE)
Eldercaps
electrical gradient
electrically excitable cell
electrochemical
e. glucose sensor
e. gradient
electroconvulsive therapy
electrode
amperometric glucose oxidase e.
H_2O_2 amperometric e.
ion-selective e.
platinum e.
electrogastrogram
electrogenic
electroimmunoassay
electrolyte
e. flux
e. therapy
electronic barostat
electron transport flavoprotein (ETF)
electroosmotic sampling procedure
electrophoresis
agarose gel e.
denaturing gradient gel e. (DGGE)
gel e.
polyacrylamide gel e.
electrophoretic gel mobility shift assay (EMSA)
electrovaporization of the prostate
eledoisin
element
activator protein-1 e.
anamnestic e.
AP-1 e.
basal promoter e. (BPE)
bone marrow e.
cAMP-response e. (CRE)
cis e.
cis-acting DNA e.
comparator e.
consensus-response e.
cyclic adenosine monophosphate
regulatory e. (CRE)
cyclic adenosine 3′,5′-
monophosphate-response e.
estrogen-receptor e. (ERE)
estrogen-response e. (ERE)
glucocorticoid response e. (GRE)

E

NOTES

element *(continued)*
    glucocorticoid-responsive e. (GRE)
    hormone response e. (HRE)
    inhibitory response e. (IRE)
    insulin response e.
    laminin B1 e.
    lysozyme F_2 e.
    negative T_3 response e. (TRE)
    negative triiodothyronine
      response e.
    NF-kappa-B e.
    nonregulatory e. (NRE)
    nuclear factor-kappa B e.
    response e.
    serum response e.
    steroid hormone-receptor hormone-
      response e.
    sterol response e.
    thyroid hormone-response e. (TRE)
    thyroid response e. (TRE)
    T_3 responsive e. (T_3RE)
    vascular e.
    vitamin D-regulatory e.
    vitamin D-response e. (VDRE)
    xenobiotic-response e. (XRE)
    Z e.
element-binding
    cAMP response e.-b. (CREB)
    cyclic arginine monophosphate
      response e.-b.
elevated
    e. intracranial pressure
    e. radioactive iodine uptake
    e. RAIU
    e. waist-to-hip ratio
elevation
    spurious e.
elfin
    e. facies
    e. facies syndrome
ELISA
    enzyme-linked immunosorbent assay
Elixomin
Elixophyllin
elliptocytosis
Ellis-van Creveld syndrome
Eltroxin
EM-652
E/M
    evaluation and management
emaciation
Embden-Meyerhof pathway
embedding
    bone e.
embolization
    arterial e.
    fat e.
    hepatic artery e.

    superselective microcoil e.
    transcatheter celiac artery e.
embolus, pl. **emboli**
    cholesterol e.
embryogenesis in pregnancy
embryologic development end-organ
   ovarian failure
embryology
embryonal
    e. adenoma
    e. carcinoma
    e. path
embryonic testicular regression
   syndrome
embryopathy
embryotoxic
embryotoxicity
embryo transfer (ET)
EMCL
    extramyocellular lipid
EMC virus
emergency
    hypocalcemic e.
EMH
    extramedullary hematopoiesis
emiglitate
eminence
    infundibular e.
    infundibulum e.
    median e.
emissary vein
emission
    nocturnal e.
emollient
    Ponaris nasal e.
emotional deprivation dwarfism
emphysematous pyelonephritis
empty
    e. sella
    e. sella syndrome
EMSA
    electrophoretic gel mobility shift assay
en
    en bloc dissection
    en face
ENaC
    epithelial sodium channel
enalapril
enanthate
    testosterone e.
encapsulated
    e. angioinvasive carcinoma
    e. islet transplant
encapsulation
    islet e.
encephalitis
    experimental allergic autoimmune e.
    (EAAE)

e. pandemic
St. Louis e.

encephalocele
basal e.
forebrain basal e.
frontoethmoidal e.
sphenoethmoidal e.
sphenoorbital e.
transethmoidal basal e.
transsphenoidal e.

encephalomyocarditis
e. virus
e. virus gene identification
e. virus-induced diabetes mellitus
e. virus islet

encephalopathy
Hashimoto e.
hypertonic e.
hyponatremic e.
hypoxic e.
spongiform e.
Wernicke e.

enclomiphene
endemia
goiter e.

endemic
e. colloid goiter
e. cretinism
e. fluorosis
e. iodine-deficiency goiter

ending
terminal nerve e.

ENDIT
European Nicotinamide Diabetes
Intervention Trial

endobone
endochondral
e. bone formation
e. bone maturation
e. ossification

endocrine
e. abnormality
e. anomaly
e. axis
e. disease
e. disorder
e. disrupting chemical (EDC)
e. disruptor
e. effect
e. effector cell
e. gene
e. gland

e. hyperfunction
e. hypertension
e. ophthalmopathy
e. pancreas
pulmonary neuroepithelial e. (PNEE)
e. remission
e. rhythm
e. therapy
e. tumor
e. tumor syndrome

endocrine-inactive pituitary adenoma
endocrine-to-exocrine ratio
endocrinologic
endocrinologist
American Association of
Clinical E.'s
pediatric e.

endocrinoma
endocrinopathy
autoimmune polyglandular e.
hyperprolactinemic e.
secondary e.

endocytose
endocytosis
absorptive e.
GLUT-4 e.
receptor-mediated e.

endoderm
endodermal sinus tumor
endo-exocrine tumor
endogenous
e. circadian pacemaker
e. cyclicity
e. estrogen
e. estrogen bioassay
e. fecal calcium
e. glucose production (EGP)
e. gonadal hormone
e. growth hormone
e. hypercortisolism
e. insulin
e. morphine
e. opioid
e. opioid peptide (EOP)
e. progesterone
e. rhythm
e. testosterone

endoglycosidase H
endolymph
endolymphatic cyst

E

NOTES

endometrial
> e. cancer
> e. cavity
> e. cycle
> e. gland
> e. stroma
> e. thickness

endometrioid tumor
endometrioma
> leaking e.

endometriosis
endometriotic implant
endometritis
> tuberculous e.

endometrium
> ectopic e.
> eutopic e.
> uterine e.

endomysial connective tissue
endonasal
> e. endoscopic pituitary surgery
> e. endoscopic technique
> e. endoscopic transsphenoidal approach
> e. hemitransfixion incision
> e. transseptal approach

endoneurial blood vessel
endopeptidase
> cysteine e.
> neutral e.

endoplasmic
> e. reticulum (ER)
> e. reticulum cisternae
> e. reticulum-Golgi network

endoprotease
> aspartyl e.
> serum e.
> subtilisin-related e.

endorectal
> e. magnetic resonance imaging
> e. MRI

end-organ
> e.-o. resistance
> e.-o. response

endorphin
endoscopic
> e. lithotripsy
> e. pituitary surgery technique
> e. sphincterotomy
> e. transsphenoidal hypophysectomy
> e. ultrasound

Endoscrub
endosome
endostatin
endosteal
> e. envelope
> e. fibrosis
> e. hyperostosis
> e. membrane

endosteum
endothelial
> e. cell (EC)
> e. cell dysfunction
> e. cell-stimulating angiogenesis factor (ESAF)
> e. function
> e. growth factor (EGF)
> e. layer
> e. nitric oxide synthase (eNOS)
> e. PAS-domain protein-1 (EPAS1)
> e. tight junction

endothelial-leukocyte adhesion
endothelin (ET)
> e. immunostaining
> e. isopeptide
> e. level
> e. receptor
> e. receptor density
> e. receptor expression
> e. release

endothelin-1 (ET-1)
endothelin-induced protein synthesis
endothelium
> capillary e.
> continuous capillary e.
> discontinuous capillary e.
> fenestrated capillary e.
> GLUT-4 e.
> luminal e.
> tumor-derived e.

endothelium-derived relaxing factor (EDRF)
endotoxemia
endotoxin contamination
endozepine
end-product
> advanced glycation e.-p. (AGE)
> advanced glycosylation e.-p. (AGE, AGEP)
> receptor for advanced glycation e.-p. (RAGE)

end-stage renal disease (ESRD)
end-systolic
> e.-s. stress
> e.-s. volume

Enduron
Enemol
Ener-B
energy
> activation e.
> e. balance
> e. charge
> e. consumption
> e. expenditure
> e. homeostasis
> e. pathway

e. requirement
e. store
energy-dispersive x-ray analysis (EDXA)
Engelmann disease
englitazone
engraftment
enhanced
e. oxidative state
e. proximal tubular salt absorption
enhancer
pleiotrophin/midkine growth e. (PTN/MK)
Enisyl
enkephalin
leucine e. (LE)
methionine e. (ME)
Met and Leu e.
e. system
enlargement
acral e.
facial feature e.
hand e.
pituitary e.
stromal e.
thyroid e.
enolase
e. enzyme
neuron-specific e.
enophthalmos
eNOS
endothelial nitric oxide synthase
Enovid
enoxaparin
ENS
enteric nervous system
Ensure Glucerna OS
enteral aluminum absorption
enteric
e. drainage
e. fever
e. hyperoxaluria
e. nervous system (ENS)
e. neuropathy
enterically drained simultaneous pancreas and kidney transplant
enteric-coated sodium fluoride
enteritidis
Salmonella e.
Enterobacter
enterochromaffin cell (EC)
enterochromaffin-like (ECL)

e.-l. cell
e.-l. cell hyperplasia
enterocolitica
Yersinia e.
enteroglucagon
enterohepatic
e. circulation
e. tumor
enteroinsular axis (EIA)
enterokinase
enteropathy
diabetic e.
gluten-sensitive e.
Entero-Vioform
enterovirus
Enterra therapy
enthesopathy
degenerative e.
entity
neonatal diabetes mellitus genetic e.
entrainment
nonphotic e.
photic e.
entrapment/compression neuropathy
entrapment syndrome
entropy
approximate e. (ApEn)
enucleation
enuresis
envelope
endosteal e.
glial e.
periosteal e.
Schwann e.
environment
photoperiodic e.
environmental trigger
enzootic goiter
enzyme
acrosomal e.
5-alpha-reductase e.
amidating e.
angiotensin-converting e.
branching e.
brush-border alpha-glucosidase e.
carbonic anhydrase e.
cathepsin B e.
circulating lipolytic e.
cytochrome P450 e. (CYP)
cytochrome P450 e. 19
cytochrome P450 e. 27 (CYP27)

E

NOTES

enzyme *(continued)*
    cytochrome P450 e. 1A1
    cytochrome P450 e. 11A
    cytochrome P450 e. 21B
    cytochrome P450 family of e.'s
    cytosolic e.
    e. defect
    e. deficiency
    deiodinase e.
    delta-5-desaturase e.
    delta-6-desaturase e.
    e. DNase I
    dopamine e.
    enolase e.
    extrapancreatic digestive e.
    furin e.
    galactosyltransferase e.
    e. gene expression
    e. glucokinase
    glycolytic e.
    guanylate cyclase e.
    hepatocellular e.
    hexokinase e.
    11-hydroxylase e.
    e. immunoassay (EIA)
    e. inhibitor
    insulin-degrading e. (IDE)
    insulin-sensitive e.
    intracellular effector e.
    iodinase e.
    laminin e.
    lipogenic e.
    liver e.
    e. lysyl oxidase
    malic e.
    mitochondrial e.
    muscle e.
    oligosaccharide transferase e.
    pancreatic e.
    paraoxonase e.
    P450c17 e.
    phosphatase e.
    phospholipase C e.
    phosphorylase e.
    proinsulin conversion processing e.
    prolyl hydroxylase e.
    proteolytic e.
    P450SCC e.
    P450 side chain cleavage e.
    *Pst*I restriction e.
    pulmonary angiotensin I
      converting e.
    restriction e.
    SCC e.
    side chain cleavage e.
    steroidogenic e.
    sulfotransferase e.
    *Taq*I restriction e.

    telomerase e.
    tyrosine aminotransferase e.
    urea cycle e.
    e. urease
enzyme-linked
    e.-l. immunoassay
    e.-l. immunosorbent assay (ELISA)
EOP
    endogenous opioid peptide
EORTC
    European Organization for Research and
      Treatment of Cancer
eosin
eosinopenia
eosinophil
eosinophilia myalgia syndrome
eosinophilic
    e. colloid
    e. pancreatitis
EPA
    eicosapentaenoic acid
epalrestat
EPAS1
    endothelial PAS-domain protein-1
ependymoma
EPF
    early pregnancy factor
ephedra
ephedrine
EPI
    epinephrine
    exocrine pancreatic insufficiency
epiandrosterone
epiblast
EPIC
    European Prospective Investigation of
      Cancer
epicanthus
epidemic hemorrhagic fever
**Epidemiology of Diabetes Interventions
and Complications (EDIC)**
epidermal
    e. cyst
    e. growth factor (EGF)
    e. growth factor receptor
    e. hyperplasia
    e. necrolysis
epidermic distress
epidermidis
    Staphylococcus e.
epidermoid cyst
epidermolysis bullosa
epididymal cystadenoma
epididymis, pl. **epididymides**
    caput e.
    ductus e.
epididymitis
epididymoorchitis

epilepsy
 catamenial e.
 diencephalic e.
epilepticus
 status e.
EPILOG
 Evaluation of PTCA to Improve Long-
 Term Outcome by C7E3 GpIIb/IIIa
 Receptor Blockade
 EPILOG trial
epimysium
epinephrine (EPI)
 e. provocation test
epinephrine-to-norepinephrine ratio
epinephros
epineurial blood vessel
epiphenomenon
epiphrenic diverticulum
epiphyseal
 e. closure
 e. dysgenesis
 e. fusion
 e. growth plate
 e. maturation
epiphysis, pl. **epiphyses**
 e. cerebri
 fused e.
 stippled e.
episode
 metabolic stress e.
 myopathy, encephalopathy, lactic
  acidosis, stroke-like e.'s (MELAS)
epistasis
 diabetogenic e.
EPISTENT
 Evaluation of Platelet IIb/IIIa
 Inhibitor for Stenting
 EPISTENT trial
epitaxial
 e. crystal proliferation
 e. growth
epithalamic region
epithelia (*pl. of* epithelium)
epithelial
 e. sodium channel (ENaC)
 e. thyroid carcinoma
epithelioid giant cell
epithelium, pl. **epithelia**
 coelomic e.
 germinal e.
 hormone-responsive e.
 maceration of e.

 retinal pigment e. (RPE)
 seminiferous e.
 squamous follicular e.
epitode
epitope
 antibody e.
 conformational dependent e.
 T-cell e.
Eplerenone
EPO
 erythropoietin
epoetin alfa
Epogen
epostane
epoxymextrenone
Epstein-Barr
 E.-B. transformed lymphocyte
 E.-B. virus (EBV)
EPT
 estrogen-progesterone therapy
equation
 Goldman-Hodgkin-Katz e.
 Harris-Benedict e.
 Henderson-Hasselbalch e.
 Nernst e.
equilenin
Equilet
equilibrium
 e. association constant (K_a)
 e. dissociation constant (K_d)
 dynamic e.
 osmotic e.
 e. tracer dialysis
equilin
equine conjugated estrogen
equipotent
equivalent
 bioengineered living-skin e.
equol
ER
 endoplasmic reticulum
 estrogen receptor
 ER alpha
 ER beta
erb
 e. B2/HER2 ligand
 E. palsy
erb **oncogene**
Erdheim-Chester disease
ERE
 estrogen-receptor element
 estrogen-response element

E

NOTES

113

erectile
> e. dysfunction (ED)
> e. impairment
> e. impotence
> e. tissue

erection
> nonsustained e.

erectogenic agent
erect penile length
ergocalciferol
ergogenic acid
ergoline derivative
ergonovine
Ergoset tablet
ergosterol
ergot
> e. alkaloid
> E. Alkaloid and Derivative

ergotamine
erigentes
> parasympathetic nervi e.

ERK
> extracellularly regulated kinase
> extracellular signal-regulated kinase
> extracellular signal-related kinase

ERK1
> extracellular signal-related kinase 1

ERK2
> extracellular signal-related kinase 2

Erlenmeyer flask deformity
erosio interdigitalis blastomycetica
erosion
> e. depth (EDe)
> e. surface per bone surface
> (ES/BS)

ERP-CT
> computed tomography under endoscopic
> retrograde pancreatography

ERT
> estrogen replacement therapy

eruption
> acneiform e.

eruptive xanthoma
erythema
> conjunctival e.
> lid e.
> e. multiforme
> necrolytic migrating e.
> necrolytic migratory e. (NME)
> e. nodosum

erythematosus
> lupus e.
> systemic lupus e. (SLE)

erythrasma
erythroblastosis fetalis
erythrocyte sedimentation rate (ESR)
erythrocytosis
erythrogenin

erythroid
> colony-forming unit e. (CFU-E)
> e. differentiation factor (EDF)
> e. hyperplasia
> e. precursor
> e. series

erythroleukemia
erythromelalgia
erythromycin
erythropoiesis
erythropoietin (EPO)
> recombinant e.
> serum e.

erythrosin
ESAF
> endothelial cell-stimulating angiogenesis
> factor

ES/BS
> erosion surface per bone surface

escalator
> mucous e.

escape
> aldosterone e.
> e. phenomenon

eschar
> pathognomonic black e.

Escherichia coli
Esclim transdermal
escutcheon
E-selectin ligand
esmolol
esodeviation
esophageal dysmotility
esophagography
> barium contrast e.

esotropia
ESR
> erythrocyte sedimentation rate

ESRD
> end-stage renal disease

ESS
> euthyroid sick syndrome

essential
> e. fatty acid (EFA)
> e. hypernatremia
> e. hypertension

EST
> expressed sequence tag

ester
> cholesteryl e.
> L-nitro-L-arginine methyl e.
> phorbol e.
> phthalate e.'s
> plant stanol e.
> retinyl fatty acid e.
> testosterone e.

esterification

esterified
> e. estrogen
> e. estrogen-methyltestosterone

estetrol

esthesiometer
> monofilament pressure e.

Estinyl

Estrace Oral

Estracomb TTS

Estraderm transdermal

Estraderm-TTS

estradiol (E_2)
> 17B e.
> cyclical ethinyl e.
> ethinyl e.
> e. matrix
> micronized e.
> nonestrogenic stereoisomer 17-
>   alpha e.
> e. and norethindrone
> e. peak
> serum e.
> e. and testosterone
> transdermal e.

estradiol/norethindrone acetate

estradiol-norethisterone phase

estradiol/norgestimate

estradiol/testosterone ratio

Estra-L Injection

estrane derivative

Estratab

Estratest H.S.

Estring vaginal insert

estriol (E_3)

Estro-Cyp Injection

EstroGel

estrogen
> conjugated equine e. (CEE)
> continuous conjugated equine e.
> e. C_{19} steroid
> cyclic conjugated e.
> cytoplasmic e.
> e. deficiency
> e. deprivation
> designer e.
> endogenous e.
> equine conjugated e.
> esterified e.
> exogenous e.
> intravaginal e.
> low-dose vaginal e.
> e. and medroxyprogesterone

> menopausal e.
> e. metabolism
> e. monotherapy
> noncontraceptive e.
> nonsteroidal e.
> e. receptor (ER)
> e. receptor alpha
> e. receptor antihormone
> e. receptor beta
> e. receptor B-variant
> e. receptor dimerization
> e. receptor phosphorylation
> e. receptor-positive breast cancer
> e. replacement therapy (ERT)
> e. synthase
> e. synthesis
> synthetic conjugated e.
> systemic e.
> e. therapy (ET)
> transdermal e.
> unopposed e. (UNE)

estrogen/androgen therapy

estrogenic effect

estrogenization

estrogen-methyltestosterone
> esterified e.-m.

estrogen-producing tumor

estrogen-progesterone
> e.-p. contraceptive
> e.-p. therapy (EPT)

estrogen-receptor
> e.-r. element (ERE)
> e.-r. modulator

estrogen-related receptor gamma

estrogen-response element (ERE)

estrone (E_1)
> e. hypothesis
> serum e.
> e. sulfate

estropipate

estroprogestin

Estrostep
> E. 21
> E. Fe

estrous cycle

ET
> embryo transfer
> endothelin
> estrogen therapy

ET-1
> endothelin-1

etanercept

E

NOTES

ETDRS
>Early Treatment Diabetic Retinopathy
>Study

ETF
>electron transport flavoprotein

ethacrynic acid
ethanol hypoglycemia
ethanthate
>norethindrone e.

ethaverine
ether
>e. bridge substitution
>ethinyl estradiol-3-methyl e.

ether-link cleavage
ether-stimulation test
ethinyl
>e. estradiol
>e. estradiol and desogestrel
>e. estradiol and ethynodiol
> diacetate
>e. estradiol and levonorgestrel
>e. estradiol-3-methyl ether
>e. estradiol and norethindrone
>e. estradiol and norgestimate
>e. estradiol and norgestrel
>e. testosterone

ethinylestradiol
Ethiofos
ethionamide
ethmoidal
ethnicity
ethylene
>e. glycol
>e. thiourea

ethylenediaminetetraacetic acid (EDTA)
ethylene thiourea
ethylene-vinyl acetate copolymer
ethynodiol diacetate
etidronate
>disodium e.
>e. disodium

etiocholanedoine
etiocholanolone
etiology
>monogenic e.

etodolac
etomidate
etonogestrel
etoposide
etrogenic
Ets motif
eucalcemic
euchromatin
EUCLID
>EURODIAB Controlled Trial of
>Lisinopril in Insulin Dependent
>Diabetes
>>EUCLID study

eucortisolemic

eucortisolism
Euflex
Euglucon
euglycemia
>posthyperglycemic e.

euglycemic
>e. clamp study
>e. diet
>e. glucose clamp technique
>e. insulin clamp

eugonadal infertility
eugonadism
eugonadotrophic anovulation
eugonadotropic hypogonadism
eukaryote
eukaryotic cell
Eulexin
eumelanin
eumenorrheic hirsute woman
eumetabolic state
eunuchism
>female e.
>hypothalamic e.

eunuchoidal body proportion
eunuchoid body habitus
eunuchoidism
euphoria
EURODIAB
>E. Controlled Trial of Lisinopril in
>Insulin Dependent Diabetes
>(EUCLID)
>E. Controlled Trial of Lisinopril in
>Insulin Dependent Diabetes study
>E. Insulin-Dependent Diabetes
>Mellitus Complications Study

Euro-Ficoll solution
European
>E. Association for the Study of
>Diabetes
>E. Nicotinamide Diabetes
>Intervention Trial (ENDIT)
>E. Organization for Research and
>Treatment of Cancer (EORTC)
>E. Prospective Investigation of
>Cancer (EPIC)

euthyroid
>biochemically e.
>e. brain glucose transporter
>clinically e.
>e. diffuse goiter
>e. Graves disease
>e. hyperthyroxinemia
>e. hypothyroxinemia
>e. nodular goiter
>e. ophthalmopathy
>e. sick
>e. sick syndrome (ESS)
>e. state

euthyroidism
    compensated e.
Euthyrox
eutopic endometrium
euvolemic patient
evaluation
    Acute Physiology and Chronic
      Health E. (APACHE II)
    Heart Outcome Prevention E.
      (HOPE)
    e. and management (E/M)
    E. of PTCA to Improve Long-
      Term Outcome by C7E3
      GpIIb/IIIa Receptor Blockade
      (EPILOG)
evening primrose oil
event
    Cholesterol and Recurrent E.'s
      (CARE)
    hypoglycemic e.
Everone Injection
Evista
E-Vitamin
ExacTech
    E. blood glucose meter
    E. RSG glucose meter
examination
    dilated eye e.
    dilated fundus e.
    dilated pupil e.
    funduscopic e.
    histomorphometric e.
    PPJ cytologic e.
    pure pancreatic juice cytologic e.
    visual e.
Excedrin
    E., Extra Strength
    E. IB
    E. P.M.
Excel
    E. GE
    E. GE electrochemical glucose
      monitoring test strip
excess
    e. acral growth
    adrenal androgen e.
    androgen e.
    apparent mineralocorticoid e.
      (AME)
    glucocorticoid e.
    glucocorticoid-suppressible
      mineralocorticoid e.

    LH-dependent androgen e.
    luteinizing hormone-dependent
      androgen e.
    mineralocorticoid e.
    parathyroid hormone e.
    prolactin e.
    sodium e.
    syndrome of apparent
      mineralocorticoid e.
    TBG e.
    thyroxine-binding globulin e.
    unilateral aldosterone e.
    vasopressin e.
excessive
    e. body odor
    e. seborrhea
    e. stature
    e. sweating
exchange
    amiloride-sensitive proton e.
    e. list
    plasma e.
exchanger
    urate-hydroxyl e.
    urate-lactate e.
excitability
    membrane e.
excitable tissue
excitatory
    e. amino acid
    e. input
    e. transmitter
exclusion chromatography
excretion
    aldosterone e.
    basal 24-hour UFC e.
    basal 24-hour urine free cortisol e.
    24-hour urinary aldosterone e.
    increased aldosterone e.
    renal e.
    urinary genistein e.
    urinary hydroxyproline e.
    urinary pyridinoline cross-link e.
    urine phosphorus e.
excretory duct
excurrent duct system
excursion
    mean amplitude of glycemic e.
      (MAGE)
    postprandial glucose e.
exemestane

E

NOTES

exemption
    humanitarian device e.
exenatide
exendin
exercise
    Jun N-terminal kinase e.
exercise-induced
    e.-i. hyperglycemia
    e.-i. hypoglycemia
    e.-i. ketosis
exercise-related amenorrhea
exertional training
exhaustion atrophy
exocoelomic fluid
exocrine
    e. cell
    e. gland
    e. pancreas
    e. pancreas disease
    e. pancreatic dysfunction
    e. pancreatic insufficiency (EPI)
    e. response
exocytosis
    misplaced e.
exodeviation
exogenous
    e. estrogen
    e. glucocorticoid
    e. glucocorticoid therapy
    e. gonadotropin
    e. hypercortisolism
    e. hyperinsulinemia
    e. obesity
    e. progesterone
    e. thyroid hormone
    e. thyrotoxicosis
exon
    XL-alpha-s e.
exopeptidase dipeptidyl peptidase I, II
exophthalmic
    e. cachexia
    e. goiter
exophthalmometer
    Hertel e.
    Luedde e.
exophthalmos
    idiopathic e.
exostosis, pl. **exostoses**
    bony e.
    metaphyseal e.
exotropia
expander
    plasma e.
expansion
    beta-cell e.
    clonal e.
    retrobulbar tissue e.

expenditure
    energy e.
    resting energy e. (REE)
experimental
    e. allergic autoimmune encephalitis
    (EAAE)
    e. autoimmune thyroiditis (EAT)
exposure keratitis
expressed sequence tag (EST)
expression
    aberrant e.
    beta-cell cytokine transgenic e.
    biallelic e.
    calcitonin gene e.
    cardiac gene e.
    e. cloning
    ectopic e.
    endothelin receptor e.
    enzyme gene e.
    growth factor e.
    monoallelic e.
    non-beta-cell regulated insulin
     gene e.
    pendrin e.
    protooncogene e.
    ras gene protooncogene e.
    receptor e.
    surfactant protein gene e.
    thyroglobulin e.
    thyroid-stimulating hormone
     receptor e.
    TSH receptor e.
exstrophy
    bladder e.
    cloacal e.
extended release metformin
extension
    alarlike e.
    extrathyroidal e.
    suprasellar e.
externa
    membrana limitans e.
    theca e.
external
    e. beam radiation
    e. genitalia
    e. ophthalmoplegia
    e. sex steroid ingestion
    e. subcutaneous insulin infusion
     pump
extirpate
extirpation
    surgical e.
extorsion
extra
    Precision E.
extraadrenal
    e. paraganglioma
    e. pheochromocytoma

extracellular
- e. calcification
- e. cathepsin action
- e. domain
- e. fluid (ECF)
- e. fluid dehydration
- e. fluid osmolarity
- e. fluid volume (EFV)
- e. iodide pool
- e. matrix (ECM)
- e. matrix protein
- e. pH
- e. receptor
- e. signal-regulated kinase (ERK)
- e. signal-related kinase (ERK)
- e. signal-related kinase 1 (ERK1)
- e. signal-related kinase 2 (ERK2)

extracellularly regulated kinase (ERK)
extracellular-regulated kinase
extracorporeal
- e. shock wave lithotripsy
- e. ultrafiltration

extract
- red clover e.
- soy phytoestrogen e. (SPE)
- thyroid e.

extraction
- testicular sperm e. (TESE)

extradural space
extraembryonic somatic mesoderm
extraglandular lesion
extraglomerular mesangium
extragonadal
- e. germ cell tumor (EGGCT)
- e. site

extrahepatic
- e. bile duct
- e. effect

extrahypophyseal portal vessel

extrahypothalamic
- e. nervous system
- e. site

extramedullary hematopoiesis (EMH)
extramitochondrial compartment
extramyocellular lipid (EMCL)
extraneuronal amine transport system
extraocular muscle dysfunction
extrapancreatic digestive enzyme
extrapituitary prolactin
extrasellar
extraskeletal calcification
extrasplanchnic area
extrathyroidal
- e. extension
- e. immunological process
- e. manifestation of Graves disease
- e. primary
- e. thyrotoxicosis

extrathyroid autoantigen
extravascular
extravillus
extreme insulin resistance
extrusion
- granule e.
- supradiaphragmatic e.

exuberant
- e. neutrophilic infiltrate
- e. thrombosis

exudate
- hard e.

ex vivo gene transfer insulin replacement
eye
- Orphan Annie e.
- raccoon e.'s

ezetimibe
Ezide
E-Z Lets II lancing device

E

NOTES

119

F

cortisol
F body
F cell
F glucosidase inhibitor and body weight
hepatitis F

FA

Natabec FA
Pramet FA
Pramilet FA

FA-1

fertilization antigen-1

$F_{1\text{-alpha}}$

prostaglandin $F_{1\text{-alpha}}$ ($PGF_{1\text{-alpha}}$)

$F_{2\text{-alpha}}$

prostaglandin $F_{2\text{-alpha}}$ ($PGF_{2\text{-alpha}}$)

Fab

fragment antigen binding

FABP

fatty acid-binding protein

FABP2

fatty acid-binding protein 2

FABP$_{pm}$

plasma membrane fatty acid binding protein

Fabricius
Fabry disease
face

en f.
moon f.
myxedematous f.

facial

f. clefting
f. feature enlargement
f. hirsutism
f. plethora

facies

adenoid f.
bird-like f.
dysmorphic f.
elfin f.
moon f.
plethoric f.
Potter f.
triangular f.

facilitative glucose transporter
F-actin
factitia

thyrotoxicosis f.

factitial hypoglycemia
factitious

f. hyperthyroidism
f. hypoglycemia

factor

abiotic environmental f.
activated Hageman f.
activating f.
activator protein-1 transcription f.
amplification f.
androgen-induced growth f. (AIGF)
angiogenic growth f.
antiapoptotic f.
antithrombotic f.
AP-1 transcription f.
atrial natriuretic f. (ANF)
autocrine motility f. (AMF)
azoospermia f. (AZF)
basic fibroblast growth f. (bFGF)
basic helix-loop-helix transcription f.
B-cell growth f. (BCGF)
beta-nerve growth f.
bHLH transcription f.
bone-derived growth f. (BDGF)
brain-derived neurotropic f. (BDNF)
calcium homeostatic f.
C/EBP transcription f.
chemotactic f.
ciliary neurotrophic f. (CNTF)
cis-acting f.
clotting f. II, V, VII, X
colony-stimulating f.
connective tissue growth f. (CTGF)
corticotropin-releasing f. (CRF)
coupling f.
decapacitation f.
dialyzable f.
early pregnancy f. (EPF)
EGF-like growth f.
endothelial cell-stimulating angiogenesis f. (ESAF)
endothelial growth f. (EGF)
endothelium-derived relaxing f. (EDRF)
epidermal growth f. (EGF)
erythroid differentiation f. (EDF)
fibroblast growth f. (FGF)
fibroblastic growth f. (FGF)
Forkhead domain transcription f.
genetically predisposing f.
genetic risk f.
GH-releasing f. (GHRF)
glia-activating f. (GAF)
glial cell line-derived neurotrophic f. (GDNF)
glia maturation f. (GMF)
glucose-sensitive transcription f. (GSTF)

F

factor *(continued)*

glycosylation-inhibiting f. (GIF)

G&M colony-stimulating f. (GM-CSF)

granulocyte colony-stimulating f. (G-CSF)

granulocyte-macrophage colony-stimulating f. (GM-CSF)

growth differentiation f. (GDF)

growth hormone-releasing f. (GHRF)

growth hormone-releasing hormone-growth hormone-insulinlike growth f. (GHRH-GH-IGF)

Hageman f.

hematopoietic cell growth f.

heparin-binding epidermal growth f.

heparin-bound growth f.

hepatocyte growth f. (HGF)

hepatocyte nuclear f. (HNF)

hepatocyte nuclear f.-1 (HNF-1)

hepatocyte nuclear f.-3 (HNF-3)

hepatocyte nuclear f.-4 (HNF-4)

f. Hesx1

HNF3 transcription f.

HNF4 transcription f.

homeodomain f.

humoral f.

hypophysiotropic f.

hypothalamic-releasing f.

f. II mutation

inhibitory f.

insulin correction f.

insulin gene transcription f.

insulin growth f.

insulinlike growth f. (IGF)

invasion suppressive f.

islet transcription f.

f. IX

juxtacrine f.

Kaposi sarcoma human growth f. (hFGF)

keratinocyte growth f. (KGF)

leukemia inhibitory f. (LIF)

LIM homeodomain transcription f.

liver-enriched transcription f.

luteinization-inhibiting f.

macrophage-activating f.

macrophage colony-stimulating f. (M-CSF)

macrophage migration-inhibiting f.

macrophage migration inhibitory f.

melanocyte-stimulating f. (MSF)

metabolic f.

migration inhibitory f. (MIF)

myeloid leukemia inhibitory f.

nerve growth f. (NGF)

neural f.

neurotrophic f.

NF-1 transcription f.

nongenomic f.

nonsuppressible insulinlike activity f.

nuclear transcription f.

octamer-binding transcription f.

Oct-1 transcription f.

oocyte maturation-inhibiting f.

opioid growth f. (OGF)

osteoclast differentiation f. (ODF)

osteoclastogenesis inhibitory f. (OCIF)

osteoprotegerin f. (OPGF)

ovarian growth f. (OGF)

pancreatic transcription f. 1 (PTF-1)

paracrine f.

PAX8 f.

pelvic infertility f.

peptide growth f.

permissive f.

pigment epithelium-derived f. (PEDF)

Pitx homeodomain f.

platelet-activating f. (PAF)

platelet-derived growth f. (PDGF)

POU-homeodomain transcription f.

predisposing f.

prolactin-inhibiting f. (PIF)

prolactin inhibitory f.

prolactin-releasing f. (PRF)

prophet of Pit-1 transcription f.

PROP-1 transcription f.

Rathke pouch homeobox transcription f. (Rpx)

recombinant human insulinlike growth f. (rhIGF)

renal erythropoietic f.

rheumatoid f.

satiety f.

schwannoma-derived growth f.

serum thymic f.

signal transducer and activator of transcription-4 transcription f.

signal transducer and activator of transcription-5 transcription f.

somatotropin release f. (SRF)

somatotropin release-inhibiting f. (SRIF)

SP-1 transcription f.

SRY transcription f.

Stat4 transcription f.

Stat5 transcription f.

stem cell f. (SCF)

Stuart f.

sulfation f.

T-cell growth f. (TCGF)

testis-determining f. (TDF)

thyroid transcription f. (TTF)

thyroid transcription f. 1 (TTF-1)
thyroid transcription f. 2 (TTF-2)
thyrotroph embryonic f. (TEF)
thyrotropin release f. (TRF)
tissue necrosis f. (TNF)
trans-acting f.
transactivation f. (TAF)
transcriptional intermediary f. 2 (TIF2)
transforming growth f. (TGF)
trophic f.
T-suppressor f. (TsF)
tumor necrosis f. (TNF)
tumor necrosis factor receptor-associated f. (TRAF)
vaccinia virus growth f.
vascular endothelial growth f. (VEGF)
vascular permeability f. (VPF)
vasoconstricting f.
vasodilating f.
f. V deficiency Leiden mutation
f. VIII
f. VIII, IX deficiency
f. VIII-related antigen
f. VIII ristocetin cofactor antigen
vitamin D-binding protein macrophage-activating f.
f. V Leiden gene
von Willebrand f. (vWF)
Wilms tumor 1 transcription f.
WTI transcription f.
f. X
f. XI
f. XIIa

factor-1
adipocyte determination and differentiation f.-1 (ADD1)
antifertility f.-1 (AF-1)
colony-stimulating f.-1
hepatocyte transcription f.-1
human stomach cancer-transforming f.-1 (hst-1)
hypoxia-inducible f.-1 (HIF-1)
insulinlike growth f.-1 (IGF-1)
insulin promoter f.-1 (IPF-1)
pituitary-specific transcription f.-1 (Pit-1)
preadipocyte f.-1 (Pref-1)
sensitive transcription f.-1 (STF-1)
serum insulinlike growth f.-1
steroidogenic f.-1 (SF-1)

factor-2
heparin-binding growth f.-2 (HBGF-2)
human stomach cancer-transforming f.-2 (hst-2)
insulinlike growth f.-2
factor-9
growth differentiation f-9. (GDF-9)
factor-κkB
nuclear f.-κB (NF-kB)
factor-4a
hepatocyte nuclear f.-4a (HNF-4a)
factor-alpha
beta-cell tumor necrosis f.-a.
PPAR-gamma tumor necrosis f.-a.
tumor necrosis f.-a. (TNF-alpha)
factor-1-alpha
hypoxia-inducible f.-1-a, (HIF-1alpha)
factor-beta
tumor necrosis f.-b. (TNF-beta)
factor-I
insulinlike growth f.-I (IGF-I)
factor-II
insulinlike growth f.-II
factor-kappa-B
nuclear f.-κB (NF-kappa-B)
Factrel
facultative
f. heterochromatin
f. thermogenesis
FAD
familial autoimmunity in diabetes
fadrozole
fa **gene**
failure
adult Leydig cell f.
autoimmune polyglandular f.
cartilage calcification f.
chronic renal f. (CRF)
embryologic development end-organ ovarian f.
glucocorticoid-induced growth f.
gonadal f.
hepatic f.
hypoglycemia-associated autonomic f.
kidney f.
liver f.
mild thyroid f.
organ f.
ovarian f.

F

NOTES

failure *(continued)*
    polyglandular endocrine f.
    premature gonadal f.
    premature ovarian f.
    primary adrenal f.
    primary gonadal f.
    regulatory f.
    renal f.
    secondary gonadal f.
    f. to thrive (FTT)
    type II multiple endocrine
      glandular f.
falciform
    f. fold
    f. ligament
Falck-Hillarp histofluorescence method
falling height velocity
fallopian tube
Fallot
    tetralogy of F.
familial
    f. adenomatous polyposis
    f. adrenoleukodystrophy
    f. amyloidotic polyneuropathy
    f. amyloid polyneuropathy (FAP)
    f. atypical multiple mole-melanoma
      (FAMMM)
    f. atypical multiple mole-melanoma
      syndrome
    f. autoimmunity in diabetes (FAD)
    f. C-cell hyperplasia
    f. central diabetes insipidus
    f. cerebral ataxia
    f. colorectal cancer
    f. combined hyperlipidemia (FCH)
    f. defective apolipoprotein B100
    f. Down syndrome
    f. dysalbuminemia
    f. dysalbuminemic
      hyperthyroxinemia (FDH)
    f. dysalbuminemic
      hypertriiodothyroninemia
    f. dysautonomia
    f. dysbetalipoproteinemia
    f. euthyroid hyperthyroxinemia
    f. expansile osteolysis (FEO)
    f. gastric cancer
    f. glucocorticoid deficiency (FGD)
    f. glucocorticoid resistance
    f. growth hormone deficiency
    f. hyperaldosteronism
    f. hypercholesterolemia (FH)
    f. hyperinsulinism
    f. hyperkalemia
    f. hyperphosphatasemia
    f. hypertriglyceridemia
    f. hypoalphalipoproteinemia
    f. hypocalciuric hypercalcemia
      (FHH)

    f. hypoparathyroidism
    f. hypospadias
    f. isolated primary
      hyperparathyroidism (FIPH)
    f. lipid disorder
    f. male-limited gonadotrophin-
      independent sexual precocity
    f. male precocious puberty
    f. Mediterranean fever
    f. medullary thyroid cancer
      (FMTC)
    f. medullary thyroid carcinoma
      (FMTC)
    f. multiple endocrine neoplasia
    f. multiple endocrine neoplasia type
      1
    f. nephrogenic diabetes insipidus
    f. nonautoimmune hyperthyroidism
    f. nonmedullary thyroid cancer
    f. oculoleptomeningea amyloidosis
    f. ovarian cancer
    f. partial lipodystrophy
    f. periodic paralysis
    f. pheochromocytoma
    f. polyposis coli
    f. testitoxicosis
    f. thyroglossal duct cyst
    f. thyroid carcinoma
    f. X-linked hypophosphatemic
      rickets
family
    Forkhead f. (FHF)
    G_q f.
    helix-loop-helix f.
    insulin receptor f.
    leucine zipper gene f.
    sodium-dependent glucose
      transporter f. (SGLT)
    T-box gene f.
    V-gene f.
    winged helix f.
FAMMM
    familial atypical multiple mole-melanoma
    FAMMM syndrome
Fanconi
    F. anemia
    F. syndrome
Fanconi-type idiopathic hypercalcemia
FAP
    familial amyloid polyneuropathy
Faraday constant
Farber disease
farnesyl-transferase (FTase)
    f.-t. inhibitor
Farré
    line of F.
FAS
    fatty acid synthetase
    fetal alcohol syndrome

Fas
> F. ligand (Fas-L)
> F. receptor

fascia
> cremasteric f.
> pectoralis f.
> prethyroidal f.
> superficial f.

fasciculata
> adrenal zona f.
> f. reticularis
> zona f.

fasciculation

fasciculus
> mammillary f.
> mammillotegmental f.
> medial longitudinal f.

fasciitis
> necrotizing f.
> nodular f.

fascioscapulohumeral muscular dystrophy

FASE sequence

Fas-L
> Fas ligand

fast
> f. asymmetric spin echo
> f. asymmetric spin echo sequence
> protein-sparing modified f. (PSMF)
> f. spin-echo technique

fast-acting insulin

fast-food guidelines

Fastin

fasting
> f. blood glucose (FBG)
> f. glucose level
> f. growth hormone
> f. hyperglycemia
> f. hypoglycemia
> f. hypophosphatemia
> f. plasma glucose (FPG)

FastTake blood glucose monitoring system

fast-twitch muscle fiber

FAT
> fatty acid translocase

fat
> brown f.
> f. catabolism
> f. embolization
> f. maldigestion/malabsorption
> f. mass (FM)
> f. necrosis
> orbital f.
> perinephric f.
> perithymic f.
> sparse body f.

fate
> pancreatic cell f.

fat-free mass (FFM)

fatigue
> quadriceps f.

FATP
> fatty acid transport protein

fatty
> f. acid
> f. acid-binding protein (FABP)
> f. acid-binding protein 2 (FABP2)
> f. acid oxidation
> f. acid synthase
> f. acid synthetase (FAS)
> f. acid translocase (FAT)
> f. acid transport protein (FATP)
> f. acylcarnitine
> f. liver
> f. meal
> f. streak

FBG
> fasting blood glucose

FBP
> fructose-bisphosphatase

FCH
> familial combined hyperlipidemia

FCPD
> fibrocalculous pancreatic diabetes

FD
> fibrous dysplasia
> > monostotic FD
> > polystotic FD

FDG
> fluorodeoxyglucose

FDG-F-18
> ^{18}F-labeled fluorodeoxyglucose

FDG-PET
> ^{18}F-fluorodeoxyglucose positron emission tomography
> > FDG-PET study

FDH
> familial dysalbuminemic hyperthyroxinemia

Fe
> iron
> > Estrostep Fe
> > Slow Fe

F

NOTES

feature
    acromegalic f.
    coarsened facial f.
    histomorphic f.
    neuropsychiatric f.'s
    tinctorial f.
    ultrastructural f.
fecal chymotrypsin test
fecundability
fecundity
federation
    International Diabetes F.
feedback
    compensatory f.
    f. control
    f. inhibition
    long-loop f.
    f. loop
    monofollicular f.
    monoovarial f.
    negative f.
    positive f.
    short-loop f.
    tubuloglomerular f. (TGF)
    ultrashort-loop f.
feeding
    f. artery
    high-fat f.
    f. jejunostomy
feet (*pl. of* foot)
Felig insulin pump
female
    f. climax
    f. eunuchism
    f. infertility
    f. orgasm
    f. phenotype
    f. pseudohermaphrodite
    f. pseudohermaphroditism (FPH)
    f. sexual dysfunction (FSD)
    f. sexual function diagnostic
    (FSFD)
    F. Sexual Function Index (FSFI)
    f. sperm
Femara
FemHRT
feminization
    complete testicular f.
    incomplete testicular f.
    testicular f.
feminizing
    f. adrenal syndrome
    f. testis
Femiron
Femogen
femora
femoral neck bone density
FemPatch
FemSeven

FemSoy
femur length
Fenesin
fenestra, pl. **fenestrae**
fenestrated capillary endothelium
fenestration
fenofibrate
    simvastatin with f.
fenoprofen
fentanyl
    f. citrate
    droperidol and f.
    F. Oralet
FEO
    familial expansile osteolysis
Feosol
Feostat
Ferancee
Feratab
Fergon
Ferguson reflex
Fer-In-Sol drops
Fer-Iron
Fero-Grad 500
Fero-Gradumet
Ferospace
Ferralet
Ferralyn Lanacaps
Ferra-TD
ferredoxin
    renal f.
ferric chloride test
Ferriman-Gallwey score
Ferriman scale of hirsutism
ferritin
ferromagnetic
Ferro-Sequels
ferrous
    f. fumarate
    f. gluconate
    f. salt and ascorbic acid
    f. sulfate
    f. sulfate, ascorbic acid, and
    vitamin B complex
    f. sulfate, ascorbic acid, vitamin B
    complex, and folic acid
fertile
    f. eunuch syndrome
    f. eunuch variant
fertilin
fertilization
    f. antigen-1 (FA-1)
    in vitro f. (IVF)
Fertinex
fetal
    f. adenoma
    f. adrenal cortisol
    f. alcohol syndrome (FAS)
    f. allograft

f. catecholamine
f. endocrine rhythm
f. hormone rhythm
f. hydantoin syndrome
f. hyperthyroidism
f. hypothyroidism
f. hypothyroxinemia
f. hypoxemia
f. hypoxia
f. lung maturity
f. macrosomia
f. mineral homeostasis
f. origin
f. pancreas transplant
f. plasma cortisol
f. steroid rhythm
f. zone
fetal-hypothalamic-pituitary-adrenal axis
fetalis
erythroblastosis f.
fetal/neonatal
f. adrenal crisis
f. rhythm
fetectomy
fetomaternal circulation
fetopathy
diabetic f.
fetoplacental
f. blood flow
f. unit
fever
enteric f.
epidemic hemorrhagic f.
familial Mediterranean f.
rheumatic f.
Feverall
FFA
free fatty acid
^{18}F-fluorodeoxyglucose
^{18}F-f. positron emission tomography (FDG-PET)
^{18}F-f. positron emission tomography study
FFM
fat-free mass
FGD
familial glucocorticoid deficiency
FGF
fibroblast growth factor
fibroblastic growth factor
FGFR
fibroblast growth factor receptor

FH
familial hypercholesterolemia
FHA
functional hypothalamic amenorrhea
FHF
Forkhead family
FHH
familial hypocalciuric hypercalcemia
FHIT
fragile histidine triad
FHIT gene
fiber
angiotensinergic f.
f. atrophy
collagen f.
crossing nasal retinal f.
dietary f.
fast-twitch muscle f.
GABAergic f.
gamma-aminobutyric acidergic f.
glutamatergic f.
f. hypertrophy
nonviscous particulate f.
f. pebble
postganglionic sympathetic f.
preganglionic sympathetic nerve f.
reciprocal peptidergic f.
secretomotor f.
slow-twitch oxidative f.
soluble f.
temporal f.
terminal nerve f.
type 1, 2 f.
type II muscle f.
unmyelinated nerve f.
urocortin f.
vasopressinergic f.
viscous dietary f.
fiberoptic headlight
fibrates
fibric
f. acid
f. acid derivative
fibril
actin f.
amyloid f.
birefringent collagen f.
collagen f.
hydrolyzed lithostathine f.
fibrillar collagen strip
fibrillary gliosis

NOTES

F

fibrillation
  atrial f.
  ventricular f.
fibrin glue
fibrinogen
fibrinolysin
fibrinolysis
  increased f.
fibrinolytic activity
fibroadenoma
  benign prostatic f.
  mammary f.
fibroadenomatous hyperplasia of breast
fibroblast
  f. growth factor (FGF)
  f. growth factor receptor (FGFR)
  orbital f.
  perimysial f.
  SV40-transformed human f.
fibroblastic
  f. growth factor (FGF)
  f. phenotype
fibrocalculous
  f. pancreatic diabetes (FCPD)
  f. pancreatopathy
fibrocystic breast disease
fibrodysplasia ossificans progressiva (FOP)
fibrogenesis
  f. imperfecta
  f. imperfecta ossium
fibroglandular tissue
fibro-inflammatory disease
fibrolipoma
fibromatosis
Fibromyalgia Impact Questionnaire (FIQ)
fibromyositis
fibronectin
  f. gene
  f. peptide isoform
  serum f.
fibroneuroma
fibroplasia
fibrosa
  osteitis f.
fibrosarcoma
fibrosclerosis
fibrosis
  cardiac f.
  cystic f.
  endosteal f.
  hypocellular marrow without f.
  interlobular f.
  intralobular f.
  pancreatic f.
fibrous
  f. atrophy
  f. dysplasia (FD)

  f. dysplasia of bone
  f. plaque
FIC
  growth factor-inducible chemokine
Fick principal
7-field stereoscopic fundus photography
filament
  actin f.
filarial infection
Filmtabs
  Cefol F.
  Surbex-T F.
  Surbex With C F.
fimbria, pl. **fimbriae**
  ovarian f.
final menstrual period (FMP)
finasteride
fine-needle
  f.-n. aspiration (FNA)
  f.-n. aspiration biopsy (FNAB)
finger
  steroid hormone receptor zinc f.
  zinc f.
fingerprints
  DNA f.
fingerstick blood sugar
Finnish
  F. Diabetes Prevention Study
  F. DIPP Study
Fiorinal with Codeine
FIPH
  familial isolated primary
  hyperparathyroidism
FIQ
  Fibromyalgia Impact Questionnaire
fire
  St. Anthony f.
firefly luciferase
firm goiter
first-generation agent
first-passage phenomenon
first-phase
  f.-p. insulin release
  f.-p. insulin response (FPIR)
first-year growth velocity response
Fischer
  F. rat thyroid line-5
  F. rat thyroid line-5 cell
FISH
  fluorescence in situ hybridization
  FISH method
fish oil
fissure
  choroidal f.
  lid f.
  f. of Santorini
  widened palpebral f.
fistula, pl. **fistulae, fistulas**
  biliary f.

cerebrospinal fluid f.
intestinal f.
pyriform sinus f.

FIT
Fracture Intervention Trial
Fitzgerald trait
FK506
FK-binding
F.-b. protein (FKBP)
F.-b. protein 12 (FKBP12)
FKBP
FK-binding protein
FKBP-rapamycin-associated protein (FRAP)
FKBP12
FK-binding protein 12
FKBP-rapamycin-associated protein (FRAP)
FKHR
Forkhead box protein O1A
FOXO1a
^{18}F-labeled fluorodeoxyglucose (FDG-F-18)
flaccid penile length
flagellar movement
flagellum
Flagyl Oral
flame
osteolytic f.
f. photometry
FLAP
5-lipoxygenase activating protein
flap
Karydakis f.
right frontal osteoplastic f.
flare
tumor f.
flashes
hot f.
Flatbush diabetes
flat-field collimator
flattened lumbar spine
flattening
posterior skull f.
Flaujeac trait
flavone
flavonoid
flavoprotein
electron transport f. (ETF)
f. NADPH-cytochrome P450 reductase

f. nicotinamide adenine dinucleotide phosphate-cytochrome P450 reductase
Flavorcee
flavum
ligamentum f.
flavus
Aspergillus f.
Fleet Phospho-Soda
FlexiGard
floating beta band
floor
pharyngeal f.
Florical
Florida Sexual Questionnaire
Florinef Acetate
flour
chupatti f.
flow
anterograde f.
bile f.
cerebral blood f. (CBF)
coronary blood f.
f. cytometric analysis
fetoplacental blood f.
hepatofugal f.
hepatopetal f.
placental blood f.
renal plasma f. (RPF)
uteroplacental blood f.
flowmetry
laser Doppler f.
flow-volume loop spirometry
floxuridine
fluasterone
fluconazole
flucytosine
fludarabine
fludrocortisone
f. acetate
f. replacement therapy
f. suppression testing (FST)
flufenemic acid
fluid
f. absorption
amniotic f.
bone f.
cerebrospinal f. (CSF)
exocoelomic f.
extracellular f. (ECF)
follicular f.
f. intake

F

NOTES

fluid *(continued)*
>   interstitial f. (ISF)
>   intracellular f. (ICF)
>   nonpurulent f.
>   pancreatitis-associated ascites f. (PAAF)
>   perilymph f.
>   peritoneal f. (PF)
>   preseminal f.
>   f. secretion
>   f. shear stress
>   subarachnoid f.
>   testicular f.
>   f. therapy
>   tubule f.
>   turbid f.
>   xanthochromic f.

flunisolide
flunitrazepam
fluochrome
fluocinolone acetonide cream
fluorenylmethoxycarbonyl-L-leucine (FMOC-Leu)
fluorescein dye
fluorescein-labeled
>   f.-l. pea agglutinin
>   f.-l. peanut agglutinin

fluorescence
>   f. imaging
>   f. microlymphography
>   f. polarization
>   f. quencing spectroscopy
>   f. in situ hybridization (FISH)

fluorescent
>   f. iodide
>   f. in situ hybridization method

fluoride
>   bioavailable f.
>   enteric-coated sodium f.
>   serum f.
>   skeletal f.
>   sodium f.
>   sustained-release sodium f. (SR-NaF)

fluorine
fluorochrome
fluorodeoxyglucose (FDG)
> ^{18}F-labeled f. (FDG-F-18)
>   f. uptake

fluorohydrocortisone
fluorosis
>   endemic f.

fluorotic change
fluorouracil
5-fluorouracil (5-FU)
fluoxetine hydrochloride
fluoxymesterone
fluphenazine
flurbiprofen

flush
>   vasomotor f.

flushing
>   cutaneous f.

flutamide
flutter
>   atrial f.

fluvastatin
fluvoxamine
flux
>   calcium f.
>   electrolyte f.
>   mineral f.
>   transmucosal calcium f.

FM
>   fat mass

FMOC-Leu
>   fluorenylmethoxycarbonyl-L-leucine
>   N-(9-fluorenylmethoxycarbonyl)-L-leucine

FMP
>   final menstrual period

FMTC
>   familial medullary thyroid cancer
>   familial medullary thyroid carcinoma

FNA
>   fine-needle aspiration
>   FNA biopsy

FNAB
>   fine-needle aspiration biopsy

foam
>   f. cell
>   f. cell formation

foamy cell
focal
>   f. dermal hypoplasia
>   f. epithelial hyperplasia
>   f. glomerulitis
>   f. photocoagulation
>   f. segmental glomerulosclerosis (FSGS)
>   f. tumor necrosis

focus, pl. **foci**
>   anechoic f.
>   F. glucose monitoring system
>   F. test strip

focusing
>   isoelectric f.

fodrin
foenum-graecum
>   *Trigonella f.-g.*

folate receptor (FR)
fold
>   falciform f.
>   urogenital f.

foliaceus
>   toxic pemphigus f.

folic acid
Folin-Wu method

follicle
  androgenic f.
  antral f.
  dominant f.
  graafian f.
  hair f.
  lymphoid f.
  mature f.
  ovarian f.
  ovulatory f.
  preantral f.
  preovulatory f.
  primary f.
  primordial f.
  secondary f.
  tertiary f.
  thyroid f.
  vesicular f.
follicle-stimulating
  f.-s. hormone (FSH)
  f.-s. hormone-beta gene
  f.-s. hormone deficiency
  f.-s. hormone receptor
  f.-s. hormone-releasing hormone
    (FSH-RH)
follicular
  f. adenoma
  f. arrest
  f. atresia
  f. cell
  f. cyst
  f. epithelial carcinoma
  f. fluid
  f. hyperthecosis
  f. lumen
  f. mucinosis
  f. neoplasm
  f. phase
  f. stage
  f. thyroid cancer
  f. thyroid carcinoma
folliculi (*pl. of* folliculus)
folliculitis
  perforating f.
folliculogenesis
folliculostatin
folliculostellate cell
folliculus, pl. **folliculi**
  liquor folliculi
  theca folliculi
follistatin protein

Follistim
follitropin (FSH)
  f. alpha
  f. beta
Follutein
Folvite
Fontana-Masson procedure
Fontan procedure
food
  f. diary
  junk f.
  f. pyramid
  thermic effect of f.
food-dependent Cushing syndrome
food-related hypercortisolism
foot, pl. **feet**
  Charcot f.
  diabetic f.
  insensate feet
  rocker-bottom f.
  f. ulcer
FOP
  fibrodysplasia ossificans progressiva
foramen, pl. **foramina**
  f. caecum linguae
  f. cecum
  foramina of Magendie and Luschka
  f. of Monro
  f. ovale
  f. rotundum
  f. spinosum
Forbes disease
force
  Starling f.
forced gate analysis scan
forceps
  Cushing f.
  transsphenoidal bipolar f.
forebrain basal encephalocele
foregut
Forkhead
  F. box protein O1A (FKHR)
  F. domain transcription factor
  F. family (FHF)
form
  alimentary f.
  dimeric f.
  gadolinium in chelated f. (Gd-
    EDTA)
  monostotic f.
  nonhistocompatibility locus antigen-
    associated f.

F

NOTES

131

form *(continued)*
    non-HLA-associated f.
    nonhuman leukocyte antigen
      associated f.
    polyostotic f.
formation
    advanced glycation end-product f.
    brainstem reticular f.
    endochondral bone f.
    foam cell f.
    hippocampal f.
    marrow cavity f.
    osteoblast-mediated bone f.
    pseudopapillary f.
    thrombus f.
formation-stimulating agent
formation-stimulation agent
formed visual hallucination
formes fruste
formestane
formication
forming-unit
formononetin
formula, pl. **formulae, formulas**
    Diabetic Tussin Children's F.
    isoosmolar semielemental f.
fornix, pl. **fornices**
    vaginal f.
forskolin
    adenylyl cyclase agonist f.
    iodo-4-azidophenetylamido-7-O-
      succinyldeacetyl f. (IAPS-forskolin)
fortuitum
    Mycobacterium f.
Fosamax
foscarnet therapy
FOS **gene**
fossa, pl. **fossae**
    interpeduncular f.
    pituitary f.
    superior orbital f.
foundation
    Insulin-Free World F.
    Juvenile Diabetes Research F.
    National Osteoporosis F. (NOF)
    Osteogenesis Imperfecta F.
four-compartment model
Fournier gangrene
Fox gene
FOXL2 gene
FOXO1a (FKHR)
FPG
    fasting plasma glucose
FPH
    female pseudohermaphroditism
FPIR
    first-phase insulin response
FQ
    nociceptin/orphanin FQ (N/OFQ)

FR
    folate receptor
fraction
    oxytocic f.
    S-phase f.
    very low density lipoprotein f.
    VLDL f.
fractional
    f. shortening
    f. urine
fractionated
    f. linear accelerator-based irradiation
    f. radiation therapy
    f. urinary catecholamine
fracture
    Charcot f.
    F. Intervention Trial (FIT)
    stress f.
    Study of Osteoporotic F.'s (SOF)
fragile
    f. histidine triad (FHIT)
    f. X-E
    f. X-E syndrome
    f. X syndrome
fragilis
    Bacteroides f.
fragment
    f. antigen binding (Fab)
    Klenow f.
    luteinizing hormone beta core f.
    major proglucagon f. (MPF)
fragmentation
    osseous f.
frame
    Leksell model G stereotactic f.
    open reading f. (ORF)
    relocatable stereotactic f.
frameless stereotaxy
frameshift
Framingham Nutrition Study
frank
    f. basilar impression
    f. necrosis
FRAP
    FKBP-rapamycin-associated protein
Fraser syndrome
Frataxin gene
FRAXE syndrome
**Fredrickson classification of lipid
  disorders**
free
    f. androgen index assay
    f. Ca^{2+}
    f. cortisol
    f. fatty acid (FFA)
    f. hormone
    f. levothyroxine
    f. Mg^{2+}
    f. radical

f. T_3
f. T_4
f. testosterone
f. testosterone level
f. thyroxine (FT_4)
f. thyroxine index (FTI, FT4I, FT_4I, FT4i)
f. T_4 index (FT4I, FT_4I, FT4i)
f. triiodothyronine (FT_3)
f. water clearance
f. water deficit

freedom
Accu-Chek II F.

Freeman-Sheldon syndrome
free-radical scavenger
free-running melatonin cycle
FreeStyle
F. Flash blood glucose meter
F. test strip
Therasense F.
F. Tracker glucose meter

freeze-dried allograft
frenulum clitoridis
frequency
gonadotropin-releasing hormone pulse f.
pulse f.

frequent blood sampling
Frey operation
friable
Friedewald calculation
Friedreich ataxia
frog skin sauvagine
Fröhlich syndrome
frond
neovascular f.

frondosum
chorion f.

front
mineralization f.

frontal
f. bossing
f. neocortex

frontoethmoidal encephalocele
frontooccipital prominence
frontotemporal
f. balding
f. headache

FRTL-5 cell
fructosamine test
fructose-bisphosphatase (FBP)
fructose-2,6-bisphosphate

fructose intolerance
fructose-6-phosphate
fruity breath
fruste
formes f.

F-scan
FSD
female sexual dysfunction

FSFD
female sexual function diagnostic

FSFI
Female Sexual Function Index

FSGS
focal segmental glomerulosclerosis

FSH
follicle-stimulating hormone
follitropin
FSH deficiency
FSH receptor
urinary FSH (uFSH)

FSH-beta gene
FSH-RH
follicle-stimulating hormone-releasing hormone

FST
fludrocortisone suppression testing

FT$_4$
free thyroxine

FT$_3$
free triiodothyronine

FTase
farnesyl-transferase

FTI
free thyroxine index

FT4I, FT$_4$I, FT4i
free thyroxine index
free T_4 index

FTT
failure to thrive

5-FU
5-fluorouracil

fuchsin
aldehyde f.

fucose
fucosidosis
fucosylation
fuel
f. homeostasis
f. metabolism
f. reservoir

Fujiwara trait

F

NOTES

133

fullness
    supraclavicular f.
full pulse
fulminant
    f. hyperthermia
    f. Letterer-Siwe disease
fumarate
    ferrous f.
fumarylacetoacetate hydrolase type Ia
Fumasorb
Fumerin
fumigatus
    Aspergillus f.
function
    adrenocortical f.
    anorectal f.
    anterior pituitary f.
    autonomic f.
    B-cell f.
    beta-cell f.
    bone marrow f.
    endothelial f.
    gastric reservoir f.
    gonadal f.
    HPA f.
    hypophysiotropic hormonal f.
    hypothalamic-pituitary-adrenal f.
    intestinal f.
    intracellular f.
    iodide trapping f.
    juxtaglomerular f.
    nodule f.
    osteoclastic f.
    phosphorylated rhodopsin f.
    pituitary-adrenal f.
    pituitary-gonadal f.
    pituitary hormone f.
    pituitary-thyroid f.
    pleiotropic f.
    renal glomerular f.

    renal tubular f.
    steroidogenic enzyme f.
    sudomotor sympathetic f.
    target gland f.
    thyroid f.
    transactivation f. 1, 2
functional
    f. genomics
    f. hypoglycemia
    f. hypothalamic amenorrhea (FHA)
    f. hypothalamic hypogonadism
    f. impotence
    f. ovarian hyperandrogenism
    f. sensitivity
functionale
    stratum f.
functioning
    f. nodule
    sexual f.
funduscopic examination
fungal
    f. infection
    f. septicemia
fungiform papilla
fungus, pl. fungi
fura-2 fluorescent Ca^{2+} chelator
furin enzyme
furosemide
furunculosis
fused epiphysis
fusiform dilatation
fusion
    delayed epiphyseal f.
    epiphyseal f.
    f. gene
    partial labioscrotal f.
futile cycle
fuzzy logic model
Fyn protein

G

G band
G cell
immunoglobulin G (IgG)
G&M colony-stimulating factor (GM-CSF)
G protein
G protein activation
G protein-coupled receptor (GPCR)
G protein dysfunction
protein kinase G (PKG)
G protein-linked receptor
G spot

G_2

cyclic endoperoxide prostaglandin G_2
prostaglandin G_2 (PGG$_2$)

G_s

G-stimulating protein

G_i

G-inhibiting protein

Ga-67

gallium citrate

GAA

glutamic acid codon

Gab-1

Grb2-associated binder-1

GABA

gamma-aminobutyric acid

GABA/BZD

gamma-aminobutyric acid/benzodiazepine
GABA/BZD system

GABAergic

G. fiber
G. projection

gabapentin
gabexate
^{67}Ga-citrate
GAD

glutamic acid decarboxylase

GAD65

glutamic acid decarboxylase 65
GAD65 antibody
GAD65 autoantibody

gadolinium-chelated compound
gadolinium in chelated form (Gd-EDTA)
gadolinium-diethylenetriaminepentaacetic acid contrast medium
gadolinium-enhanced MRI
GAF

glia-activating factor

GAFT

glutamine-fructose-6-phosphate-amidotransferase

GAG

glycosaminoglycan

Gagel disease
gain

weight g.

gain-of-function

g.-o.-f. alteration
g.-o.-f. mutation

gait

g. ataxia
waddling g.

galactitol
galactocele
galactopoiesis
galactorrhea

idiopathic g.

galactorrhea-amenorrhea

g.-a. syndrome

galactosamine
galactose intolerance
galactose-l-phosphate uridyltransferase deficiency
galactosemia
galactosialidosis
galactosyltransferase enzyme
4-galactosyltransferase isoenzyme II
galanin
Galen loop
gallium

g. citrate (Ga-67)
g. nitrate

G_s-alpha-coupled receptor
GALT

gut-associated lymphoid tissue

gamete intrafallopian transfer (GIFT)
gametogenesis
gamma

estrogen-related receptor g.
g. glutaryl transferase
interferon g. (INF-gamma)
G. Knife
G. Knife beam radiotherapy
neuropeptide g.
g. unit

gamma-aminobutyric

g.-a. acid (GABA)
g.-a. acid/benzodiazepine (GABA/BZD)
g.-a. acid/benzodiazepine system
g.-a. acidergic fiber
g.-a. acidergic projection
g.-a. acid transaminase inhibitor

G

gamma-carboxyglutamic
  g.-c. acid
  g.-c. acid protein
gamma-carboxylated glutamic acid
gamma-carboxylation
gamma-emitter
gamma-glutamylcysteine
gamma-glutamyltranspeptidase
gamma-hydroxybutyrate (GHB)
gamma-linolenic acid (GLA)
gamma-melanocyte-stimulating hormone
  (gamma-MSH)
gamma-MSH
  gamma-melanocyte-stimulating hormone
Gammaplan software
gamma-preprotachykinin A
ganciclovir
ganglia (*pl. of* ganglion)
gangliocytoma
  adenohypophysial g.
  intrasellar g.
gangliocytoma-pituitary adenoma
ganglioglioma
ganglion, pl. **ganglia**
  basal ganglia
  sympathetic ganglia
ganglioneuroblastoma
ganglioneuroma
ganglionic synapse
ganglioside
gangliosidosis
  GM1 g.
gangrene
  acute streptococcal g.
  Fournier g.
  major g.
gangrenosis
  ecthyma g.
ganirelix
GAP
  GnRH-associated peptide
  GTPase-activating protein
  guanosine triphosphate-activating protein
gap
  anion g.
  g. junction
  osmolar g.
GAPDH
  glyceraldehyde-3-phosphate
    dehydrogenase
Gardnerella vaginalis
Gardner syndrome
gargoylism
garment
  gradient pressure g.
GAS
  gene-activating sequence
gas
  g. chromatography

  g. chromatography of plasma
  g. dysbetalipoproteinemia
gas-containing abscess
gastrectomy
gastric
  g. achlorhydria
  g. acid secretion
  g. aspiration
  g. bypass
  g. carcinoid variant syndrome
  g. decompression
  g. electrical stimulation
  g. epithelioid leiomyosarcoma
  g. impedance measurement
  g. inhibitory peptide (GIP)
  g. inhibitory polypeptide (GIP)
  g. motor abnormality
  g. motor activity
  g. myoelectric abnormality
  g. parietal cell antibody screening
  g. prokinetic agent
  g. pylorus
  g. resection
  g. reservoir function
gastrin
  g. analog
  g. receptor
gastrinoma triangle
gastrin-releasing peptide (GRP)
gastritis
  atrophic g.
Gastrocrom
gastroduodenal artery (GDA)
gastrohepatic ligament
gastrointestinal (GI)
  g. autonomic neuropathy
  g. calcium absorption
  g. effect
  g. hamartoma
  g. hormone
  g. mucormycosis
  g. polyposis
  g. signal
gastroparesis
  diabetic g.
  g. diabeticorum
gastropathy
gastroplasty
  vertical banded g.
  vertical ring g.
gastroprokinetic
gastroschisis
Gastrosed
gate
  biochemical g.
gating
  circadian g.
Gaucher disease
Gaur method

Gaussian distribution
gaze
    impaired medial g.
GC300
    GluControl G.
Gc
    group-specific component
GCRH
    glucose counterregulatory hormone
G-CSF
    granulocyte colony-stimulating factor
GCT
    germ-cell tumor
GD
    Graves disease
GDA
    gastroduodenal artery
Gd-EDTA
    gadolinium in chelated form
GDF
    growth differentiation factor
GDF-9
    growth differentiation factor-9
GDM
    gestational diabetes mellitus
GDNF
    glial cell line-derived neurotrophic factor
GDP
    guanosine 5′ diphosphate
GE
    Excel GE
ge
    Novolin ge
Gee
    Gee G.
Geiger counter
gel
    aluminum g.
    clonidine g.
    Crinone bioadhesive progesterone g.
    DHT g.
    dihydrotestosterone g.
    g. electrophoresis
    g. filtration chromatography
    H.P. Acthar G.
    IPM wound g.
    Regranex g.
    transdermal hydroalcoholic g.
gelastic seizure
Gelfilm
Gelfoam sponge
Gelpirin

gelsolin
gemcitabine
gemfibrozil
Genahist Oral
Genapap
Genatuss
Gencalc 600
gender
    g. assignment
    g. identity
gene
    AIRE g.
    AKR g.
    aldo-keto reductase g.
    androgen receptor g.
    antibiotic resistance g.
    apolipoprotein B g.
    aromatase g.
    ataxia telangiectasia mutated g.
    ATM g.
    autoimmune regulator g.
    Becker muscular dystrophy g.
    beta-thyroid-stimulating hormone g.
    beta-TSH g.
    BRCA g.
    BRCA1 g.
    BRCA2 g.
    breast cancer g.
    Bruton tyrosine kinase g.
    BTK g.
    CA II g.
    CALCA g.
    calcitonin g.
    calpain-10 g.
    candidate g.
    carbonic anhydrase II g.
    catecholamine receptor g.
    cathepsin K g.
    cationic trypsinogen g.
    c-erbA-beta thyroid hormone
      receptor g.
    c-*fos* g.
    CFTR g.
    chromosome 11 insulin g.
    cJun g.
    CLOCK g.
    collagen g.
    cyclin D g.
    CYP17 g.
    CYP19 g.
    CYP1A1 g.
    CYP11A g.

NOTES

G

gene *(continued)*

cystic fibrosis transmembrane regulator g.
cytokine g.
DAX-1 g.
db g.
g. deletion
diastrophic dystrophia g.
dosage-sensitive sex reversal g.
DPC4 g.
DSS g.
DTD g.
endocrine g.
fa g.
factor V Leiden g.
FHIT g.
fibronectin g.
follicle-stimulating hormone-beta g.
FOS g.
Fox g.
FOXL2 g.
Frataxin g.
FSH-beta g.
fusion g.
genome-screen g.
GH-1, -2 g.
GH-2 g.
GH-releasing hormone receptor g.
GHRH-R g.
glucagon g.
g. glucagon
glucagon glycolytic/gluconeogenic enzyme-encoding g.
glucokinase g.
glycolytic/gluconeogenic enzyme-encoding g.
GNAS g.
GNAS1 g.
gonadotropin g.
growth hormone-1, -2 g.
H4 g.
H19 g.
hemochromatosis g.
hexokinase B g.
hexokinase II g.
hGH-N g.
hGH-V g.
histocompatibility complex g.
hKGK1 g.
housekeeping g.
Hox g.
Hoxa3 homeobox g.
human growth hormone g.
human kidney glandular kallikrein-1 g. (hKGK1)
human proCHR g.
human prokaryotic chromosome g.
human X chromosome, g. 1
21-hydroxylase g.

g. identification
Ig g.
IGF2 g.
IGF-II g.
IGF-IIR g.
immunoglobulin G g.
immunoglobulin V g.
insulin g.
insulinlike growth factor-II receptor g.
insulin receptor g.
integration g. 2 (int2)
islet g.
KAL g.
Kallmann syndrome interval g. 1 (KALIG-1)
KCNJ1 g.
Knudson model of tumor suppression g.
Krev-1 g.
lactase g.
Lep g.
leptin receptor g.
lipoprotein lipase g.
luciferase g.
malic enzyme g.
measles virus nucleocapsid g.
melanocortin receptor g.
MEN1 g.
menin g.
multiexonic g.
murine g.
n-myc g.
ob g.
obesity g.
g. overexpression
P21 g.
p53 g.
P450arom g.
PAX3 g.
Pax4 paired domain homeobox g.
Pax6 paired domain homeobox g.
PDGF g.
PDS g.
Pendred syndrome g.
PER g.
period g.
peroxisome proliferator-activated receptor g.
PHEX g.
phosphoenolpyruvate-carboxykinase g.
Pit-1 g.
pituitary tumor-transforming g. (PTTG)
p57KIP2 g.
platelet-derived growth factor g.
pleiotropic g.
polypeptide hormone g.

POMC 8-kb g.
potassium$_{ATP}$ channel g.
potassium inwardly-rectifying
 channel, subfamily J, member
 1 g.
Pou1F1 g.
PPAR-gamma target g.
preproglucagone g.
preproinsulin g.
preproPTH g.
preprotachykinin A g.
procollagen g.
proenkephalin g.
proglucagon g.
proopiomelanocortin g.
PROP-1 g.
p53 tumor-suppressor g.
p21^{WAF1} tumor-suppressor g.
putative tumor-suppressor g.
Rad g.
Rb g.
REG1 alpha g.
g. regulatory protein
reporter g.
retinoblastoma g. (Rb)
seipin g.
sex-determining region Y g. (SRY)
short-stature homeobox-containing g.
 (SHOX)
SHOX g.
SLC12A1 g.
SLC12A3 g.
sodium/iodine cotransporter g.
somatostatin g.
SOX9 g.
SRY g.
sulfonylurea receptor g.
SV40 large T-antigen g.
Tabby g.
g. targeting
g. therapy
Thra g.
Thrb g.
thrifty g.
thyroglobulin g.
thyroid hormone target g.
TIM g.
tissue nonspecific alkaline
 phosphatase g.
g. transcription
g. transfer
TSH-R g.

tumor necrosis factor g.
tumor-suppressor g. (TSG)
ubiquitin fusion degradation 1 g.
VHL tumor suppressor g.
von Hippel-Lindau tumor-
 suppressor g.
v-*sis* transforming g.
wild-type K-ras g.
Wilms tumor 1 g.
WTI g.
Xist g.
Zeitgeber g.
ZFP g.
zinc finger Y g.
gene-activating sequence (GAS)
Genebs
**Genentech biosynthetic human growth
 hormone**
generalized
 g. hyperpigmentation
 g. pruritus
 g. resistance to thyroid hormone
  (GRTH)
 g. thyroid hormone resistance
  (GTHR)
generation
 malonaldehyde g.
 thrombin g.
generator
 pulse g.
genetic
 g. counseling
 g. heterogeneity
 g. hormone resistance syndrome
 g. mapping
 g. marker
 g. mutations PPAR-gamma
 g. obesity
 g. polymorphism
 g. predisposition
 g. risk factor
genetically predisposing factor
gene-transfer technology
Gen-Glybe
geniculohypothalamic tract (GHT)
genistein
Genistin
genital atrophy
genitalia
 ambiguous g.
 external g.
 virilized external g.

NOTES

G

genitogram
genitography
genitourinary autonomic neuropathy
Gen-Minoxidil
genome
    haploid g.
    g. scan
    simian sarcoma virus g.
genome-screen gene
genome-wide screen
genomic imprinting
genomics
    functional g.
Genora
    G. 0.5/35
    G. 1/35
    G. 1/50
Genotropin
    G. Intra-Mix
    G. Mixer
    G. Pen
    G. Pen 5
    G. Pen 5 growth hormone delivery
    device
    G. Peri 12
    G. powder
    G. system
    G. two-chamber cartridge
genotype
    apo E g.
    thrifty g.
genotype-phenotype relationship
genotyping
    Kell antigen g.
    platelet antigen g.
    Rh C, D, E g.
Genpril
Gentle-Lance lancet device
genu
    g. valgum
    g. varum
geranylgeranyltransferase (GGTase)
Geref
geriatric
    g. hypogonadism
    g. hypoparathyroidism
German Multicenter BABY-DIAB study
germ-cell
    g.-c. neoplasm
    g.-c. tumor (GCT)
germinal
    g. arrest
    g. cell aplasia
    g. center
    g. epithelium
germinoma
    suprasellar g.
germline
    g. amplification

    g. deletion
    g. PTEN mutation
    g. putative protein-tyrosine
    phosphatase mutation
    g. TP53 mutation
gestagen treatment
gestational
    g. diabetes
    g. diabetes mellitus (GDM)
    g. diabetes mellitus oral glucose
    load
    g. goitrogenesis
    g. transient thyrotoxicosis (GTT)
    g. trophoblastic disease
    g. trophoblastic neoplasm (GTN)
gestodene
gestrinone
get up and go test
Gevrabon
G$_q$ family
GFR
    glomerular filtration rate
    growth factor receptor
GG
    Slo-Phyllin GG
GG/DM
    Kolephrin GG/DM
GGTase
    geranylgeranyltransferase
GH
    growth hormone
        GH cell adenoma
        GH insensitivity syndrome
        GH insulin
        pentameric GH
        placental GH
GHB
    gamma-hydroxybutyrate
GHb
    glycosylated hemoglobin
GHBP
    growth hormone-binding protein
GH-1, -2 gene
GHIH
    growth hormone-inhibiting hormone
    growth hormone inhibitory hormone
GH-N
    growth hormone (normal)
ghost
    g. cell
    g. nucleus
GH-releasing
    G.-r. factor (GHRF)
    G.-r. hormone
    G.-r. hormone receptor (GHRH-R)
    G.-r. hormone receptor gene
    G.-r. peptide (GHRP)
    G.-r. peptide receptor

ghrelin
> acylated g.
> g. hormone
> humoral g.

GHRF
> GH-releasing factor
> growth hormone-releasing factor

GHRH
> growth hormone-releasing hormone

GHRH-GH-IGF
> growth hormone-releasing hormone-
> growth hormone-insulinlike growth
> factor
>> GHRH-GH-IGF axis

GHRH-mRNA transcript
GHRH-R
> GH-releasing hormone receptor
>> GHRH-R gene

GHRH-secreting tumor
GHRP
> GH-releasing peptide
> growth hormone-releasing peptide
>> GHRP receptor

GHRP-5
> growth hormone-releasing peptide-5

GHS
> growth hormone secretagogue

GH-secreting pituitary adenoma
GHSR
> growth hormone secretagogue receptor

GHT
> geniculohypothalamic tract

GH-V
> growth hormone (variant)

GI
> gastrointestinal

giant
> g. carotid aneurysm
> g. cell carcinoma
> g. cell tumor
> g. invasive pituitary adenoma
> g. invasive prolactinoma

giant-cell
> g.-c. arteritis
> g.-c. granuloma
> g.-c. granulomatous hypophysitis
> g.-c. thyroiditis

giardiasis
Gierke disease
GIF
> glycosylation-inhibiting factor

GIFT
> gamete intrafallopian transfer

gigantism
> cerebral g.
> pituitary g.

GIH
> glucose-dependent insulinotropic
> hormone

G-inhibiting protein (G$_i$)
GIP
> gastric inhibitory peptide
> gastric inhibitory polypeptide
> glucose-dependent insulinotrophic
> polypeptide
> glucose-dependent insulinotropic peptide

GIT
> glutathione-insulin transhydrogenase

Gitelman syndrome
GK
> glucokinase

GL13 gene mutation
GLA
> gamma-linolenic acid

gland
> abnormal parathyroid g.
> acinar g.
> adenomatous adrenal g.
> adrenal g.
> anterior pituitary g.
> apocrine sweat g.
> autonomous nodular hyperplastic g.
> Bartholin g.
> Bowman g.
> Brunner g.
> bulbourethral g.
> Cowper g.
> eccrine sweat g.
> endocrine g.
> endometrial g.
> exocrine g.
> greater vestibular g.
> great vestibular g.
> high-lying thyroid g.
> hyperplastic adrenal g.
> hyperplastic parathyroid g.
> hypoplastic g.
> inferior parathyroid g.
> lacrimal g.
> lingual thyroid g.
> lymphoepithelial endocrine g.
> mammary g.
> merocrine g.

G

NOTES

gland *(continued)*
    neurosecretory g.
    parathyroid g.
    parotid g.
    percutaneous alcohol ablation of the parathyroid g. (PAAP)
    pineal g.
    pituitary g.
    posterior pituitary g.
    preputial g.
    prostate g.
    radiation-damaged thyroid g.
    salivary g.
    sebaceous sweat g.
    Skene paraurethral g.
    somatotroph adenoma of pituitary g.
    superior parathyroid g.
    thymus g.
    thyroid g.
    tubuloalveolar salivary g.
    ultimobranchial g.
    urethral g.
    uterine g.
glandular
    g. acini
    g. hypophysis
    g. kallikrein
    g. lesion
    g. pattern
glandulocavernosal shunt
glans
    g. clitoridis
    g. penis
Glanzmann disease
Gla protein
glargine
    insulin g.
glaucoma
    low-tension g.
    neovascular g.
GlcN
    glucosamine
GlcNAc
    N-acetylglucosamine
    GlcNAc receptor
glia-activating factor (GAF)
glial
    g. cell
    g. cell line-derived neurotrophic factor (GDNF)
    g. envelope
    g. reaction
    g. tumor
glia maturation factor (GMF)
glibenclamide
glicentin
glicentin-related pancreatic polypeptide (GRPP)

gliclazide
glimepiride
glioblastoma multiforme
glioma
    benign optic g.
    chiasmal g.
    hypothalamic g.
    hypothalamic/chiasmic g.
    optic apparatus g.
    opticochiasmatic g.
glioneural tumor
gliosis
    fibrillary g.
gliotic brain
GLIP-1
    glucagonlike peptide-1
glipizide GITS
glitazone
globe subluxation
globoid cell leukodystrophy
globulin
    antihemophilic g. (AHG)
    antithymocyte g.
    corticosteroid-binding g. (CBG)
    cortisol-binding g. (CBG)
    intramuscular immune g.
    lymphocyte immune g.
    plasma sex hormone-binding g.
    retinol-binding g. (RBG)
    serum thyroxine-binding g.
    sex-binding g.
    sex hormone-binding g. (SHBG)
    sex steroid-binding g. (SSBG)
    testosterone-binding g. (TeBG)
    testosterone estradiol-binding g.
    thyroid-binding g. (TBG)
    thyroid hormone-binding g. (THBG)
    thyroxine-binding g. (TBG)
    vitamin D-binding g.
globulin-vitamin D binding protein
globus pallidus
glomangioma
glomerular
    g. disease
    g. filtration rate (GFR)
glomeruli
glomerulitis
    focal g.
glomerulonephritis
    immune complex g.
    membranous g.
glomerulopathy
glomerulopressin
glomerulosa
    adrenal zona g.
    zona g.
glomerulosclerosis
    focal segmental g. (FSGS)
glomerulotubular balance

glomerulus
glomus jugulare tumor
glossitis
glove-and-stocking distribution
GLP
glucagonlike peptide
GLP-1
glucagonlike peptide-1
GLP-2
glucagonlike peptide-2
glubionate
calcium g.
GlucaGen
glucagon
g. C peptide
g. gene
gene g.
g. glycolytic/gluconeogenic enzyme-encoding gene
insulin-induced suppression of g.
g. receptor
g. stimulation test
g. storage disease
glucagon-gene promotor
glucagonlike
g. peptide (GLP)
g. peptide-1 (GLIP-1, GLP-1)
g. peptide-2 (GLP-2)
g. peptide-1 pancreatic endocrine cell
glucagonoma syndrome
glucagon-producing tumor
glucagon-related peptide hormone
glucagon-secreting tumor
glucaneogenic amino acids
glucoamylase
glucocerebrosidase deficiency
glucocorticoid
g. action
g. excess
exogenous g.
g. hormone
g. insensitivity
g. interaction
g. receptor (GR)
g. receptor deficiency
g. receptor dimer
g. receptor-interacting protein 1 (GRIP 1)
g. remediable hypertension
g. replacement
g. replacement therapy

g. resistance
g. response element (GRE)
synthetic g.
glucocorticoid-free immunosuppressive regimen
glucocorticoid-induced
g.-i. diabetes mellitus
g.-i. growth failure
g.-i. osteoporosis
glucocorticoid-regulated gluconeogenesis
glucocorticoid-remediable
g.-r. aldosteronism (GRA)
g.-r. hyperaldosteronism (GRH)
g.-r. hyperandrogenism
glucocorticoid-remedial hyperaldosteronism
glucocorticoid-resistant depressive disorder
glucocorticoid-responsive element (GRE)
glucocorticoid-suppressible
g.-s. aldosteronism
g.-s. hyperaldosteronism
g.-s. mineralocorticoid excess
glucogenesis
glucogen metabolism
glucoheptonate
calcium g.
glucokinase (GK)
enzyme g.
g. gene
g. regulatory protein
Glucolet Automatic lancing device
glucometer
Ascensia Breeze g.
Bayer g.
G. DEX blood glucose monitor
G. DEX diabetes care system
G. Elite R meter
G. II
G. II home glucose monitoring system
gluconate
calcium g.
ferrous g.
gluconeogenesis
glucocorticoid-regulated g.
hepatic g.
renal g.
GlucoNIR glucose sensor
GluControl GC300
Glucophage

G

NOTES

Gluco-Protein
- G.-P. OTC self-test
- G.-P. over-the-counter self-test

glucoregulatory neural reflex

glucosamine (GlcN)
- g. sulfate

glucose
- g. autoregulation
- B-D G.
- blood g. (bG)
- g. challenge test
- g. clamp method
- g. clamp study
- g. clearance
- g. concentration
- g. counterregulatory hormone (GCRH)
- fasting blood g. (FBG)
- fasting plasma g. (FPG)
- g. homeostasis
- impaired fasting g. (IFG)
- g. infusion rate
- instant g.
- insulin-induced g.
- g. intolerance
- g. measurement
- g. metabolism
- g. meter
- g. monitor
- g. oxidase inhibitor
- g. oxidase test
- g. oxidation
- g. phosphatase
- g. phosphate
- g. polymer
- g. polymer challenge test
- portohepatic g.
- postprandial g. (PG)
- g. receptor
- g. response
- g. sensing
- g. threshold
- g. tolerance
- g. tolerance impairment
- g. tolerance test (GTT)
- total available g. (TAG)
- g. toxicity
- g. toxicity hypothesis
- g. transport
- g. transport of diacylglycerol-sensitive protein kinase C
- g. transporter (GLUT)
- g. transporter 2 autoantibodies
- g. transporter translocation
- g. uptake
- uridine diphosphate g.
- urinary g.

glucose-dependent
- g.-d. insulinotrophic polypeptide (GIP)
- g.-d. insulinotropic hormone (GIH)
- g.-d. insulinotropic peptide (GIP)
- g.-d. insulinotropic polypeptide

glucose-fatty acid cycle

glucose-induced
- g.-i. activation of diacylglycerol-sensitive protein kinase
- g.-i. insulin secretion

glucosensor
- amperometric g.

glucose-6-phosphatase (G6Pase)
- g.-p. catalytic subunit
- g.-p. deficiency

glucose-1-phosphate

glucose-6-phosphate (G6P)
- g.-p. dehydrogenase (G6PD, G6PDH)

glucose-sensitive transcription factor (GSTF)

glucose-stimulated insulin secretion (GSIS)

glucose-transport
- g.-t. protein 1 (GLUT-1)
- g.-t. protein 2 (GLUT-2)
- g.-t. protein 3 (GLUT-3)
- g.-t. protein 4 (GLUT-4)
- g.-t. protein 5 (GLUT-5)
- g.-t. protein 6 (GLUT-6)
- g.-t. protein 7 (GLUT-7)
- g.-t. protein 6 pseudogene

glucosidase inhibitor

glucoside
- cyanogenic g.

glucostatic hypothesis

glucosuria

glucosyltransferase

glucotoxicity

Glucotrol XL

Glucovance

GlucoWatch
- G. Biographer
- G. Biographer meter
- G. Biographer transdermal sensor
- G. G2 Biographer diabetes monitoring system
- G. glucose monitor
- G. glucose monitoring device

glucuronic acid

glucuronidation

glucuronide
- 5-alpha-androstane-3-alpha,17-beta-diol g.
- androstanediol g.
- androsterone g. (AoG)
- g. conjugate

glue
 fibrin g.
Glukor
GLUT
 glucose transporter
GLUT-1
 glucose transporter 1
 glucose-transport protein 1
GLUT-2
 glucose transporter 2
 glucose-transport protein 2
GLUT-3
 glucose transporter 3
 glucose-transport protein 3
GLUT-4
 glucose transporter 4
 glucose-transport protein 4
  Cold GLUT-4
  GLUT-4 endocytosis
  GLUT-4 endothelium
  GLUT-4 vanadate
GLUT-5
 glucose transporter 5
 glucose-transport protein 5
GLUT-6
 glucose transporter 6
 glucose-transport protein 6
  GLUT-6 pseudogene
GLUT-7
 glucose transporter 7
 glucose-transport protein 7
GLUT-8
 glucose transporter 8
GLUT-9
 glucose transporter 9
GLUT-10
 glucose transporter 10
GLUT-11
 glucose transporter 11
GLUT-12
 glucose transporter 12
glutahione compound
glutamate
glutamate-cysteine ligase
glutamatergic fiber
glutamic
 g. acid
 g. acid codon (GAA)
 g. acid decarboxylase (GAD)
 g. acid decarboxylase 65 (GAD65)
glutamine

glutamine-fructose-6-phosphate-amidotransferase (GAFT)
glutamyl transferase
glutaric
 g. acidemia type II
 g. aciduria type II
glutathione
 g. peroxidase
 reduced g. (GSH)
 g. reductase
glutathione-insulin transhydrogenase (GIT)
glutathione-S-transferase (GST)
gluten-sensitive enteropathy
glutethimide
Glutose
Glu-X-Tyr
Glyate
glyburide
 Albert G.
glycan
glycated
 g. hemoglobin
 g. hemoglobin A_{1c}
 g. protein
glycation
 g. end product
 nonenzymatic protein g.
glycemia
 basal g.
 protein g.
glycemic
 g. control
 g. imprinting
 g. index
 g. load
 g. response
glyceraldehyde-3-phosphate dehydrogenase (GAPDH)
glycerol
 g. administration
 iodinated g.
 g. kinase
 g. kinase deficiency
glycerol-3-phosphate dehydrogenase
glycerol-3-PO4 acyltransferase (G3PAT)
Glycerol-T
glycerophosphate
glycine
 g. cleavage complex
glycine-rich RNA-binding protein (GRP)
glycinuria

G

NOTES

glycitein
glycobiology
glycocalyx
glycogen
g. concentration
g. content
liver g.
g. phosphorylase
g. storage
g. storage disease, types I/Ia, 1I,
III, IV, V, VI, VII, VIII
g. store
g. synthase
g. synthase kinase-3 (GSK3)
g. synthesis
g. synthesis
glycogenesis
glycogenic precursor
glycogenin-1
glycogenin-interacting protein (GNIP)
glycogenization
glycogenolysis
hepatic g.
glycohemoglobin assay
glycol
ethylene g.
salicylic acid and propylene g.
glycolated hemoglobin
glycolipid
glycolysis
anaerobic g.
glycolytic enzyme
glycolytic/gluconeogenic enzyme-encoding
gene
glycopeptide hormone
glycoprotein
alpha$_1$-acid g. (AGP)
carbohydrate-deficient g. (CDG)
g. crystal growth inhibitor (CGI)
g. crystal growth-inhibitor protein
heterodimeric g.
homodimeric g.
g. hormone
g. hormone receptor
g. IIb and IIIb blocker
g. neuraminidase deficiency
zona pellucida receptor for g. 3
glycoproteinosis
glycoprotein-producing adenoma
glycoprotein-secreting pituitary tumor
glycopyrrolate
Glycosal diabetes test
glycosaminoglycan (GAG)
g. deposition
polysulfated g.
g. synthesis
glycosuria
overt g.
glycosylasparaginase deficiency

glycosylated
g. hemoglobin (GHb)
g. serum protein
glycosylation
g. consensus motif
N-linked g.
nonenzymatic g.
thyroglobulin g.
glycosylation-inhibiting factor (GIF)
glycosylphosphatidylinositol-anchored
heparan sulfate proteoglycan
glycosyltransferase
glycotropic hormone
glycyrrhetinic acid
glycyrrhizin
glycyrrhizinic acid
glydiazinamide
Glynase PresTab
glypican-1
Glyset
Glytuss
GM1 gangliosidosis
Gm allotypes
GM-CFU
granulocyte-macrophage colony-forming
unit
G&M colony-stimulating factor (GM-
CSF)
GM-CSF
G&M colony-stimulating factor
granulocyte-macrophage colony-
stimulating factor
GMF
glia maturation factor
GMP
guanosine monophosphate
cyclic GMP
GNAS1
G. gene
G. locus
GNAS gene
gnawing pain
GNIP
glycogenin-interacting protein
GnRH
gonadotropin-releasing hormone
GnRH agonist
GnRH analog
GnRH mRNA
GnRH receptor
GnRHa
gonadotropin-releasing hormone agonist
GnRH-associated peptide (GAP)
GnRH-dependent precocious puberty
GnRH-independent precocious puberty
GnRH-R
gonadotropin-releasing hormone receptor
GNRP
guanine nucleotide regulatory protein

GO
   Graves ophthalmopathy
goal
      nutrition g.'s
      serum phosphorus g.
goblet cell
goiter
      adenomatous g.
      amyloid g.
      benign nodular g.
      cervical g.
      colloid g.
      diffuse toxic g.
      dyshormonogenetic g.
      g. endemia
      endemic colloid g.
      endemic iodine-deficiency g.
      enzootic g.
      euthyroid diffuse g.
      euthyroid nodular g.
      exophthalmic g.
      firm g.
      Himalayan g.
      hypothyroid g.
      idiopathic colloid g.
      intrathoracic g.
      iodide g.
      iodine-deficiency g.
      iodine-deficient g.
      lobulated g.
      multinodular euthyroid g.
      neonatal g.
      nodular g.
      nonautoimmune nontoxic diffuse g.
      nontoxic multinodular g.
      nontoxic nodular g.
      nontoxic sporadic g.
      ovarian g.
      g. reduction
      g. regrowth
      retrosternal g.
      sequestered g.
      simple nonendemic g.
      small g.
      sporadic g.
      substernal g.
      toxic diffuse g.
      toxic multinodal g.
      toxic multinodular g. (TMG)
      toxic nodular g. (TNG)
      uninodular g.
      g. volume

goiter-deafness syndrome
goitrin
goitrogen
goitrogenesis
      gestational g.
goitrogenic
      g. agent
      g. substance
goitrous
      g. chronic autoimmune thyroiditis
      g. cretinism
      g. Hashimoto thyroiditis
      g. hyperthyroidism
      g. tissue
gold
      Medtronic MiniMed CGMS system g.
      g. thyroglucase
gold-198
      colloidal g.
      g. radioactive isotope
Goldberg-Hogness box
Goldman-Hodgkin-Katz equation
Golgi
      G. apparatus
      G. complex
      G. network
      G. phase
      G. stack
Goltz syndrome
Gomori
      G. chromalum-hematoxylin
      G. staining method
gonad
      bipotential g.
      dysgenetic g.
      indifferent g.
      streak g.
gonadal
      g. agenesis
      g. axis
      g. dysfunction
      g. dysgenesis
      g. failure
      g. function
      g. mosaicism
      g. peptide
      g. ridge
      g. steroid
      g. steroid level
      g. steroidogenesis
      g. steroid replacement

G

NOTES

gonadal *(continued)*
    g. suppression
    g. suppression treatment
    46,XY g. dysgenesis
gonadarche
gonadectomy cell
gonadoblastoma
gonadorelin
gonadostat
gonadotoxicity
gonadotrope adenoma
gonadotroph
    g. cell
    g. cell adenoma
    g. cell hyperplasia
    g. cell origin
    g. hormone (GTH)
    g. pituitary adenoma
gonadotropic adenoma
gonadotropin
    alpha-human chorionic g. (alpha-hCG)
    asialo-human chorionic g.
    beta-human chorionic g. (beta-hCG)
    g. bioinactivity
    chorionic g. (CG)
    g. deficiency
    exogenous g.
    g. gene
    human chorionic g. (hCG)
    human menopausal g. (hMG)
    human pituitary g. (hPG)
    g. hypersecretion
    idiopathic g.
    luteinizing hormone/human chorionic g. (LH/hCG)
    g. receptor
    g. secretion
    sialylated human chorionic g.
gonadotropin-associated peptide
gonadotropin-independent precocious puberty
gonadotropinoma
gonadotropin-producing pituitary adenoma
gonadotropin-releasing
    g.-r. hormone (GnRH)
    g.-r. hormone activation
    g.-r. hormone agonist (GnRHa)
    g.-r. hormone-agonist therapy
    g.-r. hormone analog
    g.-r. hormone deficiency
    g.-r. hormone pulse frequency
    g.-r. hormone receptor (GnRH-R)
    g.-r. hormone test
gonadotropin-secreting
    g.-s. adenoma
    g.-s. tumor
Gonal-F

gonarche
gondii
    Toxoplasma g.
Gonic
gonorrhea
gonorrhoeae
    Neisseria g.
Goodpasture syndrome
Goody's Headache Powder
Gordon syndrome
Gorham massive osteolysis
Gorlin syndrome
Gormel Creme
goserelin
gossypol
gourd-shaped sella
gout
G6P
    glucose-6-phosphate
G6Pase
    glucose-6-phosphatase
G3PAT
    glycerol-3-PO4 acyltransferase
GPCR
    G protein-coupled receptor
    GPCR mutation
G6PD
    glucose-6-phosphate dehydrogenase
    G6PD deficiency
G6PDH
    glucose-6-phosphate dehydrogenase
G-protein
    heterotrimeric G.-p.
    G.-p. intermediary
    G.-p. signaling pathway
    G.-p. trimer
    G.-p. trimeric complex
GR
    glucocorticoid receptor
GRA
    glucocorticoid-remediable aldosteronism
graafian follicle
gracile
grade
    Ki67 g.
    PAHO g. 0, 1, 2
    Pan American Health Organization g. (0–2)
gradient
    calcium g.
    chemical g.
    corticomedullary osmotic g.
    corticopupillary osmolality g.
    electrical g.
    electrochemical g.
    hydrostatic pressure g.
    negative arterial-portal glucose g.
    Percoll g.

g. pressure garment
voltage g.
gradient-echo sequence
gradient-recalled
Graefenberg spot
Graefe sign
graft
dermal/epidermal composite g.
segmental g.
g. versus host (GVH)
graft-versus-host
g.-v.-h. disease
g.-v.-h. reaction
granidinium thiocyanate
granin
beta g.
granular
g. cell tumor
g. chromophil cell
granulated cell
granulation tissue
granule
beta cell secretory g.
Birbeck g.
calcium bilirubinate g.
chromaffin g.
g. extrusion
keratohyaline g.
neurosecretory g. (NSG)
secretory g.
Snaplets-FR G.
zymogen g.
granulocyte colony-stimulating factor (G-CSF)
granulocyte-macrophage
g.-m. colony-forming unit (GM-CFU)
g.-m. colony-stimulating factor (GM-CSF)
granulocytopenia
iatrogenic g.
granulocytosis
granuloma
g. annulare
caseating g.
giant-cell g.
noncaseating g.
reparative g.
sperm g.
granulomatosa
struma g.

granulomatosis
bronchocentric g.
Wegener g.
granulomatous
g. disease
g. histiocytosis
g. hypophysitis
g. inflammation
g. sarcoidosis
g. thyroiditis
granulosa
g. cell death
g. cell defect
g. cell tumor
g. cell tumor of the ovary
g. lutein
g. lutein cell
granulosa-theca cell tumor
granulosus
Echinococcus g.
granzyme
Graves
G. disease (GD)
G. ophthalmopathy (GO)
gravidarum
chloasma g.
thyrotoxicosis of hyperemesis g.
gravis
myasthenia g.
gravity
specific g.
gray patch
Grb2-associated binder-1 (Gab-1)
Grb-2 protein
GRE
glucocorticoid response element
glucocorticoid-responsive element
greater vestibular gland
great vestibular gland
Greenberg
G. bar
G. retractor mounting system
green birefringent amyloid protein
Greulich and Pyle growth measurement standard
Grey Turner sign
GRH
glucocorticoid-remediable hyperaldosteronism
growth-releasing hormone
Griffiths Scales of Infant Development
Grimelius stain technique

G

NOTES

GRIP 1
    glucocorticoid receptor-interacting
      protein 1
    GRIP 1 coactivator
groove
    Harrison g.
    hydrophobic g.
    g. pancreatitis
ground substance
group
    5-amino g.
    arylmethyl g.
    g. A *Streptococcus*
    g. B coxsackievirus
    5-cyano g.
    high mobility g. (HMG)
    International Diabetes
      Immunotherapy G.
    iodophenoxyl g.
    keto g.
    National Diabetes Data G. (NDDG)
    perikaryal g.
    thioureylene g.
group-specific component (Gc)
growth
    abnormal fetal g.
    appositional g.
    biometric assessment of fetal g.
    bone g.
    chondrocytic g.
    g. differentiation factor (GDF)
    g. differentiation factor-9 (GDF-9)
    g. disorder
    epitaxial g.
    excess acral g.
    g. factor expression
    g. factor-inducible chemokine (FIC)
    g. factor receptor (GFR)
    g. factor therapy
    g. hormone (GH)
    g. hormone-binding protein (GHBP)
    g. hormone cell
    g. hormone cell adenoma
    g. hormone cell hyperplasia
    g. hormone deficiency
    g. hormone-deficient adult
    g. hormone-deficient child
    g. hormone dose
    g. hormone dose-response curve
    g. hormone-expressing cell
    g. hormone-1, -2 gene
    g. hormone-inhibiting hormone
      (GHIH)
    g. hormone inhibitory hormone
      (GHIH)
    g. hormone insensitivity
    g. hormone insulin
    g. hormone/insulin-like growth
      factor axis

    g. hormone (normal) (GH-N)
    g. hormone-producing giant invasive
      adenoma
    g. hormone-producing tumor
    g. hormone-prolactin cell
    g. hormone-prolactin cell adenoma
    g. hormone protein-sparing effect
    g. hormone release-inhibiting
      hormone
    g. hormone-releasing factor (GHRF)
    g. hormone-releasing hormone
      (GHRH)
    g. hormone-releasing hormone-
      growth hormone-insulinlike growth
      factor (GHRH-GH-IGF)
    g. hormone-releasing hormone-
      growth hormone-insulin-like
      growth hormone axis
    g. hormone-releasing hormone-
      secreting tumor
    g. hormone-releasing peptide
      (GHRP)
    g. hormone-releasing peptide-5
      (GHRP-5, peptide-5)
    g. hormone replacement
    g. hormone resistance
    g. hormone resistance syndrome
    g. hormone response
    g. hormone secretagogue (GHS)
    g. hormone secretagogue receptor
      (GHSR)
    g. hormone-secreting pituitary
      adenoma
    g. hormone-secreting pituitary tumor
    g. hormone secretion
    g. hormone synthesis
    g. hormone therapy
    g. hormone (variant) (GH-V)
    hypothalamic hamartomatous g.
    longitudinal g.
    pituitary tumor cell g.
    prolactinoma g.
    g. rate
    g. retardation
    g. spurt
    g. suppressor
    g. velocity (GV)
growth-blocking antibody
growth-releasing hormone (GRH)
growth-stimulating antibody
growth-velocity chart
GrowTrak Plus
GRP
    gastrin-releasing peptide
    glycine-rich RNA-binding protein
GRPP
    glicentin-related pancreatic polypeptide
GRTH
    generalized resistance to thyroid hormone

Gs-cAMP pathway
GSH
　　reduced glutathione
GSIS
　　glucose-stimulated insulin secretion
GSK3
　　glycogen synthase kinase-3
gsp-positive somatotroph tumor
GST
　　glutathione-S-transferase
GSTF
　　glucose-sensitive transcription factor
G-stimulating protein (G_s)
GTH
　　gonadotroph hormone
GTHR
　　generalized thyroid hormone resistance
GTN
　　gestational trophoblastic neoplasm
GTP
　　guanosine 5′ triphosphate
GTPase
　　guanosine triphosphatase
GTPase-activating protein (GAP)
GTP-binding protein
GTP-dependent regulatory protein
　　complex
GTT
　　gestational transient thyrotoxicosis
　　glucose tolerance test
guanabenz
guanethidine
guanine
　　g. nucleotide binding protein
　　g. nucleotide regulatory protein
　　　(GNRP)
guanosine
　　g. 5′ diphosphate (GDP)
　　g. diphosphate-binding
　　g. monophosphate (GMP)
　　g. triphosphatase (GTPase)
　　g. 5′ triphosphate (GTP)
　　g. triphosphate-activating protein
　　　(GAP)
　　g. triphosphate-binding protein
　　g. triphosphate-dependent regulatory
　　　protein complex
　　g. trophosphate
guanylate
　　g. cyclase
　　g. cyclase enzyme
guanylin

guanyl nucleotide
guanylyl
　　g. cyclase
　　g. cyclase-linked receptor
guar gum
gubernaculum
guevodoces
guidelines
　　American Diabetes Association g.
　　California Diabetes and Pregnancy
　　　Sweet Success G.
　　Canadian Diabetes Association
　　　Clinical Practice G.
　　fast-food g.
　　National Cholesterol Education g.
Guillain-Barré syndrome
Gull disease
gum
　　guar g.
gumma, pl. **gummata**
　　syphilitic g.
　　gummata of the thyroid
gummatous lesion
gustatory
　　g. neurosensory process
　　g. sweating
gut
　　g. hormone
　　g. peptide
　　g. tube
gut-associated lymphoid tissue (GALT)
gut-brain peptide
gut-peptide hypothesis
guttering
GV
　　growth velocity
GVH
　　graft versus host
　　　GVH disease
　　　GVH reaction
gynandroblastoma
gynecoid obesity
gynecomastia
　　late-onset g.
Gynogen L.A. Injection
gynoid fat distribution
gyrata
　　cutis verticis g.
gyrate atrophy
gyrus, pl. **gyri**
　　cingulate g.
　　paraterminal g.

G

NOTES

gyrus *(continued)*
    parolfactory g.

H

carboxypeptidase H (CPH)
cathepsin H
Margesic H

H₂

prostaglandin H_2 (PGH_2)

H19 gene
H4 gene
habenular commissure
Habitrol Patch
habitus

body h.
eunuchoid body h.
marfanoid h.

Haemolance

H. lancet
H. Plus lancet device

Hagedorn

neutral protamine H. (NPH)

Hageman factor
hair

axillary h.
h. effect
h. follicle
parallel development of axillary h.
parallel development of pubic h.
pubic h.
terminal h.
vellus h.

HAIRAN

hyperandrogenism, insulin resistance,
acanthosis nigricans
HAIRAN syndrome

hairless woman syndrome
hairpin loop
Haldrone
half-life

biologic h.-l.
effective h.-l.
physical h.-l.

hallucination

formed visual h.
unformed visual h.
visual h.

halo

hypoechoic band
sonographic h.

halofenate
haloperidol
Halotestin
Haltran
HAM

hypoparathyroidism, adrenal
insufficiency, mucocutaneous
candidiasis

hamartoblastoma

hypothalamic h.

hamartoma

cutaneous h.
gastrointestinal h.
hypothalamic neuronal h.
neuronal h.
oral h.
retinal h.
tuber cinereum h.
h. of tuber cinereum

hamartomatous nodule
hamburger

h. thyroiditis
h. thyrotoxicosis

hamster oocyte penetration test
hand

h. enlargement
h. grip strength

Hand-Schüller-Christian disease
Hansen disease
haploidentical sibling
haploid genome
haploinsufficiency
haplotype

diabetogenic h.
h. linkage
h. tagging

HAPO

Hyperglycemia and Adverse Pregnancy
Outcome

hard exudate
Hardy

H. classification of pituitary tumor
H. ring curette

Hardy-Weinberg law
Harpenden stadiometer
Harris-Benedict equation
Harrison groove
Hartnup syndrome
Harvey-Ras oncogene
Hashimoto

H. disease
H. encephalopathy
H. thyroiditis

hashitoxicosis
Hassall corpuscle
HAT

histone acetyltransferase

H⁺-ATPase

hydrogen adenosine triphosphatase

haversian

h. canal
h. system

H

Hb
hemoglobin
HbA₁c
hemoglobin A_{1c}
HBD
hormone-binding domain
HBGF-2
heparin-binding growth factor-2
HBP
helix-bundle peptide
HC
Bancap HC
HCB
hexachlorobenzene
HCF
high-carbohydrate high-fiber
HCF diet
hCG
human chorionic gonadotropin
hCG pregnancy test
sialylated hCG
hCG-modulated thyroid activity
hCG-secreting hepatoblastoma
HCl
hydrochloride
pioglitazone HCl
HCMA
hyperchloremic metabolic acidosis
Hcrtr1 receptor
Hcrtr2 receptor
hCS
human chorionic somatomammotropin
HCT-116 colorectal cancer cell line
HDAC
histone deacetylase
HDDS
high-dose dexamethasone suppression
H-dexamethasone
HDL
high-density lipoprotein
HDL-C
high-density lipoprotein C
high-density lipoprotein cholesterol
HDL-C insulin resistance syndrome
headache
frontotemporal h.
headlight
fiberoptic h.
head of pancreas
healing
poor wound h.
wound h.
health
National Institutes of H. (NIH)
h. status counseling
heart
H. and Estrogen/Progestin
Replacement Study (HERS)

H. Outcome Prevention Evaluation
(HOPE)
Raloxifene Use for The H.
(RUTH)
heat
h. intolerance
h. shock protein (HSP, Hsp)
h. shock protein autoantibody
heating
radiofrequency capacitive h.
heat-stable protein
heavy metal poisoning
Hectorol Injection
hedgehog
Indian h.
H. protein
heel-to-pubis measurement
Heidenhain pouch
height
h. loss
midparental h. (MPH)
target h.
helical
h. computed tomography
h. CT
helicine artery
Helicobacter pylori
helix-bundle peptide (HBP)
helix-loop-helix
basic h.-l.-h. (bHLH)
h.-l.-h. family
h.-l.-h. structure
HELLP
hemolysis, elevated liver enzymes, and
low platelets
HELLP syndrome
helper/inducer T-lymphocyte
helper T cell
hemachromatosis
hereditary h. (HH)
hemadsorption
hemangioblastoma
retinal h.
hemangioblastomatosis
cerebelloretinal h.
retinal cerebellar h.
hemangioendothelioma
malignant h.
hemangioma
cavernous h.
hemangiopericytoma
Hematinic
Theragran H.
hematocrit
hematogenous
hematopoiesis
extramedullary h. (EMH)
hematopoiesis-supporting stroma

hematopoietic
 h. cell growth factor
 h. compartment
 h. stem cell precursor
 h. system
hematoxylin
 lead h.
heme-binding protein
hemiagenesis
hemianopia
 bitemporal h.
hemianopic
 h. defect
 h. scotoma
hemianopsia
 bilateral h.
 bitemporal h.
hemicastration
hemichoreoathetosis
hemifield slide phenomenon
hemigastrectomy
hemihypophysectomy
 blind h.
hemiplegia
 hypoglycemic h.
hemithyroidectomy
hemizona
 h. assay
 h. assay index (HZI)
hemizygosity
hemizygous
hemochorial placenta
hemochromatosis gene
hemoconcentration
hemocrine action
HemoCue blood glucose system
Hemocyte
hemocytoblastoma
hemodialysis
 chronic h.
 h. membrane bioincompatibility
 h. therapy
hemodilution
hemodynamic monitoring
hemofiltration
hemoglobin (Hb)
 h. A
 h. A_0
 h. A_{1c} (HbA$_1$c)
 h. A_1a
 h. A_1b
 h. C

 h. E
 glycated h.
 glycolated h.
 glycosylated h. (GHb)
 h. Raleigh
 h. Russ
 h. S
hemoglobinopathy
hemoglobinuria
 paroxysmal nocturnal h.
hemolysis
 h., elevated liver enzymes, and low platelets (HELLP)
 h., elevated liver enzymes, and low platelets syndrome
hemolytic anemia
hemolyticus
 Streptococcus h.
hemoperfusion
 charcoal h.
 resin h.
hemoperitoneum
hemophilia A
hemopoietin
hemoprotein
 cytochrome P450 h.
hemorheology
hemorrhage
 active variceal h.
 adrenal h.
 apoplectic h.
 dot and blot h.'s
 vitreous h.
hemorrhagic
 h. diathesis
 h. nodule
hemorrhagicum
 corpus h.
hemosiderin
hemosiderosis
 thyroid h.
hemostasis
 metabolic h.
 osmotic h.
Henderson-Hasselbalch equation
Henle
 loop of H.
 H. loop
 medullary thick ascending limb of H.
hentermine

NOTES

H

heparan
> h. sulfate
> h. sulfate proteoglycan

heparin
> low-dose h.
> low-molecular-weight h.

heparin-binding
> h.-b. EGF
> h.-b. epidermal growth factor
> h.-b. growth factor-2 (HBGF-2)

heparin-bound growth factor

hepatectomy

hepatic
> h. artery
> h. artery embolization
> h. artery occlusion
> h. cirrhosis
> h. cryosurgery
> h. disease
> h. effect
> h. failure
> h. fibrogenic activity
> h. free fatty acid uptake
> h. gluconeogenesis
> h. glucose efflux
> h. glucose output (HGO)
> h. glucose production (HGP)
> h. glycogenolysis
> h. glycogen synthesis
> h. hydroxymethylglutaryl coenzyme A reductase inhibitor
> h. insufficiency
> h. insulin sensitivity
> h. lipase
> h. lipase activity
> h. lipase deficiency
> h. metabolism
> h. necrosis
> h. neoplasm
> h. somatomedin
> h. steatosis
> h. tumor
> h. vein

hepatis
> peliosis h.

hepatitis
> h. A, B, C, D, E, F
> acute infectious h.
> autoimmune h.
> h. A virus
> h. C-associated osteosclerosis
> cholestatic h.
> chronic active h.

hepatoblastoma
> hCG-secreting h.
> human chorionic gonadotropin-secreting h.

hepatocellular
> h. enzyme

> h. rickets
> h. tumor

hepatocyte
> h. growth factor (HGF)
> h. nuclear factor (HNF)
> h. nuclear factor-1 (HNF-1)
> h. nuclear factor-3 (HNF-3)
> h. nuclear factor-4 (HNF-4)
> h. nuclear factor 6 (HNF-6)
> h. nuclear factor-4a (HNF-4a)
> h. nuclear factor 1 alpha
> h. nuclear factor 4 alpha
> h. nuclear factor 1 beta
> h. phosphodiesterase 3B
> h. transcription factor-1

hepatofugal flow

hepatoma cell insulin receptor

hepatomegaly

hepatopetal flow

hepatotoxicity

Heptavax-B vaccine

herbal preparation

Hercules syndrome

hereditary
> h. angioneurotic edema
> h. ataxia
> h. end-organ resistance
> h. fructose intolerance
> h. hemachromatosis (HH)
> h. hemorrhagic telangiectasia
> h. nephrogenic diabetes insipidus
> h. neuropathy with liability to pressure palsy (HNPP)
> h. nonpolyposis colon cancer (HNPCC)
> h. nonpolyposis colon cancer/ovarian cancer syndrome
> h. pancreatitis (HP)
> h. panhypopituitarism
> h. pseudovitamin D deficiency rickets
> h. thyrotoxicosis
> h. vitamin D resistance

heredofamilial disorder

heregulin

heritable

Hermansky-Pudlak syndrome

hermaphrodite

hermaphroditism
> true h.

herpes
> h. simplex virus (HSV)
> h. simplex virus thymidine kinase (HSV-TK)
> h. zoster

herpetiformis
> dermatitis h.

Herring body

Herrmann syndrome

HERS
> Heart and Estrogen/Progestin
> Replacement Study

Hers disease

Hertel exophthalmometer

HESX1
> homeobox gene expressed in ES cells

Hesx1
>> factor H.

HETE
> hydroxyeicosatetraenoic acid

5-HETE
> 5-hydroxyeicosatetraenoic acid

12-HETE
> 12-hydroxyeicosatetraenoic acid

15-HETE
> 15-hydroxyeicosatetraenoic acid

heterochromatic nucleus

heterochromatin
> constitutive h.
> facultative h.

heterochromia iridium

heterodimer
> cFos-cJun h.
> diabetogenic h.
> RelA-p50 h.
> TR-RXR h.

heterodimeric
> h. glycoprotein
> h. luteinizing hormone (hLH)
> h. structure

heterodimerization

heterodimerize

heterodisomic chromosome

heterogeneity
> genetic h.

heterogenicity
> osteoblast h.

heterologous

heterooligomer

heterophilic antibody

heteroplasmy

heteroplasty

heterosexual precocity

heterotaxy

heterotetramer
> hybrid h.

heterotetrameric molecule

heterotrimer
> type I collagen h.

heterotrimeric
> h. G-protein
> h. protein

heterozygosity
> compound h.
> loss of h. (LOH)

heterozygote

heterozygous cystathione beta synthase deficiency

heuristic

hexachlorobenzene (HCB)

Hexadrol

hexameric domain

hexarelin

hexokinase
> h. B gene
> h. enzyme
> h. II gene
> h. IV

hexosamine
> biosynthetic h.
> h. pathway

hexose phosphate

hFGF
> Kaposi sarcoma human growth factor

HGF
> hepatocyte growth factor

hGH
> human growth hormone
> somatotropin

hGH-N gene

hGH-V gene

HGM
> home glucose monitoring

HGO
> hepatic glucose output

HGP
> hepatic glucose production

H-graft
>> portacaval H-g.

HH
> hereditary hemachromatosis
> hypogonadotropic hypogonadism

H$_1$ histone

HHM
> humoral hypercalcemia of malignancy

HHPS
> hypothalamohypophysial portal system

HHRH
> syndrome of hereditary
> hypophosphatemic rickets with
> hypercalciuria

NOTES

H

HHS
    hyperglycemic hyperosmolar syndrome
5-HIAA
    5-hydroxyindoleacetic acid
hibernoma
Hibistat germicidal hand rinse
hidrosis
HIF-1
    hypoxia-inducible factor-1
HIF-1alpha
    hypoxia-inducible factor-1-alpha
high
    h. circulating parathyroid hormone
    h. glycemic index diet
    h. impact activity
    h. jugular vein sampling
    h. mobility group (HMG)
    h. mobility group box
high-arched palate
high-attenuation iodinated contrast media
high-calcium dialysate
high-carbohydrate
    h.-c. high-fiber (HCF)
    h.-c. high-fiber diet
high-density
    h.-d. lipoprotein (HDL)
    h.-d. lipoprotein C (HDL-C)
    h.-d. lipoprotein cholesterol (HDL-C)
high-dose
    h.-d. corticosteroid
    h.-d. dexamethasone suppression (HDDS)
    h.-d. dexamethasone suppression test
    h.-d. intraperitoneal aprotinin
    h.-d. statin treatment
high-fat feeding
high-fiber
    high-carbohydrate h.-f. (HCF)
high-K$_M$isoenzyme
high-lying thyroid gland
high-mannose
    h.-m. oligosaccharide
    h.-m. precursor
high-performance liquid chromatography (HPLC)
high-phosphorus diet
high-pressure baroreceptor
high-resolution coronal axis imaging
high-risk proliferative retinopathy
high-salt diet
high-sensitivity C-reactive protein (hs-CRP)
HI-K$_{IR}$6.2 beta cell
hilar cell
hilus cell
Himalayan goiter

Himbin
    Dayto H.
^{3}H-imipramine binding
hindgut
HIOMT
    hydroxyindole-O-methyltransferase
Hippel-Lindau
    von H.-L. (VHL)
hippocampal
    h. formation
    h. neuron
hippocampus
hippurate
Hirata syndrome
Hirschsprung disease
hirsute
hirsutism
    androgen-type h.
    facial h.
    Ferriman scale of h.
    idiopathic h. (IH)
hirsutism-anovulation syndrome
His-Pro-DKP
    histidyl-proline-diketopiperazine
histamine (H$_2$) antagonist
histamine-N-methyltransferase
histaminergic afferent
Histerone Injection
histidase
histidine
histidinemia
    ocular h.
histidine-rich calcium-binding protein (HRC)
histidyl-proline-diketopiperazine (His-Pro-DKP)
histiocyte
    Langerhans cell h.
histiocytic neoplasm
histiocytosis, histcytosis
    granulomatous h.
    Langerhans cell h.
    malignant h.
    h. X
histochemistry
    hybridization h.
histocompatibility
    h. class I
    h. complex gene
    h. locus antigen (HLA)
    major h.
histocytosis (*var. of* histiocytosis)
histofluorescence
histology
    bone h.
    mineralized bone h.
histomorphic feature
histomorphometric
    h. assessment

h. examination
h. study
h. technique
histomorphometry
dynamic h.
quantitative bone h.
histone
h. acetylation
h. acetyltransferase (HAT)
h. deacetylase (HDAC)
h. deacetylase activity
h. deacetylation
H_1 h.
Histoplasma capsulatum
histoplasmosis
histrelin
HIT-T15 cell
HIV
human immunodeficiency virus
Hi-Vegi-Lip
hKGK1
human kidney glandular kallikrein-1 gene
hKGK1 gene
HLA
histocompatibility locus antigen
human leukocyte antigen
HLA allele
HLA allele molecular typing
HLA autoantibody
chromosome 6 HLA
HLA DQ8
HLA DR antigen association
HLA restricted
HLA-A antigen
HLA-B35
HLA-B8 antigen
HLA-B antigen
HLA-C antigen
HLA-D antigen
HLA-DP antigen
HLA-DQ-alpha-501
HLA-DQ antigen
HLA-DR3 antigen
HLA-DR4 antigen
HLA-DR5 antigen
HLA-DR antigen
HLA-DRB1 autoimmune polyendocrine syndrome
HLA-Dw3 antigen
³H-leucine
hLH
heterodimeric luteinizing hormone

HMG
high mobility group
HMG box
hMG
human menopausal gonadotropin
HMG-CoA
beta-hydroxy-beta-methylglutaryl-coenzyme A
HMG-CoA reductase inhibitor
HNF
hepatocyte nuclear factor
HNF-1
hepatocyte nuclear factor-1
HNF-1 alpha
HNF-1 beta
HNF-3
hepatocyte nuclear factor-3
HNF3 transcription factor
HNF-4
hepatocyte nuclear factor-4
HNF-4 alpha
HNF4 transcription factor
HNF-6
hepatocyte nuclear factor 6
HNF-4a
hepatocyte nuclear factor-4a
HNK-1 antigen
HNP-4
human neutrophil peptide-4
HNPCC
hereditary nonpolyposis colon cancer
HNPP
hereditary neuropathy with liability to pressure palsy
H_2O_2 amperometric electrode
13-HODE
13-hydroxyoctadecadienoic acid
Hodgkin disease
Hofbauer cell
Hoffmann syndrome
hOKT3g1
HOKT3-gamma1
H.-g. nonmitogenic anti-CD3 antibody (Ala-Ala)
hOKT3y1
holder
Bra Pocket pump h.
Leg Thing pump h.
Pump-N-Shorts pump h.
Thigh Thing pump h.
Waist It pump h.
hole zone

NOTES

H

Holmes-Adie syndrome
holoenzyme
Hologic QDR 4500 DXA bone densitometer
holoprosencephaly
homatropine
home glucose monitoring (HGM)
homeobox
    h. gene expressed in ES cells (HESX1)
    short stature h. (SHOX)
homeobox-1
    pancreatic and duodenal h. (PDX-1)
homeodomain factor
homeostasis
    calcium h.
    energy h.
    fetal mineral h.
    fuel h.
    glucose h.
    intracellular h.
    lipid h.
    mineral h.
    osmotic h.
    phosphorus h.
    potassium h.
    potassium$_{ATP}$ channel glucose h.
    skeletal h.
    sleep-wake h.
    sodium h.
    water h.
homeotherm
homeothermia
homeotic
    paired box h. 3 (PAX3)
    paired box h. 6 (PAX6)
    paired box h. 8 (PAX8)
hominis
    Mycoplasma h.
homocarnosinase
homocarnosine
homocarnosinosis
homocysteine level
homocystinemia
    methylmalonic acidemia with h.
homocystinuria
    classic h.
homodimer
    catalytic h.
    regulatory h.
    thyroid hormone receptor h.
    TR h.
homodimeric glycoprotein
homodimerization
homogenate
    xanthoma h.
homogentisic acid

homologous
    h. pseudogene
    h. recombination
    h. thyroid antigen
homologue
    phosphatase and tensin h. (PTEN)
    tensin h.
    TNF-weak h. (TWEAK)
homology
homonymous
homoplasty
homotetramer
homovanillic acid (HVA)
homozygote
homozygous
    h. cystinuric
    h. missense mutation
Honolulu Asia Aging Study
Honvol
HOPE
    Heart Outcome Prevention Evaluation
    HOPE trial
hormogenesis
hormonal
    h. add-back therapy
    h. hyperfunction
    h. milieu
    h. regulator
    h. signal
    h. study
    h. symphony
hormone
    activational h.
    adenohypophysial h.
    adipokinetic h.
    adrenal androgen-stimulating h. (AASH)
    adrenal medullary h.
    adrenocortical h.
    adrenocorticotrophin h. (ACTH)
    adrenocorticotropic h. (ACTH)
    adrenomedullin h.
    aldosterone-stimulating h. (ASH)
    alpha-melanocyte-stimulating h. (alpha-MSH)
    alpha-MSH h.
    altered degradation of parathyroid h.
    amino acid-peptide h.
    angiotensin II antidiuretic h.
    antidiuretic h. (ADH)
    anti-müllerian h. (AMH)
    antiobesity h.
    antisteatotic h.
    antithyroid-stimulating h.
    atrial natriuretic h. (ANH)
    beta-cell melanin concentrating h.
    beta-melanocyte-stimulating h. (beta-MSH)

beta-thyroid-stimulating h. (beta-TSH)
bioactive parathyroid h.
bioidentical h.
h. biosynthesis
biosynthetic growth h.
bound h.
bovine parathyroid h. (bPTH)
brain h.
calciotropic peptide h.
calcitonin gene-related h. (CGRH)
calcitropic h.
calcium-lowering h.
calcium-regulating h.
contrainsulin h.
cortical androgen-stimulating h. (CASH)
corticotropin-releasing h. (CRH)
corticotropin-releasing h. 1R (CRH1R)
corticotropin-releasing h. 2R (CRH2R)
counterregulatory h.
C-terminal assay for parathyroid h.
h. degradation
dexamethasone-suppressed bovine corticotropin-releasing h.
eclosion h.
endogenous gonadal h.
endogenous growth h.
exogenous thyroid h.
fasting growth h.
follicle-stimulating h. (FSH)
follicle-stimulating hormone-releasing h. (FSH-RH)
free h.
gamma-melanocyte-stimulating h. (gamma-MSH)
gastrointestinal h.
Genentech biosynthetic human growth h.
generalized resistance to thyroid h. (GRTH)
GH-releasing h.
ghrelin h.
glucagon-related peptide h.
glucocorticoid h.
glucose counterregulatory h. (GCRH)
glucose-dependent insulinotropic h. (GIH)
glycopeptide h.

glycoprotein h.
glycotropic h.
gonadotroph h. (GTH)
gonadotropin-releasing h. (GnRH)
growth h. (GH)
growth hormone-inhibiting h. (GHIH)
growth hormone inhibitory h. (GHIH)
growth hormone release-inhibiting h.
growth hormone-releasing h. (GHRH)
growth h. (normal) (GH-N)
growth-releasing h. (GRH)
growth h. (variant) (GH-V)
gut h.
heterodimeric luteinizing h. (hLH)
high circulating parathyroid h.
human corticotropin-releasing h.
human growth h. (hGH)
human parathyroid h. (hPTH)
human placental uterotropic h. (hPUTH)
hydrophilic h.
hydrophobic h.
hyperglycemic h.
hypocalcemic h.
hypophyseotropic h.
hypothalamic inhibitory h.
hypothalamic-releasing h.
immunoradiometric assay of circulating parathyroid h.
immunoreactive parathyroid h. (iPTH)
inappropriate secretion of thyroid-stimulating h.
indole h.
inhibin h.
inhibitory h.
intact parathyroid h.
interstitial cell-stimulating h. (ICSH)
lactogenic h.
lactotropic h.
LH-releasing h. (LHRH, LH-RH, LRH)
lipophilic h.
"little" h.
luteinizing h. (LH)
luteinizing hormone-releasing h. (LHRH, LH-RH, LRH)
luteotropic h.

NOTES

H

hormone *(continued)*
    magnocellular h.
    melanin-concentrating h. (MCH)
    melanocyte-concentrating h.
    melanocyte-inhibiting h.
    melanocyte-releasing h. (MRH)
    melanocyte-stimulating h. (MSH)
    mineralocorticoid h.
    mini h.
    müllerian-inhibiting h. (MIH)
    müllerian inhibitory h. (MIH)
    myotropic h.
    natriuretic h.
    neurohypophysial h.
    neurotrophic h.
    nuclear accessory h.
    orexigenic h.
    ouabain-like h.
    ovine corticotropin-releasing h.
    paraneoplastic growth h.
    parathyroid h. (PTH)
    parotid h.
    pentameric growth h.
    peptide h.
    peptide-amino acid h.
    peripheral tissue resistance to thyroid h. (PTRTH)
    pituitary glycoprotein h.
    pituitary growth h.
    pituitary resistance to thyroid h. (PRTH)
    polypeptide h.
    posterior lobe h.
    primary adrenal medullary h.
    prolactin-inhibiting h. (PIH)
    prolactin inhibitory h. (PIH)
    prolactin release-inhibiting h. (PIH)
    prolactin-releasing h. (PRH)
    ProLease encapsulated sustained-release growth h.
    proparathyroid h. (proPTH)
    prothoracotropic h. (PTTH)
    h. receptor
    h. receptor-ligand complex
    h. receptor-mediated response
    h. receptor-negative tumor
    h. receptor-positive tumor
    recombinant follicle-stimulating h. (rFSH)
    recombinant human growth h. (RHGH, rhGH)
    recombinant human thyroid-stimulating h. (rhTSH)
    release-inhibiting h.
    releasing h.
    h. replacement therapy (HRT)
    h. resistance
    resistance to thyroid h. (RTH)
    h. response element (HRE)
    h. response unit (HRU)
    h. rhythm
    SciTojet needle-free injector for human growth h.
    h. secretion
    secretory burst of growth h.
    selective peripheral resistance to thyroid h.
    selective pituitary resistance to thyroid h.
    serotonin thyroid h.
    h. serum level
    sex steroid h.
    sine qua nonsuppressed thyroid-stimulating h.
    somatomammotropic h.
    somatotroph h. (STH)
    somatotropic h.
    somatotropin release-inhibiting h. (SRIH)
    steroid h.
    sterol h.
    stress h.
    syndrome of bioinactive growth h.
    syndrome of inappropriate secretion of antidiuretic h. (SIADH)
    syndrome of inappropriate thyroid-stimulating h.
    synthetic corticotropin-releasing h.
    thyroid h. (TH)
    thyroid-stimulating hormone-releasing h.
    thyrotropin-releasing h. (TRH)
    thyrotropin-stimulating h. (TSH)
    total h.
    trophic h.
    tropic anterior pituitary h.
    urinary follicle-stimulating h.
    water-soluble h.
    Y h.

hormone-beta
    luteinizing h.-b. (LH-beta)

hormone-binding
    h.-b. domain (HBD)
    h.-b. negative
    h.-b. protein

hormone-dependency effect

hormone-fuel interrelationship

hormone-resistant
    h.-r. breast cancer
    h.-r. state

hormone-responsive epithelium

hormone-secreting
    h.-s. adrenal tumor
    h.-s. cell
    h.-s. pituitary tumor

hormone-sensitive
    h.-s. adenylate cyclase system
    h.-s. lipase (HSL)

hormone-specific neurophysin
hormonogenesis
    thyroid h.
horn
    temporal h.
Horner syndrome
horny cell
hospital-acquired hyponatremia
host
    h. cell
    graft versus h. (GVH)
HOT
  Hypertensive Optimal Treatment
  Hypertensive Optimal Treatment Trial
    HOT Trial
hot
    h. flashes
    h. nodule
    h. spot
hour
    Acutrim 16 H.
24-hour
    24-h. fractionated metanephrine
    24-h. urinary aldosterone excretion
    24-h. urinary fractionated
    metanephrine
    24-h. urine collection
    24-h. urine free cortisol
hourglass constriction
housekeeping gene
Houssay phenomenon
Howell aspiration needle
Hoxa3 homeobox gene
Hox gene
HP
  hereditary pancreatitis
    Ku-Zyme HP
    Profasi HP
HPA
  hypothalamic-pituitary-adrenal
  hypothalamopituitary adrenal
    HPA axis
    HPA axis suppression
    HPA function
H.P. Acthar Gel
hPASP
  human pancreas-specific protein
5-HPETE
  5-hydroperoxyeicosatetraenoic acid
12-HPETE
  12-hydroperoxyeicosatetraenoic acid

HPG
  hypothalamic-pituitary-gonadal
    HPG axis
hPG
  human pituitary gonadotropin
hPL
  human placental lactogen
HPLC
  high-performance liquid chromatography
HPRT
  hypoxanthine-guanine
    phosphoribosyltransferase
    HPRT deficiency
HPT
  hyperparathyroidism
    HPT axis
hPTH
  human parathyroid hormone
hPUTH
  human placental uterotropic hormone
H-*ras*
HRC
  histidine-rich calcium-binding protein
HRE
  hormone response element
HRT
  hormone replacement therapy
HRU
  hormone response unit
H.S.
    Estratest H.S.
hs-CRP
  high-sensitivity C-reactive protein
HSD
  hydroxysteroid dehydrogenase
HSDD
  hypoactive sexual desire disorder
HSG
  hysterosalpingogram
HSL
  hormone-sensitive lipase
HSP, Hsp
  heat shock protein
HSPG
hst-1
  human stomach cancer-transforming
    factor-1
hst-2
  human stomach cancer-transforming
    factor-2
HSV
  herpes simplex virus

NOTES

H

HSV-TK
herpes simplex virus thymidine kinase
5HT, 5-HT
5-hydroxytryptamine
monoamine serotonin
HTA
hypophysiotropic area
hTg
human thyroglobulin
HTLV-1
human T-cell leukemia virus type I
5HTP
5-hydroxy-L-tryptophan
hTR
human thyroid hormone receptor
5HT$_2$ receptor antagonist
H-TRON
H.-T. insulin pump
H-TRONplus insulin pump
huang
ma h.
Humalog
H. Mix 50/50
H. Mix 75/25
H. Pen
human
h. allograft
h. calcitonin
h. chorionic adrenocorticotropin
h. chorionic gonadotropin (hCG)
h. chorionic gonadotropin-modulated thyroid activity
h. chorionic gonadotropin-secreting hepatoblastoma
h. chorionic somatomammotropin (hCS)
h. chorionic thyrotropin
h. corticotropin-releasing hormone
h. demineralized bone matrix
H. Genome Project
h. growth hormone (hGH)
h. growth hormone gene
h. immunodeficiency virus (HIV)
h. insulin
h. karyotype
h. kidney glandular kallikrein-1
h. kidney glandular kallikrein-1 gene (hKGK1)
h. leukocyte antigen (HLA)
h. leukocyte antigen allele
h. leukocyte antigen DR antigen association
h. leukocyte antigen restricted
h. malignant osteopetrosis
h. menopausal gonadotropin (hMG)
h. neutrophil peptide-4 (HNP-4)
h. pancreas-specific protein (hPASP)
h. parathyroid hormone (hPTH)
h. pituitary gonadotropin (hPG)
h. placental lactogen (hPL)
h. placental uterotropic hormone (hPUTH)
h. pluripotent stem cell
h. proCHR gene
h. prokaryotic chromosome gene
h. stomach cancer-transforming factor-1 (hst-1)
h. stomach cancer-transforming factor-2 (hst-2)
h. T-cell leukemia virus type I (HTLV-1)
h. thyroglobulin (hTg)
h. thyroid hormone receptor (hTR)
h. X chromosome, gene 1
h. zona binding assay
h. zona pellucide binding test
humanitarian device exemption
Humatrope
HumatroPen
Humegon
Humibid Sprinkle
humor
aqueous h.
humoral
h. factor
h. ghrelin
h. hypercalcemia of malignancy (HHM)
h. immune response
h. immunity
h. signal
h. symptom
hump
buffalo h.
dowager h.
Humulin
H. 50/50
H. 70/30
H. L
H. Mix 75/25 Pen
H. N
H. 70/30 pen
H. R
H. R pen
H. U
hunger
bone h.
hungry
h. bone
h. bone syndrome
Hunter syndrome
Huntington
H. chorea
H. disease
Hurler-Scheie syndrome
Hurler syndrome

Hürthle
    H. cell
    H. cell adenoma
    H. cell neoplasm
    H. cell tumor
Hutchinson-Gilford syndrome
HVA
    homovanillic acid
hyaline
    h. body
    h. cartilage
    h. membrane disease
hyalinization
    afferent arteriole h.
    Crooke h.
hyalinizing
    h. trabecular adenoma
    h. trabecular neoplasm
hyaluronan
hyaluronic acid
hyaluronidase
H-Y antigen
Hybolin
    H. Decanoate
    H. Improved Injection
hybrid
    h. heterotetramer
    h. steroid
hybridization
    allele-specific oligonucleotide h.
    fluorescence in situ h. (FISH)
    h. histochemistry
    h. histochemistry probe
    molecular probe h.
    in situ h.
hybridoma cell
hydatidiform mole
hydoxylase
hydradenitis
    suppurative h.
hydralazine
hydramnios
hydramnios-polyhydramnios
hydrate
    H. Injection
    terpin h.
hydremia
hydrocarbon
    polyaromatic h.
hydrocele
hydrocephalus
    X-linked h.

Hydrocet
hydrochloride (HCl)
    clonidine h.
    cyproheptadine h.
    desipramine h.
    eflornithine h.
    fluoxetine h.
    hydromorphone h.
    metformin h.
    metoclopramide h.
    oxymetazoline h.
    ranitidine h.
hydrochlorothiazide
hydrocortisone
    h. replacement therapy
    h. sodium succinate
Hydrocortone
    H. Acetate Injection
    H. Oral
    H. Phosphate Injection
HydroDIURIL
hydroflumethiazide
hydrogen
    h. adenosine triphosphatase (H^+-ATPase)
    h. breath test
    h. ion
    h. ion buffering
    h. peroxide
hydrogenase
    3-hydroxysteroid h.
hydrogen-bonding effect
Hydrogesic
hydrolase
    fumarylacetoacetate h. type Ia
    maleylacetoacetate h.
    maleylacetoacetate h. type Ib
hydrolysate
    aluminum-contaminated casein h.
    casein h.
hydrolysis
    phosphoinositide h.
    thyroglobulin h.
hydrolyzed lithostathine fibril
Hydromet
hydrometry
hydromorphone hydrochloride
hydronephrosis
Hydro-Par
hydroperiodide
    tetraglycine h.

NOTES

H

hydroperoxyeicosatetraenoic
5-hydroperoxyeicosatetraenoic acid (5-HPETE)
12-hydroperoxyeicosatetraenoic acid (12-HPETE)
Hydrophed
hydrophilic
    h. hormone
    h. macromolecule
hydrophobic
    h. amino acid
    h. groove
    h. hormone
    h. protein
hydrophobicity
hydrostatic
    h. pressure
    h. pressure gradient
hydroxide
    aluminum h.
    magnesium h.
3-hydroxy-3-methylglutaryl-CoA carboxylase deficiency
4-hydroxyandrostenedione
11-hydroxyandrostenedione
hydroxyapatite crystal
hydroxyapatite/tricalcium phosphate particle
hydroxychloroquine
hydroxycorticoid
hydroxycorticosteroid
17-hydroxycorticosteroid (17-OHCS)
    urinary 17-h.
18-hydroxycorticosterone
18-hydroxydeoxycorticosterone
15-hydroxyeicosatetraenoic acid (15-HETE)
12-hydroxyeicosatetraenoic acid (12-HETE)
5-hydroxyeicosatetraenoic acid (5-HETE)
hydroxyeicosatetraenoic acid (HETE)
2-hydroxyestrone
4-hydroxyestrone
2-hydroxyglutaric acid
5-hydroxyindoleacetic acid (5-HIAA)
hydroxyindole-*O*-methyltransferase (HIOMT)
3-hydroxyisovalerate
hydroxyisovaleric acid
hydroxylase (Ohase)
    h. deficiency
    steroid h.
    tryptophan h.
    tyrosine h.
11-hydroxylase
    11-h. deficiency
    11-h. enzyme
18-hydroxylase

21-hydroxylase
    21-h. deficiency
    21-h. gene
24-hydroxylase
    vitamin D 24-h. (24-OHase)
17-hydroxylase deficiency
17-hydroxylation
25-hydroxylation
hydroxylation deficiency rickets
hydroxyl radical
hydroxylysine (OHL)
6-hydroxymelatonin
hydroxymethylglutarate
hydroxymethylglutaryl-coenzyme A carboxylase
13-hydroxyoctadecadienoic acid (13-HODE)
4-hydroxyphenylpyruvate dioxygenase
17-hydroxypregnenolone
17-hydroxyprogesterone (17-OHP)
hydroxyprogesterone caproate
hydroxyproline
    h. oxidase
    urinary h.
hydroxypropyl-beta-cyclodextrin
11-hydroxysteroid dehydrogenase
hydroxysteroid dehydrogenase (HSD)
3-hydroxysteroid hydrogenase
5-hydroxytryptamine (5HT, 5-HT)
    5-h. subtype 2 receptor antagonist
5-hydroxytryptophan
5-hydroxy-L-tryptophan (5HTP)
hydroxyvitamin D
25-hydroxyvitamin D (25OH-VitD)
25-hydroxy-vitamin D 1-alpha-hydroxylase (1-alpha-OHase)
hydroxyzine
hygroma
    cystic h.
Hygroton
Hylutin
hyoid bone
hyoscyamine
Hyosophen
hypadrenia
Hy-Pam Oral
hypatocyte
hyperabsorptive hypercalciuric stone disease
hyperactivity
    airway h.
hyperadrenal state
hyperadrenocorticism
hyperaldosteronism
    bilateral idiopathic h.
    dexamethasone-suppressible h.
    familial h.
    glucocorticoid-remediable h. (GRH)
    glucocorticoid-remedial h.

glucocorticoid-suppressible h.
idiopathic h. (IHA)
secondary h.
syndrome of primary h.
tertiary h.
hyperalimentation
hyperaminoacidemia
hyperammonemia
hyperammonemic coma
hyperamylasemia
hyperandrogenemia
cryptic h.
hyperandrogenesis
ovarian h.
hyperandrogenic
h. anovulation
h. state
hyperandrogenism
early pubertal h.
functional ovarian h.
glucocorticoid-remediable h.
h., insulin resistance, acanthosis
nigricans (HAIRAN)
ovarian h.
hyperandrogen state
hyperapobetalipoproteinemia
hyperargininemia
hyper-beta-alaninemia
hyperbilirubinemia
hyperbradykininism
hypercalcemia
benign hypocalciuric h.
calcitriol-mediated h.
drug-induced h.
familial hypocalciuric h. (FHH)
Fanconi-type idiopathic h.
immobilization-related h.
infantile h.
malignancy-associated h. (MAH)
theophylline-induced h.
hypercalcemic
hypercalcinemia
hypercalcitonemia
hypercalciuria
absorptive h.
benign familial h.
idiopathic h.
normocalcemic h.
syndrome of hereditary
hypophosphatemic rickets with h.
(HHRH)

hypercalciuric
h. hypophosphatemic rickets
h. hypophosphatemic state
hypercapnia
hypercarnosinuria
hypercarotenemia
hyperchloremia
**hyperchloremic metabolic acidosis
(HCMA)**
hypercholesterolemia
familial h. (FH)
polygenic h.
hyperchylomicronemic syndrome
hypercontractile state
hypercortisolemia
pathologic h.
hypercortisolism
chronic h.
endogenous h.
exogenous h.
food-related h.
iatrogenic h.
metyrapone-induced h.
hypercytokinemia
hyperdefecation
hyperdeviation
hyperdibasicaminoaciduria
hyperechogenicity
hyperechoic
hyperestrinism
hyperestrogenic state
hyperestrogenism
hyperextensibility
joint h.
hyperfibrinogenemia
hyperfractionated radiotherapy
hyperfunction
autoimmune thyroid h.
autonomous h.
endocrine h.
hormonal h.
primary adrenal h.
secondary adrenal h.
hyperfunctioning tissue
hypergastrinemia
hyperglucagonemia
hyperglycemia
H. and Adverse Pregnancy
Outcome (HAPO)
beta-cell h.
exercise-induced h.
fasting h.

NOTES

H

hyperglycemia *(continued)*
    hypoinsulinemic h.
    intrauterine h.
    isolated postchallenge h. (IPH)
    persistent h.
    postprandial h.
    premeal h.
    rebound h.
    symptomatic h.
hyperglycemic
    h. coma
    h. crisis
    h. glucose clamp
    h. hormone
    h. hyperosmolar syndrome (HHS)
    h. memory
hyperglycinemia
    nonketotic h.
hypergonadotrophic hypogonadism
hypergonadotropic
    h. hypogonadism
    h. state
hyperhidrosis
    central h.
hyperhomocystinemia
    resistant h.
hyperhomocyteinemia
hyperhydroxyprolinemia
hyperimidodipeptiduria
hyperinsulinemia
    compensatory h.
    de novo h.
    exogenous h.
    islet beta-cell h.
    maternal hyperglycemia-induced
      fetal h.
    plasma glucose h.
hyperinsulinemic
    h. hypoglycemia
    h. hypoglycemia marker
    h. polycystic ovary syndrome
hyperinsulinemic-euglycemic clamp technique
hyperinsulinism
    congenital h.
    familial h.
    potassium$_{ATP}$ channel h.
hyperinsulinoma
hyperintense
hyperirritability
hyperkalemia
    familial h.
hyperkeratosis
    plantar h.
hyperkinesia
hyperlactemia
hyperleptinemia
hyperleucine-isoleucinemia

hyperlipasemia
hyperlipidemia
    combined h.
    familial combined h. (FCH)
    type IV h.
hyperlipoproteinemia
    type III h.
hyperlysinemia
hypermagnesemia
hypermelatoninism
hypermenorrhea
hypermethioninemia
hypermethylation
hypermineralocorticoidism
    licorice-induced h.
    renin-independent h.
hypermotility
hypernatremia
    essential h.
hypernatremic
hyperoral behavior
hyperornithinemia
hyperosmolality
hyperosmolar nonketotic coma
hyperosmotic
hyperostosis
    h. corticalis
    diaphyseal cortical h.
    diffuse idiopathic skeletal h.
      (DISH)
    endosteal h.
    h. frontalis interna
    infantile cortical h.
hyperoxaluria
    enteric h.
hyperoxia
hyperparathyroid bone disease
hyperparathyroidism (HPT)
    acute primary h.
    h. axis
    compensatory h.
    familial isolated primary h. (FIPH)
    neonatal severe h. (NSHPT)
    normocalcemic primary h.
    persistent h.
    phosphorus-induced h.
    primary h. (PHPT)
    secondary h.
    tertiary h.
hyperphagia
hyperphenylalaninemia
hyperphosphatasemia
    familial h.
    idiopathic h.
hyperphosphatasia
    osteoectasia with h.
hyperphosphatemia
hyperphosphaturia

hyperpigmentation
    cutaneous h.
    generalized h.
hyperpigmented skin
hyperpituitarism
hyperplacentosis
hyperplasia
    ACTH-independent bilateral
      macronodular h. (AIBH)
    adenomatous h.
    adrenal medullary h.
    adrenomedullary h.
    autonomous adrenal h.
    autosomal dominant toxic
      thyroid h.
    beta cell h.
    bilateral adrenal h. (BAH)
    bilateral macronodular h.
    C cell h.
    chronic lobular h.
    congenital adrenal h. (CAH)
    congenital lipoid adrenal h.
    congenital virilizing adrenal h.
    corticotroph cell h.
    cystic h.
    ECL cell h.
    enterochromaffin-like cell h.
    epidermal h.
    erythroid h.
    familial C-cell h.
    focal epithelial h.
    gonadotroph cell h.
    growth hormone cell h.
    iatrogenic h.
    intraductal mucinous h.
    Kupffer cell h.
    lactotroph h.
    Leydig cell h.
    lipoid congenital adrenal h.
    lymphoid h.
    macronodular adrenal h.
    massive macronodular h.
    micronodular h.
    neointimal h.
    non-salt-wasting congenital
      adrenal h.
    paraadenomatous corticotroph h.
    parathyroid gland h.
    pineal h.
    pituitary h.
    primary macronodular h.
    prolactin cell h.

    stromal h.
    thecal h.
    thymic h.
    thyroid h.
    thyrotroph cell h.
    type I, II, IV, V congenital
      adrenal h.
hyperplastic
    h. adrenal gland
    h. parathyroid gland
hyperpneumatization
hyperproinsulinemia
hyperprolactinemia
    idiopathic h.
    radiation-induced h.
    secondary h.
hyperprolactinemic
    h. disorder
    h. endocrinopathy
hyperprolinemia
hyperprostaglandin E syndrome
hyperreactio luteinalis
hyperreflexia
hyperreninemia
hyperreninemic hypoaldosteronism
hyperreninism
hyperrespond
hypersarcosinemia
hypersecretion
    ACTH h.
    adrenocorticotrophic hormone h.
    adrenocorticotropic hormone h.
    gonadotropin h.
    pituitary h.
hypersensitivity response
hypersexuality
    paroxysmal h.
hypersomnia
hypertelorism
hypertension
    benign intracranial h.
    endocrine h.
    essential h.
    glucocorticoid remediable h.
    idiopathic intracranial h.
    intracranial h. (IH)
    licorice-induced h.
    low-renin essential h.
    pregnancy-induced h. (PIH)
    pulmonary arterial h. (PAH)
    renovascular h.
    systemic arterial h.

NOTES

H

hypertensive
　　h. cardiomyopathy
　　H. Optimal Treatment (HOT)
　　H. Optimal Treatment Trial (HOT)
hyperthecosis
　　follicular h.
　　ovarian h.
　　stromal h.
hyperthermia
　　cyclic h.
　　fulminant h.
　　malignant h.
　　microwave h.
　　paroxysmal h.
　　thyroid storm h.
hyperthyroid
　　clinically h.
　　h. periodic paralysis
hyperthyroidism
　　apathetic h.
　　autoimmune h.
　　central h.
　　congenital h.
　　factitious h.
　　familial nonautoimmune h.
　　fetal h.
　　goitrous h.
　　iatrogenic h.
　　iodine-induced h. (IIH)
　　masked h.
　　monosymptomatic h.
　　monosystemic h.
　　neonatal Graves h.
　　nonautoimmune familial h.
　　non-Graves disease h.
　　painless h.
　　postpartum h.
　　pregnancy h.
　　primary h.
　　secondary h.
　　subacute h.
　　subclinical h.
hyperthyrotropinemia
hyperthyroxinemia
　　complex h.
　　dysalbuminemic h.
　　euthyroid h.
　　familial dysalbuminemic h. (FDH)
　　familial euthyroid h.
　　prealbumin-associated h. (PAH)
hypertonic
　　h. encephalopathy
　　h. syndrome
　　h. volume depletion
hypertonicity
　　impaired medullary h.
　　plasma h.
hypertrichosis
　　villous h.

hypertriglyceridemia
　　carbohydrate-induced h.
　　familial h.
hypertriiodothyroninemia
　　familial dysalbuminemic h.
hypertrophic
　　h. cardiomyopathy
　　h. lichen planus
　　h. osteoarthropathy
　　h. state
hypertrophied
　　h. corneal nerve
　　h. thyroglossal duct remnant
hypertrophy
　　benign prostatic h.
　　compensatory h.
　　fiber h.
　　periosteal h.
　　thymus h.
hyperuricemia
hyperuricosuria
hypervalinemia
hypervitaminosis
　　h. A
　　h. D
hypervolemia
hypha, pl. **hyphae**
　　aseptate h.
　　thick-walled h.
Hy-Phen
hypnosedation
hypoactive sexual desire disorder (HSDD)
hypoactivity
hypoadrenalism
　　central h.
　　primary h.
　　secondary h.
hypoadrenal state
hypoadrenocorticism
hypoalbuminemia
hypoaldosteronism
　　congenital h.
　　hyperreninemic h.
　　hyporeninemic h.
　　syndrome of hyporeninemic h. (SHH)
hypoalphalipoproteinemia
　　familial h.
hypoaminoacidemia
　　postprandial h.
hypoandrogenic milieu
hypoandrogenism
　　ovarian h.
hypoatremia
hypobetalipoproteinemia
hypocalcemia
　　anticonvulsant-associated h.
　　autosomal dominant h.

cardiac abnormality, abnormal facies, thymic hypoplasia, cleft palate, h. (CATCH)
early h.
late h.
neonatal h.
optic h.
phosphorus-induced h.
symptomatic h.
hypocalcemic
h. emergency
h. hormone
h. tetany
hypocalciuria
hypocalciuric-hypomagnesemic variant
hypocaloric diet
hypocapnia
hypocellular
h. bone surface
h. marrow without fibrosis
hypochlorhydria
hypochondroplasia
hypochromic microcytic red blood cell
hypocitraturia
primary h.
secondary h.
hypocorticotropic state
hypocortisolemia
hypocortisolism
postadenomectomy h.
hypocretin
hypodipsia
hypodipsic disorder
hypoechogenicity
hypoechoic band (halo)
hypoestrogenemia
hypoestrogenic
hypoestrogenism
hypofunction
autoimmune polyglandular h.
pituitary hormone h.
hypofunctioning
hypogammaglobulinemia
hypogeusia
hypoglossal nerve
hypoglycemia
acarbose h.
acute h.
alcohol-induced h.
alimentary h.
artifactual h.
autoimmune h.

h. biguanide
chronic h.
clinical h.
counterregulation of h.
h. crisis
drug-induced h.
ethanol h.
exercise-induced h.
factitial h.
factitious h.
fasting h.
functional h.
hyperinsulinemic h.
idiopathic reactive h.
insulin factitial h.
insulin-induced systemic h.
ketotic h.
late h.
maternal h.
nadir h.
neonatal h.
nocturnal h.
noninsulinoma pancreatogenous h.
non-islet-cell tumor-induced h.
postabsorptive h.
postexercise h.
postprandial h.
PPAR h.
problematic h.
reactive h.
secretagogue-induced h.
substrate-limited h.
h. syndrome
transient neonatal h.
tumor-associated h.
h. unawareness
h. unawareness syndrome
h. unresponsiveness
hypoglycemia-associated autonomic failure
hypoglycemic
h. agent
h. clamp
h. coma
h. disorder
h. event
h. hemiplegia
h. shock
hypoglycin
hypoglycorrhachia
hypogonadal hypogonadism

NOTES

H

171

hypogonadism
 acquired hypogonadotropic h.
 central h.
 central h. type IA, IB, IIA, III
 eugonadotropic h.
 functional hypothalamic h.
 geriatric h.
 hypergonadotrophic h.
 hypergonadotropic h.
 hypogonadal h.
 hypogonadotrophic h.
 hypogonadotropic h. (HH)
 hypothalamic hypogonadotropic h.
 idiopathic hypogonadotropic h.
  (IHH)
 neurogenic h.
 primary h.
 secondary h.
 tertiary h.
hypogonadotrophic hypogonadism
hypogonadotropic hypogonadism (HH)
Hypoguard
 H. Advance glucose meter
 H. Advance test strip
hypoinsulinemia
 relative h.
hypoinsulinemic hyperglycemia
hypokalemia
 licorice-induced h.
 spontaneous h.
hypokalemic
 h. metabolic alkalosis
 h. periodic paralysis
hypoleptinemia
 relative h.
hypolipidemic agent
hypomagnesemia
hypomagnesiuria
hypomelatoninism
hypomenorrhea
hypometabolic
hypomineralization
hyponatremia
 asymptomatic h.
 hospital-acquired h.
 iatrogenic h.
 symptomatic h.
hyponatremic encephalopathy
hypoosmolality
hypoparathyroidism
 h., adrenal insufficiency,
  mucocutaneous candidiasis (HAM)
 autoimmune h.
 autosomal dominant h.
 familial h.
 geriatric h.
 idiopathic h.
 pathological h.
 permanent h.

 postsurgical h.
 primary h.
 secondary h.
 transient h.
hypophosphatasia
hypophosphatemia
 congenital h.
 fasting h.
 X-linked h. (XLH)
hypophosphatemic
 h. bone disease
 h. osteomalacia
 h. rickets
hypophysectomized
hypophysectomy
 endoscopic transsphenoidal h.
 stereotactic h.
 transsphenoidal h.
hypophyseotropic hormone
hypophysial
 h. artery
 h. cleft
 h. lesion
 h. portal system
 h. stalk
 h. stalk circulation
hypophysial-hypothalamic portal system
hypophysial-portal circulation
hypophysiotropic
 h. area (HTA)
 h. factor
 h. hormonal function
 h. neuron
 h. system
hypophysis
 chromophilic h.
 glandular h.
 pharyngeal h.
hypophysitis
 autoimmune h.
 chronic lymphocytic h.
 giant-cell granulomatous h.
 granulomatous h.
 idiopathic granulomatous h.
 lymphocytic h.
 purulent h.
hypopituitarism
 complete h.
 idiopathic h.
 isolated h.
 partial h.
 postpartum h.
 radiotherapy-induced h.
 selective h.
hypopituitary adult
hypoplasia
 congenital lipoid adrenal h.
 cytomegalic-type congenital
  adrenal h.

focal dermal h.
Leydig cell h.
miniature-type congenital adrenal h.
h. of nipples
pituitary h.
somatotroph h.
hypoplastic
    h. gland
    h. left heart syndrome
    h. mandible
    h. nail
    h. vulva
    h. zygoma
hypoprolactinemia
hypoproliferative anemia
hypoproteinemia
hypoprothrombinemia
hyporeflexia
hyporeninemic hypoaldosteronism
hyporesponsiveness
    partial thyroid-stimulating
      hormone h.
    partial TSH h.
hyposmia
hyposmotic
hyposomatotropism
    obesity-related h.
hypospadias
    familial h.
    penoscrotal h.
    perineoscrotal h.
hypospermatogenesis
hyposthenuria
hypotelorism
    orbital h.
hypotension
    idiopathic orthostatic h.
    orthostatic h.
    postprandial h.
    postural h.
    primary orthostatic h.
    secondary orthostatic h.
hypothalamic
    h. acromegaly
    h. amenorrhea
    h. anovulation
    h. astrocytoma
    h. center
    h. diabetes insipidus
    h. dysregulation
    h. eunuchism
    h. glioma

    h. gonadotropin-releasing hormone
      deficiency
    h. hamartoblastoma
    h. hamartomatous growth
    h. hypogonadotropic hypogonadism
    h. hypothyroidism
    h. inhibitory hormone
    h. neuroendocrine regulation
    h. neuronal hamartoma
    h. obesity
    h. opioidergic tone
    h. paraventricular nucleus
    h. regulatory mechanism
    h. sulcus
    h. tumor
    h. zone
hypothalamic/chiasmic glioma
hypothalamic-hypophyseal portal vessel
hypothalamic-midbrain junction
hypothalamic-pituitary
    h.-p. axis
    h.-p. control
    h.-p. disease
    h.-p. disorder
    h.-p. response
    h.-p. tumor
hypothalamic-pituitary-adrenal (HPA)
    h.-p.-a. axis
    h.-p.-a. axis suppression
    h.-p.-a. function
hypothalamic-pituitary-gonadal (HPG)
    h.-p.-g. axis
hypothalamic-pituitary-ovarian axis
hypothalamic-pituitary-thyroid axis
hypothalamic-releasing
    h.-r. factor
    h.-r. hormone
hypothalamohypophyseal complex
hypothalamohypophysial
    h. nerve tract
    h. portal system (HHPS)
hypothalamoneurohypophysial tract
hypothalamopituitary adrenal (HPA)
hypothalamopituitary-adrenocortical axis
hypothalamus
    arcuate nucleus of the h. (ARC)
    dorsomedial nucleus of the h.
    lateral h.
    medial basal h.
    paraventricular nucleus of the h.
    preoptic area of the h. (POA)
    PVN of the h.

NOTES

H

hypothalamus (*continued*)
  rostral h.
  SCN of the h.
  suprachiasmatic nucleus of the h.
  supraoptic nucleus of the h. (SON)
  ventromedial nucleus of the h.
    (VMN)
hypothalmo-neurohypophyseal neuron
hypothermia
  cyclic h.
  paroxysmal h.
hypothermic cold adaptation
hypothesis, pl. **hypotheses**
  Barker h.
  beta-cell h.
  bystander T-cell proliferation h.
  estrone h.
  glucose toxicity h.
  glucostatic h.
  gut-peptide h.
  lipostatic h.
  Lyon h.
  null h.
  overworked B-cell h.
  Pedersen h.
  single gateway h.
  SNARE h.
  somatomedin h.
  Somogyi h.
  thermostatic h.
  thrifty genotype h.
hypothyroid
  h. drug
  h. goiter
  h. mononeuropathy
  h. myopathy
  h. polyneuropathy
  h. rhabdomyolysis
hypothyroidism
  acquired h.
  amiodarone-induced h.
  atrophic autoimmune h.
  biochemical h.
  central h.
  childhood h.
  clinical h.
  congenital h.
  fetal h.
  hypothalamic h.
  hypothyrotropic h.
  idiopathic hypothalamic h.
  iodine-induced h.
  juvenile h.
  lithium-induced h.
  maternal h.
  minimally symptomatic h. (MSH)
  neonatal h.
  pituitary h.
  postablative h.

  posttherapeutic h.
  preclinical h.
  pregnancy h.
  primary thyroidal h.
  secondary h.
  spontaneous primary h.
  sporadic congenital h.
  subclinical h.
  tertiary h.
  thyroidal h.
  transient neonatal h.
  transient postradioiodine h.
hypothyrotropic hypothyroidism
hypothyroxinemia
  euthyroid h.
  fetal h.
  maternal h.
  h. of prematurity
hypotonia
hypotonic
  h. duodenography
  h. saline
  h. syndrome
  h. urine
hypotriglyceridemic action
hypouricemia
hypovascular islet cell tumor
hypoventilation
hypovolemia
hypovolemic shock
hypoxanthine-guanine
  h.-g. phosphoribosyltransferase
    (HPRT)
  h.-g. phosphoribosyltransferase
    deficiency
hypoxanthine phosphoribosyltransferase
hypoxemia
  fetal h.
hypoxia
  fetal h.
hypoxia-inducible
  h.-i. factor-1 (HIF-1)
  h.-i. factor-1-alpha (HIF-1alpha)
hypoxic
  h. brain injury
  h. encephalopathy
Hyprogest 250
hysterectomy
hysteria
hystericus
  syndrome of globus h.
hysterosalpingogram (HSG)
hysterosalpingography
hystidyl-methionine-27
  peptide h.-m. (PHM-27)
Hytakerol
Hytinic
Hyzine-50 Injection

HZI
hemizona assay index

NOTES

^{123}I
   iodine-123
^{125}I
   iodine-125
^{127}I
   iodine-127
^{131}I
   iodine-131
   radioactive iodine
      ^{131}I isotope
      ^{131}I therapy
      thyroid ablation with ^{131}I
I$_2$
   prostaglandin I$_2$ (PGI$_2$)
[^{131}I]-19-iodocholesterol scintigraphy
IAA
   insulin autoantibody
   islet antigen autoantibody
IAK
   islet after kidney
IAPP
   islet amyloid polypeptide
IAPS-forskolin
   iodo-4-azidophenetylamido-7-O-
      succinyldeacetyl forskolin
iatrogenic
      i. Cushing syndrome
      i. granulocytopenia
      i. hypercortisolism
      i. hyperplasia
      i. hyperthyroidism
      i. hyponatremia
      i. thyrotoxicosis
      i. type 1 diabetes mellitus
IB
      Excedrin IB
      Midol IB
      Pamprin IB
Iberet-Folic-500
Iberet-Liquid
Ibuprin
ibuprofen
Ibuprohm
Ibu-Tab
ICA
   islet cell antigen
ICAM
   intercellular adhesion molecule
ICAM-1
   intercellular adhesion molecule-1
Icaps
ICARUS
   Islet Cell Antibody Registry of Users
      Study

ICCIDD
   International Council for Control of
      Iodine Deficiency Disorder
I-cell disease
ICER
   inducible cAMP early repressor
   inducible cyclic adenosine
      monophosphate early repressor
ICF
   intracellular fluid
ichthyosis
      congenital i.
      X-linked i.
ICMA
   immunochemiluminescence assay
   immunochemiluminescent assay
   immunochemiluminometric assay
ICSA
   islet cell surface antibody
ICSH
   interstitial cell-stimulating hormone
ICSI
   intracytoplasmic sperm injection
ICTP
   carboxyterminal cross-linked telopeptide
      of type I collagen
IDC
   invasive ductal carcinoma
IDD
   insulin-dependent diabetes
   iodine-deficiency disorder
IDDM
   insulin-dependent diabetes mellitus
IDE
   insulin-degrading enzyme
identical sibling
identification
      encephalomyocarditis virus gene i.
      gene i.
identity
      gender i.
idiogenic osmole
idiopathic
      i. Addison disease
      i. adrenal insufficiency
      i. aldosteronism
      i. colloid goiter
      i. complete precocious puberty
      i. diabetes
      i. diabetes insipidus
      i. exophthalmos
      i. galactorrhea
      i. gonadotropin
      i. granulomatous hypophysitis
      i. growth hormone deficiency

idiopathic *(continued)*
    i. hirsutism (IH)
    i. hyperaldosteronism (IHA)
    i. hypercalcemia of infancy
    i. hypercalciuria
    i. hyperphosphatasemia
    i. hyperprolactinemia
    i. hypogonadotropic hypogonadism (IHH)
    i. hypoparathyroidism
    i. hypopituitarism
    i. hypothalamic hypothyroidism
    i. intracranial hypertension
    i. ischemic necrosis
    i. juvenile osteoporosis
    i. myxedema
    i. orthostatic hypotension
    i. osteolysis
    i. osteoporosis in men
    i. pancreatitis
    i. panhypopituitarism
    i. parkinsonism
    i. paroxysmal myoglobinuria
    i. postprandial syndrome
    i. reactive hypoglycemia
    i. sexual precocity
    i. short stature (ISS)
    i. thrombocytopenic purpura (ITP)
    i. true precocious puberty
idioventricular pacemaker
IDL
    intermediate-density lipoprotein
IDO
    indoleamine 2,3-dioxygenase
Idox
idoxifene
IDUS
    intraductal ultrasound
IFG
    impaired fasting glucose
IFN
    interferon
IFN-alpha
    interferon-alpha
IFN-alpha$_1$
    interferon-alpha$_1$
IFN-beta
    interferon-beta
IFN-epsi
    interferon-epsilon
IFN-gamma
    interferon-gamma
IFN-omega
    interferon-omega
ifosfamide
Ig
    immunoglobulin
      Ig gene

IgA
    immunoglobulin A
IgD
    immunoglobulin D
IgE
    immunoglobulin E
IGF
    insulinlike growth factor
IGF-1
    insulinlike growth factor-1
IGF2 gene
IGF-binding
    I.-b. protein (IGFBP)
    I.-b. protein-1
IGFBP
    IGF-binding protein
    insulinlike growth factor-binding protein
IGFBP-1
    insulinlike growth factor-binding protein-1
IGFBP-2
    insulinlike growth factor-binding protein-2
IGFBP-3
    insulinlike growth factor-binding protein-3
IGFBP-4
    insulinlike growth factor-binding protein-4
IGFBP-5
    insulinlike growth factor-binding protein-5
IGFBP-6
    insulinlike growth factor-binding protein-6
IGF-I
    insulinlike growth factor-I
IGF-II
    IGF-II gene
IGF-IIR
    insulinlike growth factor-II receptor
    IGF-IIR gene
IGF-1R
    insulinlike growth factor-1 receptor
IgG
    immunoglobulin G
      aggregated human IgG (AHuG)
IGHD
    isolated growth hormone deficiency
IGHD-IB
    isolated growth hormone deficiency type IB
IGHD-II
    isolated growth hormone deficiency type II
IGHD-III
    isolated growth hormone deficiency type III

IgM
immunoglobulin M
IGT
impaired glucose tolerance
IH
idiopathic hirsutism
intracranial hypertension
IHA
idiopathic hyperaldosteronism
bilateral IHA
IHC
immunohistochemical
IHH
idiopathic hypogonadotropic
hypogonadism
IIH
iodine-induced hyperthyroidism
IITR
International Islet Transplant Registry
IJV
internal jugular vein
IJV sampling
IL
interleukin
IL-1
interleukin-1
IL-2
interleukin-2
IL-3
interleukin-3
IL-4
interleukin-4
IL-5
interleukin-5
IL-6
interleukin-6
IL-7
interleukin-7
IL-8
interleukin-8
IL-9
interleukin-9
IL-10
interleukin-10
IL-11
interleukin-11
IL-12
interleukin-12
IL-13
interleukin-13
IL-14
interleukin-14

IL-16
interleukin-16
IL-17
interleukin-17
IL-18
interleukin-18
ILA
insulinlike activity
^{131}I-labeled
^{131}I-l. iodocholesterol
^{131}I-l. metaiodobenzylguanidine (^{131}I-labeled MIBG)
^{131}I-l. MIBG
IL-1-alpha
interleukin-1-alpha
IL-1-beta
interleukin-1-beta
ileal-brake effect
Iletin
I. I
I. II Pork
Lente I. I, II
Pork Regular I. II
ileus
myxedema i.
paralytic i.
iliac artery
ill-defined nodule
illicit hormone receptor
illness
affective i.
nonthyroidal i. (NTI)
Ilozyme
IL-1RA
interleukin-1 receptor antagonist
IMA
immunometric assay
image
i. intensifier
midsagittal i.
T1-weighted i.
T2-weighted spin-echo i.
imaging
diagnostic i.
endorectal magnetic resonance i.
fluorescence i.
high-resolution coronal axis i.
intraoperative magnetic resonance i. (iMRI)
magnetic resonance i. (MRI)
radioiodine thyroid i.
radionuclide i.

NOTES

imaging *(continued)*
    sentinel node i.
    i. technique
    i. thermography
    thyroid magnetic resonance i.
imbalance
    postural i.
IMD
    immune-mediated diabetes
^{131}I-metaiodobenzylguanidine scan
^{131}I-MIBG
    iodine 131-metaiodobenzylguanidine
        ^{131}I-MIBG scan
imidazole
    i. derivative
    i. dioxolone
imidodipeptide
imiglucerase
imipramine
IMLC
    intramyocellular lipid content
immitis
    Coccidioides i.
immobilization-related hypercalcemia
immortalization
    beta-cell reversible i.
immune
    i. amyloid
    i. cell-mediated cytotoxicity
    i. complex
    i. complex glomerulonephritis
    i. dysregulation
    i. marker
    i. response antigen
    i. surveillance pathway
    i. system
immune-mediated diabetes (IMD)
immunity
    acquired i.
    active i.
    cell-mediated i.
    cellular i.
    humoral i.
    iodide-induced i.
    maternal i.
    passive i.
immunization
    paternal leukocyte i.
    peptide i.
immunoassay
    chemiluminescent i. (CLIA)
    Crosslaps i.
    enzyme i. (EIA)
    enzyme-linked i.
    Pyrilinks-D i.
    sandwich i.
    two-site sandwich i.
immunobead test
immunoblastic lymphoma

immunoblotting
immunochemiluminescence assay (ICMA)
immunochemiluminescent assay (ICMA)
immunochemiluminometric assay (ICMA)
immunocompetence
immunocytochemical
    i. analysis
    i. staining
immunocytochemistry
    neuropeptide i.
immunocytology
immunodeficiency
    combined i.
    secondary i.
    severe combined i.
immunodominant serologic determinant
immunodysregulation,
    polyendocrinopathy, enteropathy, X-
    linked syndrome
immunoelectrophoresis
immunogenetics
immunogenic glucose oxidase
immunogenicity
immunoglobulin (Ig)
    i. A (IgA)
    i. D (IgD)
    i. E (IgE)
    i. G (IgG)
    i. G gene
    intravenous i. (IVIg)
    iodothyronine-binding i.
    i. M (IgM)
    stimulatory i.
    i. synthesis
    thyroid growth i. (TGI)
    thyroid growth-blocking i. (TGBI)
    thyroid-stimulating i. (TSI)
    thyroid-stimulating hormone-binding
      inhibitor immunoglobulin i.
    thyrotropin-binding inhibitory i.
      (TBII)
    TSH-binding inhibitory i. (TBII)
    i. V gene
immunogold-labeling technique
immunogold staining
immunoheterogeneity
immunohistochemical (IHC)
    i. analysis
    i. staining
    i. staining technique
immunohistochemistry technique
immunoliposome
immunometric assay (IMA)
immunomodulator
immunomodulatory
immunoneutralization
immunopathogenesis
immunoperoxidase technique
immunophilin

immunoprecipitation assay
immunoradiometric
    i. assay (IRMA)
    i. assay of circulating calcium
    i. assay of circulating parathyroid
      hormone
immunoradiometric assay (IRMA)
immunoreactive
    i. insulin
    i. parathyroid hormone (iPTH)
immunoreactivity
    insulinlike i.
immunoregulation
immunoregulatory effect
immunoscreening
immunosenescence
immunostain
immunostaining
    endothelin i.
immunosuppression
immunosuppressive drug
immunotherapy
impaired
    i. downgaze
    i. fasting glucose (IFG)
    i. glucose counterregulation
    i. glucose tolerance (IGT)
    i. medial gaze
    i. medullary hypertonicity
    i. thirst
impairment
    beta-cell i.
    erectile i.
    glucose tolerance i.
    mineralization i.
    neurocognitive i.
impedance
    bioelectrical i.
imperfecta
    amelogenesis i.
    dentinogenesis i.
    fibrogenesis i.
    osteogenesis i. (OI)
    osteogenesis i. types I, II, III, IV
implant
    breast silicone i.
    endometriotic i.
    islet cell i.
    levonorgestrel rod i.
    LNG rod i.
    penile i.
    testosterone i.

    Uniplant contraceptive i.
    Zoladex I.
implantable
    i. biosensor
    i. glucose sensor
    i. intraperitoneal pump
    i. programmable insulin infusion
      pump
impotence
    erectile i.
    functional i.
    psychogenic i.
    stuttering i.
impression
    frank basilar i.
imprinting
    genomic i.
    glycemic i.
iMRI
    intraoperative magnetic resonance
    imaging
Imuran
in
    In Charge Diabetes Control System
    in situ hybridization
    in utero
    in vitro
    in vitro bioassay
    in vitro collagen invasion assay
    in vitro fertilization (IVF)
    in vivo
    in vivo assessment
    in vivo bioassay
    in vivo insulin gene transfer
In-111 octreotide
inactivating mutation
inactivation
    X chromosome i.
inactive
    i. agent
    i. renin concentration
inanition
inappropriate
    i. dieting
    i. hormone receptor
    i. secretion of thyroid-stimulating
     hormone
    i. secretion of TSH
Inapsine
incerta
    zona i.
incidental adrenal mass

NOTES

incidentaloma
    adrenal i.
    pituitary i.
incision
    endonasal hemitransfixion i.
incisura
    tentorial i.
inclusion cell disease
incomplete
    i. androgen resistance
    i. cell basement membrane
    i. isosexual precocity
    i. precocious puberty
    i. testicular feminization
    i. XY gonadal dysgenesis
increased
    i. adenyl cyclase activity
    i. aldosterone excretion
    i. fibrinolysis
incretin effect
incubation
    chase i.
    pulse i.
indapamide
indentation
    clival i.
Inderal
index
    baseline body mass i.
    body mass i. (BMI)
    cardiac i.
    cholecystokinin glycemic i.
    Female Sexual Function I. (FSFI)
    free T_4 i. (FT4I, FT_4I, FT4i)
    free thyroxine i. (FTI, FT4I, FT_4I, FT4i)
    glycemic i.
    hemizona assay i. (HZI)
    karyopyknotic i. (KPI)
    Ki67 i.
    Kupperman i.
    maturation i. (MI)
    penile brachial i.
    ponderal i.
    Psychological Well Being I.
    quantitative insulin sensitivity check i.
Indian hedgehog
indifferent gonad
indium-111
    i. octreotide imaging
    i. pentetreotide
Indocin
    I. I.V. Injection
    I. SR Oral
Indocollyre
indoleamine 2,3-dioxygenase (IDO)
indole hormone
indomethacin

Indotec
indoxyl sulfate
induced hypermetabolic state
inducer T lymphocyte
inducible
    i. cAMP early repressor (ICER)
    i. cyclic adenosine monophosphate early repressor (ICER)
induction
    ovulation i.
infancy
    diencephalic syndrome of i.
    idiopathic hypercalcemia of i.
    minipuberty of i.
    persistent hyperinsulinemic hypoglycemia of i. (PHHI)
infantile
    i. agranulocytosis
    i. cortical hyperostosis
    i. cystinosis
    i. embryonic carcinoma
    i. hypercalcemia
    i. osteopetrosis
infantilism
    sexual i.
infantility
    sexual i.
infarction
    Diabetes Mellitus Insulin-Glucose Infusion in Acute Myocardial I. (DIGAMI)
    diabetic muscle i.
    diabetic myocardial i.
    pituitary i.
    postpartum pituitary i.
    skeletal muscle spontaneous i.
infected pancreatic necrosis
infection
    Aspergillus i.
    bacterial i.
    congenital cytomegalovirus i.
    cryptococcal i.
    cutaneous i.
    dermatophyte i.
    filarial i.
    fungal i.
    mycotic i.
    phycomycetes i.
    sexually transmitted i. (STI)
    soft-tissue i.
    i. stone
    urinary tract i.
    viral i.
infectious
    i. adrenalitis
    i. mononucleosis
    i. thyroiditis
InFeD

inferior
- i. pancreaticoduodenal artery
- i. parathyroid artery
- i. parathyroid gland
- i. petrosal sinus
- i. petrosal sinus sampling (IPSS)
- i. phrenic artery
- i. thyroid artery

infertile
- i. male
- i. male syndrome

infertility
- anovulatory i.
- cervical factor i.
- eugonadal i.
- female i.
- male i.
- primary i.
- secondary i.

INF-gamma
- interferon gamma

infiltrate
- exuberant neutrophilic i.
- inflammatory cell i.

infiltrating
- i. ductal carcinoma
- i. lobular carcinoma

infiltration
- lymphocytic i.

infiltrative
- i. dermopathy
- i. disorder
- i. eye sign
- i. ophthalmopathy
- i. orbitopathy

inflammation
- granulomatous i.
- plica i.
- sarcoidlike noncaseating granulomatous i.
- vascular i.

inflammatory
- i. cell
- i. cell infiltrate
- i. cytokine
- i. lesion
- i. response

infliximab

influence
- inotropic i.

influx
- iodide i.
- net calcium i.

infra
- vide i.

infraclavicular fat pad

infradian rhythm

infrahyoid muscle

infundibular
- i. eminence
- i. pouch
- i. process
- i. recess
- i. stalk

infundibularis
- pars i.

infundibulohypophysial region

infundibulum
- i. eminence
- pars i.

infuser
- button i.

infusion
- bombesin i.
- continuous regional arterial i. (CRAI)
- continuous subcutaneous insulin i. (CSII)
- intracarotid artery i.
- somatostatin i.

INGAP
- islet-cell neogenesis-associated protein

ingestion
- external sex steroid i.

inhaled insulin

inhaler
- metered-dose i. (MDI)

inheritance
- Mendelian i.
- sex-linked i.
- X-linked i.

inherited
- i. disorder of ureagenesis
- i. hormone resistance syndrome

inhibin
- i. A, B
- i. hormone

inhibition
- aromatase i.
- feedback i.
- oligonucleotide i.
- short-loop i.

NOTES

inhibitor
aldose reductase i. (ARI)
allosteric i.
alpha-glucosidase i.
angiotensin-converting enzyme i.
aromatase i.
calcineurin i.
carbonic anhydrase i.
enzyme i.
farnesyl-transferase i.
gamma-aminobutyric acid
transaminase i.
glucose oxidase i.
glucosidase i.
glycoprotein crystal growth i.
(CGI)
hepatic hydroxymethylglutaryl
coenzyme A reductase i.
HMG-CoA reductase i.
iNOS i.
ionic i.
luteinization i.
mammary-derived growth i.
(MDGI)
methylglutaryl coenzyme A
reductase i.
monoamine oxidase i.
nonergot long-acting prolactin i.
oocyte meiotic i.
phosphodiesterase i.
plasminogen activator i. (PAI)
postreceptor i.
prereceptor i.
prostaglandin synthase i.
protease i.
protein kinase C i.
selective serotonin reuptake i.
(SSRI)
serine protease i. (SERPIN)
vascular endothelial cell growth i.
(VEGI)
wheat amylase i. (WAI)
inhibitor-1
plasminogen activator i.-1 (PAI-1)
inhibitor-2
plasminogen activator i.-2 (PAI-2)
inhibitory
i. factor
i. guanine nucleotide binding
regulatory protein
i. hormone
i. receptor (R_i)
i. response element (IRE)
i. transmitter
inhomogeneity
inhomogeneous texture
INIT
Intranasal Insulin Trial

initiative
The Diabetes A1C I.
injectable multiple vitamin
injection
Adlone I.
A-hydroCort I.
Amcort I.
A-methaPred I.
Andro-L.A. I.
Andropository I.
AquaMEPHYTON I.
Aristocort Forte I.
Aristocort Intralesional I.
Aristospan Intraarticular I.
Aristospan Intralesional I.
Astramorph PF I.
Ben-Allergin-50 I.
botulinum i.
Celestone Phosphate I.
Cel-U-Jec I.
Cleocin Phosphate I.
Decadron I.
Delatestryl I.
depAndro I.
depGynogen I.
depMedalone I.
Depo-Estradiol I.
Depogen I.
Depoject I.
Depo-Medrol I.
Depopred I.
Depo-Provera I.
Depotest I.
Depo-Testosterone I.
Dihyrex I.
Dilaudid I.
Dilaudid-HP I.
Dinate I.
Dioval I.
D-Med I.
Dramilin I.
Duralone I.
Duramorph I.
Duratest I.
Durathate I.
Dymenate I.
Estra-L I.
Estro-Cyp I.
Everone I.
Gynogen L.A. I.
Hectorol I.
Histerone I.
Hybolin Improved I.
Hydrate I.
Hydrocortone Acetate I.
Hydrocortone Phosphate I.
Hyzine-50 I.
Indocin I.V. I.
intracavernosal i.

intracytoplasmic sperm i. (ICSI)
Kenaject I.
Kenalog I.
Key-Pred I.
Key-Pred-SP I.
Konakion I.
Lyphocin I.
Marmine I.
Medralone I.
M-Prednisol I.
multiple daily i.'s (MDI)
multiple dose i. (MDI)
Neucalm-50 I.
Orinase Diagnostic I.
Osmitrol I.
paricalcitol i.
pegvisomant for i.
percutaneous bone marrow i.
percutaneous fine-needle ethanol i.
  (PFNEI)
Phenazine I.
Phenergan I.
Prednisol TBA I.
Prorex I.
Quiess I.
i. site
i. site rotation
Solu-Cortef I.
Solu-Medrol I.
Sublimaze I.
Tac-3, -40 I.
Tesamone I.
Triam-A I.
Triam Forte I.
Triamonide I.
Tri-Kort I.
Trilog I.
Trilone I.
Triostat I.
Trisoject I.
Ureaphil I.
Vancocin I.
Vancoled I.
Vistacon-50 I.
Vistaquel I.
Vistaril I.
Vistazine I.
zoledronic acid for i.

injector
jet i.
injury
demyelination i.

hypoxic brain i.
osmotic cell i.
parenchymal brain i.
pituitary-hypothalamic i.
radiation i.
thermal i.
vascular i.
innervate
innervated
innervation
somatostatinergic i.
InnoLet
Novolin N I.
Novolin R I.
innominate vein
Innovar
inorganic
i. iodide
i. orthophosphate (P_i)
i. phosphate
i. pyrophosphate (PPi)
iNOS inhibitor
inositol
i. diphosphate
i. 5-phosphatase
i. phosphate (IP)
i. phosphate pathway
i. triphosphate (IP3)
i. 1,4-5-triphosphate receptor (IP3R)
inositol-phospho-glycan (IPG)
i.-p.-g. headgroup mediator
inositophosphoglycan
inotropic
i. bipyridine
i. glutamate receptor antagonist
i. influence
^{111}In-pentetreotide
input
excitatory i.
insemination
intrauterine i. (IUI)
therapeutic donor i. (TDI)
insensate feet
insensitivity
congenital androgen i.
glucocorticoid i.
growth hormone i.
partial androgen i.
insert
Estring vaginal i.
insertional mutagenesis
insidious proptosis

NOTES

insipidus
>
> acquired nephrogenic diabetes i.
> central diabetes i. (CDI)
> controlled diabetes i. (CDI)
> cranial diabetes i.
> diabetes i.
> dipsogenic diabetes i.
> familial central diabetes i.
> familial nephrogenic diabetes i.
> hereditary nephrogenic diabetes i.
> hypothalamic diabetes i.
> idiopathic diabetes i.
> nephrogenic diabetes i. (NDI)
> neurogenic diabetes i.
> neurohypophysial diabetes i.
> peripheral diabetes i.
> permanent diabetes i.
> prolonged diabetes i.
> renal form of diabetes i.
> transient diabetes i.
> triphasic diabetes i.
> X-linked diabetes i.

insole
>
> Plastazote i.

instability
>
> chromosomal i.
> microsatellite i.

Insta-Glucose
instant glucose
InstantPlus
>
> Accu-Chek I.

instrumentation
>
> antegrade i.
> retrograde i.

insufficiency
>
> acute adrenal i.
> adrenal i.
> 3-beta-hydroxysteroid
>   dehydrogenase i.
> central adrenocortical i.
> chronic renal i. (CRI)
> corpus luteum i. (CLI)
> exocrine pancreatic i. (EPI)
> hepatic i.
> idiopathic adrenal i.
> Leydig cell i.
> luteal phase i.
> panadrenal i.
> pancreatic exocrine i.
> pancreatis i.
> parathyroid i.
> primary adrenocortical i.
> pseudocorpus luteum i.
> renal i.
> secondary adrenal i.
> tertiary adrenal i.

Insuflon

insular
>
> i. carcinoma
> i. pattern

insulin
>
> i. absorption
> acarbose plasma i.
> acarbose with i.
> i. action
> i. allergy
> i. analog
> i. antagonism
> i. antagonist
> i. aspart
> aspart i.
> atypical protein kinase C and i.
> autoantibodies against i.
> i. autoantibody (IAA)
> i. B
> basal i.
> bedtime i.
> beef i.
> i. binding
> i. binding affinity
> biosynthetic human i.
> biphasic i.
> bovine i.
> i. calcium transport
> i. Chicago (Phe-B25-Leu)
> i. clamp
> i. clearance
> i. compliance
> i. concentration
> i. correction factor
> crystalline zinc i. (CZI)
> i. deficiency
> i. degradation
> i. deprivation
> i. detemir
> endogenous i.
> i. factitial hypoglycemia
> fast-acting i.
> i. gene
> i. gene regulation
> i. gene transcription
> i. gene transcription factor
> i. gene transfer
> GH i.
> i. glargine
> i. growth factor
> i. growth factor-binding protein
> i. growth factor-binding protein
>   type 1–6
> growth hormone i.
> human i.
> immunoreactive i.
> i. infusion pump
> i. infusion rate
> i. infusion specialist
> inhaled i.

intermediate-acting i.
intranasal i.
intraperitoneal i.
isophane i.
i. lack
Lente i.
i. level
i. lipoatrophy
i. lipodystrophy
i. lipogenesis
i. lipohypertrophy
lispro I.
i. lispro
long-acting i.
long-lasting i.
nasal i.
neutral protamine Hagedorn i.
NPH i.
Omnican Piston syringe for i.
ophthalmic administration of i.
oral administration of i.
i. pen
phosphatidylcholine hydrolysis i.
i. phosphorylation cascade
PI3K i.
plasma i.
porcine i.
pork i.
premixed i.
i. preparation
i. preprohormone
i. promoter factor-1 (IPF-1)
protamine zinc i.
i. protease
i. pump therapy
purified pork i. (PPI)
i. receptor antibody
i. receptor family
i. receptor gene
i. receptor kinase (IRK)
i. receptor knockout (IRKO)
i. receptor-related receptor (IRR)
i. receptor substrate (IRS)
i. receptor substrate-1 (IRS-1)
i. receptor substrate-2 (IRS-2)
i. receptor substrate protein (IRS-protein)
i. receptor transmembrane domain
i. receptor tyrosine kinase (IRTK)
recombinant human i.
rectal administration of i.
Regular Purified Pork I.

i. resistance
i. response element
i. response sequence
i. secretagogue
i. secretion
i. secretory defect
i. secretory response (ISR)
semisynthetic i.
i. sensitivity
i. sensitizer
i. shock
short-acting i.
i. signaling pathway
subcutaneous i.
i. surrogate
i. surrogate value
synthetic human i.
i. target tissue
i. tolerance test (ITT)
Ultralente i.
unit of i. (U-100)
Velosulin BR i.
i. Wakayama
insulinase
insulin-autoimmune syndrome
insulin-combination regimen
insulin/C-peptide molar ratio
insulin-degrading enzyme (IDE)
insulin-dependent
    i.-d. diabetes (IDD)
    i.-d. diabetes mellitus (IDDM)
insulinemia
Insulin-Free World Foundation
insulin-IGF signaling system
insulin-induced
    i.-i. glucose
    i.-i. neuropathy
    i.-i. receptor downregulation
    i.-i. suppression of glucagon
    i.-i. systemic hypoglycemia
insulinitis
insulinlike
    i. activity (ILA)
    i. growth factor (IGF)
    i. growth factor-1 (IGF-1)
    i. growth factor-2
    i. growth factor-binding protein (IGFBP)
    i. growth factor-binding protein-1 (IGFBP-1)
    i. growth factor-binding protein-2 (IGFBP-2)

NOTES

insulinlike *(continued)*
>   i. growth factor-binding protein-3 (IGFBP-3)
>   i. growth factor-binding protein-4 (IGFBP-4)
>   i. growth factor-binding protein-5 (IGFBP-5)
>   i. growth factor-binding protein-6 (IGFBP-6)
>   i. growth factor-binding protein protease
>   i. growth factor-I (IGF-I)
>   i. growth factor-II
>   i. growth factor-II receptor (IGF-IIR)
>   i. growth factor-II receptor gene
>   i. growth factor-1 receptor (IGF-1R)
>   i. immunoreactivity

insulin-mediated glucose uptake
insulinogenesis
insulinoma
>   calcified malignant i.
>   i. cell
>   malignant i.
>   Whipple trial of i.

insulinomimetic effect
insulinopathy
insulinopenia
insulinopenic
>   i. diabetes mellitus
>   i. impaired glucose tolerance

insulinotrophic glucagonlike peptide
insulin-producing
>   i.-p. cell
>   i.-p. cell line
>   i.-p. tissue

insulin-receptor autoantibody
insulin-resistance syndrome
insulin-resistant
>   i.-r. diabetes
>   i.-r. state
>   i.-r. syndrome X

insulin-responsive aminopeptidase (IRAP)
insulin-sensitive
>   i.-s. enzyme
>   i.-s. signaling system

insulin-stimulated
>   i.-s. autophosphorylation
>   i.-s. glucose transport
>   i.-s. sympathetic activation

insulitic process
insulitis
insuloacinar portal system
insuloductular portal system
insulysin
int2
>   integration gene 2

intact
>   i. parathyroid hormone
>   i. thirst mechanism

intake
>   caloric i.
>   dietary calcium i.
>   fluid i.

Intal
integration gene 2 (int2)
integrative model of seasonality
integrin
>   i. alpha v beta 3
>   alpha v beta 3 vitronectin receptor i.

integrin-laminin interaction
intense thirst
intensified conventional therapy
intensifier
>   image i.

intensive
>   i. insulin administration
>   i. intermittent claudication
>   i. therapy

intention tremor
interaction
>   adrenocortical thyroid i.
>   agonist-receptor i.
>   cell-bone matrix i.
>   glucocorticoid i.
>   integrin-laminin i.
>   ligand-receptor i.
>   sperm-cervical mucus i.

interassay
intercalated
>   i. cell
>   i. lamella

intercellular
>   i. adhesion molecule (ICAM)
>   i. adhesion molecule-1 (ICAM-1)

interception
interconversion
intercostal nerve
interdental spacing
interdigitate
interferon (IFN)
>   i. gamma (INF-gamma)
>   i. gamma beta-cell
>   i. therapy

interferon-alpha (IFN-alpha)
>   recombinant i.-a. (rIFN-alpha)

interferon-alpha$_1$ (IFN-alpha$_1$)
interferon-alpha-induced thyroiditis
interferon-beta (IFN-beta)
interferon-epsilon (IFN-epsi)
interferon-gamma (IFN-gamma)
interferon-omega (IFN-omega)
interfollicular stroma

interieur
    milieu i.
interleukin (IL)
    i. growth factor I
    i. type 2 receptor
interleukin-1 (IL-1)
    i. receptor antagonist (IL-1RA)
interleukin-2 (IL-2)
interleukin-3 (IL-3)
interleukin-4 (IL-4)
interleukin-5 (IL-5)
interleukin-6 (IL-6)
interleukin-7 (IL-7)
interleukin-8 (IL-8)
interleukin-9 (IL-9)
interleukin-10 (IL-10)
interleukin-11 (IL-11)
interleukin-12 (IL-12)
interleukin-13 (IL-13)
interleukin-14 (IL-14)
interleukin-16 (IL-16)
interleukin-17 (IL-17)
interleukin-18 (IL-18)
interleukin-1-alpha (IL-1-alpha)
interleukin-1-beta (IL-1-beta)
interlobular fibrosis
intermedia
    massa i.
    pars i.
intermediary
    G-protein i.
intermediate
    i. lymphocytic lymphoma
    i. nucleus
    phosphorylated glycolytic i.
    i. pituitary lobe
    postreceptor signaling i.
    i. trophoblast
intermediate-acting insulin
intermediate-density lipoprotein (IDL)
intermediolateral
    i. cell column
    i. gray column
intermolecular dityrosine bridge
interna
    hyperostosis frontalis i.
    theca i.
internal
    i. capsule
    i. intraperitoneal insulin infusion
    pump

    i. jugular vein (IJV)
    i. jugular vein sampling
    i. milieu
    i. ophthalmoplegia
    i. urethra
international
    I. Council for Control of Iodine
      Deficiency Disorder (ICCIDD)
    I. Diabetes Federation
    I. Diabetes Immunotherapy Group
    I. Islet Transplant Registry (IITR)
    i. unit (IU)
interosseous atrophy
interpeduncular
    i. chiasmatic cistern
    i. fossa
interphase
Interpore
interposition method
interpositum
    velum i.
interrelationship
    hormone-fuel i.
interruption
    aortic arch i.
interstitial
    i. cell-stimulating hormone (ICSH)
    i. edema
    i. fluid (ISF)
    i. fluid compartment
    i. hyperthermic technique
    i. osmolality
    i. urea
interstitium
    renal medullary i.
intertrabecular space
intertrigo
interval
    QKd i.
    QT i.
intervening peptide (IP)
intervention
    office-based i.
interventional radiology
intervillous space
intestinal
    i. absorption
    i. bypass
    i. disease
    i. fistula
    i. function

NOTES

intestinal *(continued)*
    i. lymphectasia
    i. motility
intimal wall thickness (IWT)
intolerance
    alcohol i.
    carbohydrate i.
    cold i.
    fructose i.
    galactose i.
    glucose i.
    heat i.
    hereditary fructose i.
    lysinuric protein i.
intorsion
intoxication
    acute water i.
    aluminum i.
    chronic water i.
    syndrome of water i.
    theophylline i.
    vitamin A, D i.
    water i.
intoxification
    metal i.
intraabdominal
    i. adiposity
    i. testis
intraadrenal pressure
intraamniotic
intracarotid artery infusion
intracavernosal injection
intracavernous venous connection
intracellular
    i. calcium
    i. cAMP level
    i. cyclic adenosine monophosphate level
    i. effector enzyme
    i. fluid (ICF)
    i. function
    i. homeostasis
    i. insulin storage
    i. killing
    i. lipotoxicity
    i. lysosomal membrane
    i. messenger
    i. metabolic process
    i. receptor
    i. signaling
    i. signaling pathway
    i. solute
    i. store
intracellulare
    Mycobacterium i.
intracranial hypertension (IH)
intracrine action

intracystic
    i. radiation therapy
    i. radiotherapy
intracytoplasmic
    i. oncocytic change
    i. sperm injection (ICSI)
intraductal
    i. mucinous hyperplasia
    i. oncocytic papillary neoplasm (IOPN)
    i. pancreatic adenoma
    i. papillary mucinous neoplasm (IPMN)
    i. papilloma
    i. ultrasound (IDUS)
intraglandular
    i. fibrous septa
    i. lymphatic network
intrahepatic
    i. bile duct
    i. cholestasis
intrahepatocellular triglyceride accumulation
intra-HLA recombination
intrahypophyseal
    i. portal vessel
    i. pressure
intralesional fluorinated steroid
intralobular
    i. duct
    i. fibrosis
intramembranous
    i. bone
    i. ossification
intramitochondrial compartment
Intra-Mix
    Genotropin I.-M.
intramural uterine part
intramuscular
    i. immune globulin
    i. testosterone
intramyocellular lipid content (IMLC)
intranasal
    i. desmopressin
    i. insulin
    I. Insulin Trial (INIT)
intraocular pressure
intraoperative
    i. magnetic resonance imaging (iMRI)
    i. radiotherapy
    i. ultrasound (IOUS)
intraovarian
    i. regulator
    i. rest
intrapancreatic calculus
intrapenile nitric oxide
intraperitoneal
    i. insulin

i. lavage
i. reinfusion
intrapituitary adenoma
intrasellar
i. adenohypophyseal neuronal choristoma
i. adenoma
i. cavity
i. cystic lesion
i. gangliocytoma
i. hydatid cyst
i. pressure
i. tuberculoma
intratesticular adrenal rest
intrathoracic
i. goiter
i. goitrous component
intrathyroglobulin iodotyrosine coupling reaction
intrathyroid
B-cell i.
i. iodide concentration
intrathyroidal primary
intrauterine
i. device (IUD)
i. growth chart
i. growth retardation (IUGR)
i. hyperglycemia
i. insemination (IUI)
intravaginal
i. dose
i. estrogen
intravascular
i. compartment
i. volume
intravenous
i. glucose tolerance test (IVGTT)
i. immunoglobulin (IVIg)
i. pamidronate
i. urography
intraviral microscopy
intrinsic
i. gut neuron
i. response
intron
invasion
basophilic cell i.
i. suppressive factor
invasive
i. ductal carcinoma (IDC)
i. fibrous thyroiditis

i. hormonally active pituitary adenoma
i. hormonally inactive pituitary adenoma
i. macroprolactinoma
i. prolactinoma
inversus
situs i.
involute
involution
lymph node i.
splenic i.
thymic i.
involutional osteoporosis
inward-directed voltage-gated Ca^{2+} channel
inward-rectifying K$^+$-channel 6.2 (K$_{ir}$6.2)
iodide
calcium i.
i. channel
i. deficiency
i. efflux
fluorescent i.
i. goiter
i. influx
inorganic i.
i. organification defect
potassium i.
i. pump
saturated solution of potassium i. (SSKI)
supersaturated potassium i. (SSKI)
i. symporter
i. transport
i. transport defect
i. trap
i. trapping
i. trapping function
iodide-127
iodide-induced
i.-i. autoimmunity
i.-i. immunity
iodinase enzyme
iodinated
i. contrast dye
i. contrast media
i. glycerol
iodination
thyroglobulin i.
iodine
butanol-extractable i.
i. deficiency

NOTES

iodine *(continued)*
  i. 131-metaiodobenzylguanidine (^{131}I-MIBG)
  i. organification defect
  polyvinylpyrrolidone i.
  radioactive i. (^{131}I, RAI)
  i. release
  i. tincture
iodine-123 (^{123}I)
iodine-125 (^{125}I)
iodine-127 (^{127}I)
iodine-131 (^{131}I)
  i.-131 isotope
  i.-131 therapy
  i.-131 total body scan (^{131}I-TBS)
iodine-deficiency
  i.-d. disorder (IDD)
  i.-d. goiter
iodine-deficient goiter
iodine-induced
  i.-i. hyperthyroidism (IIH)
  i.-i. hypothyroidism
  i.-i. thyrotoxicosis
iodine-perchlorate discharge test
iodine-replete goitrous population
iodine-trapping defect
iodism
iodization
  universal salt i. (USI)
iodized oil
iodo-4-azidophenetylamido-7-O-succinyldeacetyl forskolin (IAPS-forskolin)
iodoacetate
iodoalbumin
iodoamino acid
iodocholesterol
  ^{131}I-labeled i.
  i. scan
iodoglibenclamide
iodolipid compound
Iodo-Niacin
Iodopen
iodophenoxyl group
iodophor
iodoprotein
iodothyronine
  i. coupling
  i. deiodinase
  i. metabolism
  i. ring
iodothyronine-binding immunoglobulin
iodothyronine metabolism
iodotyrosine
  i. coupling
  i. coupling defect
  i. dehalogenase
  i. dehalogenase defect
  radioiodinated i.

iodotyrosine-specific deiodinase
iodotyrosyl
ion
  calcium i.
  carbonate i.
  i. channel
  citrate i.
  divalent i.
  i. exchange chromatography
  hydrogen i.
  isocitrate i.
  phosphate i.
  potassium i. (K^+)
Ionamin
ion-exchange resin
ionic
  i. calcium
  i. inhibitor
  i. strength
  i. transport
ionized
  i. calcium concentration
  i. calcium level
ionizing radiation
ionomycin
ionophore
  calcium i.
ion-selective electrode
iontophoretic sampling procedure
iopanoate
  sodium i.
iopanoic acid
Iophen
IOPN
  intraductal oncocytic papillary neoplasm
IOUS
  intraoperative ultrasound
ioxaglate
  meglumine i.
IP
  inositol phosphate
  intervening peptide
IP3
  inositol triphosphate
IPEX
  I. disorder
  I. syndrome
IPF-1
  insulin promoter factor-1
IPG
  inositol-phospho-glycan
IPH
  isolated postchallenge hyperglycemia
IPMN
  intraductal papillary mucinous neoplasm
IPM wound gel
ipodate
  sodium i.

IP3R
  inositol 1,4-5-triphosphate receptor
ipratropium and albuterol
ipriflavone
ipsilateral paramesonephric duct
IPSS
  inferior petrosal sinus sampling
iPTH
  immunoreactive parathyroid hormone
IRAP
  insulin-responsive aminopeptidase
Ircon
IRE
  inhibitory response element
iridis
  rubeosis i.
iridium
  heterochromia i.
IRK
  insulin receptor kinase
IRKO
  insulin receptor knockout
IRMA
  immunoradiometric assay
iron (Fe)
  i. clearance
  i. deposition
  i. dextran complex
  i. overload
  Prussian blue stain for i.
  i. storage disease
  i. turnover
iron-binding protein
IRR
  insulin receptor-related receptor
irradiation
  childhood head and neck i.
  cranial i.
  fractionated linear accelerator-
    based i.
  pituitary i.
irrigation
  therapeutic i.
IRS
  insulin receptor substrate
IRS-1
  insulin receptor substrate-1
IRS-2
  insulin receptor substrate-2
IRS-protein
  insulin receptor substrate protein

IRTK
  insulin receptor tyrosine kinase
ISAtx247
ischemia
  diffuse renal i.
  mesenteric i.
  nonocclusive mesenteric i. (NOMI)
  skeletal muscle i.
ischemia-induced retinopathy
ischemic necrosis
ischiocavernosus muscle
ISF
  interstitial fluid
islet
  i. after kidney (IAK)
  i. allograft
  i. alpha-cell
  i. amyloid
  i. amyloid polypeptide (IAPP)
  i. antigen autoantibody (IAA)
  i. antigen 2 autoantibody
  i. antigen autoantibody microassay
  i. autoantigen
  i. autograft
  i. autoimmunity
  i. beta-cell
  i. beta-cell hyperinsulinemia
  capsule of i.
  i. cell
  i. cell adenoma
  i. cell adenomatosis
  I. Cell Antibody Registry of Users
    Study (ICARUS)
  i. cell antigen (ICA)
  i. cell autoantibody
  i. cell carcinoma
  i. cell cytoplasmic antibody
  i. cell implant
  i. cell surface antibody (ICSA)
  i. cell transplant
  i. cell transplantation
  i. cell tumor
  cytokine studies in isolated
    pancreatic i.'s
  i. encapsulation
  encephalomyocarditis virus i.
  i. gene
  i. of Langerhans
  mantle i.
  i. microscopy
  pseudoatrophic i.
  i. transcription factor

NOTES

islet *(continued)*
  i. transplantation alone (ITA)
  i. xenograft
islet-cell neogenesis-associated protein (INGAP)
Isletest ICA kit
isletitis
Ismotic
isoandrosterone
isobologram analysis
iso-B prolactin
isobutyric acid
isocalorically substituted diet
isocaproate
isochromosome
isocitrate ion
isodisomic chromosome
isoechoic
isoelectric focusing
isoenzyme
  brain i.
  carbonic anhydrase II i.
  4-galactosyltransferase i. II
  GalTase i. II
isoetharine
  Arm-a-Med i.
  Dey-Lute i.
isoflavone
  red clover-derived i.
  soy i.
isoform
  fibronectin peptide i.
  melanocortin receptor i.
  protein kinase C i.
  thyroid hormone nuclear receptor i.
isoform-specific thyroid hormone receptor
isohormone
isointense
isokinetic dynamometer
isolated
  i. familial somatotropinoma
  i. gonadotropin deficiency
  i. growth hormone deficiency (IGHD)
  i. growth hormone deficiency type IB (IGHD-IB)
  i. growth hormone deficiency type II (IGHD-II)
  i. growth hormone deficiency type III (IGHD-III)
  i. hypopituitarism
  i. peripheral nerve lesion
  i. postchallenge hyperglycemia (IPH)
isoleucine
  peptide histidine i. (PHI)
  i. transaminase

isomerase
  i. dehydrogenase deficiency
  disulfide i.
  protein disulfide i. (PDI)
  triose isomerase
isoniazid
isoosmolar semielemental formula
isopeptide
  endothelin i.
isophane insulin
isoprenoid
isoproterenol
  Arm-a-Med i.
  Dey-Dose i.
  i. phosphodiesterase 3B regulation
Isoptin
isopycnic centrifugation
isosexual
  i. precocious puberty
  i. precocity
  i. pubertal development
isosmotic
isosorbide
isothiocyanate
4,4′-di-isothiocyanatostilbene-2,2′-disulfonic acid (DIDS)
isotonicity
isotonic saline
isotope
  i. dilution
  gold-198 radioactive i.
  ^{131}I i.
  iodine-131 i.
  i. scanning
  yttrium-90 radioactive i.
isotopic glucose tracer
isotretinoin
isovaleric
  i. acid
  i. acidemia
isovaleryl-CoA dehydrogenase
isovalerylglycine
isoxsuprine
isozyme
ISR
  insulin secretory response
ISS
  idiopathic short stature
isthmectomy
isthmus
  thyroid i.
  i. uterus
Isuprel
ITA
  islet transplantation alone
^{131}I-TBS
  iodine-131 total body scan
ITP
  idiopathic thrombocytopenic purpura

itraconazole
I-Tropine
ITT
    insulin tolerance test
IU
    international unit
IUD
    intrauterine device
        Progestasert IUD
IUGR
    intrauterine growth retardation
IUI
    intrauterine insemination

IV
    hexokinase IV
IVF
    in vitro fertilization
IVGTT
    intravenous glucose tolerance test
IVIg
    intravenous immunoglobulin
IWT
    intimal wall thickness

NOTES

Jaa-Prednisone
Jackson-Weiss syndrome
Jadelle
JAK, Jak
 Janus kinase
Jak1 kinase
Jak2
 Janus kinase 2
 Jak2 kinase
Jakob-Creutzfeldt disease
Jamaican vomiting disease
Jansen metaphyseal chondrodysplasia
 (JMC)
Janus
 J. kinase (JAK, Jak)
 J. kinase 1
 J. kinase 2 (Jak2)
 J. kinase STAT
jaundice
 cholestatic j.
jejunocolic anastomosis
jejunoileal bypass
jejunostomy
 feeding j.
 needle catheter j.
jejunum
jelly
 Wharton j.
Jenest-28
Jerusalem syndrome
jet injector
Jew
 Ashkenazi J.
JG
 juxtaglomerular
 JG cell
JGA
 juxtaglomerular apparatus
JMC
 Jansen metaphyseal chondrodysplasia
JMV1155 gastrin receptor antagonist
JNK
 cJunN-terminal kinase
 Jun kinase
 Jun N-terminal kinase
JOD
 juvenile-onset diabetes
Jod-Basedow, jodbasedow
 J.-B. disease
 J.-B. effect
 J.-B. mechanism
 J.-B. phenomenon
Joffroy sign
Johanson-Blizzard syndrome
joint
 apophyseal j.

 Charcot j.
 cricothyroid j.
 j. hyperextensibility
Joslin Diabetes Center
Jost model
J-shaped sella
J-type diabetes
jugular
 j. bulb
 j. chain
juice
 pancreatic j.
 pure pancreatic j. (PPJ)
Jun
 J. kinase (JNK)
 J. N-terminal kinase (JNK)
 J. N-terminal kinase exercise
 J. N-terminal kinase serine
  phosphorylation
junction
 adherens j.
 beta-cell gap j.
 endothelial tight j.
 gap j.
 hypothalamic-midbrain j.
 mesodiencephalic j.
 ribosome-membrane j.
 tight j.
 ureteropelvic j.
 ureterovesical j.
junctional scotoma
junk food
Jurkat cell
juvenile
 j. Austin-type sulfatidosis
 j. cystinosis
 j. diabetes
 J. Diabetes Research Foundation
 j. hypothyroidism
 j. papillomatosis
 j. pilocytic astrocytoma
juvenile-onset
 j.-o. diabetes (JOD)
 j.-o. diabetes mellitus
juxtacrine factor
juxtaglomerular (JG)
 j. afferent arteriole
 j. apparatus (JGA)
 j. cell
 j. function
 j. stretch receptor
juxtamembrane
juxtathyroidal tissue
juxtathyroid node

J

K
    potassium
        cathepsin K
        neuromedin K
        Pen-Vee K
        substance K
K$^+$
    potassium ion
K$_1$
    vitamin K$_1$
K$_2$
    vitamin K$_2$
K$_5$
    vitamin K$_5$
K$_6$
    vitamin K$_6$
K$_7$
    vitamin K$_7$
K$_a$
    equilibrium association constant
Kabi International Growth Study (KIGS)
Kahn syndrome
kainate receptor channel
KAL gene
Kalgutkar
KALIG-1
    Kallmann syndrome interval gene 1
kaliuresis
kaliuretic stimulus
kallidin
    desArg k.
kallikrein
    k. activator
    glandular k.
    plasma k.
    k. protease
    tissue k.
kallikrein-1
    human kidney glandular k.-1
kallikrein-kinin system
Kallmann
    K. syndrome
    K. syndrome interval gene 1 (KALIG-1)
kansasii
    Mycobacterium k.
kaolin
Kaposi
    K. sarcoma
    K. sarcoma human growth factor (hFGF)
Kapseals
    Thera-Combex H-P K.

kaput
    circadian locomotor output cycles k. (CLOCK)
Kartagener syndrome
Karydakis
    K. flap
    K. operation
    K. technique
karyopyknotic index (KPI)
karyotype
    classical XO k.
    human k.
karyotyping
katacalcin (KC)
K$_{ATP}$
    potassium$_{ATP}$
Kaybovite-1000
Kayexalate
kb
    kilobase
KC
    katacalcin
Kcal
    kilocalorie
KCNJ1
    potassium inwardly-rectifying channel, subfamily J, member 1
    KCNJ1 gene
^{40}K counting
K$_d$
    equilibrium dissociation constant
kd
    adipocyte complement related protein of 30 k. (ACPR30)
9-kDA
    calbindin 9-k.
kDa
    kilodalton
    185 kDa phosphoprotein (pp185)
8-kDa protein
37-kDa protein
150-kDa ternary complex
Kearns-Sayre
    K.-S. disease
    K.-S. syndrome
Kell antigen genotyping
Kelly clamp
keloid formation
Kenacort Oral
Kenaject Injection
Kenalog Injection
Kennedy
    K. disease
    K. syndrome
Kenny Caffey syndrome

K

keratan sulfate
keratin
    acellular desquamated k.
    k. content
    wet k.
keratinization
keratinocyte growth factor (KGF)
keratitis
    exposure k.
keratoconjunctivitis
    superior limbic k.
keratography
keratohyaline granule
keratopathy
    band k.
keratosis
    palmar k.
    palmoplantar k.
    k. pilaris
    plantar k.
Kestrone
ketamine adduct
ketoacid disorder
ketoacidosis
    alcoholic k. (AKA)
    diabetic k. (DKA)
ketoaciduria
    branch chain k.
ketoconazole
3-keto-desogestrel
ketogenesis
17-ketogenic steroid
ketogenic steroid
keto group
ketone body
ketonemia
ketonuria
ketoprofen
17-ketoreductase
ketorolac tromethamine
ketosis
    exercise-induced k.
    starvation k.
ketosis-prone diabetes
ketosis-resistant diabetes
KetoSite test
ketosteroid
17-ketosteroid
    17-k. reductase (17-KR)
    17-k. reductase deficiency
    urinary 17-k.
3-ketothiolase deficiency
ketotic hypoglycemia
Key-Pred Injection
Key-Pred-SP Injection
kg
    kilogram
KGF
    keratinocyte growth factor

Ki
    antibody Ki
Ki67
    K. grade
    K. index
kidney
    k. failure
    islet after k. (IAK)
    pancreas after k. (PAK)
    simultaneous pancreas and k.
     (SPK)
    k. threshold
KIGS
    Kabi International Growth Study
killer
    lymphokine-activated k. (LAK)
    natural k. (NK)
    natural k. T (NKT)
killing
    bactericidal k.
    intracellular k.
kilobase (kb)
kilocalorie (Kcal)
kilodalton (kDa)
kilogram (kg)
    osmoles per k. (Osm/kg)
Kimmelstiel-Wilson
    K.-W. nodular lesion
    K.-W. nodule
kinase
    activinlike receptor k.
    adenosine monophosphate-activated
     protein k. (AMPK)
    Akt oncogenic serine-threonine k.
    AMP-activated protein k. (AMPK)
    beta-adrenergic receptor k. (beta-
     ARK)
    Bruton tyrosine k.
    calcium-dependent protein k.
    calmodulin-dependent protein k.
     (CaM-kinase)
    carboxyl k.
    casein k. I, II
    cGMP-dependent protein k.
    cJunN-terminal k. (JNK)
    conserved helix-loop-helix
     ubiquitous k. (CHUK)
    creatine k. (CK)
    cyclic adenosine monophosphate
     dependent protein k.
    cyclic guanosine 3′,5′-
     monophosphate-dependent
     protein k.
    cyclin-dependent k. (CDK, Cdk)
    cytokinin-regulated k.
    cytokinin-regulated k. I, II
    cytokinin-regulated k. L
    extracellularly regulated k. (ERK)
    extracellular-regulated k.

K

NOTES

Knudson
    K. model of tumor suppression gene
    K. two-hit model of tumorigenesis
Kobberling-Dunnigan syndrome
Kocher-Debré-Sémélaigne syndrome
Kolephrin GG/DM
Konakion Injection
Kornchenzellen cell
Korotkoff sound
Kozak consensus translation initiation sequence
K-Phos Neutral tablet
KPI
    karyopyknotic index
17-KR
    17-ketosteroid reductase
Krabbe disease
Krebs cycle
Krebs-Ringer solution
Krev-1 gene

kringle domain
KT
    Orudis KT
Kulchitsky cell
Kumetrix microneedle technology
Kupffer
    K. cell
    K. cell hyperplasia
Kupperman index
kuru
Kussmaul sign
Ku-Zyme HP
Kveim test
kwashiorkor
    k. disease
    k. syndrome
Kwelcof
Kyrle disease
kystis
Kyte-Doolittle hydropathy analysis

L
liter
cathepsin L
L cell
Humulin L
L₁
vitamin L_1
L₂
vitamin L_2
LA
laparoscopic adrenalectomy
label
luminescent l.
labeling
tetracycline l.
labetalol
labial fusion agglutination
labile
l. diabetes
l. previtamin D_3
lability
lack
insulin l.
lacrimal
l. gland
l. nucleus
l. system
lactacidosis
lactalbumin
lactase gene
lactate
calcium l.
l. dehydrogenase (LDH)
sodium l.
lactational amenorrhea
lactation optic neuritis
lactic
l. acid
l. acidosis
l. dehydrogenase
lactiferous
l. duct
l. sinus
lactobacillus
l. acidophilus
l. bifidus
lactoferrin
lactogen
human placental l. (hPL)
placental l.
lactogenesis
lactogenic hormone
lactogogue
lactose synthase
lactotrope

lactotroph
l. adenoma
l. hyperplasia
l. tumor
lactotropic hormone
lacuna, pl. **lacunae**
osteoclastic resorption l.
resorption l.
LADA
latent autoimmune diabetes of adults
laeve
chorion l.
laevis
Xenopus l.
lag
l. effect
lid l.
lagophthalmos
LAK
lymphokine-activated killer
LAK cell
lambdoidal suture
lamella, pl. **lamellae**
circumferential l.
intercalated l.
lamellar bone
lamina, pl. **laminae**
basal l.
dental l.
l. dura
l. propria
l. terminalis
laminated calcification
laminin (LN)
l. B1 element
l. deposition
l. enzyme
laminography
lampbrush state
Lanacaps
Ferralyn L.
Lanaphilic Topical
lancet
Haemolance l.
MPD Pro l.
Safe-T-Lance Plus l.
TechLite l.
Langerhans
L. cell
L. cell histiocyte
L. cell histiocytosis
islet of L.
Langer mesomelic dysplasia
Langhans cytotrophoblast
lanosterol

L

lanreotide
> slow-release l.

lansoprazole

lanthanum-containing compound

Lantus

LAP
> latency-associated peptide
> liver-enriched activating protein

LAP-1
> Los Angeles preservation solution 1

laparoscopic adrenalectomy (LA)

laparoscopy
> lateral transabdominal l.

LAR
> long-acting release
>> octreotide LAR
>> Parlodel LAR
>> Sandostatin LAR

large
> l. cell calcifying Sertoli cell tumor
> l. fiber neuropathy
> l. for gestational age (LGA)

large-needle aspiration biopsy (LNAB)

large-volume paracentesis (LVP)

L-arginine:nitric oxide pathway

Larodopa

Laron
> L. disease
> L. dwarfism
> L. syndrome

Laron-type dwarfism (LTD)

laryngeal nerve

laryngomalacia

laryngospasm

laser
> Altea MicroPor l.
> argon l.
> l. Doppler flowmetry
> l. photocoagulation
> l. prostatectomy
> pulsed dye l.

Lasette
> L. laser lancing device
> Personal L.
> L. Plus assisted blood sampling device

Lasix

lasofoxifene

L-asparaginase

last menstrual period (LMP)

late
> l. distal tubule
> l. dumping syndrome (LDS)
> l. hypocalcemia
> l. hypoglycemia
> l. luteal phase
> l. luteal phase disorder
> l. onset hydroxylase deficiency

latency-associated peptide (LAP)

late-night salivary cortisol test

latent
> l. autoimmune diabetes
> l. autoimmune diabetes of adults (LADA)
> l. tetany

late-onset
> l.-o. gynecomastia
> l.-o. idiopathic chronic pancreatitis

lateral
> l. aberrant thyroid
> l. aberrant thyroid tissue
> l. cricoarytenoid
> l. hypothalamus
> l. rectus palsy
> l. retrochiasmatic area
> l. sellar compartment
> l. thyroid anlage
> l. tibial prominence
> l. transabdominal laparoscopy
> l. zone

lateralization
> pituitary tumor l.

LATS
> long-acting thyroid stimulator
>> LATS protector

LATS-P
> long-acting thyroid stimulator-protector

Laurence-Moon-Biedl syndrome

Laurence-Moon syndrome

LAV
> lymphadenopathy-associated virus

lavage
> bronchial l.
> intraperitoneal l.

law
> Hardy-Weinberg l.

Lawrence syndrome

layer
> endothelial l.
> Nitabuch l.

LBD
> ligand-binding domain

LBM
> lean body mass

LBW
> low birth weight

LCAcoA
> long chain acyl CoAs

LCAD
> long chain acyl-CoA dehydrogenase
>> LCAD deficiency

L-Carnitine

LCAT
> lecithin-cholesterol acyltransferase
>> LCAT deficiency

LC-CoAs
> long chain acyl CoAs

LCED
    liquid chromatography with
    electrochemical detection
LCFA-CoA
    long chain fatty acyl-CoA
LCHAD
    long chain 3-hydroxyacyl-CoA
    dehydrogenase
        LCHAD deficiency
LCMV
    lymphocytic choriomeningitis virus
LDH
    lactate dehydrogenase
LDL
    low-density lipoprotein
        LDL deficiency
        dense LDL
        LDL direct test
        LDL receptor-related protein (LRP)
LDL-C
    low-density lipoprotein cholesterol
L-dopa test
LDS
    late dumping syndrome
LDSST
    low-dose short synacthen test
LE
    leucine enkephalin
leader
    aminoterminal l.
lead hematoxylin
leafy chorion
leaking endometrioma
leaky splice mutation
lean
    l. body mass (LBM)
    l. physique
    l. tissue
Leber hereditary optic neuropathy
lecithin
lecithin-cholesterol acyltransferase
  (LCAT)
lecithin/sphingomyelin (L/S)
    l. ratio
Lederplex
left
    l. anterior mediastinal adenoma
    l. temporal projection
leg
    bow l.
    l. glucose uptake (LGU)
    L. Thing pump holder

Legionella pneumophila **pneumonia**
Leiden mutation
Leigh disease
leiomyoma
    early-onset uterine l.
    spermatic cord l.
    uterine l.
leiomyosarcoma
    gastric epithelioid l.
Leishmania major
Leksell
    L. Gamma Knife
    L. model G stereotactic frame
Lemmel syndrome
length
    erect penile l.
    femur l.
    flaccid penile l.
    penile l.
    stretched penile l.
Lente
    L. Iletin I, II
    L. insulin
lentiginosis syndrome
lentis
    ectopia l.
Lenz-Majewski syndrome
Lep gene
leprae
    Mycobacterium l.
leprechaunism
    l. syndrome
leptin
    l. concentration
    l. deficiency
    l. deficiency/resistance
    l. paradox
    l. receptor gene
leptomeninges
Leri-Weill dyschondrosteosis (LWD)
LES
    lower esophageal sphincter
Lesch-Nyhan
    L.-N. disease
    L.-N. syndrome
lesion
    adynamic bone l.
    aplastic bone l.
    benign cystic l.
    blade-of-grass l.
    blueberry l.
    café au lait l.

L

NOTES

lesion *(continued)*
    cortisol-secreting l.
    cystic bone l.
    extraglandular l.
    glandular l.
    gummatous l.
    hypophysial l.
    inflammatory l.
    intrasellar cystic l.
    isolated peripheral nerve l.
    Kimmelstiel-Wilson nodular l.
    lipid-rich l.
    low-turnover bone l.
    mixed bone l.
    neoplastic pathologic l.
    nonneoplastic pathologic l.
    osteolytic l.
    pagetic bone l.
    polyostotic l.
    polypoid l.
    rachitic-like l.
    strawberry l.
    suprasellar cystic l.
    trophoblastic l.
lethal paroxysm
letrozole
Letterer-Siwe disease
leu-7 antigen
leucine
    l. enkephalin (LE)
    l. rich repeat (LRR)
    l. zipper gene family
leucine-zipper domain
leucovorin
leu-enkephalin
leukemia
    acute lymphoblastic l.
    acute lymphocytic l. (ALL)
    acute myelogenous l.
    adult T-cell l. (ATL)
    chronic granulocytic l. (CGL)
    chronic myelogenous l. (CML)
    l. inhibitory factor (LIF)
    radiation-induced l.
leukemoid reaction
leukocyte
    l. antigen-related phosphatase (LRP)
    l. common antigen
leukocytosis
    polymorphonuclear l.
leukodystrophy
    globoid cell l.
    metachromatic l. (MLD)
    sudanophilic l.
leukoencephalitis
leukoerythroblastic anemia
leukoma
    acromegaly, cutis verticis, l. (ACL)
    corneal l.

leukomalacia
    periventricular l. (PVL)
leukopenia
leukorrhea
leukosis
leukotriene (LT)
    l. A_4 (LTA_4)
    l. B_4 (LTB_4)
    l. C_4 (LTC_4)
    l. D_4 (LTD_4)
    l. E_4 (LTE_4)
leukovirus
leuprolide acetate
levalbuterol
levamisole
Levbid
LeVeen shunt
level
    albumin-bound testosterone l.
    aldolase l.
    aluminum bone l.
    antithrombin III l.
    antithyroperoxidase l.
    apo-AI l.
    basal aluminum l.
    basal plasma GH l.
    basal plasma growth hormone l.
    basal serum prolactin l.
    bioavailable testosterone l.
    cerebrospinal fluid ACE l.
    cerebrospinal fluid angiotensin-
      converting enzyme l.
    circulating estrogen l.
    complement l.
    C-peptide l.
    cryoglobulin l.
    elastase-1 l.
    endothelin l.
    fasting glucose l.
    free testosterone l.
    gonadal steroid l.
    homocysteine l.
    hormone serum l.
    insulin l.
    intracellular cAMP l.
    intracellular cyclic adenosine
      monophosphate l.
    ionized calcium l.
    Lp(a) l.
    normal gonadal steroid l.
    Osteocalcin l.
    out-of-target blood glucose l.
    plasma ACTH l.
    plasma aluminum l.
    plasma endothelin l.
    plasma galanin l.
    plasma growth hormone-releasing
      hormone l.
    plasma homocysteine l.

plasma insulin l.
plasma ketone l.
plasma testosterone l.
postchallenge glucose l.
preinfusion l.
procollagen l.
proinsulin l.
P-selectin l.
random cortisol l.
salivary cortisol l.
serum C-peptide l.
serum dehydroepiandrosterone
 sulfate l.
serum fructosamine l.
serum growth hormone l.
serum parathyroid hormone l.
sex steroid l.
somatomedin C l.
supranormal gonadal steroid l.
thyroglobulin l.
urine glucose l.
urine hydroxyproline l.
Levi-Lorain dwarf
Levitra
Levlen
Levlite
levoamphetamine
levodopa and carbidopa
Levo-Dromoran
levonorgestrel
ethinyl estradiol and l.
l. rod implant
Levoprome
Levora
levormeloxifene
levorphanol
Levo-T
Levothroid
levothyroxine
free l.
l. sodium
l. suppression therapy
Levoxyl
Levsin
Levsinex
Levsin/SL
Lewis
axon response of L.
triple response of L.
Lewis[a]
sialyl L.

Leydig
L. cell
L. cell agenesis
L. cell aplasia
L. cell hyperplasia
L. cell hypoplasia
L. cell insufficiency
L. cells of the testis
L. cell tumor
LFA-1
lymphocyte function-associated antigen-1
LGA
large for gestational age
LGU
leg glucose uptake
LH
luteinizing hormone
lutropin
LH interpulse secretion
LH-androstenedione
LH-beta
luteinizing hormone-beta
LH-dependent androgen excess
Lhermitte-Duclos disease
LH/hCG
luteinizing hormone/human chorionic
 gonadotropin
LH-leptin
**LH-releasing hormone (LHRH, LH-RH,
 LRH)**
LHRH, LH-RH, LRH
LH-releasing hormone
luteinizing hormone-releasing hormone
LHRH deficiency
LH-testosterone
LHX gene mutation
libido
decreased l.
libitum
ad l.
Librax
lichen
l. myxedematosus
l. sclerosus
lichenified dermatitis
licorice-induced
l.-i. hypermineralocorticoidism
l.-i. hypertension
l.-i. hypokalemia
lid
l. erythema

NOTES

lid *(continued)*
l. fissure
l. lag
Liddle
L. syndrome
L. test
LIF
leukemia inhibitory factor
LifeGuide
L. glucose meter
L. System
LifeScan
L. Profile
L. Ultra
lifestyle
sedentary l.
type 2 diabetes mellitus l.
life-years
quality-adjusted l.-y. (QALYs)
Li-Fraumeni syndrome
ligament
Berry l.
broad l.
falciform l.
gastrohepatic l.
ovarian l.
round l.
ligamentum
l. arteriosum
l. flavum
ligand
A proliferation-inducing l. (APRIL)
4-1BB l. (4-1BBL)
l. binding determinant
CD 27 l. (CD 27L)
CD 30 l. (CD 30L)
CD 40 l.
c-*mpl* l.
erb B2/HER2 l.
E-selectin l.
Fas l. (Fas-L)
osteoprotegerin l. (OPGL)
peroxisome proliferator-activated
receptor-gamma l.
polypeptide l.
PPAR l.
PPAR-alpha l.
PPAR-delta l.
PPAR-gamma retinoid X
receptor l.
radioactive l.
TNF-related apoptosis inducing l.
(TRAIL)
ligand-binding domain (LBD)
ligand-dependent
l.-d. action of thyroid hormone
receptor
l.-d. transcriptional activation
PPAR-gamma

l.-d. transcriptional repression
PPAR-gamma
ligand-directed modulator
ligand-gated channel
ligand-independent
l.-i. action of thyroid hormone
receptor
l.-i. stimulation
ligand-receptor
l.-r. complex
l.-r. interaction
ligase
glutamate-cysteine l.
light
psoralen and ultraviolet A l.
(PUVA)
lignan
lignin
Liliequist membrane
limb
adrenal gland l.
l. ataxia
thick ascending l. (TAL)
thickened adrenal l.
limbic
l. lobe
l. system
limbus
nasal l.
LIM homeodomain transcription factor
limitans
sulcus l.
limited
l. fragment proteolysis
l. joint mobility (LJM)
Limitrol-DM
linamarin
lindane
line
AtT20 pituitary cell l.
canthomeatal l.
cement l.
Colo-205 colorectal cancer cell l.
colorectal cancer cell l.
DLD-1 colorectal cancer cell l.
l. of Farré
Fischer rat thyroid l.-5
HCT-116 colorectal cancer cell l.
insulin-producing cell l.
milk l.
Muercke l.
multiple myeloma cell l.
pituitary cell l.
thyroid T-cell l. (TCL)
Lineac particle beam radiotherapy
lineage
chondrocytic l.
linear nevus sebaceous syndrome

linguae
>foramen caecum l.

lingual
>l. thyroid
>l. thyroid gland

linkage
>diphenyl ether l.
>l. disequilibrium
>haplotype l.
>phosphodiester l.
>X-chromosome l.

linoleic acid
linomide
liothyronine sodium
liotrix
LIP
>liver-enriched inhibiting protein

lipase
>hepatic l.
>hormone-sensitive l. (HSL)
>lipoprotein l. (LPL)
>preduodenal l.

lipectomy
lipemia
>postprandial l.
>l. retinalis

lipid
>l. abnormality
>l. cholesterol
>l. derivative
>l. disorder
>extramyocellular l. (EMCL)
>l. homeostasis
>l. metabolism
>l. myopathy
>l. panel
>l. peroxidation
>l. peroxide
>l. phosphatase
>l. phosphorus
>l. profile
>l. raft
>l. tumor

lipid-containing tumor
lipid-laden
>l.-l. clear cell
>l.-l. homogeneous adrenocortical carcinoma
>l.-l. lysosome

lipid-lowering
>l.-l. agent

>l.-l. drug
>l.-l. therapy

lipidosis
lipid-rich lesion
Lipitor
lipoapoptosis
lipoapoptotic pathway
lipoatrophic diabetes
lipoatrophy
>congenital generalized l.
>diabetic l.
>insulin l.

lipoblast
lipocalin protein
lipocortin
lipocortin-1
lipodystrophic syndrome
lipodystrophy
>congenital generalized l. (CGL)
>familial partial l.
>insulin l.
>l. syndrome

lipofuscin
lipogenesis
>insulin l.

lipogenic enzyme
lipogranulomatosis
lipohypertrophy
>diabetic l.
>insulin l.

lipoid
>l. cell
>l. cell tumor
>l. congenital adrenal hyperplasia

lipolysis
>perilipin l.

lipoma
lipomatosis
>retroperitoneal l.

lipophilic
>l. drug
>l. hormone
>l. molecule

lipopolysaccharide (LPS)
lipoprotein
>l. alteration
>high-density l. (HDL)
>intermediate-density l. (IDL)
>l. lipase (LPL)
>l. lipase deficiency
>l. lipase gene
>low-density l. (LDL)

NOTES

L

lipoprotein *(continued)*
    l. remnant
    very low density l. (VLDL)
lipoprotein(a) (Lp(a))
liposarcoma
liposomal amphotericin B
liposome vector
lipostatic hypothesis
lipostat mechanism
liposuction
lipotoxicity
    intracellular l.
    l. metabolic syndrome
lipotropin (LPH)
Lipovite
lipoxin
12-lipoxygenase
5-lipoxygenase activating protein (FLAP)
lipoxygenase pathway
lips
    bumpy l.
Liquibid
Liqui-Caps
liquid chromatography with electrochemical detection (LCED)
Liquid Pred
Liqui-E
Liquiprin
liquor folliculi
Lisch nodule
lisinopril
lisofylline (LSF)
lispro
    l. Insulin
    insulin l.
lissencephaly
list
    exchange l.
    menopause symptom l. (MSL)
Listeria
listeriosis
liter (L)
    osmoles per l. (Osm/L)
Lite Touch lancing device
lithiasis
    renal l.
lithium-associated thyrotoxicosis
lithium carbonate
lithium-induced hypothyroidism
litholysis
lithostathine assay
lithotripsy
    endoscopic l.
    extracorporeal shock wave l.
    shock wave l.
"little" hormone
livedo reticularis
liver
    l. cancer

l. disease
l. enzyme
l. failure
fatty l.
l. glucose production
l. glycogen
l. glycogen cycling
l. peroxisome proliferator-activated receptor-gamma
l. phosphorylase
l. pyruvate kinase (LPK)
l. pyruvate kinase promoter
l. volume
liver-enriched
    l.-e. activating protein (LAP)
    l.-e. inhibiting protein (LIP)
    l.-e. transcription factor
living
    l. segmental donor pancreas transplantation
    l. segmental donor survival
LJM
    limited joint mobility
LKV-Drops
L-leucine
l-lysine
LMP
    last menstrual period
lmx1.1 protein
lmx1.2 protein
LN
    laminin
LNAB
    large-needle aspiration biopsy
LNG rod implant
L-nitro-L-arginine methyl ester
load
    gestational diabetes mellitus oral glucose l.
    glycemic l.
    phenytoin l.
    phosphate l.
loading
    aluminum l.
    calcium l.
    salt l.
lobe
    anterior pituitary l.
    conical l.
    contralateral l.
    intermediate pituitary l.
    limbic l.
    neural l.
    pyramidal l.
lobectomy
    unilateral l.
lobulated goiter
lobule
    breast l.

localized myxedema
local symptom
lochia
 red l.
 l. rubra
Locilex
 L. pexiganan acetate cream
 L. topical cream
locus, pl. **loci**
 adenosine deaminase l.
 aggressive insulin-dependent
  diabetes l.
 l. ceruleus
 chromosome 7 T-cell receptor beta
  chain l.
 class II HLA l.
 class II human leukocyte antigen l.
 diabetogenic l.
 GNAS1 l.
 quantitative trait l. (QTL)
Lodine XL
Loestrin
 L. 1.5/30
 L. 1/20
log
 l. dose-response relationship
 sugar l.
logarithm
LOH
 loss of heterozygosity
lomefloxacin
long
 l. bone
 l. chain acyl-CoA dehydrogenase
  (LCAD)
 l. chain acyl-CoA dehydrogenase
  deficiency
 l. chain acyl CoAs (LCAcoA, LC-
  CoAs)
 l. chain fatty acyl-CoA (LCFA-
  CoA)
 l. chain 3-hydroxyacyl-CoA
  dehydrogenase (LCHAD)
 l. chain 3-hydroxyacyl-CoA
  dehydrogenase deficiency
long-acting
 l.-a. insulin
 l.-a. release (LAR)
 l.-a. thyroid stimulator (LATS)
 l.-a. thyroid stimulator-protector
  (LATS-P)

longitudinal
 l. growth
 l. relaxation time
long-lasting insulin
long-loop
 l.-l. feedback
 l.-l. feedback signal
long-term complication
loop
 advanced insulin infusion with a
  control l. (ADICOL)
 disulfide l.
 l. diuretic
 feedback l.
 Galen l.
 hairpin l.
 Henle l.
 l. of Henle
 negative feedback l.
 neuroendocrine control l.
looping
 cardiac l.
Looser
 L. fissure
 L. pseudofracture
 L. zone
Lo/Ovral
loperamide
Lorcet
 L. 10/650
 L. Plus
Lorcet-HD
Lortab
Los Angeles preservation solution 1
 (LAP-1)
losartan
loss
 bone l.
 distal motor axonal l.
 height l.
 l. of heterozygosity (LOH)
 male pattern hair l.
 nerve-fiber l.
 postimplantation embryofetal l.
 receptor l.
 sensorineural hearing l.
 visual l.
 weight l.
loss-of-function mutation
Louis-Bar and Nijmegen breakage
 syndrome
lovastatin

L

NOTES

low
    l. birth weight (LBW)
    l. bone density
    l. bone turnover syndrome
    l. glycemic index diet
low-calcium dialysate
low-density
    l.-d. lipoprotein (LDL)
    l.-d. lipoprotein cholesterol (LDL-C)
    l.-d. lipoprotein cholesterol and
      insulin-resistance syndrome
    l.-d. lipoprotein receptor
    l.-d. lipoprotein receptor-related
      protein (LRP)
low-dose
    l.-d. dexamethasone test
    l.-d. heparin
    l.-d. short synacthen test (LDSST)
    l.-d. vaginal estrogen
Lowe
    L. disease
    L. syndrome
lower esophageal sphincter (LES)
low-grade astrocytoma
low-molecular-weight
    l.-m.-w. heparin
    l.-m.-w. PTPase (low-Mr PTP)
low-Mr PTP
low-phosphorus diet
low-pressure baroreceptor
low-protein diet
low-renin essential hypertension
low-tension glaucoma
low-triiodothyronine syndrome
low-T$_3$ syndrome
low-turnover
    l.-t. bone lesion
    l.-t. disease
    l.-t. osteoporosis
Lozol
Lp(a)
    lipoprotein(a)
    Lp(a) level
LPH
    lipotropin
LPK
    liver pyruvate kinase
LPL
    lipoprotein lipase
LPS
    lipopolysaccharide
LRH (*var. of* LHRH)
LRP
    LDL receptor-related protein
    leukocyte antigen-related phosphatase
    low-density lipoprotein receptor-related
      protein
LRR
    leucine rich repeat

L/S
    lecithin/sphingomyelin
    L/S ratio
LSF
    lisofylline
LT
    leukotriene
LT$_4$
    l-thyroxine
L-T$_3$
    L-triiodothyronine
LTA$_4$
    leukotriene A$_4$
LTB$_4$
    leukotriene B$_4$
LTC$_4$
    leukotriene C$_4$
LTD
    Laron-type dwarfism
LTD$_4$
    leukotriene D$_4$
LTE$_4$
    leukotriene E$_4$
l-thyroxine (LT$_4$)
L-triiodothyronine (L-T$_3$)
    L-t. uptake
L-type calcium channel
lucent zone
luciferase
    firefly l.
    l. gene
Luedde exophthalmometer
LUFS
    luteinized unruptured follicle syndrome
Lufyllin
Lugol solution
lumbar
    l. plexopathy
    l. spine bone density
lumen
    follicular l.
    residual l.
luminal
    l. brush-border membrane
    l. compartment
    l. endothelium
    l. surface
luminescent
    l. label
    l. paint
lumisterol
Lunelle
lung
    l. disease
    Wilms l.
Lupron
    L. Depot
    L. Depot-3, -4 Month
    L. Depot-Ped

lupus
    cutaneous l.
    drug-induced l.
    l. erythematosus
Luschka
    foramina of Magendie and L.
luteal
    l. cyst
    l. dysfunction
    l. phase
    l. phase defect
    l. phase deficiency
    l. phase insufficiency
luteal-follicular transition
luteectomy
lutein
    l. cell
    granulosa l.
luteinalis
    hyperreactio l.
luteinization
    l. inhibitor
    premature l.
    l. stimulant
luteinization-inhibiting factor
luteinized
    l. theca cell
    l. unruptured follicle syndrome (LUFS)
luteinizing
    l. hormone (LH)
    l. hormone-beta (LH-beta)
    l. hormone beta core fragment
    l. hormone/chorionic gonadotropin (LH/CG) receptor
    l. hormone-dependent androgen excess
    l. hormone/human chorionic gonadotropin (LH/hCG)
    l. hormone receptor
    l. hormone-releasing hormone (LHRH, LH-RH, LRH)
    l. hormone-releasing hormone deficiency
    l. hormone-secreting tumor
luteogenesis
luteolysis
luteoma of pregnancy
luteotropic hormone
luteum
    corpus l.

Lutrepulse
lutropin (LH)
Luveris
LVP
    large-volume paracentesis
LWD
    Leri-Weill dyschondrosteosis
LY294002
    phosphatidylinositol 3-kinase
lyase
    argininosuccinate l.
    peptidyl-alpha-hydroxyglycine alpha-amidating l. (PAL)
17,20-lyase
lycopene
Lyme disease
lymph
    l. node
    l. node involution
    l. node metastasis
lymphadenitis
lymphadenoma
lymphadenopathy-associated virus (LAV)
lymphangiectasis
lymphangiogenesis
lymphangioma
lymphangiosarcoma
lymphectasia
    intestinal l.
lymphedema
    congenital hereditary l.
lymphocutaneous sporotrichosis
lymphocyte
    l. adenylate cyclase response
    B l.
    CD4 helper l.
    CD8 suppressor l.
    cytotoxic T l.
    Epstein-Barr transformed l.
    l. function-associated antigen-1 (LFA-1)
    l. immune globulin
    inducer T l.
    peripheral blood l. (PBL)
    regulatory l.
    T l.
    T-effector l.
    thymic l.
    T-suppresser l.
lymphocytic
    l. choriomeningitis virus (LCMV)
    l. hypophysitis

L

NOTES

lymphocytic *(continued)*
    l. infiltration
    l. thyroiditis
lymphocytopenia
lymphoepithelial endocrine gland
lymphoid
    l. cell
    l. follicle
    l. hyperplasia
lymphokine
    secrete l.
lymphokine-activated
    l.-a. killer (LAK)
    l.-a. killer cell
lymphoma
    aggressive hypothalamic l.
    B-cell l.
    Burkitt l.
    immunoblastic l.
    intermediate lymphocytic l.
    lymphoplasmacytoid l.
    mantle zone l.
    PCNS l.
    primary central nervous system l.
    primary pituitary l. (PPL)
    primary thyroid l.
    small cleaved l.
    small noncleaved l.
    T-cell l.
    thyroid l.
lymphomatosa
    struma l.
lymphoplasmacytoid lymphoma

lymphoproliferative disorder
lymphoreticular neoplasm
lymphoscintigraphy
lymphotoxin
lymphotoxin-beta
Lynch syndrome
lynestrenol
Lynoral
Lyon
    L. hypothesis
    L. phenomenon
lyonization
Lyphocin Injection
lypressin
Lyrica
lysine
    l. dehydrogenase
    l. vasopressin
lysinuric protein intolerance
lysis
    vitreal l.
lysophosphatidylcholine
lysosomal
    l. dense body
    l. membrane
lysosome
    lipid-laden l.
lysozyme F_2 element
lysuride
lysyl-bradykinin
lysyl oxidase
lysylpyridinoline

M
immunoglobulin M (IgM)
1/50M
Norethin 1/50M
MA
megestrol acetate
Maalox Plus
MAb, Mab
monoclonal antibody
maceration of epithelium
Machado-Joseph disease
macroadenoma
pituitary growth hormone-
secreting m.
pluripotent pituitary m.
prolactin-secreting pituitary m.
solitary unilateral m.
macroalbuminuria
macroangiopathy
dysglycemic m.
macrocephaly
macroencapsulation device
macrofollicular
m. adenoma
m. pattern
macroglossia
macrognathia
macrolipasemia
macromastia
macromolecule
hydrophilic m.
macronodular adrenal hyperplasia
macroorchidism
macrophage
m. colony-stimulating factor (M-
CSF)
m. inflammatory protein-1-alpha
(MIP-1-alpha)
m. inflammatory protein-1-beta
(MIP-1-beta)
m. migration-inhibiting factor
m. migration inhibitory factor
macrophage-activating factor
macropinocytotic
macroprolactinemia, macroprolactinaemia
macroprolactinoma
invasive m.
macrosomia
fetal m.
macrovascular disease
macula, pl. **maculae**
m. densa
m. densa cell
m. densa chemoreceptor
m. densa receptor

macular
m. degeneration
m. edema
macule
café au lait m.
mad cow disease
Madelung deformity
magaldrate and simethicone
MAGE
mean amplitude of glycemic excursion
magnesium
m. ammonium phosphate
m. carbonate
m. deficiency
m. depletion
m. hydroxide
m. oxide
m. salt
m. sulfate
magnesium-lipid salt
magnetic
m. resonance elastography (MRE)
m. resonance imaging (MRI)
m. resonance spectroscopy (MRS)
magnocellular
m. cholinergic neuron
m. hormone
m. hypothalamohypophyseal neuron
m. neurosecretory neuron
m. neurosecretory system
m. perikaryon
Magnum food scale
MAH
malignancy-associated hypercalcemia
mahogany cofactor
ma huang
Maillard
M. product
M. reaction
M. site
main
m. d'accoucheur
m. pancreatic duct (MPD)
major
m. depressive disorder (MDD)
m. gangrene
m. histocompatibility
m. histocompatibility complex
(MHC)
Leishmania m.
m. proglucagon fragment (MPF)
thalassemia m.
m. tranquilizer
malabsorption
bile-salt m.

M

malabsorption *(continued)*
    calcium m.
    carbohydrate m.
    m. syndrome
maldescent
maldevelopment
maldigestion/malabsorption
    fat m.
male
    androgen deficiency in aging m.'s
      (ADAM)
    m. climacteric
    infertile m.
    m. infertility
    m. orgasm
    m. pattern baldness
    m. pattern hair loss
    m. phenotype
    m. precocious puberty
    m. pseudohermaphrodite
    m. pseudohermaphroditism (MPH)
    m. sperm
    m. Turner syndrome
    undervirilized m.
maleate
    rosiglitazone m.
male-limited familial precocious puberty
maleylacetoacetate
    m. hydrolase
    m. hydrolase type Ib
malformation
    arteriovenous m. (AVM)
    congenital m.
    conotruncal m.
malic
    m. enzyme
    m. enzyme gene
malignancy
    humoral hypercalcemia of m.
      (HHM)
    periampullary m.
    secondary m.
malignancy-associated hypercalcemia
    (MAH)
malignant
    m. external otitis
    m. hemangioendothelioma
    m. histiocytosis
    m. hyperthermia
    m. insulinoma
    m. islet cell tumor
    m. peripheral nerve sheath tumor
      (MPNST)
Mallamint
malnutrition
    protein-calorie m.
    protein-energy m. (PEM)
malnutrition-related diabetes mellitus
malonaldehyde generation

Maloney stain for aluminum
malonyl-CoA
malonyldialdehyde (MDA)
MALT
    mucosa-associated lymphoid tissue
maltase
mammalian
    m. achaete-scute homologous
      protein-2 (Mash-2)
    m. bombesin
    m. target of rapamycin (mTOR)
mammary
    m. crest
    m. dysplasia
    m. fibroadenoma
    m. gland
    m. ridge
    m. tumor virus (MTV)
mammary-derived growth inhibitor
    (MDGI)
mammillary
    m. body
    m. fasciculus
    m. peduncle
    m. region
mammillotegmental fasciculus
mammillothalamic tract
mammography
    ultrasound m.
mammosomatotroph
    m. cell
    m. cell adenoma
mammotrope
mammotroph
management
    evaluation and m. (E/M)
mandible
    hypoplastic m.
manifestation
    morphologic m.
    neuroophthalmologic m.
mannitol administration
mannose
mannose-6-phosphate/IGF-2 receptor
    (M6P/IGF-2R)
manometry
    sphincter of Oddi m.
Mansonella perstans
mantle
    m. islet
    m. zone lymphoma
MAO
    monoamine oxidase
Maox
MAP
    mean arterial pressure
    mitogen-activated protein
      MAP kinase
      MAP kinase pathway

MAP kinase phosphatase-1 (MKP-1)

map
MHC gene m.
Mapap
MAP/ERK kinase (MEK)
MAPK
mitogen-activated protein kinase
MAPK cascade
MAPK pathway
maple syrup urine disease
mapping
c-*fos* m.
congenic m.
genetic m.
quantitative trait locus m.
transracial m.
MAR
mineral apposition rate
Maranox
marasmus syndrome
Marax
marble
m. bone disease
m. bone pattern
marcescens
Serratia m.
Marcillin
marfanoid habitus
Marfan syndrome
Margesic H
margin
adrenal gland m.
coast of California smooth m.
coast of Maine irregular m.
marginal zone/mucosa-associated lymphoid tissue
Marine-Lenhart syndrome
marine vibrios
Marinol
marker
biochemical m.
genetic m.
hyperinsulinemic hypoglycemia m.
immune m.
microsatellite m.
postreceptor m.
short tandem repeat m.
STR m.
variable number of tandem repeat m.'s
VNTR m.'s

Marmine
M. Injection
M. Oral
marrow
bone m.
m. cavity formation
m. cell vacuolization
m. hematopoietic stem cell
m. monocyte
red bone m.
yellow bone m.
marsupialization
Marthritic
MAS
McCune-Albright syndrome
masculinization
brain m.
Mash-2
mammalian achaete-scute homologous protein-2
masked
m. hyperthyroidism
m. thyroid autonomy
mask sign
mas **oncogene**
mass
beta-cell m.
body cell m.
bone m.
cold m.
decreased lean m.
density of the fat m. (d_{FF})
density of the fat-free m. (d_{FFM})
fat m. (FM)
fat-free m. (FFM)
incidental adrenal m.
m. isotopomer distribution analysis (MIDA)
lean body m. (LBM)
musculoskeletal m.
peak adult bone m. (PABM)
protein m.
pseudoadrenal m.
red cell m.
skeletal m.
m. spectrometry
syncytiotrophoblast m.
T- and Z- scores of bone m.
massa intermedia
mass-forming pancreatitis
massive macronodular hyperplasia
mastalgia

NOTES

M

mast cell
mastitis
    chronic cystic m.
    cystic m.
mastocytoma
mastocytosis
mastoparan
mastopathy
    diabetic m.
maternal
    m. autoimmunity
    m. blocking antibody
    m. deprivation syndrome
    m. estradiol rhythm
    m. hyperglycemia-induced fetal
      hyperinsulinemia
    m. hypoglycemia
    m. hypothyroidism
    m. hypothyroxinemia
    m. immunity
    m. morbidity
    m. mortality
    m. postpartum thyroid dysfunction
maternally
    m. expressed gene 3 (MEG3)
    m. inherited diabetes and deafness
      (MIDD)
maternotoxic effect
matrix, pl. **matrices**
    cellulose-derived m.
    estradiol m.
    extracellular m. (ECM)
    m. Gla protein (MGP)
    human demineralized bone m.
    mesangial m.
    m. metalloprotease (MMP)
    m. metalloproteinase (MMP)
    m. metalloproteinase-12 (MMP-12)
    m. mineralization
    mineralized m.
    mitochondrial m.
    noncollagen bone m.
    organic m.
    osseous m.
    porous collagen m.
    m. transdermal system
    m. vesicle
matrix-dissolution product
maturation
    endochondral bone m.
    epiphyseal m.
    m. index (MI)
    precocious m.
mature
    m. follicle
    m. teratoma
mature-onset diabetes of the young
  (MODY)

maturity
    fetal lung m.
maturity-onset
    m.-o. diabetes (MOD)
    m.-o. diabetes mellitus
    m.-o. diabetes of the young
      (MODY)
    m.-o. diabetes in the young
      (MODY)
    m.-o. diabetes of youth (MODY)
MAU
    microalbuminuria
Mauriac syndrome
maximal urinary flow rate
maximum
    m. intensity projection (MIP)
    M. Strength Dex-A-Diet
    M. Strength Dexatrim
    tubular transport m. (T_m)
Maxolon
Mayer-Rokitansky-Küster-Hauser
  syndrome
Mazanor
mazindol
MB-35 peptide
MBH
    medial basal hypothalamic region
MBP
    myelin basic protein
MCAD
    medium chain acyl-CoA dehydrogenase
      MCAD deficiency
MCAR
    melanocortin receptor type 4
McCardle syndrome
McCune-Albright syndrome (MAS)
MCD
    medullary collecting duct
mcg
    microgram
MCH
    melanin-concentrating hormone
McMaster classification
MCP
    membrane cofactor protein
    mucosal carrier protein
MCP-1
    monocyte chemotactic protein-1
    mucosal carrier protein-1
MC2-R
    melanocortin-2 receptor
MC3-R
    melanocortin-3 receptor
MC4-R
    melanocortin-4 receptor
M-CSF
    macrophage colony-stimulating factor
MCT
    medullary carcinoma of the thyroid

MDA
    malonyldialdehyde
MDC
    minimal detectable concentration
MDD
    major depressive disorder
MDGI
    mammary-derived growth inhibitor
MDI
    metered-dose inhaler
    multiple daily injections
    multiple dose injection
mDNA
    mitochondrial deoxyribonucleic acid
MDR
    multidrug resistance protein
MDRD
    Modification of Diet in Renal Disease
ME
    methionine enkephalin
MEA
    multiple endocrine abnormalities
    multiple endocrine adenopathies
meal
        carbohydrate m.
        fatty m.
        m. plan
        m. timing
meal-planning approach
mean
        m. amplitude of glycemic
          excursion (MAGE)
        m. arterial pressure (MAP)
Means-Lerman
        M.-L. scratch
        M.-L. scratch murmur
measles virus nucleocapsid gene
measurement
        capacitance m.
        Doppler-derived pressure m.
        gastric impedance m.
        glucose m.
        heel-to-pubis m.
        pubis-to-crown m.
        skin fold m.
        transrectal ultrasound m.
        TSH receptor antibody m.
Measurin
mechanism
        adipocyte lipolysis m.
        autonomic cooling m.
        cell-signaling m.

        cis m.
        counterregulation m.
        Effector m.
        hypothalamic regulatory m.
        intact thirst m.
        Jod-Basedow m.
        lipostat m.
        photoperiodic m.
        prolactin inhibitory m.
        Randle m.
        thirst m.
        trans m.
        ubiquitin m.
        urinary concentrating m.
mechanoreceptor
Meckel
        M. cartilage
        M. diverticulum
meclofenamate
Meda
        M. Cap
        M. Tab
media (*pl. of* medium)
medial
        m. anlage
        m. basal hypothalamic region
         (MBH)
        m. basal hypothalamus
        m. forebrain bundle
        m. longitudinal fasciculus
        m. zone
median
        m. anlage
        m. eminence
mediastinal parathyroid adenoma
mediastinitis
        sclerosing m.
mediastinum testis
mediator
        bioactive m.
        inositol-phospho-glycan
         headgroup m.
        molecular m.
        peptide m.
        proinflammatory m.
medical nutrition therapy
medicamentosa
        rhinitis m.
        thyrotoxicosis m.
medication
        aluminum-containing m.
        antidiabetic m.

M

NOTES

medication *(continued)*
 antithyroid m.
 atypical antipsychotic m.
medicine
 weight-loss m.
Medi-Glybe
Medihaler-Iso
Medi-Ject needle-free insulin injection system
Medi-Jector
 M.-J. Choice
 M.-J. Choice needle-free insulin injection system
mediobasal brain structure
Medipren
MediSense
 M. 2 Card glucose meter
 M. 2 Pen Sensor glucose meter
 M. Q.I.D. test strip
 M. 2 test strip
Medisense
 M. Pen 2
 M. Pen 2 self-blood glucose monitor
 M. Precision Xtra
Mediterranean diet
Medi-Tuss
medium, pl. **media**
 m. chain acyl-CoA dehydrogenase (MCAD)
 m. chain acyl-CoA dehydrogenase deficiency
 gadolinium-diethylenetriaminepentaacetic acid contrast m.
 high-attenuation iodinated contrast media
 iodinated contrast media
 radiopaque iodinated radiographic contrast media
 tunica media
Medralone Injection
medrogestone
Medrol
 M. Oral
 M. Veriderm Cream
medroxyprogesterone
 m. acetate (MPA)
 estrogen and m.
Medtronic MiniMed CGMS system gold
medulla, pl. **medullae**
 adrenal m.
 m. oblongata
 m. pons
 rostral ventrolateral m.
 ventrolateral m.
medullary
 m. carcinoma of the thyroid (MCT)

 m. cavity
 m. cell
 m. collecting duct (MCD)
 m. thick ascending limb of Henle
 m. thyroid cancer (MTC)
 m. thyroid carcinoma (MTC)
mefenamic acid
MEG3
 maternally expressed gene 3
Mega B
Megace
megakaryocyte
megalencephaly
megalin
megaloblastic anemia
Megaton
megestrol acetate (MA)
meglitinide with metformin
meglumine ioxaglate
Meige disease
meiosis
meiotic
 m. division
 m. nondysjunction
MEK
 MAP/ERK kinase
 MEK kinase (MEKK)
MEKK
 MEK kinase
Mel1a melatonin receptor
Mel1b melatonin receptor
melancholia
 syndrome of m.
melanin
melanin-concentrating hormone (MCH)
melanoblastoma
melanocortin
 m. receptor gene
 m. receptor isoform
 m. receptor system
 m. receptor type 4 (MCAR)
 m. signaling
melanocortin-2 receptor (MC2-R)
melanocortin-3 receptor (MC3-R)
melanocortin-4 receptor (MC4-R)
melanocyte-concentrating hormone
melanocyte-inhibiting hormone
melanocyte-releasing hormone (MRH)
melanocyte-stimulating
 m.-s. factor (MSF)
 m.-s. hormone (MSH)
 m.-s. hormone sequence
melanocytoma
melanoma growth stimulatory activity (MGSA)
Melanotan II
melanotropic cell

MELAS
>   myopathy, encephalopathy, lactic
>   acidosis, stroke-like episodes
>   MELAS syndrome

melatonin (MLT)
>   m. rhythm

Melfiat-105 Unicelles

meliloti
>   *Rhizobium m.*

melitensis
>   *Brucella m.*

mellitus
>   adolescent type 2 diabetes m.
>   adult-onset diabetes m.
>   Ala-Ala preventing diabetes m.
>   atypical diabetes m. (ADM)
>   autoimmune diabetes m.
>   autosomal dominant diabetes m.
>   coxsackievirus B-induced
>   diabetes m.
>   diabetes m.
>   drug-induced diabetes m.
>   encephalomyocarditis virus-induced
>   diabetes m.
>   gestational diabetes m. (GDM)
>   glucocorticoid-induced diabetes m.
>   iatrogenic type 1 diabetes m.
>   insulin-dependent diabetes m.
>   (IDDM)
>   insulinopenic diabetes m.
>   juvenile-onset diabetes m.
>   malnutrition-related diabetes m.
>   maturity-onset diabetes m.
>   neonatal diabetes m.
>   noninsulin-dependent diabetes m.
>   (NIDDM)
>   obese type 2 noninsulin-dependent
>   diabetes m.
>   posttransplant diabetes m. (PTDM)
>   pyriminil-induced diabetes m.
>   triple oral combination therapy for
>   type 2 diabetes m.
>   tropical diabetes m.
>   type 1 diabetes m.
>   type 2 diabetes m. (T2DM)
>   White classification of diabetes m.

melorheostosis

melphalan

memapsin 2

membrana
>   m. granulosa cell
>   m. limitans externa

membrane
>   apical m.
>   arachnoid m.
>   basement m.
>   basolateral plasma m.
>   brush-border m. (BBM)
>   cell basement m.
>   m. cofactor protein (MCP)
>   cricothyroid m.
>   cuprophane dialysis m.
>   dialysis m.
>   endosteal m.
>   m. excitability
>   incomplete cell basement m.
>   m. integral protein (MIP)
>   intracellular lysosomal m.
>   Liliequist m.
>   luminal brush-border m.
>   lysosomal m.
>   nitrocellulose m.
>   nuclear m.
>   parathyroid cell m.
>   periodontal m.
>   piarachnoid m.
>   plasma m.
>   postsynaptic m.
>   m. trafficking
>   tubular dialysis m.
>   vasculosyncytial m.

membrane-associated estrogen receptor

membrane-bound
>   m.-b. receptor
>   m.-b. receptor molecule

membranous
>   m. bone
>   m. glomerulonephritis
>   m. urethra

memory
>   hyperglycemic m.

MEN
>   multiple endocrine neoplasia
>   MEN syndrome

MEN 1
>   multiple endocrine neoplasia type 1

MEN 2
>   multiple endocrine neoplasia type 2

MEN 3
>   multiple endocrine neoplasia type 3

men
>   idiopathic osteoporosis in m.

MEN1 **gene**

M

NOTES

MEN 2A
multiple endocrine neoplasia type 2A
Menadol
menarche
MEN 2B
multiple endocrine neoplasia type 2B
mendelian
M. inheritance
m. obesity syndrome
Mendenhall syndrome
Menest
Mengo virus
menin gene
meningioma
parasellar m.
pituitary m.
meningitis
basilar m.
tuberculous m.
meningococcal sepsis
meningococcemia
meningoencephalitis
Menkes disease
menometrorrhagia
menopausal estrogen
menopause
precocious emotional m.
premature m.
surgical m.
m. symptom list (MSL)
menorrhagia
Menostar
menotropin
menses
oligomenorrhea with anovulatory m.
menstrual
m. cycle
m. dysfunction
menstruation
retrograde m.
MENT
7-alpha-methyl-19-nortestosterone
mental retardation
mepenzolate
Mepergan
meperidine
Mephyton Oral
meprednisone
6-mercaptopurine
Meridia
Merkel cell carcinoma
merocrine gland
21-mer phosphorothioate antisense oligodeoxynucleotide
mesangial
m. cell
m. matrix
mesangiocapillary

mesangium
extraglomerular m.
mesencephalon
mesenchymal
m. progenitor
m. stem cell
m. tumor
mesenchyme
mesenteric
m. artery
m. ischemia
mesh
titanium m.
Mesigyna
mesoderm
extraembryonic somatic m.
mesodermal cell
mesodiencephalic junction
mesomelic shortening
mesometric dysplasia
mesonephros
mesosalpinx
mesothelioma
mesovarium
messenger
chemical m.
intracellular m.
m. ribonucleic acid (mRNA)
m. RNA (mRNA)
second m.
tertiary m.
mesterolone
mestranol and norethindrone
mesylate
2-Br-alpha-ergocryptine m.
nafomostat m.
pergolide m.
metabolic
m. acidosis
m. alkalosis
m. balance
m. bone disease
m. clearance rate
m. control
m. decompensation
m. effect
m. factor
m. hemostasis
m. pathway
m. profile
m. response
m. signal
m. stone workup
m. stress episode
m. syndrome
m. thrift
m. web
metabolism
acarbose lipid m.

basal m.
bone mineral m.
calcium phosphorus m.
carbohydrate m.
cobalamin m.
disordered water m.
estrogen m.
fuel m.
glucogen m.
glucose m.
hepatic m.
iodothyronine m.
lipid m.
peripheral thyroid hormone m.
phosphorus m.
prereceptor m.
protein m.
purine m.
selenoprotein m.
sterol m.
theophylline m.
thyroid hormone m.
water m.
metabolite
calciferol m.
phosphatidylinositide m.
vitamin D m.
metabolomics
metachromatic leukodystrophy (MLD)
Metahydrin
metaiodobenzylguanidine (MIBG)
^{131}I-labeled m. (^{131}I-labeled MIBG)
131-metaiodobenzylguanidine
iodine 131-m. (^{131}I-MIBG)
^{131}metaiodobenzylguanidine
metal
m. intoxification
paramagnetic m.
trace m.
metalloprotease
matrix m. (MMP)
metalloproteinase
matrix m. (MMP)
tissue inhibitor of m. (TIMP)
zinc m.
metalloproteinase-1
tissue inhibitor of m.-1 (TIMP-1)
metalloproteinase-12
matrix m.-12 (MMP-12)
metallothionein (MT)
metamorphopsia
metamyelocyte

Metandren
metanephrine
24-hour fractionated m.
24-hour urinary fractionated m.
metanephros
metaphyseal, metaphysial
m. dysplasia
m. exostosis
m. sclerosis
metaphysis, pl. **metaphyses**
metaplasia
clear cell m.
coelomic m.
myeloid m.
oxyphilic m.
Metaprel
metaproterenol
Arm-a-Med m.
Dey-Dose m.
metastasis, pl. **metastases**
distant m.
lymph node m.
pituitary m.
prior distant m.
sellar m.
tumor m.
metastatic
m. deposit
m. extraosseal calcification
m. tumor
metatarsal-phalangeal flexion deformity
metenkephalin
meter
Accu-Chek Active glucose m.
Accu-Chek Advantage glucose m.
Accu-Chek Compact glucose m.
Accu-Chek Instant glucose m.
Accu-Chek Voicemate glucose m.
amperometric m.
blood glucose m.
Chemstrip MatchMaker blood
  glucose m.
coulometric m.
Dex series m.'s
ExacTech blood glucose m.
ExacTech RSG glucose m.
FreeStyle Flash blood glucose m.
FreeStyle Tracker glucose m.
Glucometer Elite R m.
glucose m.
GlucoWatch Biographer m.
Hypoguard Advance glucose m.

M

NOTES

meter *(continued)*
LifeGuide glucose m.
MediSense 2 Card glucose m.
MediSense 2 Pen Sensor
glucose m.
OneTouch blood glucose m.
OneTouch InDuo glucose m.
OneTouch SureStep glucose m.
Prestige IQ glucose m.
Prestige LX glucose m.
QuickTek glucose m.
reflectance m.
ReliOn glucose m.
Supreme II blood glucose m.
TD Glucose m.
metered-dose inhaler (MDI)
metformin
acarbose with m.
extended release m.
m. hydrochloride
meglitinide with m.
m. monotherapy
methacholine
methadone
methamphetamine
methandrostenolone
methanol
methantheline
methasone-suppressed corticotropin-
releasing hormone test
methemoglobinemia
methimazole (MMI)
methionine
m. adenosyltransferase
m. enkephalin (ME)
peptide histidine m. (PHM)
method
carbodiimide modified heteroduplex
screening m.
colorimetric m.
Falck-Hillarp histofluorescence m.
FISH m.
fluorescent in situ hybridization m.
Folin-Wu m.
Gaur m.
glucose clamp m.
Gomori staining m.
interposition m.
microscopic transsphenoidal m.
paracetic acid-based m.
ribonuclease A cleavage m.
sandwich enzyme immunoassay m.
Sanger dideoxy sequencing m.
Somogyi-Nelson m.
symptothermal rhythm m.
Uchida m.
uricase m.
Ziehl-Neelsen m.
methotrexate

methotrimeprazine
methoxychlor
methoxyflurane
methoxyhydroxyphenylglycol
5-methoxyindoleacetic acid
methoxyisobutylisonitrile (MIBI)
5-methoxytryptamine
5-methoxytryptophol
methscopolamine
methyclothiazide
methyl
m. chloride
Oreton M.
m. oxidase
2-methylacetoacetate
methylation
2-methylbutyric acid
3-methylcrotonyl carboxylase
3-methylcrotonyl-CoA carboxylase
deficiency
3-methylcrotonylglycine
2-methyl-d-hydroxybutyrate
methyldopa
methylene blue
methylenetetrahydrofolate reductase
3-methylglutaconate
3-methylglutarate
methylglutaryl coenzyme A reductase
inhibitor
methylglyoxal
3-methylhistidine
methylisobutylxanthine (MIX)
methylmalonic
m. acid
m. acidemia
m. acidemia with homocystinemia
m. aciduria
methylmalonyl-CoA mutase
methylmercaptoimidazole (MMI)
methylmethacrylate
methylprednisolone
methylprednisone
methyl-sulfated neostigmine
methyltestosterone
Premarin with m.
methylxanthine drug
methysergide
Meticorten
Met and Leu enkephalin
metoclopramide hydrochloride
metolazone
metoprolol
metrapone stimulation test
Metrika A1c Now
metrizamide
Metrodin
metronidazole
metrorrhagia

metyrapone
    m. test
    m. testing
    m. therapy
metyrapone-induced hypercortisolism
metyrosine
Mevacor
mexiletine
Meynert
    nucleus basalis of M.
Mg^{2+}
    free M.
    total M.
mg/dL
    milligrams per deciliter
M-Glucometer
MGP
    matrix Gla protein
MGSA
    melanoma growth stimulatory activity
MGUS
    monoclonal gammopathy of unknown
      significance
MHC
    major histocompatibility complex
    myosin heavy chain
      MHC beta-cell
      MHC class I molecule
      MHC gene map
MI
    maturation index
Miacalcin
MIB-1 antibody
MIBG
    metaiodobenzylguanidine
      ^{131}I-labeled MIBG
      ^{131}I-labeled
        metaiodobenzylguanidine
    radiolabeled MIBG
    MIBG scan
MIBG-negative pelvic pheochromocytoma
MIBI
    methoxyisobutylisonitrile
      Tc-99m MIBI
micelle
Michigan
    M. Diabetic Neuropathy Score
    M. Neuropathy Screening Test
Miconazole
Micral
    M. Chemistrip
    M. urine dipstick test

microadenoma
    nonfunctioning m.
    pituitary m.
    silent m.
microadenomectomy
    transsphenoidal m.
microalbumin
microalbuminuria (MAU)
microaneurysm
microangiopathy
    diabetic m.
microarchitectural deterioration
microarray
microassay
    islet antigen autoantibody m.
microcarcinoid
    bronchial m.
microcatheter
microcephaly
microchimerism
microclip
    dural m.
microcornea
microcyst
    subcapsular follicular m.
microcytic anemia
microcytosis
microdactyly
microdeletion
    Y chromosome m.
microdialysis probe
microelectrode
    voltammetric m.
microencapsulation
microencephaly
microfilament-mediated process
microfilaria
Microflo test strip
microfollicular pattern
micrognathia
microgram (mcg)
microhematuria
microheterogeneity
microinfusion pump
Microlet Vaculance
microlithiasis
    occult biliary m.
microlymphography
    fluorescence m.
micromelia
micrometastasis

M

NOTES

Micro-monitor
Tracer Blood Glucose M.-m.
Micronase
microNefrin
Micronesia
microneurographic
micronized
m. estradiol
m. progesterone
micronodular
m. adrenal disease
m. hyperplasia
Micronor
micronutrient
micropenis
microperfusion
microphallus
microphthalmia
microphthalmic
m. cyst
osteopetrotic m.
micropinocytosis
micropinocytotic
MicroPor
Altea M.
microprolactinoma
micropsia
micropuncture
microsatellite
m. instability
m. marker
microscissors
single-bladed Kurze m.
microscopic
m. current
m. transsphenoidal method
microscopy
intraviral m.
islet m.
Nomarski m.
polarized light m.
microsomal
m. antibody
m. antibody titer
m. antigen
microsome
microsphere
microsurgery
pituitary m.
microsurgical resection
microtome
sectioning m.
microtubule-associated protein kinase cascade
microvascular
m. complication
m. disease
microvilli

microwave
m. hyperthermia
m. hyperthermia of the prostate
Microzide
MIDA
mass isotopomer distribution analysis
Midamor
midbrain raphe nucleus
midcycle spotting
MIDD
maternally inherited diabetes and deafness
midgut
midline
m. central neuraxis
m. jugum sphenoidale
m. zone
midnight plasma cortisol concentration
Midol
M. IB
M. PM
midparental height (MPH)
midsagittal image
MIF
migration inhibitory factor
Mifegyne
mifepristone
miglitol
migration
m. inhibitory factor (MIF)
thyroid m.
migratory
m. osteolysis
m. osteolysis of the knee
MIH
müllerian-inhibiting hormone
müllerian inhibitory hormone
mild
m. overt thyrotoxicosis
m. thyroid failure
milia
multiple m.
miliary tuberculosis
milieu
androgen m.
hormonal m.
hypoandrogenic m.
m. interieur
internal m.
reproductive m.
milk
breast m.
m. ejection
m. let down
m. let-down reflex
m. line
m. protein
uterine m.
milk-alkali syndrome

Milkman syndrome
Miller-Dicker syndrome
Miller syndrome
milligrams per deciliter (mg/dL)
millimeter (mm)
Milophene
milrinone
Milroy disease
mimicry
    molecular m.
mineral
    m. apposition rate (MAR)
    bone m.
    m. deficiency
    m. flux
    m. homeostasis
mineralization
    m. defect
    m. front
    m. impairment
    m. lag time
    matrix m.
mineralized
    m. bone histology
    m. matrix
mineralocorticoid
    adrenal corticosteroid (m.)
    m. agonist
    m. excess
    m. hormone
    m. receptor (MR)
    m. replacement
    m. replacement therapy
miniature-type congenital adrenal hypoplasia
miniglucagon
minihelix
mini hormone
minimal detectable concentration (MDC)
minimally symptomatic hypothyroidism (MSH)
MiniMed
    M. continuous glucose sensor
    M. 508, 511 insulin pump
    M. Paradigm insulin pump
minipill
    progesterone-only m.
Minipress
minipuberty of infancy
minipump
    osmotic m.

minisequencing
    solid-phase m.
minocycline-associated pigment
minor
    m. mechanical debridement
    m. tranquilizer
minora
minoxidil
Minoxigaine
miosis
MIP
    maximum intensity projection
    membrane integral protein
MIP-1-alpha
    macrophage inflammatory protein-1-alpha
MIP-1-beta
    macrophage inflammatory protein-1-beta
Mirena intrauterine device
MIS
    müllerian-inhibiting substance
        MIS II receptor
misfolded protein
misoprostol
misplaced exocytosis
missense
MIT
    monoiodinated tyrosine
    monoiodotyrosine
    3-monoiodotyrosine
MIT:DIT ratio
mithramycin
mitochondria
    tubulovesicular m.
mitochondrial
    m. defect
    m. deoxyribonucleic acid (mDNA, mtDNA)
    m. diabetes
    m. DNA
    m. electron transport chain
    m. enzyme
    m. matrix
    m. myopathy
    m. P450 monooxygenase
    m. porin
mitogen
mitogen-activated
    m.-a. protein (MAP)
    m.-a. protein kinase (MAPK)
    m.-a. protein kinase cascade
    m.-a. protein kinase pathway

M

NOTES

mitogenesis
mitogenic
mitomycin C
mitosis
mitotane
MIX
    methylisobutylxanthine
mix
    antiknock m.
mixed
    m. agonist-antagonist
    m. bone lesion
    m. dose
    m. GH cell-prolactin cell adenoma
    m. GH-PRL cell adenoma
    m. GH-secreting and prolactin-secreting adenoma
    m. gonadal dysgenesis
    m. growth hormone cell-prolactin cell adenoma
    m. growth hormone-prolactin cell adenoma
    m. growth hormone-secreting and prolactin-secreting adenoma
    m. pattern
    m. phenotype tumor
    m. pituitary adenoma-gangliocytoma
    m. sclerosing bone dystrophy
    m. sensorimotor polyneuropathy
    m. uremic osteodystrophy
mixed-function oxygenase
mixer
    Genotropin M.
mixture
    racemic m.
MKP-1
    MAP kinase phosphatase-1
MLC
    myosin light chain
        MLC kinase (MLCK)
MLCK
    MLC kinase
    myosin light chain kinase
MLD
    metachromatic leukodystrophy
MLT
    melatonin
mm
    millimeter
MMC
    myelomeningocele
MMI
    methimazole
    methylmercaptoimidazole
MMP
    matrix metalloprotease
    matrix metalloproteinase
MMP-12
    matrix metalloproteinase-12

Mobenol
mobility
    limited joint m. (LJM)
mobilization
    plasmin m.
Möbius syndrome
MOD
    maturity-onset diabetes
modality
    dialysis m.
model
    four-compartment m.
    fuzzy logic m.
    Jost m.
    predictive growth m.
    three-compartment m.
    transgenic mouse m.
    tumor xenograft m.
    m. U Gamma Knife
modem
    Acculink M.
Modicon
modification
    behavior m.
    M. of Diet in Renal Disease (MDRD)
    posttranslational m.
modified
    m. University of Wisconsin (mUW)
    m. University of Wisconsin solution
modifier
    selective estrogen response m. (SERM)
Modigliani syndrome
Modual
modulator
    cAMP-response element m. (CREM)
    estrogen-receptor m.
    ligand-directed m.
    PPAR selective m.
    selective androgen-receptor m. (SARM)
    selective estrogen-receptor m. (SERM)
    selective PPAR-gamma m. (SPPARM)
    serum estrogen-receptor m.
MODY
    mature-onset diabetes of the young
    maturity-onset diabetes in the young
    maturity-onset diabetes of the young
    maturity-onset diabetes of youth
mofetil
    mycophenolate m.
moiety
    adenylate cyclase m.

asparagine-linked glycosylation m.
carbohydrate m.
diphenyl ether m.

mole

complete hydatidiform m.
hydatidiform m.
partial hydatidiform m.

molecular

m. biology
m. chaperone
m. mediator
m. mimicry
m. probe hybridization

molecule

accessory m.
adhesion m.
amphoteric m.
cell-cell adhesion m. (CAM)
cJun m.
class I major histocompatibility
complex m.
class I, II MHC m.
class II major histocompatibility
complex m.
class III major histocompatibility
complex m.
class III MHC m.
collagen m.
coregulator m.
crystallized HLA-A2 m.
heterotetrameric m.
intercellular adhesion m. (ICAM)
lipophilic m.
membrane-bound receptor m.
MHC class I m.
nascent collagen m.
neural cell adhesion m. (N-CAM)
poorly processed POMC m.
poorly processed
proopiomelanocortin m.
procollagen m.
proinsulinlike m.
proopiomelanocortin m.
proteoglycan m.
reporter m.

molecule-1

intercellular adhesion m. (ICAM-1)
vascular cell adhesion m. (VCAM-1)

mole-melanoma

familial atypical multiple m.-m.
(FAMMM)

molimina

premenstrual m.

Mol-Iron
Molypen
Monafed
monamine (*var. of* monoamine)
Monckeberg sclerosis
Mondini dysplasia
monitor

BodyGem metabolism m.
Diasensor 2000 glucose m.
Duet glucose control m.
Glucometer DEX blood glucose m.
glucose m.
GlucoWatch glucose m.
Medisense Pen 2 self-blood
glucose m.
Paradigm Link blood glucose m.
m. peptide
Rigi-Scan m.
Sof-Tact Diabetes glucose m.
SpectRx glucose m.
SureStep glucose m.
TrackEASE glucose m.

monitoring

blood glucose m.
capillary blood glucose m.
hemodynamic m.
home glucose m. (HGM)
noninvasive blood glucose m.
self-blood glucose m. (SBGM)

monoallelic

m. expression
m. transcription

monoamine, monamine

brain m.
m. oxidase (MAO)
m. oxidase inhibitor
m. pathway
m. serotonin (5HT, 5-HT)

monoclonal

m. antibody (MAb, Mab)
m. anti-T-cell antibody
m. gammopathy of unknown
significance (MGUS)

monoclonus
monocular temporal arcuate defect
monocyte

m. chemoattractant protein-1
m. chemotactic protein-1 (MCP-1)
marrow m.
peripheral blood m. (PBM)

M

NOTES

monocytopenia
5′-monodeiodinase
    5′-m. activity
    5′-m. type I
monodeiodinase activity
monodeiodination activity
monofilament
    m. pressure esthesiometer
    Semmes-Weinstein 5.07 m.
monofluorophosphate
monofollicular feedback
monogenic
    m. disorder
    m. etiology
    m. Mendelian trait
    m. obesity
Mono-Gesic
monohydrate
    sibutramine hydrochloride m.
monohydrogen phosphate
monoiodinated tyrosine (MIT)
monoiodotyrosine (MIT)
3-monoiodotyrosine (MIT)
Monojector
    M. fingerstick device
    M. fingerstick device for blood
      glucose testing
monokine
monolayer culture
monomer
    calcitonin m.
    collagen m.
    thyroid hormone receptor m.
    TR m.
    triiodothyronine m.
monomorphic
monomorphous
mononeuritis multiplex
mononeuropathy
    compressive m.
    cranial m.
    diabetic m.
    hypothyroid m.
    m. multiplex
    truncal m.
mononucleosis
    infectious m.
monoovarial feedback
monooxygenase
    mitochondrial P450 m.
    peptidylglycine alpha-amidating m.
      (PAM)
    peptidylglycine alpha-
      hydroxylating m. (PHM)
monophasic
monophosphate
    adenosine cyclic m.
    cyclic adenosine m. (cAMP)
    cyclic 3′,5′-adenosine m. (cAMP)

    cyclic arginine m. (cAMP)
    cyclic guanosine m. (cGMP)
    cyclic 3′,5′-guanosine m. (cGMP)
    5′-cyclic guanosine m. (cGMP)
    dibutyryl cyclic arginine m.
    guanosine m. (GMP)
    nephrogenous cyclic adenosine m.
monophosphate-phosphodiesterase
    cyclic guanosine m.-p.
monosaturated fatty acid
monostotic
    m. disease
    m. FD
    m. form
monosymptomatic hyperthyroidism
monosystemic hyperthyroidism
monotherapy
    adolescent metformin m.
    estrogen m.
    metformin m.
    troglitazone m.
monovalent
monozygotic
Monro
    foramen of M.
mons pubis
Month
    Lupron Depot-3, -4 M.
moon
    m. face
    m. facies
morbidity
    maternal m.
morbid obesity
Morgagni syndrome
morning
    m. corticotropin-releasing hormone
      test
    m. cortisol
    m. CRH test
    m. glory disc
morning-after pill
morphine
    endogenous m.
    m. sulfate
morphogen
morphogenesis
    thyroid m.
morphologic
    m. differentiation
    m. manifestation
morphology
    colony m.
    spindle-shaped fibroplastic m.
morphometry
Morquio syndrome
Morris syndrome
mortality
    maternal m.

morula
mosaic
    47,XXY m.
    46,XY m.
mosaicism
    chromosomal m.
    gonadal m.
    trisomy X m.
    Turner m.
    XO/XY m.
    Y chromosome m.
MOS protooncogene
Mostofi classification of testicular tumor
motif
    E-box m.
    Ets m.
    glycosylation consensus m.
    nuclear localization signal m.
     (NLS)
    ribonucleic acid-binding m. (RBM)
    RNA-binding m. (RBM)
    Sp1 m.
    splice m.
    Y chromosome RNA
     recognition m. (YRRM)
    zinc-finger m.
motilin
motility
    aberrant m.
    intestinal m.
    ocular m.
    pharyngeal m.
movement
    abnormal ocular m.
    athetoid m.
    choreiform m.
    flagellar m.
moxestrol
MPA
    medroxyprogesterone acetate
MPD
    main pancreatic duct
    MPD Pro lancet
MPF
    major proglucagon fragment
MPH
    male pseudohermaphroditism
    midparental height
M6P/IGF-2R
    mannose-6-phosphate/IGF-2 receptor
MPLV
    myeloproliferative leukemia virus

MPNST
    malignant peripheral nerve sheath tumor
MPO
    myeloperoxidase
M-Prednisol Injection
MPS I
MR
    mineralocorticoid receptor
MRE
    magnetic resonance elastography
MRFIT
    Multiple Risk Factor Intervention Trial
MRH
    melanocyte-releasing hormone
MRI
    magnetic resonance imaging
     gadolinium-enhanced MRI
mRNA
    messenger ribonucleic acid
    messenger RNA
     GnRH mRNA
     receptor mRNA
     TRH mRNA
MRS
    magnetic resonance spectroscopy
MS-8
    Pancrecarb MS-8
MS Contin Oral
MSF
    melanocyte-stimulating factor
MSH
    melanocyte-stimulating hormone
    minimally symptomatic hypothyroidism
     MSH peptide
MSIR Oral
MSL
    menopause symptom list
MT
    metallothionein
     Pancrease MT
     Ultrase MT
MTC
    medullary thyroid cancer
    medullary thyroid carcinoma
mtDNA
    mitochondrial deoxyribonucleic acid
M.T.E.-4, -5, -6
99m-technetium sestamibi
mTOR
    mammalian target of rapamycin
MTV
    mammary tumor virus

M

NOTES

mucification
mucin
mucinosis
    follicular m.
    papular m.
    reticular erythematous m.
mucinous
    m. cystadenocarcinoma
    m. cystadenoma
    m. cystic tumor
mucin-producing
    m.-p. adenocarcinoma
    m.-p. tumor of the pancreas
mucocele
mucocutaneous
    m. candidiasis
    m. rash
mucoepidermoid carcinoma
Muco-Fen-DM
Muco-Fen-LA
mucoid wedge
mucolipidosis II
Mucomyst
Mucoplex
mucopolysaccharide
mucopolysaccharidosis,
  pl. **mucopolysaccharidoses**
    m. types I, II, III, IIIB, III, IIID,
      IVA, IVB, VI, VII
mucoprotein
Mucor
mucormycosis
    bone m.
    cardiac m.
    disseminated m.
    gastrointestinal m.
    pulmonary m.
    renal m.
    rhinocerebral m.
mucosa
    cervical m.
mucosa-associated lymphoid tissue
  (MALT)
mucosal
    m. carrier protein (MCP)
    m. carrier protein-1 (MCP-1)
    m. neuroma
Mucosil
mucosulfatidosis
mucous escalator
mucus thread
Muercke line
mulibrey nanism
müllerian
    m. agenesis
    m. anomaly
    m. derivative
    m. duct
    m. duct derived structure

    m. duct syndrome
    m. inhibitory hormone (MIH)
müllerian-inhibiting
    m.-i. hormone (MIH)
    m.-i. substance (MIS)
    m.-i. substance receptor
Müller muscle
MulTE-PAK-4
MulTE-PAK-5
multiantennary
multicentric
    m. islet cell adenoma
    m. reticulohistiocytosis
multidose insulin treatment
multidrug resistance protein (MDR)
multiexon
multiexonic gene
multiforme
    erythema m.
    glioblastoma m.
multigenic
multihormonal system disorder
multinodular euthyroid goiter
multiple
    m. anterior pituitary hormone
     deficiency
    m. daily injections (MDI)
    m. dose injection (MDI)
    m. endocrine abnormalities (MEA)
    m. endocrine adenomatosis
    m. endocrine adenopathies (MEA)
    m. endocrine neoplasia (MEN)
    m. endocrine neoplasia type 1
     (MEN 1)
    m. endocrine neoplasia type 2
     (MEN 2)
    m. endocrine neoplasia type 3
     (MEN 3)
    m. endocrine neoplasia type 2A
     (MEN 2A)
    m. endocrine neoplasia type 2B
     (MEN 2B)
    m. hamartoma syndrome
    m. luteinized theca cyst
    m. milia
    m. myeloma
    m. myeloma cell line
    M. Risk Factor Intervention Trial
     (MRFIT)
    m. sclerosis
    m. sulfatase deficiency
    m. system atrophy
multiple-injection regimen
multiplex
    dysostosis m.
    mononeuritis m.
    mononeuropathy m.
multiplier effect
multiport collimated cobalt-60 therapy

multipotent
multipotential progenitor
multisynaptic pathway
mu-M
mumps
    m. orchitis
    postpubertal m.
    m. virus
Münchausen syndrome
mural trophectoderm
muramidase
murine
    m. gene
    m. L cell
    m. osteopetrosis mutation
murmur
    Means-Lerman scratch m.
muscarinic
    m. agonist carbamylcholine
    m. cholinergic receptor
muscimol
muscle
    anterior scalene m.
    bulbospongiosus m.
    m. catabolism
    cremaster m.
    cricothyroid m.
    m. effect
    m. enzyme
    infrahyoid m.
    ischiocavernosus m.
    Müller m.
    myometrial smooth m.
    omohyoid m.
    platysma m.
    posterior cricoarytenoid m.
    skeletal m.
    sternocleidomastoid m.
    sternohyoid m.
    sternothyroid m.
    strap m.
    stylohyoid m.
    superficial perineal m.
    transverse rectus abdominis m.
    (TRAM)
    transversus perinei superficialis m.
    white m.
muscle:fat ratio
muscular
    m. dystrophy
    m. pseudohypertrophy
    m. weakness

musculoskeletal
    m. mass
    m. syndrome
mutagenesis
    insertional m.
    site-directed m.
mutans
    Streptococcus m.
mutant allele
mutase
    methylmalonyl-CoA m.
mutated
    ataxia telangiectasia m. (ATM)
mutation
    AIRE gene m.
    androgen receptor gene m.
    Arg m.
    BRCA1 m.
    BRCA2 m.
    breast cancer antigen 1, 2 m.
    DEHAL1 gene m.
    EIF2AK3 gene m.
    factor II m.
    factor V deficiency Leiden m.
    gain-of-function m.
    germline PTEN m.
    germline putative protein-tyrosine
      phosphatase m.
    germline TP53 m.
    GL13 gene m.
    GPCR m.
    homozygous missense m.
    inactivating m.
    m. inhibiting tyrosine kinase
    leaky splice m.
    Leiden m.
    LHX gene m.
    loss-of-function m.
    murine osteopetrosis m.
    osteopetrotic m.
    PHF6 gene m.
    point m.
    potassium$_{ATP}$ channel
      hyperinsulinemia m.
    proopiomelanocortin m.
    Prop-a gene m.
    R257X m.
    somatic PTEN m.
    somatic RET protooncogene m.
    thyroid-stimulating hormone
      receptor m.
    TSH receptor m.

M

NOTES

mutation-enriched restriction fragment length polymorphism assay
mutism
    deaf m.
mUW
    modified University of Wisconsin
    mUW solution
M.V.C. 9 + 3
M.V.I.-12
M.V.I. Pediatric
myalgia
Myapap
myasthenia gravis
mycobacteria
    nontuberculous m.
Mycobacterium
    M. avian-intracellulare
    M. avium-intracellulare
    M. cheloni
    M. fortuitum
    M. intracellulare
    M. kansasii
    M. leprae
    M. tuberculosis
mycobacterium
    atypical m.
mycophenolate mofetil
Mycoplasma hominis
mycotic infection
mydriasis
    anisocoria with ipsilateral m.
myelinated fiber bundle
myelin basic protein (MBP)
myelinolysis
    central pontine m.
myelodysplasia
    occult m.
myelofibrosis
myeloid
    m. leukemia inhibitory factor
    m. metaplasia
    m. precursor
myelolipoma
myeloma
    multiple m.
myelomeningocele (MMC)
myelomonocytic cell
myelopathy
    diabetic m.
myeloperoxidase (MPO)
myelophthisic anemia
myeloproliferative leukemia virus (MPLV)
Mykrox
Mylicon
myocardium

myocyte
myoedema
myoepithelial cell
myofiber diameter
myofibroblast
myogenic regeneration
myogenin
myoglobin
myoglobinuria
    idiopathic paroxysmal m.
myoid cell
myoinositol
myokymia
myometrial
    m. oxytocin receptor
    m. relaxation
    m. smooth muscle
myometrium
myopathy
    m., encephalopathy, lactic acidosis, stroke-like episodes (MELAS)
    hypothyroid m.
    lipid m.
    mitochondrial m.
    thyrotoxic m.
    tRNA mitochondrial m.
    X-linked myotubular m.
myosalpinx
myosin
    m. heavy chain (MHC)
    m. light chain (MLC)
    m. light chain kinase (MLCK)
Myotonachol
myotonia dystrophica
myotonic dystrophy
myotropic hormone
myxedema
    m. ataxia
    m. coma
    idiopathic m.
    m. ileus
    localized m.
    preclinical m.
    preradial m.
    pretibial m.
    primary m.
myxedematosus
    lichen m.
myxedematous
    m. endemic cretinism
    m. face
myxoma
    atrial m.
    cutaneous m.
    ventricular m.

N
norepinephrine
Humulin N
Nabadial
nabilone
Nabolin
nabothian cyst
nabumetone
NAC
N-acetylcysteine
N-**acetylated**
N-**acetyl-beta-glucosaminidase**
N-**acetylcysteine (NAC)**
N-**acetylglucosamine (GlcNAc)**
N-a. receptor
N-**acetyl-5-methoxykynurenamine**
N-**acetyl-5-methoxytryptamine**
N-**acetylserotonin**
N-**acetyltransferase**
serotonin *N*-a.
NAD
nicotinamide-adenine dinucleotide
NAD kinase
nadir
cortisol n.
n. hypoglycemia
nadolol
NADPH
nicotinamide adenine dinucleotide
phosphate
NADPH-cytochrome P450 reductase
naeslundii
Actinomyces n.
nafarelin
nafcillin
nafenopin
nafomostat mesylate
nafoxidine
Nägele rule
Nager syndrome
Na⁺/H⁺-ion exchanger

nail
hypoplastic n.
pitting of n.
Plummer n.
Terry n.
nail-patella syndrome
naïve
cold n.
Najjar syndrome
Na+K+-ATPase
nalbuphine
Naldecon Senior DX, EX
Nalfon

nalidixic acid
naloxone
naltrexone
NAMS
North American Menopause Society
nandrolone
n. decanoate
n. phenylpropionate
nanism
mulibrey n.
Na⁺-phosphate cotransporter
Naprosyn
naproxen
NAPRTCS
North American Pediatric Renal
Transplant Cooperative Study
Naqua
narcotine analog
nasal
n. cavity
n. insulin
n. limbus
nascent
n. collagen molecule
n. protein
n. protein chain
n. thrombus
nasogastric (NG)
nasogastrojejunal tube (NGJT)
Natabec FA, Rx
Natalins Rx
nateglinide
national
N. Cardiac Surgery Database
(NCSD)
N. Center for Health Statistics
chart
N. Cholesterol Education guidelines
N. Cholesterol Education Program
(NCEP)
N. Cholesterol Education Program
Adult Treatment Panel III
N. Cholesterol Education Program
criteria
N. Cholesterol Evaluation Program
N. Cooperative Growth Study
(NCGS)
N. Diabetes Data Group (NDDG)
N. Diabetes Data Group/World
Health Organization
(NDDG/WHO)
N. Health Interview Survey (NHIS)
N. Health and Nutrition
Examination Survey (NHANES)

national *(continued)*
>> N. Institute of Diabetes and Digestive and Kidney Diseases (NIDDK)
>> N. Institutes of Health (NIH)
>> N. Osteoporosis Foundation (NOF)

native pancreas
natriuresis
> pressure n.

natriuretic
> n. hormone
> n. peptide
> n. peptide receptor (NPR)

natruresis
natural
> n. hormone therapy (NHT)
> n. killer (NK)
> n. killer cell
> n. killer T (NKT)

nature
> pleiotropic n.

Naturetin
N-CAM
> neural cell adhesion molecule

NCEP
> National Cholesterol Education Program
>> NCEP criteria

NCGS
> National Cooperative Growth Study

NCHS
Nck protein
NCoA-1, -2 coactivator
N-CoR
> nuclear receptor corepressor

NCSD
> National Cardiac Surgery Database

NDDG
> National Diabetes Data Group

NDDG/WHO
> National Diabetes Data Group/World Health Organization

NDI
> nephrogenic diabetes insipidus

NE
> norepinephrine

near-total thyroidectomy
nebenkern
neck
> n. of pancreas
> webbed n.

neck-to-thigh ratio (N/T)
necrobiosis lipoidica diabeticorum (NLD)
necrolysis
> epidermal n.
> toxic epidermal n.

necrolytic
> n. migrating erythema
> n. migratory erythema (NME)

necropsy

necrosis
> adrenal n.
> brain n.
> central n.
> disseminated fat n.
> fat n.
> focal tumor n.
> frank n.
> hepatic n.
> idiopathic ischemic n.
> infected pancreatic n.
> ischemic n.
> papillary n.
> pituitary growth hormone-secreting adenoma n.
> postischemic acute tubular n.
> postpartum pituitary n.
> pressure n.
> renal papillary n.
> spontaneous pituitary n.
> subcutaneous fat n.
> thyroid n.

necrospermia
necrotic palatal ulcer
necrotizing
> n. cellulitis
> n. fasciitis

N.E.E. 1/35
needle
> n. catheter jejunostomy
> Howell aspiration n.
> osteodysplasia of Melnick and N.'s
> Tru-Cut n.
> Vim-Silverman n.

needlescopic procedure
NEFA
> nonesterified fatty acid

negative
> n. arterial-portal glucose gradient
> n. feedback
> n. feedback loop
> n. feedback regulation
> hormone-binding n.
> n. T_3 response element (TRE)
> n. triiodothyronine response element

Neisseria gonorrhoeae
Nelova
> N. 10/11
> N. 0.5/35E
> N. 1/50M

Nelson syndrome
NEM
> N-ethylmaleimide

Neo-Calglucon
neocortex
> frontal n.

Neo-Durabolic
Neo-Estrone

neoformans
    Cryptococcus n.
neointimal hyperplasia
neologism
neonatal
    n. adrenoleukodystrophy
    n. diabetes mellitus
    n. diabetes mellitus genetic entity
    n. diabetes mellitus insulin action
    n. exchange transfusion
    n. goiter
    n. Graves hyperthyroidism
    n. hypocalcemia
    n. hypoglycemia
    n. hypothyroidism
    n. severe hyperparathyroidism
    (NSHPT)
    n. thyroid dysfunction
    n. thyrotoxicosis
neoplasia
    familial multiple endocrine n.
    multiple endocrine n. (MEN)
    multiple endocrine n. type 1
    (MEN 1)
    multiple endocrine n. type 2
    (MEN 2)
    multiple endocrine n. type 3
    (MEN 3)
    multiple endocrine n. type 2A
    (MEN 2A)
    multiple endocrine n. type 2B
    (MEN 2B)
neoplasm
    androgen-secreting n.
    clonal n.
    ectopic n.
    follicular n.
    germ-cell n.
    gestational trophoblastic n. (GTN)
    hepatic n.
    histiocytic n.
    Hürthle cell n.
    hyalinizing trabecular n.
    intraductal oncocytic papillary n.
    (IOPN)
    intraductal papillary mucinous n.
    (IPMN)
    lymphoreticular n.
    pancreatic endocrine n. (PEN)
    peripancreatic n.
    plurihormonal neuroendocrine n.
    trophoblastic n.

neoplastic
    n. adenohypophysial cell
    n. pathologic lesion
Neoral
Neosar
Neosten
neostigmine
    methyl-sulfated n.
neotenin
Neotrace-4
NeoVadrin B Complex
neovascular
    n. frond
    n. glaucoma
neovascularization
    n. of disc (NVD)
    n. elsewhere in retina (NVE)
nephrectomy
nephritis
    chronic interstitial n.
    thyroid antigen-antibody n.
Nephro-Calci
nephrocalcin
nephrocalcinosis
    papillary n.
Nephrocaps
Nephro-Fer
nephrogenic
    n. diabetes
    n. diabetes insipidus (NDI)
nephrogenous
    n. cAMP
    n. cyclic adenosine monophosphate
nephrolithiasis
nephrolithotomy
    percutaneous n.
nephron
    cortical n.
    renal n.
nephropathic cystinosis
nephropathy
    acute uric acid n.
    diabetic n.
    tubulointerstitial n.
    urate n.
nephrotic syndrome
Nephrox Suspension
neprilysin
Nernst equation
nerve
    abducent n.
    ansa cervicalis n.

N

NOTES

nerve *(continued)*
>ansa hypoglossal n.
>buffer n.
>cervical sensory n.
>n. conduction velocity
>cranial n.'s II through XII
>N. Disability Score
>n. growth factor (NGF)
>hypertrophied corneal n.
>hypoglossal n.
>intercostal n.
>laryngeal n.
>ocular motor cranial n.
>oculomotor n.
>optic n.
>n. palsy
>parasympathetic n.
>peripheral n.
>phrenic n.
>preganglionic sympathetic n.
>pudendal n.
>recurrent laryngeal n.
>spinal accessory n.
>splanchnic n.
>superior laryngeal n.
>sural n.
>sympathetic n.
>N. Symptom Score
>trigeminal n.
>trochlear n.
>vagus n.

nerve-fiber loss
nervorum
>vasa n.

nervosa
>anorexia n.
>bulimia n.
>pars n.

nesidioblastoma
nesidioblastosis
>pancreatic n.

nesidiodysplasia
NESP55
>neuroendocrine secretory protein 55
>NESP55 protein

nest
>solid cell n.
>squamous cell n.

Nestrex
NET
>norepinephrine transporter
>norethisterone

net
>n. calcium absorption
>n. calcium influx
>n. efflux
>n. hepatic glucose uptake (NHGU)

N-ethylmaleimide (NEM)

network
>cis Golgi n.
>endoplasmic reticulum-Golgi n.
>Golgi n.
>intraglandular lymphatic n.
>trans-Golgi n. (TGN)

Neucalm-50 Injection
neu **oncogene**
neural
>n. cell adhesion molecule (N-CAM)
>n. crest
>n. factor
>n. lobe
>n. plate
>n. relationship
>n. stalk
>n. tube
>n. tube defect
>n. tumor

neuraminidase treatment
neuraxis
>midline central n.

neurilemoma
>cystic n.

neurinoma
neurite outgrowth
neuritis
>chiasmal n.
>lactation optic n.

neuroanatomic technique
neuroarthropathy
>Charcot n.

neuroblast
neuroblastoma
neurocircuit
neurocognitive impairment
neurocrest
neuroD1
>neurogenic differentiation 1

neurodegenerative disease
neurodevelopmental delay
neurodiagnostic study
neuroectoderm
neuroendocrine
>n. cell
>n. control
>n. control loop
>n. programming
>n. reflex
>n. secretory protein 55 (NESP55)
>n. system
>n. tumor

neuroendocrinology
neurofibroma
neurofibromatosis, type I, II
neurofilament
neurogenic
>n. atrophy

n. diabetes insipidus
n. differentiation 1 (neuroD1)
n. hypogonadism
n. precocious puberty
n. pulmonary edema
neuroglia
    n. cell
    peripheral n.
neuroglucopenia
neuroglycopenia
neuroglycopenic symptom
neurogranin
neurohormonal cell
neurohormone
neurohumoral
neurohypophysial
    n. diabetes insipidus
    n. hormone
    n. nerve terminal
    n. peptide
    n. stalk
neurohypophysis
neuroimaging study
neuroimmunology
neuroimmunomodulation
neurokinin A, B
neuroleptic malignant syndrome
neurologic endemic cretinism
neuroma
    mucosal n.
neuromedin K
neuromodulator
neuromuscular junction disorder
neuromyotonia
    ocular n.
neuron
    cholinergic n.
    dopaminergic n.
    hippocampal n.
    hypophysiotropic n.
    hypothalmo-neurohypophyseal n.
    intrinsic gut n.
    magnocellular cholinergic n.
    magnocellular
      hypothalamohypophyseal n.
    magnocellular neurosecretory n.
    oxytocinergic n.
    paraventricular n.
    parvocellular n.
    peptidergic n.
    postganglionic sympathetic n.
    preganglionic sympathetic n.

primary afferent nociceptor n.
    (PAN)
thermosensitive n.
tuberohypophyseal dopaminergic n.
    (THDA)
tuberoinfundibular n.
tuberoinfundibular dopaminergic n.
    (TIDA)
neuronal
    n. cytosol
    n. hamartoma
    n. shock
neuronavigation
neuron-specific enolase
Neurontin
neuroophthalmologic manifestation
neuroophthalmology
neuropathic
    n. arthropathy
    n. cachexia
    n. ulcer
neuropathy
    acute painful n.
    asymmetric n.
    autonomic n.
    cardiovascular autonomic n.
    clonidine diabetic n.
    compression n.
    compressive n.
    cranial n.
    demyelinative n.
    diabetic autonomic n.
    distal sensory n.
    distal small-fiber n.
    distal symmetric diabetic n.
    enteric n.
    entrapment/compression n.
    gastrointestinal autonomic n.
    genitourinary autonomic n.
    insulin-induced n.
    large fiber n.
    Leber hereditary optic n.
    nondiabetic immune-mediated n.
    optic and chiasmal n.
    peripheral n.
    progressive multifocal axonal n.
    proximal diabetic n.
    proximal motor n.
    radiation optic n.
    sensorimotor n.
    small-fiber type of diabetic n.

NOTES

N

neuropeptide
    n. B, K
    n. gamma
    n. immunocytochemistry
    n. Y (NPY)
neuropharmacology
neurophysin
    hormone-specific n.
    n. I, II
    n. protein
    vasopressin n. II
neurophysin-positive varicosity
neurophysiology
neuropsychiatric
    n. disorder
    n. effect
    n. feature
neuroradiologic imaging procedure
neuroradiology
neurosarcoidosis
neurosecretion
neurosecretory
    n. cell
    n. gland
    n. granule (NSG)
    n. vessel
neurosis
neurosteroid
neurosurgeon
    pituitary n.
neurotensin
neurotransmitter
    bioamine n.
    primary sympathetic n.
neurotrophic
    n. factor
    n. hormone
    n. therapy
    n. tyrosine kinase receptor, type 1 (NTRK1)
neurotrophin
neurotrophin-3 (NT-3)
neurotrophin-4 (NT-4)
neurotrophin-5 (NT-5)
neurturin (NTN)
Neut
neutral
    n. endopeptidase
    n. protamine Hagedorn (NPH)
    n. protamine Hagedorn insulin
neutrophil
    n. activation
    n. chemotaxis
    n. respiratory burst activity (NRBA)
nevoid basal cell carcinoma
Newcastle bone disease
New England Diabetes and Endocrinology Center

NF-1 transcription factor
NF-kappa-B
    nuclear factor-kappa-B
        NF-kappa-B element
        receptor activator of NF-kappa-B (RANK)
NF-kB
    nuclear factor-κkB
N-(9-fluorenylmethoxycarbonyl)-L-leucine (FMOC-Leu)
NFPA
    nonfunctioning pituitary adenoma
NG
    nasogastric
NGF
    nerve growth factor
NGGCT
    nongerminomatous germ cell tumor
NGJT
    nasogastrojejunal tube
N-glycosylation
NGM
    norgestimate
NHANES
    National Health and Nutrition Examination Survey
        NHANES I, II, III
NHGU
    net hepatic glucose uptake
NHIS
    National Health Interview Survey
NHT
    natural hormone therapy
niacin
niacinamide
Niaspan
Nicobid
Nicoderm Patch
Nicolar
nicotinamide-adenine dinucleotide (NAD)
nicotinamide adenine dinucleotide phosphate (NADPH)
nicotine-stimulated pathway
Nicotinex
nicotinic
    n. acid
    n. cholinergic receptor
nicotinic-type receptor
Nicotrol Patch
NIDDK
    National Institute of Diabetes and Digestive and Kidney Diseases
NIDDM
    noninsulin-dependent diabetes mellitus
        nonobese type 2 NIDDM
        obese type 2 NIDDM
nidus
Niemann-Pick disease
nifedipine

Niferex
Niferex-PN
night-day rhythm
nigra
> substantia n.

nigrans
nigricans
> hyperandrogenism, insulin resistance, acanthosis n. (HAIRAN)

nigrostriatal bundle
NIH
> National Institutes of Health

Nilandron
Nilevar
nilutamide
nimesulide
nipple
> hypoplasia of n.'s
> supranumerous mammary glands and n.'s

NIS
> sodium-iodide symporter

Nissl substance
Nitabuch layer
nitrate
> gallium n.

nitric
> n. oxide (NO)
> n. oxide synthase (NOS)

nitrite
> sodium n.

nitroblue tetrazolium test
nitrocellulose membrane
nitrofurantoin
nitrogen
> n. balance
> blood urea n. (BUN)
> n. retention
> total body n.
> n. wasting

nitroglycerin
nitroprusside reaction
nitrosonaphthol
nitrosourea
nitrous oxide-donor drug
nizatidine
NK
> natural killer
> NK cell

NK1 receptor
NK2 receptor
NK3 receptor

NKCC2
> sodium-potassium-2 chloride cotransporter

NKH
> nonketotic hyperglycemia

NKT
> natural killer T
> NKT cell

NLD
> necrobiosis lipoidica diabeticorum

N-linked glycosylation
NLS
> nuclear localization signal motif

NMDA
> N-methyl-D-aspartate

NME
> necrolytic migratory erythema

N-methyl-D-aspartate (NMDA)
N-methyl D-aspartic acid
N-methyltransferase
> phenylethanolamine N.-m. (PNMT)

NMR
> nuclear magnetic resonance

***n-myc* gene**
NO
> nitric oxide
> NO synthase (NOS)

Nocardia asteroides
nociceptin/orphanin
> n. FQ (N/OFQ)
> n. FQ peptide

nocturnal
> n. emission
> n. hypoglycemia
> n. penile tumescence (NPT)
> n. penile tumescence testing
> n. rhythm
> n. thyroid-stimulating hormone surge
> n. TSH surge
> n. vasopressin release

node
> cervical lymph n. (CLN)
> Delphian lymph n.
> juxtathyroid n.
> lymph n.
> paraaortic lymph n.
> parasternal n.
> sentinel lymph n.
> Sister Mary Joseph n.
> upper pretracheal n.

N

NOTES

node-based malignant lymphoproliferative disease
NO-donor drug
nodosa
> periarteritis n.
> polyarteritis n.
> trichorrhexis n.

nodosum
> erythema n.

nodular
> n. autonomy
> n. fasciitis
> n. goiter

nodule
> autonomous n.
> autonomously functioning thyroid n. (AFTN)
> autonomous toxic n.
> cold n.
> cool n.
> cystic n.
> distinct n.
> dominant thyroid n.
> n. function
> functioning n.
> hamartomatous n.
> hemorrhagic n.
> hot n.
> ill-defined n.
> Kimmelstiel-Wilson n.
> Lisch n.
> single thyroid n.
> soft tissue n.
> solitary nontoxic n.
> solitary thyroid n.
> thyroid n.
> toxic solitary n.
> toxic thyroid n. (TTN)
> warm n.

NOF
> National Osteoporosis Foundation

N/OFQ
> nociceptin/orphanin FQ
> N/OFQ peptide

Nomarski microscopy
nomegestrole acetate
NOMI
> nonocclusive mesenteric ischemia

nomogram
non
> sine qua n.

nonaggressive tumor
nonandrogen
nonandrogenic progestin
nonapeptide
non-aureus
> *Staphylococcus n.-a.*

nonautoimmune
> n. familial hyperthyroidism
> n. nontoxic diffuse goiter

non-beta-cell regulated insulin gene expression
nonbeta cell tumor
noncalcareous stone
noncalcemic analog
noncaseating granuloma
noncholecystokinin substance
nonclassical
> n. hydroxylase deficiency
> n. 21-hydroxylase deficiency

nonclassic 21-hydroxylase deficiency
nonclostridial anaerobic cellulitis
noncollagen bone matrix
noncollagenous protein
noncompliance
noncontraceptive estrogen
noncontractile cell
noncornified cell
noncovalent bond
nondiabetic immune-mediated neuropathy
nondissociated acid
nondysjunction
> meiotic n.

nonencapsulated
nonendocrine disease
nonenzymatic
> n. glycosylation
> n. photolysis
> n. protein glycation

nonergot long-acting prolactin inhibitor
nonessential fatty acids
nonesterified fatty acid (NEFA)
nonestrogenic stereoisomer 17-alpha estradiol
nonfamilial parathyroid adenoma
nonfunctional pituitary adenoma
nonfunctioning
> n. microadenoma
> n. pheochromocytoma
> n. pituitary adenoma (NFPA)
> n. pituitary tumor

nongenomic
> n. action
> n. effect
> n. factor
> n. pathway

nongerminomatous germ cell tumor (NGGCT)
nongoitrous
nongranular clear chromophobe cell
non-Graves disease hyperthyroidism
nongrowth hormone-deficient short stature
nonhistocompatibility locus antigen-associated form

nonhistone protein
non-HLA-associated form
nonhomologous recombination
nonhormonal regulator
nonhuman leukocyte antigen associated form
noninsulin-dependent diabetes mellitus (NIDDM)
noninsulinoma pancreatogenous hypoglycemia
noninvasive blood glucose monitoring
nonionic
    n. contrast radiography
    n. iodinated contrast
non-islet cell tumor
non-islet-cell tumor-induced hypoglycemia
nonisotropic technique
nonketotic
    n. hyperglycemia (NKH)
    n. hyperglycinemia
    n. hyperosmolar coma
    n. hyperosmolar state
    n. hypoglycemic acidosis
nonmitogenic anti-CD3 antibody
nonneoplastic pathologic lesion
nonobese
    n. diabetic
    n. type 2 NIDDM
nonocclusive mesenteric ischemia (NOMI)
nonoral estradiol delivery system
nonosmotic stimulus
nonosteoporotic
nonpapillary thyrogenic carcinoma
nonpeptide antagonist
nonphotic
    n. cue
    n. entrainment
nonpituitary thyrotropin
nonprolactinoma
nonproliferative diabetic retinopathy (NPDR)
nonpurulent fluid
nonpyknotic nucleus
nonregulatory element (NRE)
nonresorbable resin
non-salt-wasting congenital adrenal hyperplasia
nonsecreting
    n. pituitary adenoma
    n. pituitary tumor

nonsecretory adrenal adenoma
nonshivering thermogenesis
nonsmall cell carcinoma
nonspecific binding (NSB)
nonsteroidal
    n. antiinflammatory agent
    n. antiinflammatory drug (NSAID)
    n. estrogen
nonsulfonylurea insulin secretagogues (NSIS)
nonsuppressible
    n. insulinlike activity (NSILA)
    n. insulinlike activity factor
nonsustained erection
nonsyndromic
    n. autosomal recessive disorder
    n. coronal craniosynostosis
    n. familial enlarged vestibular aqueduct
nonsyndromic deafness
nonthyroidal
    n. illness (NTI)
    n. illness syndrome
nonthyroid disease
nonthyroid illness
nonthyromimetic
nontoxic
    n. multinodular goiter
    n. nodular goiter
    n. sporadic goiter
    n. thyroid adenoma
nontropical sprue
nontropic sprue
nontuberculous mycobacteria
nonviral vector
nonviscous particulate fiber
Noonan syndrome
No Pain-HP
noradrenaline
noradrenergic
    n. afferent
    n. blocker
    n. receptor
norandrostenolone
Norcet
nor-derivative progestin
Nordette
NordiPen
Norditropin SimpleXx
norelgestromin
norepinephrine (N, NE)

NOTES

N

norepinephrine *(continued)*
    n. perikaryon
    n. transporter (NET)
norethandrolone
Norethin
    N. 1/35E
    N. 1/50M
norethindrone
    n. acetate
    estradiol and n.
    n. ethanthate
    ethinyl estradiol and n.
    mestranol and n.
norethisterone (NET)
norethynodrel
noretisterone
norfloxacin
Norgesic
norgestimate (NGM)
    ethinyl estradiol and n.
norgestrel
    conjugated equine estrogen plus n.
    (CEEP)
    ethinyl estradiol and n.
Norinyl
    N. 1+35
    N. 1+50
Norlutin
normal
    n. gonadal steroid level
    n. saline (NS)
    n. sexual differentiation
normetanephrine
normoalbuminuria
normocalcemia
normocalcemic
    n. hypercalciuria
    n. primary hyperparathyroidism
normocholesterolemia
normocortisolemia
normocytic normochromic anemia
Normodyne
normofunctioning
normoglycemia
    posthyperglycemic n.
normoglycemic
normokalemia
normolipidemic
normomagnesemic
normoprolactinemia
normoprolactinemic woman
normothermic
Norplant II
Norprolac
norpseudoephedrine
NOR-QD
Norrie disease
nortestosterone
Nor-tet Oral

north
    N. America blastomycosis
    N. American Menopause Society
    (NAMS)
    N. American Pediatric Renal
    Transplant Cooperative Study
    (NAPRTCS)
northern
    N. blot
    N. blot analysis
Norwood repair
NOS
    nitric oxide synthase
    NO synthase
notochord
Nottingham Health Profile
Novartis
novo
    de n.
Novo-Butamide
NovoFine
Novogen
Novo-Glyburide
Novolin
    N. 70/30
    N. ge
    N. L, N, R
    N. N InnoLet
    N. 85/15 PenFill cartridge
    N. R InnoLet
Novolin-Pen II
NovoLog
Novo-Metformin
Novo-Methacin
NovoNorm
NovoPen 3
Novo-Prednisolone
Novo-Prednisone
Novo-Profen
Novo-Propamide
NovoRapid
Novo-Spiroton
Now
    Metrika A1c N.
NP-59
    N. iodonocholesterol scan
    N. scintigraphy
NPDR
    nonproliferative diabetic retinopathy
NPH
    neutral protamine Hagedorn
    NPH Iletin I
    NPH insulin
    Pork NPH
NPH-N
NP-59 isotope
NPR
    natriuretic peptide receptor

NPT
  nocturnal penile tumescence
    NPT testing
NPY
  neuropeptide Y
N-3-pyridyl-methyl-N-*p*-nitrophenylurea
NRBA
  neutrophil respiratory burst activity
NRE
  nonregulatory element
NS
  normal saline
    Stadol NS
NSAID
  nonsteroidal antiinflammatory drug
NSB
  nonspecific binding
NSG
  neurosecretory granule
NSHPT
  neonatal severe hyperparathyroidism
NSILA
  nonsuppressible insulinlike activity
NSIS
  nonsulfonylurea insulin secretagogue
  nonsulfonylurea insulin secretagogues
NT-3
  neurotrophin-3
NT-4
  neurotrophin-4
NT-5
  neurotrophin-5
N/T
  neck-to-thigh ratio
    N/T ratio
N-telopeptide collagen
N-telopeptide/creatine
N-terminal
    N-t. peptide
    N-t. telopeptide of type I collagen
**N-terminus peroxisome proliferator-
  activated receptor-gamma**
NTI
  nonthyroidal illness
NTN
  neurturin
NTRK1
  neurotrophic tyrosine kinase receptor,
    type 1
    NTRK1 protooncogene

NTS
  nucleus of the tractus solitarius
  nucleus tractus solitarius
Nubain
nuclear
    n. accessory hormone
    n. atypia
    n. factor-κkB (NF-kB)
    n. factor beta
    n. factor-kappa-B (NF-kappa-B)
    n. factor-kappa B element
    n. hormone receptor
    n. localization signal motif (NLS)
    n. magnetic resonance (NMR)
    n. membrane
    n. pore complex
    n. receptor corepressor (N-CoR)
    n. runoff assay
    n. scintigraphy
    n. transcription factor
    n. translocation
nucleation
nuclei (*pl. of* nucleus)
nucleolar channel system
nucleotide
    antisense n.
    guanyl n.
    n. triphosphate
nucleus, pl. nuclei
    arcuate n.
    n. basalis of Meynert
    cortical amygdaloid n.
    dorsal motor n.
    dorsomedial n. (DMN)
    Edinger-Westphal n.
    ghost n.
    heterochromatic n.
    hypothalamic paraventricular n.
    intermediate n.
    lacrimal n.
    midbrain raphe n.
    nonpyknotic n.
    osteoclastic n.
    paramagnetic n.
    paramedian reticular n.
    paraventricular n. (PVN)
    paraventricular thalamic n. (PVT)
    premammillary n.
    pyknotic n.
    Raphe n.
    salivatory n.
    sexually dimorphic n.

N

NOTES

nucleus *(continued)*
    stress-relevant amygdalar n.
    suprachiasmatic n. (SCN)
    suprachiasmic n.
    supraoptic n.
    thalamic n.
    n. tractus solitarius (NTS)
    n. of the tractus solitarius (NTS)
    vagal n.
    n. ventralis anterior of thalamus
    ventromedial n. (VMN)
Nucofed
Nucotuss
Nu-Glyburide
Nu-Ibuprofen
Nu-Indo
Nu-Iron
null
    n. cell
    n. hypothesis
null-cell adenoma
nulliparous
numbness
    circumoral n.
Numorphan
Nuprin
Nu-Propranolol
Nurses¹ Health Study

nutans
    spasmus n.
Nutraplus Topical
NutraSweet
nutrient
    carbohydrate n.
nutrigenomics
nutrition
    n. goals
    parenteral n.
    n. requirement
    n. therapy
    total parenteral n. (TPN)
nutritional rickets
Nutropin
    N. AQ
    N. Depot
NuvaRing
NVD
    neovascularization of disc
NVE
    neovascularization elsewhere in retina
nyctohemeral rhythm
nystagmus
    roving n.
    see-saw n.
nystatin

O

cathepsin O

O₂

oxygen
O₂ disposable boot device

OA

open adrenalectomy
osteoarthritis
osteoid area

O1A

Forkhead box protein O1A
(FKHR)

OB

Chromagen OB

obese

o. type 2 NIDDM
o. type 2 noninsulin-dependent
diabetes mellitus

obesity

abdominal o.
android o.
central o.
centripetal o.
childhood o.
clinical o.
diet-induced o. (DIO)
exogenous o.
o. gene
genetic o.
gynecoid o.
hypothalamic o.
monogenic o.
morbid o.
polygenic o.
television-watching o.
truncal o.
visceral o.

obesity-related hyposomatotropism
obesity/type 2 diabetes syndrome
ob gene
obligatory thermogenesis
oblique arytenoid
oblongata

medulla o.

obstruction

airway o.
superior ophthalmic vein o.

obstructive intestinal disease
obtundation
Oby-trim
OC

Osteocalcin

OCA

oculocutaneous albinism

occludens

zone o.
zonula o.

occlusion

acute arterial o.
branch retinal vein o.
hepatic artery o.

occult

o. biliary microlithiasis
o. carcinoma
o. diabetes
o. myelodysplasia

occupancy

receptor o.

ochronosis
Ochsner clamp
OCIF

osteoclastogenesis inhibitory factor

Oct-1

octamer-binding
Oct-1 transcription factor

octacalcium phosphate
octamer-binding (Oct-1)

o.-b. transcription factor

Octamide
[13C]-octanoic acid test
octapeptide
Octostim
OctreoScan
octreotide

In-111 o.
o. LAR
o. long-acting release
o. scan
somatostatin analogue o.
o. therapy

Ocufen Ophthalmic
ocular

o. albinism
o. calcification
o. complications of diabetes
o. dysmotility
o. histidinemia
o. motility
o. motor cranial nerve
o. neuromyotonia
o. pain
o. paresis

oculocutaneous

o. albinism (OCA)
o. albinism type I

oculodentoosseous dysplasia
oculomotor

o. nerve
o. nerve palsy

O

oculopharyngeal muscular dystrophy
ODC
>ornithine decarboxylase

ODF
>osteoclast differentiation factor

odontoblast
odontohypophosphatasia
odor
>apocrine body o.
>excessive body o.

oestradiol
Oestrillin
office-based intervention
ofloxacin
Ogen
>O. Oral
>O. Vaginal

OGF
>opioid growth factor
>ovarian growth factor

OGTT
>oral glucose tolerance test

24-OHase
>vitamin D 24-hydroxylase

Ohase
>hydroxylase

17-OHCS
>17-hydroxycorticosteroid

24,25(OH)$_2$D$_3$
>24,25-dihydroxyvitamin D

25(OH)$_2$D$_3$
>25-dihydroxyvitamin D

OHL
>hydroxylysine

17-OHP
>17-hydroxyprogesterone

OHSS
>ovarian hyperstimulation syndrome

1,25(OH)$_2$-VitD
25OH-VitD
>25-hydroxyvitamin D

OI
>osteogenesis imperfecta

oil
>evening primrose o.
>fish o.
>iodized o.
>progesterone o.

ointment
>Collagenase Santyl o.

okadaic acid
OKT3
>ornithine-ketoacid transaminase

olanzapine
oleic acid
Olestra
olfaction

olfactory
>o. bulb
>o. placode

oligoanovulation
oligoanuric
oligoasthenozoospermia
oligoclonal
oligoclonality
oligodendrocyte
oligodeoxynucleotide
>o. antisense probe
>21-mer phosphorothioate
>antisense o.

oligodontia
oligomenorrhea with anovulatory menses
oligonucleotide
>allele-specific o. (ASO)
>o. inhibition
>o. probe

oligosaccharide
>o. chain
>high-mannose o.
>o. transferase enzyme

oligospermia
oligozoospermia
olivopontocerebellar atrophy
OM
>oncostatin M

omega-3 polyunsaturated fatty acid
omega-conotoxin-sensitive pathway
omentum
>Cushing disease of the o.

omeprazole
O-methylation
OMIM
>Online Mendelian Inheritance of Man
>database

Omnican Piston syringe for insulin
Omnicef
Omnipen
Omnipen-N
omohyoid muscle
omphalocele
OMS Oral
onapristone
Oncet
oncocyte
oncocytic
>o. adenoma
>o. tumor
>o. variant

oncocytoma
oncocytosis
oncogene
>B o.
>c-*fms* o.
>c-myc o.
>*erb* o.
>Harvey-Ras o.

kit o.
mas o.
neu o.
RAS o.
rearranged during transformation o.
RET o.
ros o.
v-*erb* A o.
viral o.
oncogenesis
oncogenic
    o. osteomalacia
    o. rickets
oncogenous osteomalacia
oncoretrovirus vector
oncosis
oncostatin M (OM)
oncotic pressure
ondansetron
ONDST
    overnight high-dose dexamethasone
    suppression test
One-Alpha
OneTouch
    O. Basic
    O. blood glucose meter
    O. Fast Take meter kit
    O. II hospital blood glucose
      monitoring system
    O. InDuo glucose meter
    O. Profile
    O. SureStep glucose meter
    O. Ultra test strip
Online Mendelian Inheritance of Man
database (OMIM)
ontogenesis
ontogeny
    B-cell o.
    osteoblast o.
onycholysis
oocyesis
oocyte
    o. maturation-inhibiting factor
    o. meiotic inhibitor
    primary o.
    secondary o.
oogonia
oolemma
oophorectomize
oophorectomy
oophoritis
    autoimmune o.

oophorus
    cumulus o.
OP
    osteoporosis
open
    o. adrenalectomy (OA)
    o. reading frame (ORF)
opener
    adenosine triphosphate potassium o.
opening
    diaphragmal o.
operation
    Frey o.
    Karydakis o.
    Partington o.
    Sistrunk o.
OPG
    osteoprotegerin
OPGF
    osteoprotegerin factor
OPGL
    osteoprotegerin ligand
ophthalmic
    o. administration of insulin
    o. artery
    o. Graves disease
    Ocufen O.
ophthalmopathy
    endocrine o.
    euthyroid o.
    Graves o. (GO)
    infiltrative o.
    radioiodine-induced exacerbation
      of o.
    thyroid o.
    thyroid-associated o. (TAO)
ophthalmoplegia
    external o.
    internal o.
ophthalmoscopy
opiate
opioid
    endogenous o.
    o. growth factor (OGF)
    o. peptide
opioidergic
opioid-stimulated pathway
opisthotonus
opium
    o. alkaloid
    belladonna and o.
    o. tincture

O

NOTES

opsonin receptor
opsonization
optic
- o. apparatus glioma
- o. canal
- o. chiasm
- o. and chiasmal neuropathy
- o. disc edema
- o. disc pallor
- o. hypocalcemia
- o. nerve
- o. radiation
- o. recess
- o. tract
- o. tract pituitary tumor

opticochiasmatic glioma
OptiQuant assay
OR
- ovary reserve

Oragrafin
oral
- o. administration of insulin
- AllerMax O.
- Amen O.
- o. antibiotic
- o. antidiabetic agent
- Anxanil O.
- Aristocort O.
- Atarax O.
- Atolone O.
- Atozine O.
- Banophen O.
- Belix O.
- Benadryl O.
- Calm-X O.
- Cataflam O.
- Celestone O.
- o. cholecystographic dye
- Cleocin HCl O.
- Cleocin Pediatric O.
- o. contraceptive
- Cortef O.
- Curretab O.
- Cycrin O.
- Cytomel O.
- Decadron O.
- Delta-Cortef O.
- Dilaudid O.
- Dimetabs O.
- Dormarex 2 O.
- Dormin O.
- Dramamine O.
- Durrax O.
- Estrace O.
- Flagyl O.
- Genahist O.
- o. glucose tolerance test (OGTT)
- o. hamartoma
- Hydrocortone O.

- Hy-Pam O.
- o. hypoglycemic agent
- Indocin SR O.
- Kenacort O.
- Marmine O.
- Medrol O.
- Mephyton O.
- MS Contin O.
- MSIR O.
- o. multiple vitamin
- Nor-tet O.
- Ogen O.
- OMS O.
- Oramorph SR O.
- Orinase O.
- Ortho-Est O.
- Panmycin O.
- Pediapred O.
- Phenergan O.
- o. prednisolone
- Prelone O.
- Proglycem O.
- Protostat O.
- Provera O.
- Robitet O.
- Roxanol SR O.
- Sumycin O.
- Tega-Vert O.
- Tetracap O.
- Vamate O.
- Vancocin O.
- Vistaril O.
- Voltaren O.
- Voltaren-XR O.

Oralet
- Fentanyl O.

Oralgen
Oralin
Oramorph SR Oral
Oramyd
Orasone
orbital
- o. apex syndrome
- o. cellulitis
- o. fat
- o. fibroblast
- o. hypotelorism
- o. tissue

orbitopathy
- dysthyroid o.
- infiltrative o.
- thyroid o.

orchidometer
- Prader o.

orchiectomy
orchis
orchitis
- mumps o.

tuberculous o.
viral o.
orciprenaline
Oretic
Oreton Methyl
orexigenic
o. agent
o. hormone
o. peptide
Orexin A, B
ORF
open reading frame
organ
circumventricular o. (CVO)
effector o.
o. failure
peripheral o.
o. procurement organization
subcommissural o. (SCO)
subfornical o. (SFO)
o. transplantation
ultimobranchial o.
vomeronasal o.
o. of Zuckerkandl
organic
o. impotence
o. matrix
o. osmolyte
Organidin
organification defect
organization
National Diabetes Data
Group/World Health O.
(NDDG/WHO)
organ procurement o.
Pan American Health O. (PAHO)
World Health O. (WHO)
World Health O. (type I, II, III)
organogenesis
thyroid o.
organomegaly
organotherapy
Brown-Séquard o.
organum
o. vasculosum
o. vasculosum laminae terminalis
(OVLT)
o. vasculosum of the lamina
terminalis (OVLT)
orgasm
female o.
male o.

origin
fetal o.
gonadotroph cell o.
Schwann cell o.
somatropin of rDNA o.
original
o. University of Wisconsin (oUW)
o. University of Wisconsin solution
Orinase
O. Diagnostic Injection
O. Oral
ORL-1 receptor
orlista
orlistat
Ormazine
ornithine
o. carbamoyltransferase
o. cycle
o. decarboxylase (ODC)
o. transaminase
o. transcarbamylase (OTC)
o. transcarbamylase deficiency
ornithine-ketoacid transaminase (OKT3)
orosomucoid
orotic acid
orphan
O. Annie eye
o. receptor
orphenadrine, aspirin, and caffeine
Ortho
O. Evra Patch
O. Tri-Cyclen
Ortho-Cept
Ortho-Cyclen
Ortho-Est Oral
Ortho-Novum
O.-N. 1/35
O.-N. 1/50
O.-N. 7/7/7
O.-N. 10/11
orthophosphate
inorganic o. (P_i)
Ortho-Prefest
orthorhombic
orthostasis
orthostatic hypotension
orthotic
custom-healing o.
orthotopic liver transplantation
Orudis KT
Oruvail

O

NOTES

OS
Ensure Glucerna OS
Os-Cal 500
oscillation
ultradian o.
oscillator
circadian o.
oscillatory behavior
Osler-Rendu-Weber disease
Osmitrol Injection
Osm/kg
osmoles per kilogram
Osm/L
osmoles per liter
osmolality
body fluid o.
body water o.
cytosolic o.
o. dehydration test
effective o.
interstitial o.
plasma o. (POSM)
serum o.
urine o.
osmolar
o. clearance
o. gap
osmolarity
extracellular fluid o.
osmole
idiogenic o.
o.'s per kilogram (Osm/kg)
o.'s per liter (Osm/L)
osmolyte
organic o.
osmoreceptor
osmoregulation
osmoregulatory defect
osmostat
osmotic
o. cell injury
o. demyelination
o. diarrhea
o. diuresis
o. diuretic
o. equilibrium
o. hemostasis
o. homeostasis
o. minipump
o. regulation
o. stimulus
o. threshold
osseous
o. fragmentation
o. matrix
ossification
endochondral o.
intramembranous o.
periosteal o.

ossium
fibrogenesis imperfecta o.
Ostaderm
osteitis
o. deformans
o. fibrosa
o. fibrosa cystica
o. fibrosa cystica generalisata of von Recklinghausen
osteoarthritis (OA)
osteoarthropathy
hypertrophic o.
primary hypertrophic o.
pulmonary o.
secondary hypertrophic o.
osteoarticular destruction
osteoblast
o. apoptosis
o. heterogenicity
o. ontogeny
o. phenotype
o. progenitor proliferation
o. proliferation
osteoblastic
o. phenotype
o. resorption
o. tumor
osteoblastlike osteosarcoma cell
osteoblast-mediated bone formation
Osteocalcin (OC)
O. level
O. secretion
serum O.
osteochondrodysplasia
osteoclast
o. activity
o. apoptosis
bone-resorbing o.
o. differentiation factor (ODF)
o. precursor
o. ultrastructure
osteoclast-activated bone resorption
osteoclast-driven bone resorption
osteoclastic
o. activity
o. bone
o. bone resorption
o. function
o. nucleus
o. osteolysis
o. resorption lacuna
o. stimulation
osteoclast-mediated bone resorption
osteoclastogenesis inhibitory factor (OCIF)
osteocyte
osteocytic
o. membrane system
o. osteolysis

osteodysplasia of Melnick and Needles
osteodysplastic primordial dwarfism
osteodystrophy
    Albright hereditary o. (AHO)
    aplastic uremic o.
    mixed uremic o.
    pediatric renal o.
    renal o.
    thyrotoxic o.
    uremic o.
osteoectasia with hyperphosphatasia
osteofibrosis
osteogenesis
    o. imperfecta (OI)
    O. Imperfecta Foundation
    o. imperfecta types I, II, III, IV
osteogenic protein-2
osteoid
    o. accumulation
    o. area (OA)
    o. seam
    o. seam thickness
    o. surface
    unmineralized lamellar o.
    woven o.
osteoinduction
osteolysis
    carpotarsal o.
    familial expansile o. (FEO)
    Gorham massive o.
    idiopathic o.
    migratory o.
    osteoclastic o.
    osteocytic o.
osteolytic
    o. flame
    o. lesion
osteoma
osteomalacia
    aluminum-associated o.
    aluminum-induced o.
    aluminum-related o.
    axial o.
    calvarial o.
    hypophosphatemic o.
    oncogenic o.
    oncogenous o.
    o. syndrome
    vitamin D-deficiency o.
Osteomark
osteomesopyknosis

osteomyelitis
    temporal bone o.
osteon
osteonecrosis
osteonectin
osteopathia striata
osteopathy
    diabetic o.
osteopenia
    corticoid-induced o.
    cyclosporine A-induced o.
    posttransplantation o.
    progressive o.
    trabecular o.
osteopetrosis
    human malignant o.
    infantile o.
osteopetrotic
    o. microphthalmic
    o. mutation
    o. phenotype
osteophyte
osteopoikilosis
osteopontin
osteoporosis (OP)
    age-related o.
    o. bisphosphonate
    o. circumscripta
    glucocorticoid-induced o.
    idiopathic juvenile o.
    involutional o.
    low-turnover o.
    postmenopausal o.
    posttraumatic o.
    steroid-induced o.
osteoporotic cytokine
osteoprogenitor cell
osteoprotegerin (OPG)
    o. factor (OPGF)
    o. ligand (OPGL)
osteosarcoma
osteosclerosis
    autosomal dominant o.
    hepatitis C-associated o.
osteostatin
osteotomy
    cranioorbitozygomatic o. (COZ)
Ostoforte
O'Sullivan-Mahan study
OT
    oxytocin

NOTES

OTC
>ornithine transcarbamylase
>OTC deficiency

otitis
>malignant external o.

ouabain

ouabain-like hormone

ouabain-sensitive Na⁺-K⁺ ATPase

outcome
>Hyperglycemia and Adverse Pregnancy O. (HAPO)
>visual o.

outfracture

outgrowth
>neurite o.

out-of-target blood glucose level

output
>cardiac o.
>hepatic glucose o. (HGO)
>urine o.

oUW
>original University of Wisconsin
>oUW solution

ova (*pl. of* ovum)

ovale
>foramen o.

ovarian
>o. ablation
>o. antibody
>o. cortex
>o. cycle
>o. dysgenesis
>o. endometriosis cyst
>o. failure
>o. fimbria
>o. follicle
>o. goiter
>o. granulosa cell
>o. growth factor (OGF)
>o. hyperandrogenesis
>o. hyperandrogenism
>o. hyperstimulation syndrome (OHSS)
>o. hyperthecosis
>o. hypoandrogenism
>o. ligament
>o. steroidogenesis
>o. steroidogenic dysfunction
>o. teratoma
>o. tumor
>o. venous plasma oxytocin

ovariectomy

ovarii
>struma o.

ovary
>Chinese hamster o. (CHO)
>cystic o.
>granulosa cell tumor of the o.
>polycystic o. (PCO)

>o. reserve (OR)
>resistant o.
>streak o.
>syndrome of polycystic o.

Ovcon 35, 50

overactivity
>thyroid o.

overexpressed

overexpression
>gene o.

overgrowth
>acral o.
>articular o.
>bacterial o. (BO)

overlap syndrome

overload
>aluminum o.
>iron o.

overnight
>o. high-dose dexamethasone suppression test (ONDST)
>o. metyrapone test
>o. 1-mg dexamethasone suppression test

overnutrition

oversuppression

overt
>o. diabetes
>o. glycosuria

overtreatment

overweight

overworked B-cell hypothesis

Ovidrel

oviduct

ovine corticotropin-releasing hormone

OVLT
>organum vasculosum laminae terminalis
>organum vasculosum of the lamina terminalis

Ovol

ovotestis

Ovral

Ovrette

ovulation
>o. induction
>paracyclic o.

ovulatory
>o. cycle
>o. follicle

ovum, pl. **ova**
>primordial ova

22-oxacalcitriol

oxalate
>calcium o.

Oxandrin

oxandrolone

oxaprozin

oxidase
>corticosterone methyl o. (CMO)

corticosterone methyl o. II
cytochrome o.
diamine o. (DAO)
enzyme lysyl o.
hydroxyproline o.
immunogenic glucose o.
lysyl o.
methyl o.
monoamine o. (MAO)
proline o.
terminal o.
thyroid o. (THOX)
18-oxidase
oxidation
fatty acid o.
glucose o.
oxidative
o. damage
o. phosphorylation
o. stress
oxide
intrapenile nitric o.
magnesium o.
nitric o. (NO)
phenylarsine o.
zirconium o.
oxilorphan
oximetry
OX40L
2-oxoacid
3-oxoacid-CoA transferase
18-oxocortisol
5-oxoproline

oxtriphylline
oxycodone
OxyContin
oxygen (O$_2$)
o. consumption
o. disposable boot device
o. free radical
singlet o.
o. tension
oxygenase
mixed-function o.
OxyIR
oxymetazoline hydrochloride
oxymetholone
oxymorphone
oxyntomodulin
oxyphenbutazone
oxyphil cell
oxyphilic
o. adenoma
o. change
o. metaplasia
oxytocic fraction
oxytocin (OT)
ovarian venous plasma o.
o. secretion
oxytocinergic
o. cell body
o. neuron
oxytocin-neurophysin
Oyst-Cal 500
Oystercal 500

NOTES

O

P
    progesterone
    substance P
P450
    P450 arom
    aromatase P450
    P450 aromatase (placental)
        deficiency
    cytochrome P450
    P450 side chain cleavage
        (P450SCC)
    P450 side chain cleavage enzyme
P$_i$
    inorganic orthophosphate
6p21.3
    chromosome 6p21.3
17p12-13
    chromosome 17p12-13
18p11
    chromosome 18p11
p53
    p53 gene
    p53 tumor-suppressor gene
P21 gene
p21^{WAF1} tumor-suppressor gene
P450arom gene
P450c21 deficiency
p57KIP2 gene
p75 protein
P85 subunit
PAAF
    pancreatitis-associated ascites fluid
PAAP
    percutaneous alcohol ablation of the
        parathyroid gland
PABM
    peak adult bone mass
PAC
    pancreatic adenocarcinoma
    plasma aldosterone concentration
        PAC lateralization ratio
PACAP
    pituitary adenylate cyclase-activating
        peptide
pacemaker
    endogenous circadian p.
    idioventricular p.
    sloppy p.
    universal p.
    X p.
    Y p.
pachydermoperiostosis
packing
    cotton pledget p.
paclitaxel

PAC/PRA
    plasma aldosterone concentration/plasma
        renin activity
        PAC/PRA ratio
PAD
    peripheral arterial disease
pad
        cervicodorsal fat p.
        clavicular fat p.
        dorsocervical fat p.
        infraclavicular fat p.
        supraclavicular fat p.
        thinning fat p.
PAF
    platelet-activating factor
PAG
    pineal antigonadotropin
Paget
        P. disease
        P. disease of bone
pagetic
        p. bone
        p. bone lesion
PAH
    prealbumin-associated hyperthyroxinemia
    pulmonary arterial hypertension
PAHO
    Pan American Health Organization
        PAHO grade 0, 1, 2
        PAHO stage 0, Ia, Ib, II, III
PAI
    plasminogen activator inhibitor
PAI-1
    plasminogen activator inhibitor-1
PAI-2
    plasminogen activator inhibitor-2
pain
        bone p.
        C-fiber p.
        gnawing p.
        ocular p.
painful subacute thyroiditis
Pain-HP
        No P.-H.
painless
        p. cold-sensitive digital vasospasm
        p. hyperthyroidism
        p. postpartum thyroiditis
paint
        luminescent p.
pair
        affected sibling p. (ASP)
paired
        p. box homeotic 3 (PAX3)

paired *(continued)*
> p. box homeotic 6 (PAX6)
> p. box homeotic 8 (PAX8)

PAK
> pancreas after kidney
> PAK transplantation

PAL
> peptidyl-alpha-hydroxyglycine alpha-amidating lyase
> primary aldosteronism

palate
> high-arched p.

palliative surgery
pallidus
> globus p.

Pallister-Hall syndrome
pallor
> disc p.
> optic disc p.

palmar
> p. keratosis
> p. xanthomata

Palmitate-A 5000
palmitic acid
palmitoleic acid
palmitoyltransferase
> carnitine p. I (CPTI)
> carnitine p. II (CPTII)

palmoplantar keratosis
palpation thyroiditis
palpebral aperture
palsy
> cerebral p.
> cranial nerve p.
> Erb p.
> hereditary neuropathy with liability to pressure p. (HNPP)
> lateral rectus p.
> nerve p.
> oculomotor nerve p.
> superior oblique p.

PAM
> peptidylglycine alpha-amidating monooxygenase

pamidronate
> intravenous p.

Pamine
PAMP
> proadrenomedullin N-20 terminal peptide

pampiniform plexus
Pamprin IB
PAN
> primary afferent nociceptor neuron

pan
> P. American Health Organization (PAHO)
> P. American Health Organization grade (0–2)

Panadol

panadrenal insufficiency
PANAS
> Positive and Negative Affect Scale

Panasal 5/500
PANCH
> pituitary adenoma-adenohypophyseal neuronal choristoma

pancreas
> p. after kidney (PAK)
> p. after kidney transplantation
> annular p.
> artificial endocrine p.
> bioartificial p.
> cadaver p.
> p. cancer
> cortex p.
> p. divisum
> endocrine p.
> exocrine p.
> head of p.
> mucin-producing tumor of the p.
> native p.
> neck of p.
> postnatal p.
> remnant p.
> retention cyst of the p.
> serous cystadenoma of the p.
> Starling curve of the p.
> p. transplant alone (PTA)
> p. transplantation alone (PTA)
> p. transplantation organ allocation
> p. transplant registry of living segmental donor

Pancrease MT
pancreas-kidney
> simultaneous p.-k. (SPK)

pancreastatin
pancreatectomy
> distal subtotal p.
> partial p.
> total p.

pancreatic
> p. acinar cell
> p. adenocarcinoma (PAC)
> p. alpha-cell tumor
> p. cell fate
> p. cholera
> p. denervation
> p. desmoplastic response
> p. diabetes
> p. digestive zymogen
> p. disorder
> p. duct cell carcinoma (PDC)
> p. and duodenal homeobox-1 (PDX-1)
> p. endocrine neoplasm (PEN)
> p. endocrine tissue
> p. endocrine tumor
> p. enzyme

p. exocrine deficit
p. exocrine insufficiency
p. fibrosis
p. functioning diagnostant (PFD)
p. functioning diagnostant test
p. islet beta-cell
p. islet beta-cell glucose toxicity in diabetes mellitus type 2
p. islet cell-specific enhancer sequence (PICSES)
p. islet cell tumor
p. juice
p. nesidioblastosis
p. parenchyma
p. parenchymal perfusion
p. polypeptide (PP)
p. polypeptide-secreting tumor (PPoma)
p. steatorrhea
p. stone
p. transcription factor 1 (PTF-1)
p. transcription factor 1 beta-cell
p. tuberculosis
pancreaticoblastoma
pancreaticoduodenal transplant alone
pancreaticojejunostomy
side-to-side p.
pancreatin
pancreatis insufficiency
pancreatitis
acute hemorrhagic p. (AHP)
acute necrotizing p. (ANP)
acute recurrent p.
alcohol-related chronic p.
autoimmune p. (AIP)
chronic alcoholic p. (CAP)
duct-narrowing chronic p. (DNCP)
early-onset idiopathic chronic p.
eosinophilic p.
groove p.
hereditary p. (HP)
idiopathic p.
late-onset idiopathic chronic p.
mass-forming p.
severe acute p. (SAP)
tropical calcific p. (TCP)
tumor-forming p.
pancreatitis-associated
p.-a. ascites fluid (PAAF)
p.-a. protein (PAP)

pancreatoblastoma
pancreatoduodenectomy (PD)
pylorus-preserving p. (PPPD)
pancreatogram
pancreatography
computed tomography under endoscopic retrograde p. (ERP-CT)
pancreatopathy
fibrocalculous p.
pancreatoscope
ultrathin p.
pancreatoscopy
peroral p.
Pancrecarb MS-8
pancrelipase
pancreolauryl test
pancreoprivic
pancreozymin
p. secretin (PS)
p. secretin test
pancytopenia
pandemic
encephalitis p.
panel
comprehensive metabolic p. (CMP)
lipid p.
National Cholesterol Education Program Adult Treatment P. III
panhypopituitarism
hereditary p.
idiopathic p.
panhypopituitary dwarfism
Panmycin Oral
panniculus adiposus
Panomat microinfusion pump
panophthalmitis
panoramic visualization
panretinal laser photocoagulation
Pantopon
pantothenic acid
PAP
pancreatitis-associated protein
Pap
Papanicolaou
Pap smear
Papanicolaou (Pap)
P. smear
PAPase
phosphatidate phosphohydrolase
papaverine
papilla, pl. **papillae**

NOTES

P

papilla *(continued)*
    dental p.
    dermal p.
    fungiform p.
    renal p.
papillary
    p. adenoma
    p. craniopharyngioma
    p. necrosis
    p. nephrocalcinosis
    p. renal carcinoma
    p. stenosis
    p. thyroid cancer
    p. thyroid carcinoma (PTC)
    p. tumor projection
papilledema
papilloma
    intraductal p.
papillomatosis
    diffuse p.
    juvenile p.
papillomatous papule
papillopathy
    diabetic p.
papular mucinosis
papule
    papillomatous p.
PAQUID
    Personnes Agées Quid
    PAQUID study
PAR
    plasma appearance rate
paraadenomatous corticotroph hyperplasia
paraaminobenzoic acid
paraaminosalicylic acid
paraaortic lymph node
parabasal cell
parabolic reflector
paracellular calcium resorption
paracentesis
    abdominal p.
    large-volume p. (LVP)
paracetamol
paracetic acid-based method
paracoccidioidomycosis
paracrine
    p. action
    p. agent
    p. cell
    p. effect
    p. factor
    p. regulation
    p. secretion
    p. suppressor
    p. system
paracyclic ovulation

Paradigm
    P. insulin pump
    P. Link blood glucose monitor
paradox
    leptin p.
paraendocrine
paraffin-embedded semithin section
parafollicular
    p. calcitonin-producing cell
    p. duct
paraganglia
paraganglioma
    adrenal medullary p.
    extraadrenal p.
    thyroid p.
paragonimiasis
parahormone
paralactin
parallel
    p. development of axillary hair
    p. development of pubic hair
    p. hole collimation
paralysis, pl. paralyses
    familial periodic p.
    hyperthyroid periodic p.
    hypokalemic periodic p.
    thyrotoxic periodic p.
    vocal cord p.
paralytic ileus
paramagnetic
    p. metal
    p. nucleus
paramedian reticular nucleus
paramesonephric duct
paramethasone acetate
paramyxovirus
paraneoplastic
    p. growth hormone
    p. syndrome
    p. tumor
paraneurone
paraoxonase enzyme
parapineal
parapituitary area
paraplegia
    Basedow p.
    spastic p.
paraquat
parasellar
    p. meningioma
    p. region
    p. syndrome
    p. tissue
    p. tumor
parastatin
parasternal node
parasympathetic
    p. nerve

p. nervi erigentes
p. nervous system
paraterminal gyrus
Parathar
parathion
parathormone (PTH)
parathyrin
parathyroid
p. adenoma
p. autotransplantation
p. carcinoma
p. cell membrane
p. computed tomography
congenital aplasia of the p.
p. crisis
p. cyst
p. extracellular calcium-sensing
receptor
p. gland
p. gland dysfunction
p. gland hyperplasia
p. hormone (PTH)
p. hormone assay
p. hormone excess
p. hormone gene transcription
p. hormonelike polypeptide
(PTHLP)
p. hormonelike protein
p. hormone-mediated calcium efflux
p. hormone-related peptide (PTHrP,
PTH-RP)
p. hormone-related protein (PTHrP,
PTH-RP)
p. hormone-related protein-
transfected RIN-141 cell
p. hormone resistance syndrome
p. hormone secretion
p. insufficiency
p. scintigraphy
p. ultrasound
parathyroidal abscess
parathyroidectomy (PTX)
subtotal p.
total p.
parathyroiditis
paraventricular
p. neuron
p. nucleus (PVN)
p. nucleus of the hypothalamus
p. thalamic nucleus (PVT)
parenchyma
breast p.

pancreatic p.
thyroid p.
parenchymal brain injury
parenchymography
cephalic p.
parent
consanguineous p.'s
parenteral
p. iron dextran
p. nutrition
paresis
ocular p.
paresthesia
paricalcitol injection
parietalis
decidua p.
Parinaud syndrome
Parkinson disease
parkinsonism
idiopathic p.
Parlodel LAR
parolfactory gyrus
paronychia
parotid
p. gland
p. hormone
p. sialography
parotitis
paroxetine
paroxysm
lethal p.
paroxysmal
p. hypersexuality
p. hypertension
p. hyperthermia
p. hypothermia
p. nocturnal hemoglobinuria
p. pain disorder
Parry disease
pars, pl. **partes**
p. arcuata
p. distalis
p. infundibularis
p. infundibulum
p. intermedia
p. intermedia cyst
p. nervosa
p. plana vitrectomy
p. posterior
p. recta
p. tuberalis

NOTES

P

261

part
>intramural uterine p.
>thickened acral p.

partial
>p. agonist
>p. agonist-partial antagonist
>p. androgen insensitivity
>p. androgen sensitivity
>p. hydatidiform mole
>p. 21-hydroxylase deficiency
>p. hypopituitarism
>p. insulin resistance
>p. labioscrotal fusion
>p. pancreatectomy
>p. resection
>p. thyroid-stimulating hormone hyporesponsiveness
>p. TSH hyporesponsiveness

particle
>hydroxyapatite/tricalcium phosphate p.

Partington operation

partner
>small heterodimer p. (SHP)

parturition

parvocellular
>p. division
>p. neuron

parvovirus B19

passive immunity

paste
>Critic-Aid skin p.

patch
>Androderm testosterone transdermal p.
>blue p.
>p. clamp
>gray p.
>Habitrol P.
>Nicoderm P.
>Nicotrol P.
>Ortho Evra P.
>Peyer p.
>ProStep P.
>scrotal matrix p.
>signal p.
>testosterone skin p.
>transdermal scrotum testosterone p.
>transdermal torso testosterone p.

paternal leukocyte immunization

path
>embryonal p.

Pathilon

pathogen
>blood-borne p.

pathogenesis

pathogenesis-specific therapy

pathognomic

pathognomonic
>p. Askanazy cell
>p. black eschar

pathologic
>p. calcification
>p. hypercortisolemia
>p. parathyroid disease

pathological
>p. endocrine tissue
>p. hypoparathyroidism

pathophysiological condition

pathway
>adenylyl cyclase p.
>afferent p.
>aldose reductase polyol p.
>apoptosis p.
>L-arginine:nitric oxide p.
>beta-cell secretory p.
>cholinergic p.
>ctor-kB IkK mediated signaling p.
>cyclooxygenase p.
>17-deoxy p.
>downstream signaling p.
>Embden-Meyerhof p.
>energy p.
>G-protein signaling p.
>Gs-cAMP p.
>hexosamine p.
>immune surveillance p.
>inositol phosphate p.
>insulin signaling p.
>intracellular signaling p.
>lipoapoptotic p.
>lipoxygenase p.
>MAPK p.
>MAP kinase p.
>metabolic p.
>mitogen-activated protein kinase p.
>monoamine p.
>multisynaptic p.
>nicotine-stimulated p.
>nongenomic p.
>omega-conotoxin-sensitive p.
>opioid-stimulated p.
>pentose phosphate p.
>phosphoinositide-protein kinase A p.
>phospholipase C p.
>PI3K independent p.
>polyol p.
>$potassium_{ATP}$ channel independent p.
>protein kinase A p. (AKAP)
>proteolytic p.
>Ras p.
>serine phosphorylation p.
>Shc-dependent p.
>signal-transduction p.
>steroidogenic p.
>type 2 energy p.

ubiquitin-proteasome p.
Wnt/Wingless signaling p.
patient
acromegalic p.
Bercu p.
chronic dialysis p.
euvolemic p.
Refetoff p.
testosterone-deficient p.
uremic diabetic p.
patient-provider relationship
pattern
bimodal p.
birefringent p.
bursting p.
chromophobic p.
circadian p.
glandular p.
insular p.
macrofollicular p.
marble bone p.
microfollicular p.
mixed p.
sinusoidal p.
trabecular p.
undifferentiated p.
pauciclonal
pause and squeeze technique
PAX3
paired box homeotic 3
PAX3 gene
PAX6
paired box homeotic 6
PAX8
paired box homeotic 8
PAX8 factor
Pax4 paired domain homeobox gene
Pax6 paired domain homeobox gene
PBB
polybrominated biphenyl
PBL
peripheral blood lymphocyte
PBM
peripheral blood monocyte
P-box
PBR
peripheral-type benzodiazepine receptor
PC
proprotein convertase
PC1
prohormone convertase 1

PC2
prohormone convertase 2
PC3
prohormone convertase 3
P450c17
P. deficiency
P. enzyme
PCB
polychlorinated biphenyl
p/CIP coactivator
PCNA
proliferating cell nuclear antigen
PCNS
primary central nervous system
PCNS lymphoma
PCO
polycystic ovary
PCO syndrome (PCOS)
PCOD
polycystic ovary disease
PCOS
PCO syndrome
polycystic ovarian syndrome
polycystic ovary syndrome
PCPB
procarboxypeptidase B
PC-PLD
phosphatidylcholine phospholipase D
PCR
plasma clearance rate
polymerase chain reaction
PCT
proximal convoluted tubule
PD
pancreatoduodenectomy
peritoneal dialysis
PDC
pancreatic duct cell carcinoma
PDE5
phosphodiesterase 5
PDGF
platelet-derived growth factor
PDGF gene
PDGF protein
PDGF-A
platelet-derived growth factor A
PDH
pyruvate dehydrogenase
PDI
protein disulfide isomerase
PDI-mediated disulfide bond reduction

NOTES

P

PDK
> 3-phosphoinositide-dependent protein kinase

PDM
> Bontril P.

PDR
> proliferative diabetic retinopathy

PDS
> Pendred syndrome
> PDS gene

PDX-1
> pancreatic and duodenal homeobox-1
> PDX-1 IRS-2 signaling

PE-3
> phosphatidylinositol-3

peak
> p. action
> p. adult bone mass (PABM)
> p. effect
> estradiol p.
> p. thyroid-stimulating hormone response
> p. TSH response

peakless

pearl
> P. Hypoglycemic capsule
> pheochromocytoma p.

Pearson syndrome

pebble
> fiber p.

pectoralis fascia

Pedersen hypothesis

PEDF
> pigment epithelium-derived factor
> PEDF diabetic retinopathy

Pediapred Oral

pediatric
> p. endocrinologist
> p. multiple vitamin
> M.V.I. P.
> p. renal osteodystrophy

pedicle
> superior vascular p.

pedigree
> p. analysis
> X-linked dominant p.

PedTE-PAK-4

Pedtrace-4

peduncle
> cerebral p.
> mammillary p.
> Zuckerkandl p.

pedunculus, pl. pedunculi
> basis pedunculi

PEG-ADA
> polyethylene glycol-adenosine deaminase

pegademase bovine

pegvisomant
> p. for injection
> Trovett p.

peliosis hepatis

Pelizaeus-Merzbacher disease

pellagra

pellet
> Testopel P.

pellucida
> zona p.
> zona p. 1 (ZP1)
> zona p. 2 (ZP2)
> zona p. 3 (ZP3)

pellucidum
> absent septum p.
> septum p.

pelvic
> p. infertility factor
> p. inflammatory disease
> p. rhabdomyosarcoma

pelvis, pl. pelves
> renal p.

PEM
> protein-energy malnutrition

Pemberton sign

pemphigoid
> bullous p.

pemphigus vulgaris

PEN
> pancreatic endocrine neoplasm

pen
> Disetronic P.
> Genotropin P.
> Genotropin P. 5
> Humalog P.
> Humulin Mix 75/25 P.
> Humulin R p.
> insulin p.

Pendred
> P. syndrome (PDS)
> P. syndrome gene

pendrin
> p. expression
> p. protein

PenFill

penicillamine

penicillin v potassium

penile
> p. brachial index
> p. implant
> p. length
> p. prosthesis
> p. self-injection
> p. urethra

penis
> p. at twelve syndrome
> bulbus p.
> crus p.
> glans p.

Penlet II Automatic blood sampling device
penoscrotal hypospadias
pentachlorophenol
pentaerythritol tetranitrate
pentagastrin
        p. provocation test
        p. stimulation test
pentalaminar tubular structure
pentalogy of Cantrell
pentameric
        p. GH
        p. growth hormone
pentamidine
pentapeptide
pentavalent dimercaptosuccinate (DMSA)
pentazocine compound
pentetreotide
        indium-111 p.
pentolinium tartrate
pentose phosphate pathway
pentosuria
Pentothal
pentoxifylline
Pen-Vee K
PEPCK
    phosphoenolpyruvate-carboxykinase
PEPI
    Postmenopausal Estrogen/Progestin Interventions Trial
Peptavlon
peptic ulcer disease
peptid
        signal p.
peptidase
        dipeptidyl p.
        dipeptidyl p. IV (DPIV, DPP-IV)
        exopeptidase dipeptidyl p. I, II
        pyroglutamyl p. II
        signal p.
peptide
        adipocyte-derived p.
        agouti-related p.
        amyloid p.
        atrial natriuretic p. (ANP)
        bombesin-like p.
        brain-gut p.
        brain natriuretic p. (BNP)
        C p.
        calcitonin gene-related p. (CGRP)
        circulating proinsulin-like p.

        corticotropin-like intermediate lobe p. (CLIP)
        C-type natriuretic p. (CNP)
        endogenous opioid p. (EOP)
        gastric inhibitory p. (GIP)
        gastrin-releasing p. (GRP)
        GH-releasing p. (GHRP)
        glucagon C p.
        glucagonlike p. (GLP)
        glucose-dependent insulinotropic p. (GIP)
        GnRH-associated p. (GAP)
        gonadal p.
        gonadotropin-associated p.
        p. growth factor
        growth hormone-releasing p. (GHRP)
        gut p.
        gut-brain p.
        helix-bundle p. (HBP)
        p. histidine isoleucine (PHI)
        p. histidine methionine (PHM)
        p. hormone
        p. hystidyl-methionine-27 (PHM-27)
        p. immunization
        insulinotrophic glucagonlike p.
        intervening p. (IP)
        latency-associated p. (LAP)
        MB-35 p.
        p. mediator
        monitor p.
        MSH p.
        natriuretic p.
        neurohypophysial p.
        nociceptin/orphanin FQ p.
        N/OFQ p.
        N-terminal p.
        opioid p.
        orexigenic p.
        parathyroid hormone-related p. (PTHrP, PTH-RP)
        pituitary adenylate cyclase-activating p. (PACAP)
        pituitary adenylyl cyclase-activating p.
        proadrenomedullin N-20 terminal p. (PAMP)
        procollagen-III p. (pIIIp)
        proopiomelanocortin-derived p.
        regulatory p.
        signal p.

NOTES

P

peptide *(continued)*
    thrombin receptor-activating p. 6
      (TRAP-6)
    thymosin p.
    trypsinogen-activating p. (TAP)
    type 1 procollagen p.
    p. tyrosine tyrosine
    urinary gonadotropin p. (UGP)
    vasoactive intestinal p. (VIP)
    vasodilator p.
    p. YY (PYY)
peptide-1
    glucagonlike p.-1 (GLIP-1, GLP-1)
peptide-4
    human neutrophil p.-4 (HNP-4)
peptide-5
    growth hormone-releasing peptide-5
    growth hormone-releasing p.-5
      (GHRP-5, peptide-5)
peptide-6
peptide-amino acid hormone
peptidergic neuron
peptidoglycan
peptidyl-alpha-hydroxyglycine alpha-amidating lyase (PAL)
peptidylglycine
    p. alpha-amidating monooxygenase
      (PAM)
    p. alpha-hydroxylating
      monooxygenase (PHM)
PER
    period
    PER gene
    PER protein
peracetic acid
perception
    depth p.
    thermal p.
perchlorate
    p. discharge test
    potassium p.
Percocet
Percodan
Percodan-Demi
Percogesic
Percoll gradient
Percolone
percutaneous
    p. alcohol ablation of the
      parathyroid gland (PAAP)
    p. alcohol serotherapy
    p. biopsy
    p. bone marrow injection
    p. femoral vein
    p. fine-needle ethanol injection
      (PFNEI)
    p. nephrolithotomy
perforating
    p. disorder of the skin

    p. folliculitis
    p. ulcer
perforin
perfusion
    pancreatic parenchymal p.
    peripheral p.
pergolide mesylate
Pergonal
Perheentupa syndrome
Peri
    Genotropin P. 12
Periactin
periampullary malignancy
periaqueductal gray area
periarteritis nodosa
pericardial bioprosthetic tissue
perichondrium
perifornical region
perikarya
perikaryal
    p. cytoplasm
    p. group
perikaryon
    magnocellular p.
    norepinephrine p.
perilipin lipolysis
periluminal
perilymph fluid
perimenarchal period
perimenopausal
    p. period
    p. syndrome
perimenopause
perimetric technique
perimetrium
perimysial fibroblast
perineoplastic thyroiditis
perineoscrotal hypospadias
perinephric fat
period (PER)
    final menstrual p. (FMP)
    p. gene
    last menstrual p. (LMP)
    perimenarchal p.
    perimenopausal p.
    postimplantation p.
    p. protein
    somatosensory-evoked potential
      recovery p.
periodic acid-Schiff-positive
periodically fluctuating protein kinase (PFK)
periodontal membrane
perioral dermatitis
periorbital
    p. edema
    p. puffiness
    p. swelling

periosteal
    p. envelope
    p. hypertrophy
    p. ossification
periosteocytic space
periosteum
periovarian adhesion
periovulatory phase
peripancreatic
    p. neoplasm
    p. pseudoaneurysm
peripapillary staphylomata
peripheral
    p. arterial disease (PAD)
    p. blood lymphocyte (PBL)
    p. blood monocyte (PBM)
    p. circulatory change
    p. cytotrophoblast cell
    p. diabetes insipidus
    p. glucocorticoid deficiency
    p. glucose utilization (PGU)
    p. insulin sensitivity
    p. nerve
    p. nervous system (PNS)
    p. neuroglia
    p. neuropathy
    p. organ
    p. perfusion
    p. scalloping
    p. thyroid hormone metabolism
    p. thyroxine
    p. tissue
    p. tissue resistance to thyroid hormone (PTRTH)
    p. vascular disease
    p. vascular resistance
peripheral-type benzodiazepine receptor (PBR)
peristalsis
perithymic fat
perithyroidal adventitia
peritoneal
    p. dialysis (PD)
    p. fluid (PF)
    p. oocyte and sperm transfer (POST)
peritoneovenous shunt
peritonitis
    p. carcinomatosa
    spontaneous bacterial p.
peritubular endothelial cell
peritumor glial reaction

periumbilical staining
perivasculitis
    superficial dermal p.
periventricular
    p. leukomalacia (PVL)
    p. stratum
    p. zone
perivitelline
    p. barrier
    p. space
perlecan
perleche
permanent
    p. diabetes insipidus
    p. hypoparathyroidism
Permax
permissive factor
pernicious anemia
peroral pancreatoscopy
peroxidase
    antithyroid p.
    glutathione p.
    thyroid p. (TPO)
peroxidation
    lipid p.
peroxide
    benzoyl p.
    hydrogen p.
    lipid p.
    p. tone
peroxisomal disorder
peroxisome
    p. proliferator
    p. proliferator-activated receptor (PPAR)
    p. proliferator-activated receptor-alpha (PPAR-alpha)
    p. proliferator-activated receptor-delta (PPAR-delta)
    p. proliferator-activated receptor-gamma (PPAR-gamma)
    p. proliferator activated receptor-gamma 2 (PPAR-gamma 2)
    p. proliferator-activated receptor-gamma ligand
    p. proliferator-activated receptor gene
peroxynitrite anion
perphenazine
Perrault syndrome
persephin (PSP)

NOTES

persistent
    p. hyperglycemia
    p. hyperinsulinemic hypoglycemia
      of infancy (PHHI)
    p. hyperparathyroidism
    p. müllerian duct syndrome
    p. polyuria
Personal Lasette
Personnes
    P. Agées Quid (PAQUID)
    P. Agées Quid study
perstans
    Mansonella p.
    telangiectasia macularis eruptiva p.
pertechnetate (Tc-99m-TcO4)
    p. scintigraphy
    technetium p.
    p. thyroid scan
perturbation
pertussis
    p. toxin
    p. toxin-sensitive
PET
    positron emission tomography
PET/CT
    combined P.
petrosal
    p. sinus
    p. sinus sampling
Peutz-Jeghers syndrome
PEX
    phosphate-regulating gene with
      homologies to endopeptidases found at
      the HYP locus on the X chromosome
pexiganan acetate
Peyer patch
Peyronie disease
PF
    peritoneal fluid
p160 family of coactivators
PFD
    pancreatic functioning diagnostant
    polyostotic fibrous dysplasia
      PFD test
Pfeiffer syndrome
PFK
    periodically fluctuating protein kinase
    phosphofructokinase
PFNEI
    percutaneous fine-needle ethanol
      injection
PG
    postprandial glucose
PGA-I
    polyglandular autoimmune syndrome
      type I
PGA-II
    polyglandular autoimmune syndrome
      type II

PGC
    primordial germ cell
PGD$_2$
    prostaglandin D$_2$
PGE
    prostaglandin E
PGE$_1$
    prostaglandin E$_1$
PGE$_2$
    prostaglandin E$_2$
PGF$_{2a}$
    prostaglandin F$_{2a}$
PGF$_{1\text{-alpha}}$
    prostaglandin F$_{1\text{-alpha}}$
PGF$_{2\text{-alpha}}$
    prostaglandin F$_{2\text{-alpha}}$
PGG$_2$
    prostaglandin G$_2$
PGH$_2$
    prostaglandin H$_2$
PGHS
    prostaglandin H synthase
PGI
    prostaglandin I
PGI2
    prostacyclin
PGI$_2$
    prostaglandin I$_2$
PGJ
    prostaglandin J
PGK
    phosphoglycerate kinase
      PGK deficiency
P-glycoprotein (Pgp)
Pgp
    P-glycoprotein
PGU
    peripheral glucose utilization
pH
    pH domain-interacting protein
      (PHIP)
    extracellular pH
    physiologic pH
    urine pH
PHA
    phytohemagglutinin
    posterior hypothalamic area
    pseudohypoaldosteronism
PHA I
    pseudohypoaldosteronism type I
PHA II
    pseudohypoaldosteronism type II
phagedena
phagocytic activity
phagocytosis
phagolysosome
phagosome
phakomatoses
phallic size

pharmacoepidemiologic survey
pharmacokinetics
pharmacologic
    p. estrogen administration
    p. therapy
    p. treatment
pharmakinetic
pharyngeal
    p. floor
    p. hypophysis
    p. motility
    p. pituitary
    p. pouch
phase
    acrosome p.
    cap p.
    cephalic p.
    coupling p.
    estradiol-norethisterone p.
    follicular p.
    Golgi p.
    late luteal p.
    luteal p.
    periovulatory p.
    reversal p.
    shortened luteal p.
    short luteal p.
    thyrotoxic p.
Phazyme
Phe-B25-Leu
    insulin Chicago
Phe-B24-Ser
Phenadex Senior
Phenazine Injection
phendimetrazine
phenelzine
Phenerbel-S
Phenergan
    P. Injection
    P. Oral
    P. VC with codeine
phenformin
phenobarbital
phenobarbitone
phenolic orthohydrogen atom
phenol sulfotransferase
phenomenon, pl. **phenomena**
    aldosterone escape p.
    Arthus p.
    Charcot foot p.
    dawn p.
    escape p.

    first-passage p.
    hemifield slide p.
    Houssay p.
    Jod-Basedow p.
    Lyon p.
    Somogyi p.
    thyroid cork p.
    Titanic p.
phenothiazine
phenotype
    beta-cell p.
    CD8+ p.
    female p.
    fibroblastic p.
    male p.
    osteoblast p.
    osteoblastic p.
    osteopetrotic p.
    pituicyte hormonal p.
    Reifenstein p.
    somatic p.
phenotype-genotype analysis
Phenoxine
phenoxybenzamine
phentermine
phentolamine
phenylacetate
phenylalanine
phenylalanine-restricted diet
phenylarsine oxide
phenylbutazone
Phenyldrine
phenylethanolamine N-methyltransferase
    (PNMT)
phenylhydrazine
phenylisopropyladenosine
phenylketonuria (PKU)
phenylpropionate
    nandrolone p.
phenyltoloxamine
phenytoin
    p. load
    p. sodium
pheochromoblast
pheochromocyte
pheochromocytoma
    adrenal p.
    asymptomatic p.
    benign sporadic adrenal p.
    extraadrenal p.
    familial p.
    MIBG-negative pelvic p.

NOTES

P

pheochromocytoma *(continued)*
    nonfunctioning p.
    p. pearl
    subclinical p.
pheomelanin
pheromone
    signaling p.
PHEX gene
PHF6 gene mutation
PHHI
    persistent hyperinsulinemic hypoglycemia
      of infancy
PHI
    peptide histidine isoleucine
philtrum
PHIP
    pH domain-interacting protein
      dominant-negative mutant of PHIP
      (DN-PHIP)
phlebotomy
phlorhizin, phlorizin
phloroglucinol
PHM
    peptide histidine methionine
    peptidylglycine alpha-hydroxylating
      monooxygenase
PHM-27
    peptide hystidyl-methionine-27
phogrin autoantibodies
phonocardiogram
phorbol ester
phosphatase
    p. activity
    alkaline phosphatase antialkaline p.
      (APAAP)
    bone alkaline p.
    bone-specific alkaline p.
    p. enzyme
    glucose p.
    leukocyte antigen-related p. (LRP)
    lipid p.
    phosphoprotein p.
    plasma bone alkaline p.
    protein tyrosine p. (PTPase)
    serum alkaline p.
    Src homology containing p. 1
      (SHP-1)
    Src homology containing p. 2
      (SHP-2)
    tartrate-resistant acid p. (TR-ACP,
      TRAP)
    T-cell protein tyrosine p. (TCPTP)
    p. and tensin homologue (PTEN)
    p. and tensin homologue deleted
      on chromosome (PTEN)
phosphatase-1
    MAP kinase p.-1 (MKP-1)
5-phosphatase
    inositol 5-p.

phosphate
    alpha-glycerol p.
    amorphous calcium p.
    p. balance
    p. binder
    p. binding
    calcium hydrogen p.
    cellulose sodium p.
    p. deficiency
    p. depletion
    dibasic calcium p.
    dihydrogen p.
    dolichyl p.
    glucose p.
    hexose p.
    inorganic p.
    inositol p. (IP)
    p. ion
    p. load
    magnesium ammonium p.
    monohydrogen p.
    nicotinamide adenine dinucleotide p.
      (NADPH)
    octacalcium p.
    phosphatidylinositol p.
    plasma p.
    potassium p.
    pyridoxal p.
    p. reabsorption
    p. retention
    sodium p.
    p. therapy
5′-phosphate
    pyridoxal 5′-p. (PLP)
phosphate-binding agent
phosphate-protein restriction
**phosphate-regulating gene with
  homologies to endopeptidases found
  at the HYP locus on the X
  chromosome (PEX)**
**phosphatidate phosphohydrolase
  (PAPase)**
phosphatidic acid
phosphatidylcholine
    p. hydrolysis insulin
    p. phospholipase D (PC-PLD)
phosphatidylglycerol
phosphatidylinositide-3
    p.-3 kinase
    p.-3 kinase cascade insulin receptor
      cell protein
phosphatidylinositide metabolite
phosphatidylinositol
    p. 4,5-bisphosphate (PIP$_2$)
    p. 3′-kinase (PI3-K)
    p. 3-kinase (LY294002, PI3K)
    p. phosphate
    p. signal

p. 4,5-triphosphate (PIP3)
p. 4,5-triphosphate kinase
phosphatidylinositol-3 (PE-3)
p. kinase (PI3K)
phosphatonin
phosphaturia
calcitonin-induced p.
phosphaturic
p. action
p. response
phosphodiesterase
p. 3
p. 5 (PDE5)
p. 3A, 3B
cGMP p.
cyclic nucleotide p.
p. inhibitor
phosphodiester linkage
phosphoenolpyruvate-carboxykinase (PEPCK)
p.-c. gene
phosphoethanolamine
urinary p.
phosphofructokinase (PFK)
6-phosphofructo-2-kinase
phosphoglycerate
p. kinase (PGK)
p. kinase deficiency
p. mutase deficiency
phosphohydrolase
phosphatidate p. (PAPase)
phosphoinositide
3-p.-dependent protein kinase (PDK)
p. hydrolysis
p. 3′kinase (PI3′K)
3-phosphoinositide-dependent protein kinase (PDK)
phosphoinositide-protein kinase A pathway
phosphokinase
serum creatine p.
Pholine
phospholipase
p. A$_2$ (PLA$_2$)
p. C (PLC)
p. C enzyme
p. C pathway
p. D (PLD)
phospholipid vesicle
phosphopenia
phosphopenic rickets

phosphoprotein
185 kDa p. (pp185)
p. phosphatase
phosphoribosylpyrophosphate (PRPP)
phosphoribosylpyrophosphate synthase
phosphoribosyltransferase
adenine p.
hypoxanthine p.
hypoxanthine-guanine p. (HPRT)
phosphorus
p. balance
p. binding
p. content
dietary p.
p. dietary restriction
p. distribution
p. homeostasis
lipid p.
p. metabolism
serum inorganic p.
phosphorus-induced
p.-i. hyperparathyroidism
p.-i. hypocalcemia
phosphorylase
p. *a*
p. *b*
p. b kinase
p. enzyme
glycogen p.
liver p.
purine nucleoside p. (PNP)
phosphorylated
p. glycolytic intermediate
p. rhodopsin function
p. serine 137
phosphorylate membrane protein
phosphorylation
cJunN-terminal kinase serine p.
estrogen receptor p.
Jun N-terminal kinase serine p.
oxidative p.
protein tyrosine p.
tyrosine p.
phosphoserine
Phospho-Soda
Fleet P.-S.
phosphotransferase
phosphotyrosine binding (PTB)
phosphotyrosine-binding domain (PTB)
photic entrainment
photoactivation

NOTES

P

photoactive yellow protein
photoaging
    cutaneous p.
photocoagulation
    focal p.
    laser p.
    panretinal laser p.
    scatter p.
photography
    7-field stereoscopic fundus p.
photolabel
    bis-mannose p.
photolysis
    nonenzymatic p.
photometry
    flame p.
photomotogram
photooncogene
photoperiodic
    p. environment
    p. mechanism
photoperiodism
photopsia
photosensitivity
photosensitization reaction
phototherapy
PHP
    pseudohypoparathyroidism
    PHP-1a, -1b
PH-20, -30 protein
PHPT
    primary hyperparathyroidism
phrenic nerve
phthalate esters
phycomycetes infection
phycomycosis
Phyllocontin
phylloides
    cystosarcoma p.
phylogeny
physalaemin
physical
    p. activity
    p. half-life
physiologic
    p. effect
    p. pH
    p. regulator
physiologically active calcium
physiological range
physiology
    reproductive p.
physiolysis
physique
    lean p.
Phyto-EST
phytoestrogen
phytohemagglutinin (PHA)
phytohormone

phytonadione
phytosterolemia
PI
    polyphosphoinositide
PIA
    purinergic agonist
piarachnoid membrane
PIC
    preinitiation complex
pickwickian syndrome
picogram
PICSES
    pancreatic islet cell-specific enhancer
     sequence
PID
    primary immune deficiency
Piedmont plateau
piezoelectric effect
PIF
    prolactin-inhibiting factor
pigeon
    p. breast
    p. crop sac-stimulation assay
pigment
    age p.
    cytochrome p. (CYP)
    p. epithelium-derived factor (PEDF)
    minocycline-associated p.
    p. urochrome
pigmentation
    café au lait p.
    cutaneous p.
pigmented nodular adrenocortical disease (PNAD)
pigmentosa
    retinitis p.
    urticaria p.
    xeroderma p.
pigmentosum
PIH
    pregnancy-induced hypertension
    prolactin-inhibiting hormone
    prolactin inhibitory hormone
    prolactin release-inhibiting hormone
pIIIp
    procollagen-III peptide
PI3K
    phosphatidylinositol-3 kinase
    PI3K independent pathway
    PI3K insulin
PI3′K
    phosphoinositide 3′kinase
PI3-K
    phosphatidylinositol 3′-kinase
pilaris
    keratosis p.
pill
    morning-after p.
    progesterone-only p.

pilocytic
pilosebaceous dysfunction
pimagedine
Pima Indian study
pindolol
pineal
    p. antigonadotropin (PAG)
    p. dysgerminoma
    p. gland
    p. hyperplasia
    p. recess
    p. tumor
pinealectomy
pinealocyte beta-receptor
pinealoma
    ectopic p.
pinhole
    p. collimation
    p. collimator
pinocytic vesicle
pinocytosis
pinopode
pioglitazone HCl
PIP3
    phosphatidylinositol 4,5-triphosphate
PIP$_2$
    phosphatidylinositol 4,5-bisphosphate
piperazine estrone sulfate
pirbuterol
piriform cortex
piroxicam
Pit-1
    pituitary-specific transcription factor-1
      Pit-1 gene
      prophet of Pit-1 (PROP-1)
pit
    clathrin-coated p.
    coated p.
Pitocin
pitressin tannate
pitting of nail
pituicyte hormonal phenotype
pituicytoma
pituitaire
    tige p.
pituitary
    p. abscess
    p. adenoma
    p. adenoma-adenohypophyseal neuronal choristoma (PANCH)
    p. adenoma-neuronal choristoma

p. adenylate cyclase-activating peptide (PACAP)
p. adenylate cyclase-activating polypeptide
p. adenylate cyclase-activating protein
p. adenylyl cyclase-activating peptide
p. agenesis
p. amyloid
p. aneurysm
p. aplasia
p. bright spot
p. carcinoma
p. cell line
p. cell-surface antibody
p. cell-surface receptor
p. corticotrope
p. corticotropinoma
p. craniopharyngioma
p. Cushing disease
p. cyst
p. deficiency
p. diabetes
p. disorder
p. dwarfism
p. dynamic test
p. dysfunction
p. dystopia
p. enlargement
p. fossa
p. gigantism
p. gland
p. glycoprotein hormone
p. growth hormone
p. growth hormone-secreting adenoma necrosis
p. growth hormone-secreting macroadenoma
p. hormone deficit
p. hormone function
p. hormone hypofunction
p. hyperplasia
p. hypersecretion
p. hypoplasia
p. hypothyroidism
p. incidentaloma
p. infarction
p. irradiation
p. isolation syndrome
p. lactotroph cell
p. meningioma

NOTES

P

pituitary *(continued)*
  p. metastasis
  p. microadenoma
  p. microsurgery
  p. neurosurgeon
  pharyngeal p.
  posterior p.
  p. resistance to thyroid hormone (PRTH)
  p. resistance to thyroid hormone action
  p. resistance to thyroid hormone syndrome
  p. RTH (PRTH)
  p. somatotropinoma
  p. stalk
  p. stalk interruption syndrome
  p. surgery
  p. synthesis
  p. target organ test
  p. thyroid hormone resistance (PThHR, PTHR)
  p. thyrotropin
  p. tumor
  p. tumor apoplexy
  p. tumor cell growth
  p. tumorigenesis
  p. tumor lateralization
  p. tumor-related acromegaly
  p. tumor-transforming gene (PTTG)
pituitary-adrenal function
pituitary-dependent
  p.-d. Cushing disease
  p.-d. thyrotoxicosis
pituitary-gonadal
  p.-g. axis
  p.-g. function
pituitary-hypothalamic
  p.-h. axis
  p.-h. injury
pituitary-specific transcription factor-1 (Pit-1)
pituitary-thyroid
  p.-t. axis
  p.-t. function
pituitary-thyroidal axis
pituitrin
Pitx homeodomain factor
pizotifen
PKA
  protein kinase A
PKB
  protein kinase B
PKC
  protein kinase C
  PKC-alpha
PKG
  protein kinase G
P13-kinase

PKU
  phenylketonuria
Pl3K-independent glucose transport
PLA$_2$
  phospholipase A$_2$
placenta
  definitive p.
  hemochorial p.
placental
  p. aromatase deficiency
  p. blood flow
  p. CRH
  p. GH
  p. hormone deficiency
  p. lactogen
  p. septa
  p. sulfatase deficiency
  p. transfer
  p. vasopressinase
placental-fetal aromatase deficiency
placentoma
placode
  olfactory p.
plan
  meal p.
planar
  P. gamma camera
  p. xanthoma
plane
  coronal p.
  p. radiography
planning
  preconceptional p.
  prepregnancy p.
plantar
  p. fascia syndrome
  p. hyperkeratosis
  p. keratosis
plant stanol ester
planum sphenoidale
planus
  hypertrophic lichen p.
plaque
  fibrous p.
  psoriatic p.
Plaquenil
plasma
  p. ACTH level
  p. aldosterone
  p. aldosterone concentration (PAC)
  p. aldosterone concentration/plasma renin activity (PAC/PRA)
  p. aldosterone-to-plasma renin activity ratio
  p. aluminum level
  p. appearance rate (PAR)
  p. beta-endorphin
  p. bone alkaline phosphatase

p. cell dyscrasia with polyneuropathy, organomegaly, endocrinopathy, M protein in plasma, and skin changes syndrome
p. clearance rate (PCR)
p. cortisol
p. endothelin level
p. exchange
p. expander
p. free fatty acid
p. galanin level
gas chromatography of p.
p. glucose concentration
p. glucose hyperinsulinemia
p. growth hormone-releasing hormone level
p. homocysteine level
p. hypertonicity
p. insulin
p. insulin level
p. kallikrein
p. ketone level
p. lipid profile
p. membrane
p. membrane beta-granule transport
p. membrane fatty acid binding protein (FABP$_{pm}$)
p. osmolality (POSM)
p. osmotic pressure
p. phosphate
p. polymorphonuclear elastase (PMN-3)
p. renin activity (PRA)
p. ristocetin cofactor
p. sex hormone-binding globulin
p. sodium
p. sulfonylurea
p. testosterone
p. testosterone level
plasmacytoma
thyroid p.
plasmalemma
plasmapheresis
plasmic islet cell autoantibody
plasmid
plasmin
p. mobilization
p. renin activity (PRA)
plasminogen
p. activator

p. activator inhibitor (PAI)
p. activator inhibitor-1 (PAI-1)
plasminogen-activator stimulation
Plastazote insole
plasticity
plate
alar p.
basal p.
chorionic p.
cribriform p.
epiphyseal growth p.
neural p.
pterygoid p.
trabecular p.
plateau
Piedmont p.
platelet
p. activity
p. adhesiveness
p. aggregation
p. antigen genotyping
p. consumption
hemolysis, elevated liver enzymes, and low p.'s (HELLP)
p. lipid peroxide concentration
p. protein
p. stability
platelet-activating factor (PAF)
platelet-derived
p.-d. growth factor (PDGF)
p.-d. growth factor A (PDGF-A)
p.-d. growth factor AA
p.-d. growth factor BB
p.-d. growth factor gene
platinum electrode
platybasia
platysma muscle
PLC
phospholipase C
PLD
phospholipase D
pleckstrin homology domain
Plegine
pleiotrophin/midkine growth enhancer (PTN/MK)
pleiotropic
p. domain
p. function
p. gene
p. nature
pleomorphic carcinoma
pleomorphism

NOTES

P

plethora
    facial p.
plethoric facies
plethysmography
pleuropericardial cyst
plexopathy
    lumbar p.
plexus, pl. **plexuses**
    brachial p.
    celiac p.
    choroid p.
    pampiniform p.
    p. pancreaticus capitalis
    primary capillary p.
    subependymal p.
    subtunical venous p.
    sympathetic p.
    vertebral venous p.
plica inflammation
plicamycin
PI3K
    phosphatidylinositol 3-kinase
ploidy
    DNA p.
plot
    Scatchard p.
PLP
    pyridoxal 5′-phosphate
plug
    cervical mucous p.
    protein p.
Plummer
    P. disease
    P. nail
pluriglandular endocrine deficiency
plurihormonal
    p. adenoma
    p. Cushing disease
    p. deficiency
    p. neuroendocrine neoplasm
plurimorphous
pluripotent
    p. hematopoietic cell
    p. pituitary macroadenoma
    p. stem cell
pluripotential
    p. precursor cell
    p. stromal cell
plus
    DHC P.
    GrowTrak P.
    Lorcet P.
    Maalox P.
    Riopan P.
    Tri-Tannate P.
    Vicon P.
plutonium
PM
    Midol P.

P.M.
    Excedrin P.M.
PMDD
    premenstrual dysphoric disorder
PMN
    polymorphonuclear
    PMN cell
PMN-3
    plasma polymorphonuclear elastase
PMS
    premenstrual syndrome
PMS-Cyproheptadine
PMS-Levothyroxine Sodium
PMS-Progesterone
PNAD
    pigmented nodular adrenocortical disease
PNEE
    pulmonary neuroepithelial endocrine
pneumocephalus
pneumococcal vaccine
pneumococcus
Pneumocystis
    P. carinii
    P. carinii pneumonia
    P. carinii thyroiditis
pneumoencephalography
Pneumomist
pneumonia
    Legionella pneumophila p.
    Pneumocystis carinii p.
pneumoniae
    Diplococcus p.
    Klebsiella p.
    Staphylococcus p.
    Streptococcus p.
PNMT
    phenylethanolamine N-methyltransferase
PNP
    purine nucleoside phosphorylase
    PNP deficiency
PNS
    peripheral nervous system
POA
    preoptic area of the hypothalamus
pocket
    p. P9 insulin B
    subclavian p.
POEMS
    polyneuropathy, organomegaly,
      endocrinopathy, monoclonal
      component, skin changes
    polyneuropathy, organomegaly,
      endocrinopathy, M proteins, skin
      changes
    POEMS syndrome
poikilothermia
point
    abnormal set p.
    altered set p.

beta-cell set p.

P. of Change weight management
program

p. mutation

spilling p.

pointes

torsades de p.

poisoning

heavy metal p.

polyvinyl chloride p.

polar

p. body

p. triiodothyronine syndrome

p. T_3 syndrome

polarizability

polarization

fluorescence p.

polarized

p. cell

p. light microscopy

pole

anterior p.

posterior p.

Pol II

poliomyelitis

polyacrylamide gel electrophoresis

polyadenylation

polyalcohol

polyaromatic hydrocarbon

polyarteritis nodosa

polyarthritis

polybrominated biphenyl (PBB)

polycaryon

polychlorinated biphenyl (PCB)

Polycitra

Polycitra-K

polyclonal

p. anti-T-cell antibody

p. B, T cell

Polycose

polycystic

p. kidney disease

p. ovarian disease

p. ovarian syndrome (PCOS)

p. ovary (PCO)

p. ovary disease (PCOD)

p. ovary syndrome (PCOS)

polycythemia vera

polydactyly

polydipsia

primary p.

psychogenic p.

secondary p.

polydystrophy

pseudo-Hurler p.

polyendocrine

p. deficiency syndrome

p. failure type I syndrome

polyendocrinoma

polyendocrinopathy

polyestradiol

**polyethylene glycol-adenosine deaminase
(PEG-ADA)**

polygalactia

polygenic

p. hypercholesterolemia

p. obesity

polyglandular

p. autoimmune syndrome

p. autoimmune syndrome type I
(PGA-I)

p. autoimmune syndrome type II
(PGA-II)

p. autoimmunity

p. autoimmunity type 1

p. endocrine deficiency

p. endocrine failure

polygonal cell

polyhedral cell

polyhydramnios

polykaryon

polymannose

polymastia

polymenorrhea

polymer

glucose p.

polymerase

p. chain reaction (PCR)

ribonucleic acid p.

RNA p. II

polymerization

polymerize

polymorphism

genetic p.

restriction fragment length p.
(RFLP)

simple tandem repeat p. (STRP)

single nucleotide p. (SNP)

single-strand conformation p.
(SSCP)

polymorphonuclear (PMN)

p. cell

p. leukocytosis

NOTES

P

polyneuropathy
    autonomic p.
    chronic inflammatory
      demyelinating p. (CIDP)
    distal sensory p.
    distal symmetric sensorimotor p.
    familial amyloid p. (FAP)
    familial amyloidotic p.
    hypothyroid p.
    mixed sensorimotor p.
    p., organomegaly, endocrinopathy,
      monoclonal component, skin
      changes (POEMS)
    p., organomegaly, endocrinopathy,
      M proteins, skin changes
      (POEMS)
    proximal diabetic p.
    sensory ataxic p.
    small fiber p.
    symmetrical distal p.
    symmetrical peripheral p.
    symmetric distal p.
polyol pathway
polyostotic
    p. fibrous dysplasia (PFD)
    p. form
    p. lesion
    p. Paget disease
polypeptide
    beta cell p.
    gastric inhibitory p. (GIP)
    glicentin-related pancreatic p.
      (GRPP)
    glucose-dependent insulinotrophic p.
      (GIP)
    glucose-dependent insulinotropic p.
    p. hormone
    p. hormone gene
    islet amyloid p. (IAPP)
    p. ligand
    pancreatic p. (PP)
    parathyroid hormonelike p.
      (PTHLP)
    pituitary adenylate cyclase-
      activating p.
    relaxin p.
    single-chain p.
    vasoactive intestinal p. (VIP)
polypeptide-1
    apo B mRNA-editing catalytic p.-1
      (apobec-1)
polypeptide-producing cell
polyphagia
polypharmacy
polyphosphatidylinositide
polyphosphoinositide (PI)
polyploidic cell
polypoid lesion

polyposis
    adenomatous p.
    familial adenomatous p.
    gastrointestinal p.
polyradiculopathy
polysaccharide-iron complex
polyspermy
polystotic FD
polysulfated glycosaminoglycan
polythelia
polythiazide
polytomogram
polytomography
polyunsaturated fatty acid (PUFA)
polyuria
    persistent p.
polyuric syndrome
Poly-Vi-Flor
polyvinyl
    p. chloride poisoning
    p. sponge
polyvinylpyrrolidone iodine
Poly-Vi-Sol
POMC
    proopiomelanocortin
    POMC 8-kb gene
Pompase
Pompe glycogen storage disease, type II
pona reticularis
Ponaris nasal emollient
ponderal index
pons
    medulla p.
Ponstel
pontomesencephalic sulcus
pool
    beta-cell granule p.
    beta-granule storage p.
    extracellular iodide p.
    readily releasable p. (RRP)
    steroidogenic cytoplasmic p.
    total body iodide p.
poorly
    p. processed POMC molecule
    p. processed proopiomelanocortin
      molecule
poor wound healing
popcorn calcification
population
    iodine-replete goitrous p.
porcine
    p. insulin
    p. thyroid
porin
    mitochondrial p.
pork
    Iletin II P.
    p. insulin

P. NPH
P. Regular Iletin II
porous
p. calcium phosphate cube
p. collagen matrix
porphobilinogen synthase
porphyria
congenital erythropoietic p.
p. cutanea tarda
cyclic p.
toxic p.
porphyrin
portable endocrine system
portacaval
p. H-graft
p. shunt
portal
p. circulation
p. insulin delivery
p. system
p. vein
portasystemic shunt
Porter-Silber reaction
portion
clival p.
portio vaginalis
portohepatic
p. denervation
p. glucose
positional cloning strategy
positive
p. feedback
P. and Negative Affect Scale (PANAS)
positron emission tomography (PET)
POSM
plasma osmolality
POST
peritoneal oocyte and sperm transfer
postablative hypothyroidism
postabsorptive
p. hypoglycemia
p. state
postadenomectomy hypocortisolism
postchallenge glucose level
postcoital
p. contraception
p. contraceptive
p. test
postcosyntropin plasma cortisol
posterior
p. cerebral artery
p. clinoid process
p. communicating artery
p. cricoarytenoid
p. cricoarytenoid muscle
p. gastric diverticulum
p. hypothalamic area (PHA)
p. lobe hormone
pars p.
p. pituitary
p. pituitary gland
p. pole
p. skull flattening
postexercise hypoglycemia
postfixed
postgadolinium study
postganglionic
sympathetic p.
p. sympathetic fiber
p. sympathetic neuron
postgastrectomy
posthyperglycemic
p. euglycemia
p. normoglycemia
postimplantation
p. embryofetal loss
p. period
postinflammatory testicular atrophy
postischemic acute tubular necrosis
postmeiotic spermatocyte
postmenopausal
P. Estrogen/Progestin Interventions Trial (PEPI)
p. osteoporosis
postnatal
p. pancreas
p. therapy
postpartum
p. blues
p. hyperthyroidism
p. hypopituitarism
p. lymphocytic thyroiditis
p. painless thyroiditis
p. pituitary infarction
p. pituitary necrosis
p. silent thyroiditis
p. thyroid disease (PPTD)
p. thyroid dysfunction
postpill amenorrhea
postprandial
p. glucose (PG)
p. glucose concentration
p. glucose excursion

NOTES

P

postprandial *(continued)*
    p. glucose-mediated toxicity
    p. hyperglycemia
    p. hypoaminoacidemia
    p. hypoglycemia
    p. hypotension
    p. insulin concentration
    p. insulin deficiency
    p. lipemia
    p. lipemia insulin-resistance
      syndrome
    p. state
    p. symptom
    p. syndrome
postpubertal
    p. diabetes
    p. mumps
    p. testicular atrophy
postradioiodine
postreceptor
    p. desensitization
    p. inhibitor
    p. leptin resistance
    p. marker
    p. pyruvate dehydrogenase activity
    p. signaling intermediate
postrema
    area p. (AP)
postsupraventricular tachycardia
postsurgical hypoparathyroidism
postsynaptic membrane
posttesticular defect
posttherapeutic hypothyroidism
postthyrotropin scan
posttranslational
    p. cleavage
    p. modification
posttransplantation
    p. lymphoproliferative disorder
      (PTLD)
    p. osteopenia
posttransplant diabetes mellitus (PTDM)
posttraumatic osteoporosis
postural
    p. hypotension
    p. imbalance
posture stimulation test
postvoid residual urine volume
potassium (K)
    acesulfame p.
    p. balance
    p. chloride
    p. citrate
    p. citrate and citric acid
    delayed rectifier voltage-gated beta-
      cell adenosine triphosphate p.
    p. depletion
    p. homeostasis

    p. inwardly-rectifying channel,
      subfamily J, member 1 (KCNJ1)
    p. inwardly-rectifying channel,
      subfamily J, member 1 gene
    p. iodide
    p. ion (K^+)
    p. leak channel
    penicillin v p.
    p. perchlorate
    p. phosphate
    p. spectroscopy
    p. $_{IR}6.2$
    p. $_{IR}6.2$ sulfonylurea receptor 1, 2
    p. $_{IR}6.2$ sulfonylurea receptor 1
      potassium$_{ATP}$ channel
    total body p.
potassium-32
potassium$_{ATP}$ (K$_{ATP}$)
    p. blockade
    p. channel
    p. channel blocker
    p. channel gene
    p. channel glucose homeostasis
    p. channel hyperinsulinemia
      mutation
    p. channel hyperinsulinism
    p. channel independent pathway
    p. channel independent pathway
      term-dependent potentiation
    p. channel isoform sulfonylurea
      receptor
    p. whole-cell beta-cell
potassium-sparing diuretic
potency
    uterine-stimulating p. (USP)
potential
    action p.
    adenosine triphosphate potassium
      channel hyperpolarized resting
      membrane p.
    redox p.
    resting membrane p.
    stress-generated p. (SGP)
    visual-evoked p.
potentiation
    potassium$_{ATP}$ channel independent
      pathway term-dependent p.
    time-dependent p. (TDP)
potocytosis
potomania
    beer p.
Potter facies
pouch
    branchial p.
    cleft of the Rathke p.
    Heidenhain p.
    infundibular p.
    pharyngeal p.

Rathke p.
stomodeal hypophysial p.
Pou1F1 gene
POU-homeodomain transcription factor
povidone-iodine
powder
Genotropin p.
Goody's Headache P.
Secretin-Ferring P.
PP
pancreatic polypeptide
pyrophosphate
vitamin PP
pp185
185 kDa phosphoprotein
PPAR
peroxisome proliferator-activated receptor
PPAR dimerization
PPAR DNA binding
PPAR functional domain
PPAR hypoglycemia
PPAR ligand
PPAR protein structure
PPAR selective modulator
PPAR-alpha
peroxisome proliferator-activated
receptor-alpha
PPAR-alpha ligand
PPAR-delta
peroxisome proliferator-activated
receptor-delta
PPAR-delta ligand
PPAR-gamma
peroxisome proliferator-activated
receptor-gamma
PPAR-gamma atherosclerosis
PPAR-gamma functional domain
genetic mutations PPAR-gamma
ligand-dependent transcriptional
activation PPAR-gamma
ligand-dependent transcriptional
repression PPAR-gamma
PPAR-gamma partial agonist
PPAR-gamma resistance syndrome
PPAR-gamma retinoid X receptor
ligand
PPAR-gamma target gene
PPAR-gamma therapy
PPAR-gamma tumor necrosis
factor-alpha

PPAR-gamma 2
peroxisome proliferator activated
receptor-gamma 2
PPHP
pseudoPHP
pseudopseudohypoparathyroidism
PPI
purified pork insulin
PPi
inorganic pyrophosphate
PPJ
pure pancreatic juice
PPJ cytologic examination
PPL
primary pituitary lymphoma
PPoma
pancreatic polypeptide-secreting tumor
PPPD
pylorus-preserving
pancreatoduodenectomy
PPTD
postpartum thyroid disease
pQCT
computer tomographic methods of
peripheral skeleton
PR
progesterone receptor
PRA
plasma renin activity
plasmin renin activity
Prader
P. calipers
P. orchidometer
Prader-Labhart-Willi syndrome
Prader-Willi syndrome (PWS)
Pramet FA
Pramilet FA
pramlintide acetate
Prandase
prandial
Prandin
pravastatin
prazosin
preadipocyte factor-1 (Pref-1)
prealbumin
thyroid-binding p. (TBPA)
thyronine-binding p. (TBPA)
thyroxine-binding p.
prealbumin-associated hyperthyroxinemia
(PAH)
preantral follicle
prechondrocyte differentiation

NOTES

P

281

precipitin reaction
precision
    P. Extra
    P. QID
    P. Xtra Advanced Diabetes
      Management System
    P. Xtra test strip
preclinical
    p. hypothyroidism
    p. myxedema
precocious
    p. adrenarche
    p. emotional menopause
    p. maturation
    p. pseudopuberty
    p. pubarche
    p. puberty
precocity
    contrasexual p.
    familial male-limited gonadotrophin-
      independent sexual p.
    heterosexual p.
    idiopathic sexual p.
    incomplete isosexual p.
    isosexual p.
    sexual p.
precolloid stage
preconceptional
    p. glycemic control
    p. planning
preconception counseling
Precose
precursor
    adrenal steroid p.
    arginine vasopressor p.
    p. cell
    erythroid p.
    glycogenic p.
    hematopoietic stem cell p.
    high-mannose p.
    myeloid p.
    osteoclast p.
    protein p.
precursor/product ratio
Pred
    Liquid P.
prediabetes
Predicort-50
prediction
    Roche, Wainer, and Thissen
      method of height p. (RWT)
predictive
    p. growth model
    p. value
    p. value test
predisposing factor
predisposition
    genetic p.
Prednicen-M

prednisolone
    oral p.
Prednisol TBA Injection
prednisone taper
predominant hyperparathyroid bone
    disease
preduodenal lipase
Pref-1
    preadipocyte factor-1
prefixed
pregabalin capsule
pregadolinium study
preganglionic
    p. sympathetic nerve
    p. sympathetic nerve fiber
    p. sympathetic neuron
pregestational diabetes
pregnancy
    acute fatty liver of p.
    p. cell
    diabetes in early p. (DIEP)
    diabetic p.
    ectopic p.
    embryogenesis in p.
    p. hyperthyroidism
    p. hypothyroidism
    luteoma of p.
    p. nodular thyroid disease
    p. radioiodine therapy
    p. thyroid function test
    p. thyroid underfunction
    p. thyrotoxicosis
    p. thyrotropin receptor
    toxemia of p.
pregnancy-induced hypertension (PIH)
pregnane derivative
pregnanediol
pregnanetriol
pregnenolone
Pregnyl
prehormone
preinfusion level
preinitiation complex (PIC)
prekallikrein
preleptotene primary spermatocyte
Prelone Oral
Prelu-2
Premack-C
premammillary nucleus
Premarin with methyltestosterone
premature
    p. adrenarche
    p. ejaculation
    p. epiphyseal fusion
    p. gonadal failure
    p. luteinization
    p. menopause
    p. ovarian failure
    p. sexual development

p. thelarche
p. top codon (TAA)
prematurity
hypothyroxinemia of p.
rickets of p.
Pre-Meal
Dexatrim P.-M.
premeal hyperglycemia
premenstrual
p. dysphoric disorder (PMDD)
p. molimina
p. syndrome (PMS)
premixed insulin
Prempak-C
Premphase
Prempro
prenatal
p. diagnosis
p. multiple vitamin
Stuart P.
Prenavite
prenyltransferase
preoptic
p. area of the hypothalamus
(POA)
p. region
preosseous cartilage
preosteoblast
preosteoclast
preovulatory follicle
preparation
acid resistant/coated p.
herbal p.
insulin p.
preprandially
preprandial recurrent symptom
prepregnancy planning
preprocalcitonin
preproendothelin
preprogastrin
preproglucagone gene
preprohormone
insulin p.
preprohypocretin
preproinsulin
p. gene
p. messenger ribonucleic acid
preproPTH gene
preprosomatostatin
preprotachykinin A gene
prepubertal diabetes
preputial gland

preradial myxedema
prereceptor
p. inhibitor
p. metabolism
prerenal azotemia
preseminal fluid
preservation
B-cell p.
pressor response
pressure
ankle p.
atmospheric p.
basal sphincter p.
blood p.
brachial p.
colloid osmotic p.
continuous positive airway p.
p. diuresis
elevated intracranial p.
hydrostatic p.
intraadrenal p.
intrahypophyseal p.
intraocular p.
intrasellar p.
p. natriuresis
p. necrosis
oncotic p.
plasma osmotic p.
pulmonary capillary wedge p.
toe p.
transcutaneous oxygen p.
widened pulse p.
pressure-flow study
Pressyn
PresTab
Glynase P.
Prestige
P. IQ glucose meter
P. Lite Touch lancing device
P. LX glucose meter
P. Smart System test strip
presubunit
presymptomatic diagnosis
presynaptic nerve terminal
prethyroid
prethyroidal fascia
pretibial
p. dermopathy
p. myxedema
Pretz-D
Prevacid
Preven

NOTES

P

preventive hormone therapy
previtamin
    p. D
    p. D_3
PRF
    prolactin-releasing factor
PRH
    prolactin-releasing hormone
priapism
primary
    p. adjuvant treatment
    p. adrenal failure
    p. adrenal hyperfunction
    p. adrenal medullary hormone
    p. adrenocortical insufficiency
    p. afferent nociceptor neuron
    (PAN)
    p. aldosteronism (PAL)
    p. amenorrhea
    p. antibody
    p. antiphospholipid syndrome
    p. biliary cirrhosis
    p. capillary plexus
    p. central nervous system (PCNS)
    p. central nervous system
    lymphoma
    p. cortisol resistance
    p. craniosynostosis
    p. empty sella syndrome
    extrathyroidal p.
    p. follicle
    p. gonadal failure
    p. hyperparathyroidism (PHPT)
    p. hyperthyroidism
    p. hypertrophic osteoarthropathy
    p. hypoadrenalism
    p. hypocitraturia
    p. hypogonadism
    p. hypoparathyroidism
    p. immune deficiency (PID)
    p. immunoregulatory abnormality
    p. infertility
    intrathyroidal p.
    p. macronodular hyperplasia
    p. myxedema
    p. oocyte
    p. orthostatic hypotension
    p. ovarian carcinoid
    p. ovarian choriocarcinoma
    p. pigmental nodular adrenal
    dysplasia
    p. pigmented nodular adrenal
    dysplasia
    p. pituitary lymphoma (PPL)
    p. polydipsia
    p. sclerosing cholangitis (PSC)
    p. spermatocyte
    p. spongiosa
    p. suprasellar dysgerminoma

    p. sympathetic neurotransmitter
    p. therapy
    p. thyroidal hypothyroidism
    p. thyroid lymphoma
    p. villus
primer
    sequence-specific p. (SSP)
Primobolan
primordial
    p. follicle
    p. germ cell (PGC)
    p. ova
principal
    Fick p.
Principen
prion protein
prior distant metastasis
priori
    a p.
PRISM calendar
PRL
    prolactin
PRL-cell adenoma
PRL-secreting adenoma
proadrenomedullin N-20 terminal
    peptide (PAMP)
proalbumin
proamnion
Pro-Banthine
probe
    hybridization histochemistry p.
    microdialysis p.
    oligodeoxynucleotide antisense p.
    oligonucleotide p.
    thyroid uptake p.
probenecid
probe-tissue hybridization protocol
problematic hypoglycemia
Probolin
probucol antioxidant
procalcitonin
procarbazine
procarboxypeptidase B (PCPB)
procedure
    Cushing p.
    electroosmotic sampling p.
    Fontan p.
    Fontana-Masson p.
    iontophoretic sampling p.
    needlescopic p.
    neuroradiologic imaging p.
    revascularization p.
    Sistrunk p.
process
    anterior clinoid p.
    clinoid p.
    extrathyroidal immunological p.
    gustatory neurosensory p.
    infundibular p.

insulitic p.
intracellular metabolic p.
microfilament-mediated p.
posterior clinoid p.
pterygoid p.
translocation p.
zygomatic p.
processor
signal p.
processus vaginalis
prochlorperazine
procollagen
p. gene
p. level
p. molecule
type I p.
procollagen-III peptide (pIIIp)
proconceptive
Procrit
product
Amadori p.
calcium times phosphorus p.
cleavage p.
glycation end p.
Maillard p.
matrix-dissolution p.
production
autoantibody p.
cytokine p.
ectopic hormone p.
ectopic paraneoplastic ACTH p.
endogenous glucose p. (EGP)
hepatic glucose p. (HGP)
liver glucose p.
theca cell androgen p.
thyroid hormone p.
prodynorphin
proenkephalin
p. A
p. B
p. gene
Profasi HP
profile
LifeScan P.
lipid p.
metabolic p.
Nottingham Health P.
OneTouch P.
plasma lipid p.
profunda penis artery
progenitor
bone marrow-derived myogenic p.

p. cell
mesenchymal p.
multipotential p.
progeria
progestagen
Progestasert
P. intrauterine device
P. IUD
Pro-Gest cream
progesterone (P)
p. challenge test
endogenous p.
exogenous p.
micronized p.
p. oil
p. receptor (PR)
p. resistance
p. suppository
venous ovarian plasma p.
progesterone-based contraceptive
progesterone-only
p.-o. minipill
p.-o. pill
progestin
C-19 p.
C-21 p.
p. dienogest
p. ethynodiol diacetate
nonandrogenic p.
nor-derivative p.
progestin-containing intrauterine device
progestogen
progestogenic
proglucagon gene
Proglycem Oral
prognathism
Prograf
program
Diabetes Autoantibody
Standardization P. (DASP)
diabetes education p.
Diabetes Prevention P. (DPP)
disease-management p.
National Cholesterol Education P.
(NCEP)
National Cholesterol Evaluation P.
Point of Change weight
management p.
split mixed insulin p.
University Group Diabetes P.
(UGDP)
XeniCare p.

NOTES

P

285

programmed theory of aging
programming
    neuroendocrine p.
progressiva
    fibrodysplasia ossificans p. (FOP)
progressive
    p. depigmentation
    p. diaphyseal dysplasia
    p. multifocal axonal neuropathy
    p. osteopenia
Progynon
Progynon-B
prohormone
    p. convertase
    p. convertase 1 (PC1)
    p. convertase 2 (PC2)
    p. convertase 3 (PC3)
    steroid p.
Pro-Indo
proinflammatory
    p. cytokine
    p. mediator
proinsulin
    p. conversion processing enzyme
    p. insulin ratio
    p. level
proinsulinlike molecule
project
    Captopril Prevention P. (CAPP)
    Diabetes Prediction and
      Prevention P. (DIPP)
    Human Genome P.
projection
    GABAergic p.
    gamma-aminobutyric acidergic p.
    left temporal p.
    maximum intensity p. (MIP)
    papillary tumor p.
    retinohypothalamic p.
    right temporal p.
    serotonergic p.
prokaryote
prokaryotic cell
prolactin (PRL)
    p. biosynthesis
    p. cell adenoma
    p. cell hyperplasia
    p. deficiency
    p. excess
    extrapituitary p.
    p. hormone-expressing cell
    p. inhibitory factor
    p. inhibitory hormone (PIH)
    p. inhibitory mechanism
    iso-B p.
    p. pulse amplitude
    p. release-inhibiting hormone (PIH)
    p. secretion
    p. secretion during menstrual cycle

    serum p.
    p. synthesis
    p. transcription
prolactinemia
prolactin-inhibiting
    p.-i. factor (PIF)
    p.-i. hormone (PIH)
prolactinoma
    giant invasive p.
    p. growth
    invasive p.
prolactin-producing
    p.-p. pituitary adenoma
    p.-p. pituitary tumor
prolactin-releasing
    p.-r. factor (PRF)
    p.-r. hormone (PRH)
prolactin-secreting
    p.-s. adenoma
    p.-s. pituitary macroadenoma
    p.-s. pituitary tumor
ProLease encapsulated sustained-release growth hormone
prolidase
proliferating cell nuclear antigen (PCNA)
proliferation
    appositional crystal p.
    p. assay
    autonomous parathyroid chief
      cell p.
    chondrocyte p.
    epitaxial crystal p.
    osteoblast p.
    osteoblast progenitor p.
proliferative diabetic retinopathy (PDR)
proliferator
    peroxisome p.
proline oxidase
prolonged diabetes insipidus
Proluton
prolyl hydroxylase enzyme
promegestone
Promensil
Prometa
Prometrium
prominence
    frontooccipital p.
    lateral tibial p.
prominent supraorbital ridge
promoter
    A element insulin gene p.
    CCAAT element insulin gene p.
    C1 element insulin gene p.
    C2 element insulin gene p.
    c-*fos* p.
    c-*jun* p.
    core p.

cyclic adenosine monophosphate
  regulatory element insulin gene p.
E-box element insulin gene p.
liver pyruvate kinase p.
Z element insulin gene p.
promotor
  glucagon-gene p.
Pronestyl
pronuclei
proopiomelanocortin (POMC)
  p. derivative
  p. gene
  p. molecule
  p. mutation
proopiomelanocortin-derived peptide
PROP-1
  prophet of Pit-1
  PROP-1 gene
  PROP-1 transcription factor
Propacet
Prop-a gene mutation
propanolol
propantheline
proparathyroid hormone (proPTH)
propeptide
  C-terminal p.
properdin
property
  antigenic p.
  antirachitic p.
prophet
  p. of Pit-1 (PROP-1)
  p. of Pit-1 transcription factor
prophylactic pituitary radiotherapy
propionate
  testosterone p.
propionic
  p. acidemia
  p. aciduria
propionyl-coenzyme A carboxylase
propofol
proportion
  eunuchoidal body p.
propoxyphene
propranolol
propressophysin
propria
  lamina p.
proprioception
proprotein convertase (PC)
proPTH
  proparathyroid hormone

proptosis
  insidious p.
propylthiouracil (PTU)
Propyl-Thyracil
proreceptor
prorenin
Prorex Injection
Proscar
prosencephaly
Prospective Record of the Impact and Severity of Menstrual Symptoms
prostacyclin (PGI2)
prostaglandin
  p. A
  p. B_2
  p. D_2 (PGD_2)
  p. E (PGE)
  p. E_1 (PGE_1)
  p. E_3
  p. E_2 (PGE_2)
  p. E_2 release
  p. $F_{1\text{-alpha}}$ ($PGF_{1\text{-alpha}}$)
  p. $F_{2\text{-alpha}}$ ($PGF_{2\text{-alpha}}$)
  p. F_{2a} (PGF_{2a})
  p. F receptor
  p. G_2 (PGG_2)
  p. H_2 (PGH_2)
  p. H synthase (PGHS)
  p. I (PGI)
  p. I_2 (PGI_2)
  p. J (PGJ)
  p. synthase inhibitor
  vasodilator p.
prostanoid
ProstaScint scan
prostate
  electrovaporization of the p.
  p. gland
  microwave hyperthermia of the p.
  transurethral incision of the p. (TUIP)
  transurethral resection of the p. (TURP)
prostatectomy
  laser p.
prostate-specific
  p.-s. membrane antigen (PSMA)
prostatic
  p. concretion
  p. duct
  p. urethra
  p. utricle

NOTES

P

prostatitis
prostatropin
ProStep Patch
prosthesis, pl. **prostheses**
    penile p.
Prostigmin
protamine zinc insulin
protean
protease
    p. inhibitor
    insulin p.
    insulinlike growth factor-binding
      protein p.
    kallikrein p.
protease-sensitive site
proteasome
    20S p.
    26S p.
Protectaid sponge
protector
    LATS p.
protein
    acid-stable p.
    actin-binding p.
    p. acylation
    acylation-stimulating p.
    adaptor p.
    adenovirus E1A p.
    adipocyte differentiation-related p.
      (ADRP)
    adipose tissue-uncoupling p.
    agouti p.
    agouti-related p.
    A-Kinase anchoring p. (AKAP)
    albuminoid p.
    androgen-binding p. (ABP)
    beta-arrestin p.
    beta-cell lmx1.1 p.
    BGP p.
    p. binding
    BMAL1 p.
    bone G1a p. (BGP)
    bone morphogenetic p. (BMP)
    bone morphogenic p. (BMP)
    bone-related p.
    bone-specific p.
    brain/muscle AhR nuclear
      translocator-like p. 1
    brain/muscle ARNT-like p. 1
      (BMAL1)
    calcium-binding p.
    calmodulin p.
    carrier p.
    cartilage oligomeric matrix p.
    catabolite activator p. (CAP)
    catabolite regulatory p.
    Cbl/Cbl-associated p. (CAP)
    CCAAT/enhancer binding p.
      (C/EBP)

    CGI p.
    channel-forming integral p. (CHIP)
    chimeric p.
    cholesteryl ester transfer p.
    chromogranin A, B, C p.
    chromogranin-secretogranin p.
    CLOCK p.
    cloned steroid acute respiratory p.
    c-myc p.
    coactivator p.
    cold-inducible ribonucleic acid-
      binding p. (CIRP)
    cold-inducible RNA-binding p.
      (CIRP)
    cold-shock p.
    connexin p.
    contractile p.
    contraction-associated p. (CAP)
    corticotropin-releasing hormone-
      binding p. (CRH-BP)
    COUP-TF thyroid hormone receptor
      auxillary p.
    cow's milk p. (CMP)
    C-reactive p. (CRP)
    CREB-binding p. (CBP)
    CRH-binding p. (CRH-BP)
    Crk p.
    CrkI p.
    CrkII p.
    CrkL p.
    cyclic AMP response-element
      binding p.
    cyclin D1 p.
    cytochrome p. (CYP)
    cytokinin-regulated kinase I, II p.
    cytokinin-regulated kinase L p.
    dietary p.
    p. disulfide isomerase (PDI)
    p. disulfide isomerase-mediated
      disulfide bond reduction
    docking p.
    EAAT2 p.
    E-cadherin p.
    p. efficiency ratio
    extracellular matrix p.
    fatty acid-binding p. (FABP)
    fatty acid-binding p. 2 (FABP2)
    fatty acid transport p. (FATP)
    FK-binding p. (FKBP)
    FK-binding p. 12 (FKBP12)
    FKBP-rapamycin-associated p.
      (FRAP)
    follistatin p.
    Fyn p.
    G p.
    gamma-carboxyglutamic acid p.
    gene regulatory p.
    G-inhibiting p. (G_i)
    Gla p.

globulin-vitamin D binding p.
glucocorticoid receptor-interacting p. 1 (GRIP 1)
glucokinase regulatory p.
glucose-transport p. 1 (GLUT-1)
glucose-transport p. 2 (GLUT-2)
glucose-transport p. 3 (GLUT-3)
glucose-transport p. 4 (GLUT-4)
glucose-transport p. 5 (GLUT-5)
glucose-transport p. 6 (GLUT-6)
glucose-transport p. 7 (GLUT-7)
glycated p.
p. glycemia
glycine-rich RNA-binding p. (GRP)
glycogenin-interacting p. (GNIP)
glycoprotein crystal growth-inhibitor p.
glycosylated serum p.
Grb-2 p.
green birefringent amyloid p.
growth hormone-binding p. (GHBP)
G-stimulating p. (G$_s$)
GTPase-activating p. (GAP)
GTP-binding p.
guanine nucleotide binding p.
guanine nucleotide regulatory p. (GNRP)
guanosine triphosphate-activating p. (GAP)
guanosine triphosphate-binding p.
heat shock p. (HSP, Hsp)
heat-stable p.
Hedgehog p.
heme-binding p.
heterotrimeric p.
high-sensitivity C-reactive p. (hs-CRP)
histidine-rich calcium-binding p. (HRC)
hormone-binding p.
human pancreas-specific p. (hPASP)
hydrophobic p.
IGF-binding p. (IGFBP)
inhibitory guanine nucleotide binding regulatory p.
insulin growth factor-binding p.
insulinlike growth factor-binding p. (IGFBP)
insulin receptor substrate p. (IRS-protein)
iron-binding p.

islet-cell neogenesis-associated p. (INGAP)
8-kDa p.
37-kDa p.
p. 70-kDa S6 ribosomal subunit kinase (p70S6k)
p. kinase A (PKA)
p. kinase A pathway (AKAP)
p. kinase B (Akt, PKB)
p. kinase B/Akt
p. kinase B substrate
p. kinase C (PKC)
p. kinase C cascade
p. kinase C inhibitor
p. kinase C isoform
p. kinase G (PKG)
p. kinase/phosphatase cascade
LDL receptor-related p. (LRP)
lipocalin p.
5-lipoxygenase activating p. (FLAP)
liver-enriched activating p. (LAP)
liver-enriched inhibiting p. (LIP)
lmx1.1 p.
lmx1.2 p.
low-density lipoprotein receptor-related p. (LRP)
macrophage inflammatory p.-1-alpha (MIP-1-alpha)
macrophage inflammatory p.-1-beta (MIP-1-beta)
p. mass
matrix Gla p. (MGP)
membrane cofactor p. (MCP)
membrane integral p. (MIP)
p. metabolism
milk p.
misfolded p.
mitogen-activated p. (MAP)
mucosal carrier p. (MCP)
multidrug resistance p. (MDR)
myelin basic p. (MBP)
nascent p.
Nck p.
NESP55 p.
neuroendocrine secretory p. 55 (NESP55)
neurophysin p.
noncollagenous p.
nonhistone p.
p75 p.
pancreatitis-associated p. (PAP)
parathyroid hormonelike p.

NOTES

P

protein *(continued)*
    parathyroid hormone-related p.
      (PTHrP, PTH-RP)
    PDGF p.
    pendrin p.
    PER p.
    period p.
    PH-20, -30 p.
    pH domain-interacting p. (PHIP)
    p. phosphatase 2B
    phosphatidylinositide-3 kinase
      cascade insulin receptor cell p.
    phosphorylate membrane p.
    photoactive yellow p.
    pituitary adenylate cyclase-
      activating p.
    plasma membrane fatty acid
      binding p. (FABP$_{pm}$)
    platelet p.
    p. plug
    p. precursor
    prion p.
    protein kinase regulator p.
    PTH-related p. (PTHrP, PTH-RP)
    Rab p.
    Rac p.
    Rap p.
    ras p.
    ras-like p.
    receptor-coupled membrane p.
    ret-fused p. (RFP)
    retinol-binding p.
    Rho p.
    S-100 p.
    S-14 p.
    scaffold p.
    secretory carrier membrane p.
      (SCAMP)
    serpin p.
    serum response element binding p.
      (SREBP)
    serum thyroid hormone-binding p.
    single-pass transmembrane p.
    soluble *N*-ethylmaleimide-sensitive
      factor attachment p.
    soluble *N*-ethylmaleimide-sensitive
      factor attachment p. (SNAP)
    somatomedin C p.
    soy p.
    soybean p.
    Src p.
    StAR p.
    steroid acute regulatory p. (StAR)
    steroid acute respiratory p. (StAR)
    steroidogenic acute regulatory p.
      (StAR)
    sterol regulatory element binding p.
      (SREBP)
    stimulatory G p.

    surfactant-associated p.
    syntaxin 4-interacting p. (SYNIP)
    p. synthesis
    Syp p.
    Tamm-Horsfall p.
    TATA-binding p. (TBP)
    tax p.
    thyroglobulin p.
    thyroid hormone receptor auxiliary
      antibody p.
    thyroid hormone transport p.
    thyroid-specific enhancer-binding p.
      (T/EBP)
    TIM p.
    transport p.
    triose isomerase p.
    troponin C p.
    p. truncation test (PTT)
    p. tyrosine kinase (PTK)
    p. tyrosine phosphatase (PTPase)
    p. tyrosine phosphorylation
    ubiquitinylated p.
    uncoupling p. (UCP)
    uncoupling p. 1 (UCP1)
    vascular endocrine p.
    vesicle-associated membrane p.
      (VAMP)
    vitamin D-binding p. (DBP)
    v-mpl p.
    Wnt p.
    XL-alpha p.
    Yes p.
    zinc finger p. (ZFP)
    ZOG p.
    zona glomerulosa p. (ZOG)

protein-1
    activator p.-1 (AP-1)
    endothelial PAS-domain p.-1
      (EPAS1)
    IGF-binding p.-1
    insulinlike growth factor-binding p.-
      1 (IGFBP-1)
    monocyte chemoattractant p.-1
    monocyte chemotactic p.-1 (MCP-1)
    mucosal carrier p.-1 (MCP-1)

protein-2
    bone morphogenetic p.-2
    insulinlike growth factor-binding p.-
      2 (IGFBP-2)
    mammalian achaete-scute
      homologous p.-2 (Mash-2)
    osteogenic p.-2
    sterol carrier p.-2 (SCP-2)

protein-3
    insulinlike growth factor-binding p.-
      3 (IGFBP-3)

protein-4
    bone morphogenetic p.-4

insulinlike growth factor-binding p.-4 (IGFBP-4)
protein-5
insulinlike growth factor-binding p.-5 (IGFBP-5)
protein-6
insulinlike growth factor-binding p.-6 (IGFBP-6)
protein-7
bone morphogenetic p.-7
protein-1-alpha
proteinase
protein-1-beta
protein-calorie malnutrition
protein/chymotrypsin
chymotrypsinogen-related 30-kd p.
protein-deficient pancreatic diabetes
protein-dimerizing activity
protein-energy malnutrition (PEM)
protein-sparing modified fast (PSMF)
protein-tyrosine
p.-t. binding (PTB)
p.-t. phosphatase 1B (PTP1B)
p.-t. phosphatase enzyme superfamily
proteinuria
proteoglycan
glycosylphosphatidylinositol-anchored heparan sulfate p.
heparan sulfate p.
p. molecule
proteolipid
proteolysis
limited fragment p.
p. of pancreatic zymogen
proteolytic
p. activity
p. cleavage
p. enzyme
p. pathway
thyroglobulin p.
proteomics
Proteus
Prothazine-DC
prothoracotropic hormone (PTTH)
prothrombinase
Protilase
protirelin
protocol
biotinylated-nucleotide p.
Edmonton P.

probe-tissue hybridization p.
tolerogenic p.
proton
p. beam radiation
p. beam therapy
p. buffer
p. diffusion
proton-pump
protooncogene
p. c-erbA
p. c-*fos*
c-myc p.
p. c-*src*
p. expression
MOS p.
NTRK1 p.
p. TRK
Protostat Oral
Protrophin II
Protropin
Provera Oral
provisional calcification
provitamin D
provocation test
provocative testing
Provocholine
proximal
p. convoluted tubule (PCT)
p. diabetic neuropathy
p. diabetic polyneuropathy
p. Golgi apparatus
p. motor neuropathy
p. muscle weakness
PRPP
phosphoribosylpyrophosphate
PRPP synthase
PRTH
pituitary resistance to thyroid hormone
pituitary RTH
selective PRTH
PRTH syndrome
prurigo
Besnier p.
pruritus
generalized p.
uremic p.
Prussian blue stain for iron
PS
pancreozymin secretin
PS test
psammoma body

NOTES

PSC
   primary sclerosing cholangitis
P450SCC
   P450 side chain cleavage
   P450SCC enzyme
P-selectin level
pseudoachondroplasia
pseudoacromegaly
pseudoadrenal mass
pseudoaldosteronism
pseudoaneurysm
   peripancreatic p.
pseudoatrophic islet
pseudoautosomal region
pseudocapsule
pseudocholinesterase deficiency
pseudoclubbing
pseudocorpus luteum insufficiency
pseudo-Cushing
   p.-C. state
   p.-C. syndrome
   p.-C. syndrome of alcoholism
pseudocyst
pseudodementia
pseudodiabetes
   uremic p.
pseudofracture
   Looser p.
pseudogene
   chimeric p.
   glucose-transport protein 6 p.
   GLUT-6 p.
   homologous p.
pseudogiant cell
pseudogoiter
pseudogout
pseudogranulomatous thyroiditis
pseudohermaphrodism
pseudohermaphrodite
   female p.
   male p.
pseudohermaphroditism
   female p. (FPH)
   male p. (MPH)
pseudo-Hurler polydystrophy
pseudohyperaldosteronism
pseudohypercortisoluria
pseudohypertrophy
   muscular p.
pseudohypoaldosteronism (PHA)
   type II
   p. type I (PHA I)
   p. type II (PHA II)
pseudohypoglycemia
pseudohyponatremia
pseudohypoparathyroidism (PHP)
   Aurbach p.
   p. type Ia, Ib
pseudohypoxia

Pseudomonas aeruginosa
pseudomotor cerebri
pseudomyotonia
pseudopapillary formation
pseudoparalysis
pseudoperiodic biorhythm
pseudoPHP (PPHP)
   pseudopseudohypoparathyroidism
pseudopod
   cytoplasmic p.
pseudoprecocious puberty
pseudopregnancy
pseudoprolactinoma
pseudopseudohypoparathyroidism (PPHP, pseudoPHP)
pseudopuberty
   precocious p.
pseudorosette
pseudoscleroderma
pseudothrombocytopenia
pseudotuberculous thyroiditis
pseudotumor
   adrenal p.
   p. cerebri
pseudotumorous
pseudo-Turner syndrome
pseudovagina
pseudovitamin D deficiency rickets (VDDR)
p70S6k
   protein 70-kDa S6 ribosomal subunit kinase
PSMA
   prostate-specific membrane antigen
PSMF
   protein-sparing modified fast
psoralen and ultraviolet A light (PUVA)
psoriasis
psoriatic plaque
PSP
   persephin
*Pst*I **restriction enzyme**
psychogenic
   p. amenorrhea
   p. impotence
   p. polydipsia
Psychological Well Being Index
psychoneuroimmunology
psychophysiological study
psychosexual
psychosocial dwarfism
psychosurgery
PTA
   pancreas transplant alone
   pancreas transplantation alone
PTB
   phosphotyrosine binding

phosphotyrosine-binding domain
protein-tyrosine binding
PTC
papillary thyroid carcinoma
PTDM
posttransplant diabetes mellitus
P.T.E.-4, -5
PTEN
phosphatase and tensin homologue
phosphatase and tensin homologue
deleted on chromosome
pterion
pterional approach
pterygium colli
pterygoid
p. plate
p. process
PTF-1
pancreatic transcription factor 1
PTH
parathormone
parathyroid hormone
C-terminal assay for PTH
PThHR
pituitary thyroid hormone resistance
PTHLP
parathyroid hormonelike polypeptide
PTH-mediated calcium efflux
PTHR
pituitary thyroid hormone resistance
PTH-related protein (PTHrP, PTH-RP)
PTHrP, PTH-RP
parathyroid hormone-related peptide
parathyroid hormone-related protein
PTH-related protein
PTHrP-transfected RIN-141 cell
PTK
protein tyrosine kinase
PTLD
posttransplantation lymphoproliferative
disorder
PTN/MK
pleiotrophin/midkine growth enhancer
ptosis
PTP
low-Mr P.
low-molecular-weight PTPase
PTPase
protein tyrosine phosphatase
low-molecular-weight PTPase (low-Mr PTP)

PTP1B
protein-tyrosine phosphatase 1B
PTRTH
peripheral tissue resistance to thyroid
hormone
PTT
protein truncation test
PTTG
pituitary tumor-transforming gene
PTTH
prothoracotropic hormone
PTU
propylthiouracil
PTX
parathyroidectomy
pubarche
precocious p.
pubertal
p. development
p. growth spurt
puberty
central precocious p. (CPP)
complete precocious p.
constitutional precocious p.
delayed p.
familial male precocious p.
GnRH-dependent precocious p.
GnRH-independent precocious p.
gonadotropin-independent
precocious p.
idiopathic complete precocious p.
idiopathic true precocious p.
incomplete precocious p.
isosexual precocious p.
male-limited familial precocious p.
male precocious p.
neurogenic precocious p.
precocious p.
pseudoprecocious p.
stalled p.
temporary delayed p.
true precocious p.
pubic
p. hair
p. ramus
pubis
mons p.
pubis-to-crown measurement
pudendal nerve
pudendum, pl. **pudenda**
PUFA
polyunsaturated fatty acid

NOTES

P

puffiness
    periorbital p.
pulmonary
    p. angiotensin I converting enzyme
    p. arterial hypertension (PAH)
    p. aspiration
    p. capillary wedge pressure
    p. chondroma
    p. disease
    p. edema
    p. mucormycosis
    p. neuroepithelial endocrine (PNEE)
    p. osteoarthropathy
Pulmozyme
Pulsar analysis
pulsatile
    p. gonadotropin-releasing hormone
      therapy
    p. insulin release
    p. insulin secretion
    p. pituitary hormone release
pulse
    p. amplitude
    p. dosing
    p. frequency
    full p.
    p. generator
    p. incubation
pulsed
    p. administration
    p. Doppler ultrasound
    p. dye laser
    p. progestin hormone replacement
      therapy
pulse-height analyzer
pump
    Animas R-1000 insulin p.
    Ca^{2+} p.
    calcium p.
    computerized continuous
      subcutaneous insulin infusion p.
    continuous subcutaneous insulin
      infusion p.
    Dana Diabecare insulin p.
    Disetronic Diaport p.
    Disetronic Dihedi 25 insulin p.
    Disetronic D-Tron insulin p.
    D-Tron insulin p.
    external subcutaneous insulin
      infusion p.
    Felig insulin p.
    H-TRON insulin p.
    H-TRONplus insulin p.
    implantable intraperitoneal p.
    implantable programmable insulin
      infusion p.
    insulin infusion p.
    internal intraperitoneal insulin
      infusion p.

    iodide p.
    microinfusion p.
    MiniMed 508, 511 insulin p.
    MiniMed Paradigm insulin p.
    Panomat microinfusion p.
    Paradigm insulin p.
    sodium-potassium p.
    Versaflow peristatic p.
Pump-N-Shorts pump holder
punctata
    chondrodysplasia p.
    chondrodystrophia p.
pupillary
    p. abnormality
    p. defect
    p. reaction
pure
    p. gonadal dysgenesis
    p. pancreatic juice (PPJ)
    p. pancreatic juice cytologic
      examination
purified pork insulin (PPI)
purine
    p. metabolism
    p. nucleoside phosphorylase (PNP)
    p. nucleoside phosphorylase
      deficiency
purinergic
    p. activation
    p. agonist (PIA)
Purkinje
    P. cell
    P. cell dendrite
puromycin
purple stria
purplish stria
purpura
    autoimmune thrombocytopenia p.
    idiopathic thrombocytopenic p.
      (ITP)
purulent hypophysitis
pus
    black p.
putative
    p. neural axis
    p. physiologic role
    p. regulatory sequence DNA
    p. satiety
    p. tumor-suppressor gene
putative-binding site
PUVA
    psoralen and ultraviolet A light
PVL
    periventricular leukomalacia
PVN
    paraventricular nucleus
      PVN of the hypothalamus
PVT
    paraventricular thalamic nucleus

PWS
  Prader-Willi syndrome
PYD
  pyridinoline
pyelolithotomy
pyelonephritis
  ascending p.
  emphysematous p.
pygmy
pyknodysostosis
pyknotic nucleus
Pyle disease
pylori
  Helicobacter p.
pylorus
  gastric p.
pylorus-preserving
  pancreatoduodenectomy (PPPD)
pyogenes
  Staphylococcus p.
  Streptococcus p.
pyogenic thyroiditis
pyomyositis
pyramid
  food p.
pyramidal
  p. lobe
  p. tract
  p. tract sign
pyrexic
pyridinium cross-link
pyridinoline (PYD)
  p. cross-link
pyridoglutethimide
pyridostigmine

pyridoxal
  p. phosphate
  p. 5′-phosphate (PLP)
pyridoxine
pyriform sinus fistula
Pyrilinks-D
  P.-D. deoxypyridinoline crosslinks
    urine assay
  P.-D. immunoassay
pyriminil
pyriminil-induced diabetes mellitus
pyro-Glu-His-Pro-amide
  pyroglutamyl-histidyl-prolineamide
pyroglutamic
  p. acid
  p. aciduria
pyroglutamyl-histidyl-prolineamide (pyro-Glu-His-Pro-amide)
pyroglutamyl peptidase II
pyrophosphatase
pyrophosphate (PP)
  p. arthropathy
  calcium p.
  inorganic p. (PPi)
  technetium p.
pyrophosphoric acid
pyrosequencing
pyrroline-5-carboxylate dehydrogenase
pyruvate
  p. carboxylase
  p. dehydrogenase (PDH)
  p. kinase
PYY
  peptide YY

NOTES

P

Q10
     coenzyme Q10
3q27
     chromosome 3q27
5q31
     chromosome 5q31
10q
     chromosome 10q
12q
     chromosome 12q
12q15
     chromosome 12q15
QAFT
     quantitative autonomic functioning
       testing
QALYs
     quality-adjusted life-years
Q band
QCT
     quantified computed tomography
       axial QCT
          computer tomographic methods of
            axial skeleton
QID
     Precision QID
QKd interval
1q21-q23
     chromosome 1q21-q23
6q22-q23
     chromosome 6q22-q23
11q23-q25
     chromosome 11q23-q25
QST
     quantitative sensory testing
QT interval
QTL
     quantitative trait locus
quadrantanopia
quadrantanopsia
quadriceps fatigue

Quadrinal
quality-adjusted life-years (QALYs)
quantified computed tomography (QCT)
quantitative
     q. autonomic functioning testing
       (QAFT)
     Q. Autonomic Function Test
     q. bone histomorphometry
     q. insulin sensitivity check index
     q. radiography
     Q. Sensory Test
     q. sensory testing (QST)
     q. trait locus (QTL)
     q. trait locus mapping
quantum
     bone q.
questionnaire
     Fibromyalgia Impact Q. (FIQ)
     Florida Sexual Q.
Questran
quetiapine
Quibron
Quibron-T
Quibron-T/SR
QuickLance lancing device
QuickTek
     Q. glucose meter
     Q. test strip
QuickVue UrinChek urine test strip
Quid
     Personnes Agées Q. (PAQUID)
quiescence
quiescent
Quiess Injection
quin-2 fluorescent Ca^{2+} chelator
quinagolide
quinidine
quinine
quotient
     respiratory q. (RQ)

R

Humulin R

R$_s$

stimulatory receptor

R$_i$

inhibitory receptor

R257X mutation

RAAS

renin-angiotensin-aldosterone system

rabeprazole

Rab protein

Rabson-Mendenhall syndrome

RAC3

receptor-associated coactivator 3

raccoon eyes

racemic mixture

racemization

rachitic

r. bone
r. change
r. child
r. deformity
r. disease
r. rosary

rachitic-like

r.-l. lesion
r.-l. skeletal defect

rachitis

Rac protein

Rad gene

radiata

corona r.
zona r.

radiation

external beam r.
r. injury
ionizing r.
optic r.
r. optic neuropathy
proton beam r.
r. therapy (XRT)
r. thyroiditis

radiation-associated papillary thyroid carcinoma

radiation-damaged thyroid gland

radiation-induced

r.-i. hyperprolactinemia
r.-i. leukemia
r.-i. thyroiditis

radical

free r.
hydroxyl r.
oxygen free r.

radicular dentin

radiculomyelopathy

radiculopathy

radioablation therapy

radioactive

r. glucose tracer
r. iodine (^{131}I, RAI)
r. iodine-induced carcinogenesis
r. iodine therapy
r. iodine uptake (RAIU)
r. ligand

radioautographic study

radiodense striation

radioembolization

radiofluoride uptake

radiofrequency (RF)

r. capacitive heating
r. signal

radiogallium

radiography

bone-age r.
nonionic contrast r.
plane r.
quantitative r.

radioimmunoassay (RIA)

solid-phase r.

radioimmunology

radioiodinated iodotyrosine

radioiodine (RAI)

r. ablation therapy
r. thyroid imaging
r. trapping
r. uptake (RAIU)
r. uptake test

radioiodine-induced exacerbation of ophthalmopathy

radioisotope

radiolabeled

r. analogue of norepinephrine
r. breath test
r. MIBG
r. monoclonal antibody
r. octreotide scintigraphy
r. somatostatin analog

radiology

interventional r.

radiolucency

radiolucent

radionecrosis

delayed brain r.

radionuclide

r. gastric emptying study
r. imaging
r. scintigraphy

radiopaque

r. dye

radiopaque *(continued)*
 r. iodinated radiographic contrast media
radiopharmaceutical
radioreceptor assay (RRA)
radiosensitivity
Radiostol
radiostrontium uptake
radiosurgery
 cobalt-knife r.
 stereotactic r.
radiotherapy
 conventional r.
 Gamma Knife beam r.
 hyperfractionated r.
 intracystic r.
 intraoperative r.
 Lineac particle beam r.
 prophylactic pituitary r.
 stereotactic r.
radiotherapy-induced hypopituitarism
radiothyroidectomy
radiotracer
radium
radius Z score
Raf protein kinase
raft
 lipid r.
RAGE
 receptor for advanced glycation end-product
RAI
 radioactive iodine
 radioiodine
RAI-induced carcinogenesis
rainbow coverage
RAIU
 radioactive iodine uptake
 radioiodine uptake
 thyroidal radioactive iodine uptake test
 elevated RAIU
rake
 r. defect
 Senn r.
ralaxifene
Raleigh
 hemoglobin R.
RALES
 Randomized Aldactone Evaluation Study
Raloxifene Use for The Heart Trial (RUTH Trial)
ramipril
ramus, pl. **rami**
 pubic r.
 white r.
Randle
 R. cycle
 R. mechanism

random
 r. cortisol
 r. cortisol level
 r. glucose test
randomized
 R. Aldactone Evaluation Study (RALES)
 r. controlled trial (RCT)
 r. control trial (RCT)
range
 physiological r.
ranitidine
 r. bismuth citrate
 r. hydrochloride
RANK
 receptor activator of NF-kappa-B
RANKL
 RANK-ligand
RANK-ligand (RANKL)
Ranson score
RANTES
 regulated on activation, normal T-cell expressed and secreted
rapamycin
 mammalian target of r. (mTOR)
 target of r. (TOR)
Raphe nucleus
Rap protein
RAR
 retinoic acid receptor
 trans-retinoic acid
RAS
 RAS oncogene
ras
 r. gene protooncogene expression
 R. pathway
rash
 mucocutaneous r.
ras-**like protein**
ras **protein**
rate
 absolute thyroidal uptake r.
 aldosterone secretory r.
 basal r.
 basal metabolic r. (BMR)
 bone formation r. (BFR)
 decreased mineral apposition r.
 erythrocyte sedimentation r. (ESR)
 glomerular filtration r. (GFR)
 glucose infusion r.
 growth r.
 insulin infusion r.
 maximal urinary flow r.
 metabolic clearance r.
 mineral apposition r. (MAR)
 plasma appearance r. (PAR)
 plasma clearance r. (PCR)
 sedimentation r.
 somatotroph cell proliferative r.

ultrafiltration r.
urinary paraaminobutyric acid
excretion r.

Rathke

R. cleft cyst
R. pouch
R. pouch cyst
R. pouch homeobox transcription
factor (Rpx)

rating

Sex Maturity R. (SMR)

ratio

A/C r.
adrenal vein aldosterone r.
albumin:creatinine r.
aldosterone/renin r. (ARR)
aldosterone-to-renin r.
baseline aldosterone/plasma renin
activity r.
brachial-to-penile Doppler blood
pressure r.
calcium/creatinine r.
calcium-to-creatinine r.
elevated waist-to-hip r.
endocrine-to-exocrine r.
epinephrine-to-norepinephrine r.
estradiol/testosterone r.
insulin/C-peptide molar r.
lecithin/sphingomyelin r.
L/S r.
MIT:DIT r.
muscle:fat r.
neck-to-thigh r. (N/T)
N/T r.
PAC lateralization r.
PAC/PRA r.
plasma aldosterone-to-plasma renin
activity r.
precursor/product r.
proinsulin insulin r.
protein efficiency r.
renin activity-to-aldosterone r.
thyroid hormone-binding r. (THBR)
triiodothyronine/thyroxine r.
TSH:T_4 r.
T_3:T_4 r.
urinary iodine/thiocyanate r.
VLDL cholesterol/total
triglyceride r.
waist-to-hip circumference r.
(WHR)
WHR r.

X:A r.
X chromosome to autosome ratio
X chromosome to autosome r.
(X:A ratio)

Raxar

Rb

retinoblastoma gene
Rb gene

RBC

red blood cell

RBG

retinol-binding globulin

RBM

ribonucleic acid-binding motif
RNA-binding motif

RCR

replication competent retrovirus

RCT

randomized controlled trial
randomized control trial

RDS

respiratory distress syndrome

Reabilan

reabsorption

phosphate r.
renal tubular r.

reactant

acute phase r.

reaction

acrosomal r.
acrosome r.
argentaffin r.
decreased flare r.
dystonic r.
glial r.
graft-versus-host r. (GVH reaction)
GVH r.
intrathyroglobulin iodotyrosine
coupling r.
leukemoid r.
Maillard r.
nitroprusside r.
peritumor glial r.
photosensitization r.
polymerase chain r. (PCR)
Porter-Silber r.
precipitin r.
pupillary r.
reverse transcription-polymerase
chain r. (RT-PCR)
zona r.

NOTES

reactive
>r. hypoglycemia
>r. oxygen species (ROS)

readily releasable pool (RRP)

reagent
>chemiluminescent r.
>r. strip

Rea-Lo

rearranged
>r. during transfection (RET)
>r. during transformation oncogene

rearrangement
>Amadori-type r.

Reaven syndrome

rebaudiana
>Stevia r.

rebound hyperglycemia

receptor
>r. activator of NF-kappa-B (RANK)
>activin r. (ActR)
>activin A r.
>activin r. I (ActRI)
>activin r. IB (ActRIB)
>activin r. II (ActRII)
>activin r. IIB (ActRIIB)
>adenine nucleotide sulfonylurea r.
>adrenergic r.
>r. for advanced glycation end-product (RAGE)
>Ah r.
>aldosterone r.
>alpha$_2$ r.
>alpha-adrenergic r.
>alpha$_1$-adrenergic r.
>alpha$_2$-adrenergic r.
>androgen r. (AR)
>arylhydrocarbon r. (AhR)
>asialoglycoprotein r.
>r. autoantibody
>r. autoradiography
>B-cell antigen r. (BCR)
>beta$_1$-adrenergic r.
>beta$_2$-adrenergic r.
>beta-adrenergic r.
>bone cell r.
>calcitonin r.
>calcium-sensing r. (CaR)
>CCK-A and CCK-B r.
>c-erbA-beta r.
>chemokine r.
>chimeric r.
>cholecystokinin A and cholecystokinin B r.
>cholinergic nicotinic r.
>compensatory ligand-induced upregulation of tissue r.
>corticosteroid r.
>CRH-R1 r.

>cytoplasmic r.
>r. degradation
>r. desensitization
>dioxin r.
>dopamine r.
>dopaminergic r.
>E$_2$ r.
>ecdysone r.
>ectopic hormone r.
>EGF r.
>endothelin r.
>epidermal growth factor r.
>estrogen r. (ER)
>r. expression
>extracellular r.
>Fas r.
>fibroblast growth factor r. (FGFR)
>folate r. (FR)
>follicle-stimulating hormone r.
>FSH r.
>G$_s$-alpha-coupled r.
>gastrin r.
>GH-releasing hormone r. (GHRH-R)
>GH-releasing peptide r.
>GHRP r.
>GlcNAc r.
>glucagon r.
>glucocorticoid r. (GR)
>glucose r.
>glycoprotein hormone r.
>GnRH r.
>gonadotropin r.
>gonadotropin-releasing hormone r. (GnRH-R)
>G protein-coupled r. (GPCR)
>G protein-linked r.
>growth factor r. (GFR)
>growth hormone secretagogue r. (GHSR)
>guanylyl cyclase-linked r.
>Hcrtr1 r.
>Hcrtr2 r.
>hepatoma cell insulin r.
>hormone r.
>human thyroid hormone r. (hTR)
>illicit hormone r.
>inappropriate hormone r.
>inhibitory r. (R$_i$)
>inositol 1,4-5-triphosphate r. (IP3R)
>insulinlike growth factor-1 r. (IGF-1R)
>insulinlike growth factor-II r. (IGF-IIR)
>insulin receptor-related r. (IRR)
>interleukin type 2 r.
>intracellular r.
>isoform-specific thyroid hormone r.
>juxtaglomerular stretch r.
>kinase-deficient activin r.

r. ligand binding
ligand-dependent action of thyroid hormone r.
ligand-independent action of thyroid hormone r.
r. loss
low-density lipoprotein r.
luteinizing hormone r.
luteinizing hormone/chorionic gonadotropin (LH/CG) r.
macula densa r.
mannose-6-phosphate/IGF-2 r. (M6P/IGF-2R)
Mel1a melatonin r.
melanocortin-2 r. (MC2-R)
melanocortin-3 r. (MC3-R)
melanocortin-4 r. (MC4-R)
Mel1b melatonin r.
membrane-associated estrogen r.
membrane-bound r.
mineralocorticoid r. (MR)
MIS II r.
r. mRNA
müllerian-inhibiting substance r.
muscarinic cholinergic r.
myometrial oxytocin r.
N-acetylglucosamine r.
natriuretic peptide r. (NPR)
neurotrophic tyrosine kinase r., type 1 (NTRK1)
nicotinic cholinergic r.
nicotinic-type r.
NK1 r.
NK2 r.
NK3 r.
noradrenergic r.
nuclear hormone r.
r. occupancy
opsonin r.
ORL-1 r.
orphan r.
parathyroid extracellular calcium-sensing r.
peripheral-type benzodiazepine r. (PBR)
peroxisome proliferator-activated r. (PPAR)
pituitary cell-surface r.
potassium$_{ATP}$ channel isoform sulfonylurea r.
potassium $_{IR}$6.2 sulfonylurea r. 1, 2

pregnancy thyrotropin r.
progesterone r. (PR)
prostaglandin F r.
retinoic acid r. (RAR)
retinoic acid-related orphan r. (ROR)
retinoid X r. (RXR)
retinoid Z r. (RZR)
ryanodine r.
scavenger r.
serotoninergic r.
serpentine r.
seven-transmembrane-domain r.
signal recognition particle r.
silencing mediator of retinoic acid and thyroid hormone r. (SMRT)
single-transmembrane-domain r.
SNAP r.
soluble complement r. (sCR1)
soluble N-ethylmaleimide-sensitive factor attachment protein r. (SNARE)
somatostatin r.
spare r.
steroid hormone r.
steroid/thyroid hormone r.
stimulatory r. (R_s)
stretch r.
sulfonylurea r. (SUR)
sulfonylurea r. 1 (SUR1)
sulfonylurea r. 2 (SUR2)
T_3 r. (TR)
taste r.
T-cell r. (TCR)
tethered ligand thrombin r.
thermolabile r.
thyroid hormone receptor-retinoid X r. (TR-RXR)
thyroid-stimulating hormone r. (TSH-R, TSHR)
thyrotropin r. (TSH-R)
thyrotropin-releasing hormone r. (TRH-R)
transferrin r.
TSH r. (TSH-R)
tumor necrosis factor r. (TNFR)
r. tyrosine kinase (RTK)
r. tyrosine kinase activity
tyrosine kinase domain of insulin r.
unliganded thyroid hormone r.
unmutated r.

NOTES

receptor *(continued)*
    V_1 r.
    V_{1a} r.
    V_{1b} r.
    V_2 r.
    vasoactive intestinal peptide r.
    vasopressin r. (V2R)
    VIP r.
    vitamin D r. (VDR)
    vitronectin r.
    volume r.
    wild-type r.

receptor-alpha
    peroxisome proliferator-activated r.-a. (PPAR-alpha)

receptor-associated coactivator 3 (RAC3)
receptor-binding abnormality
receptor-coupled membrane protein
receptor-delta
    peroxisome proliferator-activated r.-d. (PPAR-delta)

receptor-effector coupling
receptor-gamma
    liver peroxisome proliferator-activated r.-g.
    N-terminus peroxisome proliferator-activated r.-g.
    peroxisome proliferator-activated r.-g. (PPAR-gamma)

receptor-ligand complex
receptor-mediated endocytosis
receptors
recess
    infundibular r.
    optic r.
    pineal r.
    suprapineal r.

recessive
    r. abetalipoproteinemia
    r. adrenoleukodystrophy

reciprocal peptidergic fiber
Recklinghausen
    R. disease
    osteitis fibrosa cystica generalisata of von R.
    R. syndrome

recognition domain
recombinant
    r. adenovirus
    r. DNA technique
    r. enzyme replacement therapy
    r. erythropoietin
    r. follicle-stimulating hormone (rFSH)
    r. human growth hormone (RHGH, rhGH)
    r. human growth hormone treatment
    r. human insulin

    r. human insulinlike growth factor (rhIGF)
    r. human thyroid-stimulating hormone (rhTSH)
    r. human TSH (rhTSH)
    r. insulinlike growth factor I
    r. interferon-alpha (rIFN-alpha)

recombination
    homologous r.
    intra-HLA r.
    nonhomologous r.

reconstruction
    arterial r.
    beta-cell potassium$_{ATP}$ channel r.
    bone r.
    Suzuki duodenopancreatobiliary r.

recovery
    short T1 inversion r. (STIR)

recta
    pars r.
    vasa r.

rectal administration of insulin
rectilinear scanner
rectouterine recess of Douglas
rectus
    tubulus r.

recumbent
    r. aldosterone
    r. dyspnea

recurrent
    r. adenoma
    r. laryngeal nerve
    r. pituitary tumor

recycling
    urea r.

red
    r. blood cell (RBC)
    r. bone marrow
    r. cell coagulability
    r. cell coagulation
    r. cell mass
    r. clover-derived isoflavone
    r. clover extract
    r. lochia
    vital r.

red-green deficiency
Redisol
redox
    r. balance
    r. potential
    r. state

reduced
    r. exercise capacity
    r. glutathione (GSH)
    r. thyroid reserve

reductase
    adrenodoxin r.
    aldo-keto r.
    aldose r.

r. deficiency
dihydropteridine r.
flavoprotein NADPH-cytochrome
  P450 r.
flavoprotein nicotinamide adenine
  dinucleotide phosphate-cytochrome
  P450 r.
glutathione r.
17-ketosteroid r. (17-KR)
methylenetetrahydrofolate r.
NADPH-cytochrome P450 r.
renal ferredoxin r.
5-reductase deficiency
reduction
acarbose cardiovascular risk r.
acarbose type 2 diabetes mellitus
  risk r.
goiter r.
PDI-mediated disulfide bond r.
protein disulfide isomerase-mediated
  disulfide bond r.
Redutemp
REE
resting energy expenditure
reesterification
refeeding edema
Refetoff
R. patient
R. syndrome
refined carbohydrate
reflectance meter
reflector
parabolic r.
reflex
Bruchner r.
Ferguson r.
glucoregulatory neural r.
milk let-down r.
neuroendocrine r.
slow relaxation phase of deep
  tendon r.
suckling r.
r. sympathetic dystrophy
reflux esophagitis
refraction
cycloplegic r.
refractoriness
secretory r.
thyrotropin-releasing hormone-
  induced r.
TRH-induced r.
REG1 **alpha gene**

regeneration
adrenocortical r.
myogenic r.
skeletal r.
tissue r.
regimen
add-back r.
block-replace r.
glucocorticoid-free
  immunosuppressive r.
insulin-combination r.
multiple-injection r.
region
carboxyl-terminal r.
chromosome 11p15 insulin gene r.
epithalamic r.
infundibulohypophysial r.
mammillary r.
medial basal hypothalamic r.
  (MBH)
parasellar r.
perifornical r.
preoptic r.
pseudoautosomal r.
retrochiasmatic r.
sellar r.
suprachiasmatic r.
supraoptic r.
suprasellar r.
third complementarity
  determining r. (CDR3)
tuberal r.
untranslated r. (UTR)
5'-untranslated r. (UTR)
ventricular r.
registry
International Islet Transplant R.
  (IITR)
Regitine
Reglan
Regranex gel
regrowth
goiter r.
regular
R. (Concentrated) Iletin II U-500
R. Iletin I
R. Purified Pork Insulin
r. spin-echo technique
regulated
r. on activation, normal T-cell
  expressed and secreted (RANTES)
r. secretion

NOTES

regulation
    abnormal r. of calcium-dependent parathyroid hormone secretion
    adipocyte lipolysis r.
    adipose tissue r.
    cell-cycle r.
    hypothalamic neuroendocrine r.
    insulin gene r.
    isoproterenol phosphodiesterase 3B r.
    negative feedback r.
    osmotic r.
    paracrine r.

regulator
    autoimmune r. (AIRE)
    cystic fibrosis transmembrane r. (CFTR)
    hormonal r.
    intraovarian r.
    nonhormonal r.
    physiologic r.

regulatory
    r. failure
    r. gene defect
    r. homodimer
    r. lymphocyte
    r. peptide

regurgitation
    tricuspid r.

Reifenstein
    R. phenotype
    R. syndrome

reinfusion
    intraperitoneal r.

Reinke
    R. crystal
    R. crystalloid
    R. edema

Reiter syndrome
rejection
    clonal r.

rejuvenation
    B-cell r.

RelA-p50 heterodimer
relationship
    genotype-phenotype r.
    log dose-response r.
    neural r.
    patient-provider r.

relative
    r. hypoinsulinemia
    r. hypoleptinemia
    r. leptin deficiency
    r. leptin resistance
    r. osteoid volume

relaxation
    myometrial r.

relaxin polypeptide

release
    calcium r.
    calcium-induced calcium r. (CICR)
    endothelin r.
    first-phase insulin r.
    iodine r.
    long-acting r. (LAR)
    nocturnal vasopressin r.
    octreotide long-acting r.
    prostaglandin E_2 r.
    pulsatile insulin r.
    pulsatile pituitary hormone r.
    renal glucose r.
    tethered cord r.

release-inhibiting hormone
releasing hormone
Relefact TRH
relief
    Diabetic Tussin Allergy R.

ReliOn
    R. glucose meter
    R. test strip

relocatable stereotactic frame
Remeron
remethylation
remifentanil
remission
    biochemical r.
    endocrine r.

remnant
    r. hyperplastic tissue
    hypertrophied thyroglossal duct r.
    lipoprotein r.
    r. pancreas
    thyroglossal duct r.
    thyroid r.

remodeling
    adrenal r.
    bone r.
    r. cycle
    vascular r.

removal
    tumor r.

renal
    r. agenesis
    r. aplasia
    r. artery
    r. aspergilloma
    r. calcium wasting
    r. calculus
    r. carcinoma cell
    r. colic
    r. cyst
    r. diabetes
    r. disease
    r. erythropoietic factor
    r. excretion
    r. failure
    r. Fanconi syndrome

R

r. ferredoxin
r. ferredoxin reductase
r. form of diabetes insipidus
r. glomerular function
r. gluconeogenesis
r. glucose release
r. insufficiency
r. lithiasis
r. medullary interstitium
r. mucormycosis
r. nephron
r. osteodystrophy
r. papilla
r. papillary necrosis
r. pelvis
r. phosphate wasting
r. plasma flow (RPF)
r. rickets
r. sodium retention
r. sodium wasting
r. threshold
r. transplant
r. transplantation
r. tubular acidosis (RTA)
r. tubular function
r. tubular reabsorption

Renese
renin
active r.
r. activity-to-aldosterone ratio
total r.
upright plasma r.
renin-aldosterone axis
renin-angiotensin-aldosterone
r.-a.-a. axis
r.-a.-a. system (RAAS)
renin-angiotensin system
renin-independent
hypermineralocorticoidism
renocortin
Renografin-76
renotropic
renotropin
renovascular
r. disease
r. hypertension
Rentamine
reovirus
repaglinide
repair
Norwood r.
tissue r.

reparative granuloma
repeat
leucine rich r. (LRR)
short tandem r. (STR)
variable number of tandem r. (VNTR)
repertoire
B-cell r.
T-cell r.
repetitive stress of walking
replacement
beta cell r.
ex vivo gene transfer insulin r.
glucocorticoid r.
gonadal steroid r.
growth hormone r.
r. therapy
thyroid hormone r.
thyroxine r.
Replens
replication competent retrovirus (RCR)
Repliderm
reporter
r. gene
r. molecule
repression
apoT3R-mediated r.
basal r.
repressor
bacteriophage lambda r.
inducible cAMP early r. (ICER)
inducible cyclic adenosine monophosphate early r. (ICER)
reproductive
r. milieu
r. physiology
Repronex
requirement
energy r.
nutrition r.
RER, rER
rough endoplasmic reticulum
resection
abdominoperineal r.
duodenum-preserving pancreatic head r. (DPPHR)
gastric r.
microsurgical r.
partial r.
Resectisol irrigation solution
reserpine

NOTES

307

reserve

adrenal r.
r. capacity
decreased thyroid r.
diminished ovarian r.
ovary r. (OR)
reduced thyroid r.
thyroid r.

reservoir

bony r.
fuel r.
r. transdermal system

residual

r. adenoma
r. lumen
r. pituitary tumor

residue

tyrosyl r.

resin

bile acid r.
bile-binding r.
cholestyramine r.
r. hemoperfusion
ion-exchange r.
nonresorbable r.
r. uptake

resin-embedded semithin section

resistance

absolute leptin r.
acquired end-organ r.
ACTH r.
activated protein C r.
airway r.
aldosterone r.
androgen r.
congenital leptin r.
end-organ r.
extreme insulin r.
familial glucocorticoid r.
generalized thyroid hormone r.
  (GTHR)
glucocorticoid r.
growth hormone r.
hereditary end-organ r.
hereditary vitamin D r.
hormone r.
incomplete androgen r.
insulin r.
partial insulin r.
peripheral vascular r.
pituitary thyroid hormone r.
  (PThHR, PTHR)
postreceptor leptin r.
primary cortisol r.
progesterone r.
relative leptin r.
selective pituitary r.
severe insulin r.
skeletal r.

r. state
syndrome of complete androgen r.
syndrome of generalized thyroid
  hormone r.
syndrome of incomplete
  androgen r.
syndrome of insulin r.
systemic vascular r. (SVR)
target organ r.
temporary end-organ r.
r. to thyroid hormone (RTH)
thyroid hormone r.
total peripheral r.
type A, B, C syndrome of
  insulin r.
vascular r.
vitamin D end-organ r.

resistant

r. hyperhomocystinemia
r. ovary
r. ovary syndrome

resistin

resonance

nuclear magnetic r. (NMR)
spin-echo magnetic r.

resorcinol

resorcylic acid

resorption

bone r.
calcium r.
cyclosporine A-induced r.
r. lacuna
osteoblastic r.
osteoclast-activated bone r.
osteoclast-driven bone r.
osteoclastic bone r.
osteoclast-mediated bone r.
paracellular calcium r.
r. trench

respiratory

r. acidosis
r. alkalosis
r. compensation
r. distress syndrome (RDS)
r. quotient (RQ)
r. syncytial virus

response

acute insulin r. (AIR)
acute phase r. (APR)
adaptational r.
anamnestic antibody r.
antibody r.
calcemic r.
carbohydrate r.
catecholamine r.
r. curve decline
r. element
end-organ r.
exocrine r.

first-phase insulin r. (FPIR)
first-year growth velocity r.
glucose r.
glycemic r.
growth hormone r.
hormone receptor-mediated r.
humoral immune r.
hypersensitivity r.
hypothalamic-pituitary r.
inflammatory r.
insulin secretory r. (ISR)
intrinsic r.
lymphocyte adenylate cyclase r.
metabolic r.
pancreatic desmoplastic r.
peak thyroid-stimulating hormone r.
peak TSH r.
phosphaturic r.
pressor r.
secretory r.
T-cell r.
triphasic r.
wheal and flare r.
rest
accessory adrenocortical r.
adrenal r.
beta-cell r.
intraovarian r.
intratesticular adrenal r.
squamous cell r.
resting
r. cell
r. energy expenditure (REE)
r. membrane potential
restricted
HLA r.
human leukocyte antigen r.
restriction
r. enzyme
r. fragment length polymorphism
  (RFLP)
phosphate-protein r.
phosphorus dietary r.
restrictive lung disease
RET
rearranged during transfection
RET oncogene
RET oncogene test
retardation
growth r.
intrauterine growth r. (IUGR)
mental r.

retention
aluminum r.
r. cyst of the pancreas
nitrogen r.
phosphate r.
renal sodium r.
urinary r.
rete testis
ret-fused protein (RFP)
reticular erythematous mucinosis
reticularis
adrenal zona r.
fasciculata r.
livedo r.
pona r.
zona r.
zone r.
reticulin
reticulocytosis
reticuloendothelial system
reticuloendotheliosis
reticulohistiocytosis
multicentric r.
reticulum
endoplasmic r. (ER)
rough endoplasmic r. (RER, rER)
smooth endoplasmic r. (SER, sER)
retina
neovascularization elsewhere in r.
  (NVE)
retinal
r. angioid streak
r. capillary angioma
r. cerebellar hemangioblastomatosis
r. coloboma
r. hamartoma
r. hemangioblastoma
r. pigment epithelium (RPE)
r. tear
retinalis
lipemia r.
retinitis pigmentosa
retinoblastoma
r. gene (Rb)
r. tumor
retinohypothalamic
r. projection
r. tract
retinoic
r. acid
r. acid receptor (RAR)

NOTES

retinoic *(continued)*
    r. acid-related orphan receptor (ROR)
    r. acid X receptor beta
    9-*cis* r. acid (RXR)
    13-*cis* r. acid
retinoid
    r. X receptor (RXR)
    r. Z receptor (RZR)
retinol-binding
    r.-b. globulin (RBG)
    r.-b. protein
retinopathy
    background r.
    diabetic r.
    high-risk proliferative r.
    ischemia-induced r.
    nonproliferative diabetic r. (NPDR)
    PEDF diabetic r.
    proliferative diabetic r. (PDR)
    van Heuven anatomic classification of diabetic r.
    Wisconsin Epidemiologic Study of Diabetic R. (WESDR)
retinyl fatty acid ester
retrobulbar tissue expansion
retrochiasmatic
    r. area
    r. region
retroclavicular
retroendocytosis
retrograde
    r. ejaculation
    r. instrumentation
    r. menstruation
retroocular tissue
retroorbital
    r. adipose tissue
    r. connective tissue
    r. fat deposition
retroperitoneal lipomatosis
retrosternal goiter
retrotracheal
retroviral vector
retrovirus
    replication competent r. (RCR)
reuptake
    serotonin r.
revascularization procedure
reversal
    dosage-sensitive sex r.
    DSS r.
    r. phase
reverse
    r. cholesterol transport
    r. dot blot assay
    r. hemolytic plaque assay
    r. hemolytic plaque assay system
    r. Randle cycle

    r. T_3 (rT_3)
    r. transcriptase
    r. transcription-polymerase chain reaction (RT-PCR)
    r. triiodothyronine
Reye syndrome
Rezulin
RF
    radiofrequency
RFLP
    restriction fragment length polymorphism
RFP
    ret-fused protein
rFSH
    recombinant follicle-stimulating hormone
R-Gel
R-Gene
Rh
    R. blood group antigen
    R. C, D, E genotyping
rhabdomyolysis
    hypothyroid r.
rhabdomyosarcoma
    pelvic r.
rhenium-186
rhenium-188 DMSA
rheologic agent
Rhesus factor blood group antigen
rheumatic
    r. condition
    r. fever
    r. syndrome
rheumatism
rheumatoid factor
RHGH, rhGH
    recombinant human growth hormone
        RHGH treatment
rhIGF
    recombinant human insulinlike growth factor
rhinitis medicamentosa
rhinocerebral mucormycosis
rhinorrhea
    cerebrospinal fluid r.
    CSF r.
Rhinosyn-DMX
Rhizobium meliloti
rhizomelic shortening
Rhizomucor
Rhizopus
rhodamine
rhodopsin kinase
Rho protein
rhTSH
    recombinant human thyroid-stimulating hormone
    recombinant human TSH
rhythm
    activity r.

behavioral r.
circadian/diurnal hormonal r.
circadian hormonal r.
circannual r.
dehydroandrosterone sulfate r.
diurnal r.
endocrine r.
endogenous r.
fetal endocrine r.
fetal hormone r.
fetal/neonatal r.
fetal steroid r.
hormone r.
infradian r.
maternal estradiol r.
melatonin r.
night-day r.
nocturnal r.
nyctohemeral r.
seasonal r.
ultradian r.
uterine activity r.
uterine contractile r.

rhythmicity
uterine r.

RI
type I regulatory dimer
RI regulatory component

RIA
radioimmunoassay

ribavirin

Ribbing disease

riboflavin

ribonuclease A cleavage method

ribonucleic
r. acid (RNA)
r. acid-binding motif (RBM)
r. acid polymerase

ribonucleoprotein

ribose-5-phosphate

riboside
5-amino-4-imidazolecarboxamide r.
(AICAR)
aminoimidazole carboximide r.
(AICAR)

ribosome

ribosome-membrane junction

ribosylated

ribosylation
adenosine diphosphate r.

rich
Rolaids Calcium R.

Richner-Hanhart syndrome

ricinoleate

rickets
adult r.
autosomal recessive
hypophosphatemic r.
calciopenic r.
familial X-linked
hypophosphatemic r.
hepatocellular r.
hereditary pseudovitamin D
deficiency r.
hydroxylation deficiency r.
hypercalciuric hypophosphatemic r.
hypophosphatemic r.
nutritional r.
oncogenic r.
phosphopenic r.
r. of prematurity
pseudovitamin D deficiency r.
(VDDR)
renal r.
r. type II
type II vitamin D dependency r.
vitamin D-dependent r. type II
(VDDR-II)
vitamin D-resistant r.
XLH r.
X-linked recessive
hypophosphatemic r.

Ridenol

ridge
gonadal r.
mammary r.
prominent supraorbital r.
urogenital r.

Riedel
R. disease
R. disorder
R. struma
R. thyroiditis

Rieger syndrome

rifampicin

rifampin

rIFN-alpha
recombinant interferon-alpha

right
r. frontal osteoplastic flap
r. temporal projection

rigidity
decorticate r.

Rigi-Scan monitor

R

NOTES

RII
> type II regulatory dimer
> RII regulatory component

Riley-Day syndrome
Riley-Smith syndrome
rilopirox
ring
> bromophenolic r.
> chromosome r.
> iodothyronine r.
> Silastic r.
> vaginal r.

ring-substitution effect
rinse
> Hibistat germicidal hand r.

Riobin
Riopan Plus
rioprostil
risedronate sodium
risk
> r. factor clustering
> Trial to Reduce Incidence of Diabetes in Genetically at R. (TRIGR)

ristocetin
ritanserin
ritanserine
ritodrine
RNA
> ribonucleic acid
> > messenger RNA (mRNA)
> > RNA polymerase II
> > small interference RNA (siRNA)

RNA-binding motif (RBM)
Robinul
Robitet Oral
Rocaltrol
Roche, Wainer, and Thissen method of height prediction (RWT)
rocker-bottom foot
rod
> Silastic r.

roentgenography
Rogaine Topical
Rokitansky-Kuster-Hauser syndrome
Rokitansky-Küster syndrome
Rolaids Calcium Rich
role
> putative physiologic r.

roll
> absorbable gelatin film r.

roller coaster glucose control
Romozin
root
> dilatation of aortic r.

ROR
> retinoic acid-related orphan receptor

ROS
> reactive oxygen species

rosary
> acromegalic r.
> rachitic r.

rose bengal drops
rosiglitazone maleate
ros **oncogene**
rostral
> r. area
> r. hypothalamus
> r. ventrolateral medulla

rostrum
rotation
> injection site r.

Rotocaps
> Ventolin R.

rotundum
> foramen r.

rough endoplasmic reticulum (RER, rER)
round ligament
Roux-en-Y gastric bypass
Roux stasis syndrome
roving nystagmus
Roxanol SR Oral
Roxicet 5/500
Roxicodone
Roxilox
Roxiprin
RPE
> retinal pigment epithelium

RPF
> renal plasma flow

Rpx
> Rathke pouch homeobox transcription factor

RQ
> respiratory quotient

RRA
> radioreceptor assay

RRP
> readily releasable pool

rT$_3$
> reverse T$_3$

RTA
> renal tubular acidosis
> > type 4 RTA

RTH
> resistance to thyroid hormone
> pituitary RTH (PRTH)

RTK
> receptor tyrosine kinase

RT-PCR
> reverse transcription-polymerase chain reaction

rubella
> r. syndrome
> r. virus

rubeosis iridis
Rubinstein-Taybi syndrome

ruboxistaurin
rubra
    lochia r.
Rubramin-PC
ruffled border
rugger jersey appearance of vertebra
rugger-jersey spine
rule
    1500 r.
    Bayes r.
    Nägele r.
    r. of 10s
runt disease
Russ
    hemoglobin R.
Russell-Silver syndrome

RUTH
    Raloxifene Use for The Heart
      RUTH Trial
RWT
    Roche, Wainer, and Thissen method of
      height prediction
Rx
    Natabec Rx
    Natalins Rx
RXR
    9-*cis* retinoic acid
    retinoid X receptor
ryanodine receptor
Ryna-CX
RZR
    retinoid Z receptor

R

NOTES

S

Bercu patient of Kindred S
Betalin S
cathepsin S
compound S
hemoglobin S
S test

4S

Scandinavian Simvastatin Survival Study

10s

rule of 10s

S-100 protein
S-14 protein
saber shin
sac

chorionic s.

saccharin
sacral

s. agenesis
s. autonomic area

sacrococcygeal chordoma
sacrosidase
SAD

seasonal affective disorder

saddle

Turkish s.

saddlenose deformity
S-adenosyl-L-methionine (SAM)
Saethre-Chotzen syndrome
Safe-T-Lance Plus lancet
Saizen
Sakamoto

carcinoma of S.

salbutamol
Saleto-200, -400
Salflex
Salgesic
salicylate

choline s.
sodium s.

salicylic acid and propylene glycol
salicylism
saline

BES buffered s. (BBS)
hypotonic s.
isotonic s.
normal s. (NS)
s. suppression study
s. suppression test

salivary

s. cortisol
s. cortisol concentration
s. cortisol level
s. gland
s. ultrafiltrate

salivatory nucleus
Salla disease
salmeterol
salmon calcitonin
Salmonella

S. brandenberg
S. enteritidis
S. typhi

Salmonine
salpinges (*pl. of* salpinx)
salpingitis
salpingo-oophorectomy

bilateral s.-o. (BSO)
unilateral s.-o.

salpinx, pl. salpinges
salt

s. absorption
aluminum s.
s. appetite
calcium s.
s. craving
s. delivery
s. loading
magnesium s.
magnesium-lipid s.
s. and pepper appearance of skull
s. sensitivity
trifluoroacetate s.
urate s.
s. wasting

salt-losing

s.-l. crisis
s.-l. deficiency

salt-wasting

s.-w. crisis
s.-w. hydroxylase deficiency variant

saluresis
Saluron
salute

allergic s.

salvage therapy
SAM

S-adenosyl-L-methionine

sampling

adrenal vein s.
adrenal venous s. (AVS)
arterial stimulation and venous s.
  (ASVS)
blood s.
cavernous sinus s. (CSS)
chorionic villus s. (CVS)
frequent blood s.
high jugular vein s.
IJV s.
inferior petrosal sinus s. (IPSS)

S

sampling *(continued)*
>internal jugular vein s.
>petrosal sinus s.
>transhepatic portal venous s.
>venous s.

San Antonio Heart Study
Sandhoff disease
Sandimmune
Sandostatin
>S. LAR
>S. LAR Depot

sandwich
>s. enzyme immunoassay method
>s. immunoassay

Sanfilippo syndrome
SangCya
Sanger dideoxy sequencing method
Sangstat
Sanorex
Santorini
>S. duct system
>fissure of S.

Santyl
SAP
>severe acute pancreatitis

SAPK2
>stress-activated protein kinase 2

saponification
sarafotoxin
saralasin
sarcoid
sarcoidlike noncaseating granulomatous inflammation
sarcoidosis
>granulomatous s.

sarcoma
>Kaposi s.
>undifferentiated s.

sarcomatous
>s. bone
>s. degeneration

sarcomere
sarcopenia
sarcoplasma
sarcoplasmic/endoplasmic reticulum calcium ATPase (SERCA)
sarcosine dehydrogenase
sarcosinemia
SARM
>selective androgen-receptor modulator

SAT
>spontaneous autoimmune thyroiditis

Satietrol
satiety
>early s.
>easy s.

s. factor
>putative s.

saturated solution of potassium iodide (SSKI)
sauvagine
>frog skin s.

Savage syndrome
SBGM
>self-blood glucose monitoring

SBS
>short bowel syndrome

SC
>sclerosing cholangitis
>sickle cell
>SC disease

SCAD
>short chain acyl-CoA dehydrogenase deficiency

scaffold protein
scale
>Attache food s.
>Clyde mood s.
>Magnum food s.
>Positive and Negative Affect S. (PANAS)
>sliding s.

scalenus anticus
scalloping
>peripheral s.

SCAMP
>secretory carrier membrane protein

scan
>bone s.
>color Doppler s.
>DEXA s.
>forced gate analysis s.
>genome s.
>^{131}I-metaiodobenzylguanidine s.
>^{131}I-MIBG s.
>iodine-131 total body s. (^{131}I-TBS)
>iodocholesterol s.
>MIBG s.
>NP-59 iodonocholesterol s.
>octreotide s.
>pertechnetate thyroid s.
>postthyrotropin s.
>subtraction thyroid s.
>technetium bone s.
>technetium pertechnetate s.
>Thyrogen radioiodine s.
>thyroid s.
>total body s. (TBS)
>whole-body radioiodine s.

Scandinavian Simvastatin Survival Study (4S)
scanner
>rectilinear s.
>UltraSure DTU-one ultrasound s.

scanning
  isotope s.
  technetium/thallium subtraction
    nuclear s.
  whole-body s. (WBS)
19S cap complex
scaphocephalic skull
scaphocephaly
scapula, pl. **scapulae**
  winged scapulae
Scatchard plot
scatter photocoagulation
scavenger
  free-radical s.
  s. receptor
SCC
  side chain cleavage
  SCC enzyme
SCF
  stem cell factor
Scheie syndrome
scheme
  dosimetric s.
  Sillence classification s.
schenckii
  Sporothrix s.
Schilling test
Schindler disease
Schirmer test
schizophreniform
Schmidt syndrome
Schmid-type
  S.-t. metaphyseal chondrodysplasia
  S.-t. metaphyseal dysplasia
Schultze sign
Schumann body
Schwabing Insulin Prophylaxis Trial
Schwann
  S. cell
  S. cell origin
  S. cell system
  S. envelope
schwannoma
  trigeminal s.
schwannoma-derived growth factor
Schwartz-Bartter syndrome
SCID
  severe combined immunodeficiency
  disease
scintigram
scintigraphy
  adrenal s.

  11-C-hydroxyephedrine s.
  [^{131}I]-19-iodocholesterol s.
  NP-59 s.
  nuclear s.
  parathyroid s.
  pertechnetate s.
  radiolabeled octreotide s.
  radionuclide s.
  sestamibi-pertechnetate subtraction s.
  skeletal s.
  somatostatin receptor s. (SRS)
  Tc-99m sestamibi s.
  ^{99m}Tc sestamibi s.
  technetium sestamibi s.
  thallium-pertechnetate subtraction s.
  thallium-technetium dual isotope s.
  thyroid s.
  whole-body s.
scintiscan
  thyroid s.
SciTojet needle-free injector for human growth hormone
sclera, pl. **sclerae, scleras**
  blue tinge s.
scleredema diabeticorum
scleroderma
scleroderma-like syndrome (SLS)
sclerosing
  s. adenosis
  s. cholangitis (SC)
  s. mediastinitis
  s. mucoepidermoid carcinoma
sclerosis
  amyotrophic lateral s. (ALS)
  cranial s.
  diaphyseal s.
  metaphyseal s.
  Monckeberg s.
  multiple s.
  seminiferous tubule s.
  skeletal s.
  tuberous s.
  tuberous s. complex 1 (TSC1)
  tuberous s. complex 2 (TSC2)
sclerostenosis
sclerosus
  lichen s.
SCN
  suprachiasmatic nucleus
  SCN of the hypothalamus
SCO
  subcommissural organ

S

NOTES

Scop
    Transderm S.
scopolamine
score
    American Urologic Association
      symptom s.
    APACHE II s.
    AUA symptom s.
    coronary artery calcium s. (CACS)
    Ferriman-Gallwey s.
    Michigan Diabetic Neuropathy S.
    Nerve Disability S.
    Nerve Symptom S.
    radius Z s.
    Ranson s.
    Z s.
scotoma, pl. **scotomata**
    cecocentral s.
    central s.
    hemianopic s.
    junctional s.
SCP-2
    sterol carrier protein-2
sCR1
    soluble complement receptor
scrapie
scratch
    Means-Lerman s.
screen
    genome-wide s.
screening
    adrenal s.
    autoimmune nervous system s.
    diabetic s.
    gastric parietal cell antibody s.
    thyroid s.
    universal s.
scrotal matrix patch
scrotum
    bifid s.
SCT
    solid cystic tumor
SCTAT
    sex cord tumor with annular tubule
scurvy
5-S-cysteinyldopa
seam
    osteoid s.
    wide osteoid s.
seasonal
    s. affective disorder (SAD)
    s. rhythm
seasonality
    integrative model of s.
sebaceous sweat gland
seborrhea
    excessive s.
sebum

Seckel
    S. bird-headed dwarfism
    S. syndrome
second
    s. attack theory
    s. hormone syndrome
    s. messenger
    S. National Health and Nutrition
      Examination Survey
secondary
    s. adrenal hyperfunction
    s. adrenal insufficiency
    s. amenorrhea
    s. antibody
    s. arteritis
    s. diabetes
    s. empty sella
    s. empty sella syndrome
    s. endocrinopathy
    s. follicle
    s. gonadal failure
    s. hyperaldosteronism
    s. hyperparathyroidism
    s. hyperprolactinemia
    s. hyperthyroidism
    s. hypertrophic osteoarthropathy
    s. hypoadrenalism
    s. hypocitraturia
    s. hypogonadism
    s. hypoparathyroidism
    s. hypothyroidism
    s. immunodeficiency
    s. infertility
    s. interstitial cell
    s. malignancy
    s. oocyte
    s. orthostatic hypotension
    s. polydipsia
    s. spermatocyte
    s. villus
second-generation agent
secosteroid
secosterol
Secran
secretagogue
    growth hormone s. (GHS)
    insulin s.
    nonsulfonylurea insulin s. (NSIS)
secretagogue-induced hypoglycemia
secreted
    regulated on activation, normal T-
      cell expressed and s. (RANTES)
secrete lymphokine
secretin
    pancreozymin s. (PS)
    s. stimulation test
Secretin-Ferring Powder
secreting pituitary adenoma

secretion
- abnormal regulation of calcium-dependent parathyroid hormone s.
- apocrine s.
- autocrine s.
- basal catecholamine s.
- basal insulin s.
- biphasic insulin s.
- chronic hyperglycemia impaired insulin s.
- circadian rhythm of hormone s.
- constitutive s.
- cortisol s.
- ectopic ACTH s.
- ectopic adrenocorticotropic hormone s.
- ectopic growth hormone-releasing hormone s.
- fluid s.
- gastric acid s.
- glucose-induced insulin s.
- glucose-stimulated insulin s. (GSIS)
- gonadotropin s.
- growth hormone s.
- hormone s.
- insulin s.
- LH interpulse s.
- Osteocalcin s.
- oxytocin s.
- paracrine s.
- parathyroid hormone s.
- prolactin s.
- pulsatile insulin s.
- regulated s.
- semiautonomous basal insulin s.
- serotonin s.
- set point for insulin s.
- spontaneous s.
- sterol s.
- syndrome of inappropriate antidiuretic hormone s.
- syndrome of inappropriate somatotropin s.
- thyroglobulin s.
- thyroid s.
- thyroidal autoantibody s.

secretomotor fiber

secretory
- s. burst of growth hormone
- s. carrier membrane protein (SCAMP)
- s. granule
- s. refractoriness
- s. response
- s. vacuole
- s. vesicle

section
- paraffin-embedded semithin s.
- resin-embedded semithin s.
- silver-impregnated semithin s.

sectioning microtome

SED
- spondyloepiphyseal dysplasia

sedentary
- s. death syndrome (SeDS)
- s. lifestyle

sedimentation rate

Sedlackova syndrome

SeDS
- sedentary death syndrome

see-saw nystagmus

segmental
- s. graft
- s. pancreas donation
- s. pancreas and kidney transplant
- s. transplantation

Seip-Berardinelli syndrome

seipin gene

seizure
- catamenial s.
- gelastic s.

Select GT blood glucose system

selectin

selective
- s. aldosterone antagonist
- s. androgen-receptor modulator (SARM)
- s. arterial calcium stimulation study
- s. estrogen-receptor modulator (SERM)
- s. estrogen response modifier (SERM)
- s. $5HT_2$ receptor antagonist
- s. hypopituitarism
- s. peripheral resistance to thyroid hormone
- s. pituitary resistance
- s. pituitary resistance to thyroid hormone
- s. PPAR-gamma modulator (SPPARM)
- s. PRTH
- s. serotonin reuptake inhibitor (SSRI)

NOTES

Select-Lite lancing device
selegiline
selenium
selenocysteine
selenodeiodinase
selenoenzyme
    type III s.
selenoprotein metabolism
selenosulfide bond
Sele-Pak
Selepen
Selestoject
self-blood glucose monitoring (SBGM)
self-injection
    penile s.-i.
self-management
    diabetes s.-m.
self-test
    Gluco-Protein OTC s.-t.
    Gluco-Protein over-the-counter s.-t.
self-tolerance
sella
    diaphragma s.
    dorsum s.
    empty s.
    gourd-shaped s.
    J-shaped s.
    secondary empty s.
    s. turcica
sellar
    s. cyst
    s. disease
    s. metastasis
    s. region
    s. tumor
    s. volume
Selye
    stress response of S.
semen
    s. analysis
    s. culture
    s. fructose test
semenogelin I, II
semiautonomous basal insulin secretion
seminalis
    colliculus s.
seminal vesicle
seminiferous
    s. epithelium
    s. tubule
    s. tubule dysgenesis
    s. tubule sclerosis
seminoma
semisynthetic
    s. ergot alkaloid
    s. insulin
Semmes-Weinstein 5.07 monofilament

senescence
    cell s.
    tissue s.
senile
    s. purpura
    s. systemic amyloidosis
senilis
    arcus s.
Senior
    Phenadex S.
Senn rake
sensate focus exercise
sensation
    sexual s.
    vibratory s.
sense
    time s.
sensing
    glucose s.
sensitive
    s. transcription factor-1 (STF-1)
    s. transcription factor 1 antibody
sensitivity
    acarbose insulin s.
    analytical s.
    androgen s.
    beta-cell glucose s.
    clinical insulin s.
    complete androgen s.
    functional s.
    hepatic insulin s.
    insulin s.
    partial androgen s.
    peripheral insulin s.
    salt s.
    s. test
sensitizer
    insulin s.
sensor
    Animas R-1000 s.
    calcium s.
    Diasensor 1000 s.
    electrochemical glucose s.
    GlucoNIR glucose s.
    GlucoWatch Biographer
     transdermal s.
    implantable glucose s.
    MiniMed continuous glucose s.
    Therasense subcutaneous glucose s.
    TouchTrak glucose s.
sensoria (*pl. of* sensorium)
sensorimotor neuropathy
sensorineural
    s. deafness
    s. hearing loss
sensorium, pl. **sensoria, sensoriums**
    clouded s.

sensory
> s. ataxic polyneuropathy
> s. nerve conduction velocity

sentinel
> s. lymph node
> s. node imaging

Sentry
> Sleep S.

sepsis
> meningococcal s.

septa (*pl. of* septum)

septal pushover technique

septicemia
> fungal s.

septicum
> *Clostridium s.*

septooptic dysplasia

septum, pl. **septa**
> intraglandular fibrous septa
> s. pellucidum
> placental septa
> sphenoid s.
> transverse vaginal s.

sequence
> adenoma-carcinoma s.
> consensus s.
> DiGeorge s.
> DQ alpha s.
> FASE s.
> fast asymmetric spin echo s.
> gene-activating s. (GAS)
> gradient-echo s.
> insulin response s.
> Kozak consensus translation
>   initiation s.
> melanocyte-stimulating hormone s.
> pancreatic islet cell-specific
>   enhancer s. (PICSES)
> short time inversion recovery s.
> SPGR pulse s.
> spoiled gradient-recalled acquisition
>   pulse s.
> STIR s.

sequence-specific primer (SSP)

sequencing
> DNA s.

sequential
> s. deiodination
> s. hormone replacement therapy

sequestered
> s. goiter
> s. vesicle

sequestrant
> bile acid s.

sequestration

SER, sER
> smooth endoplasmic reticulum

sera (*pl. of* serum)

SERCA
> sarcoplasmic/endoplasmic reticulum
>   calcium ATPase

series
> amine precursor uptake and
>   decarboxylation s.
> anion of the Hofmeister s.
> APUD s.
> erythroid s.

serine
> phosphorylated s. 137
> s. phosphorylation pathway
> s. protease inhibitor (SERPIN)

serine/threonine (Ser/Thr)
> s. kinase

SERM
> selective estrogen-receptor modulator
> selective estrogen response modifier

sermorelin acetate

Serophene

Serostim

serotherapy
> percutaneous alcohol s.

serotogenic agonist

serotonergic
> s. agent
> s. axis
> s. projection
> s. system
> s. therapy

serotonin
> monoamine s. (5HT, 5-HT)
> s. *N*-acetyltransferase
> s. reuptake
> s. secretion
> s. syndrome
> s. thyroid hormone

serotoninergic receptor

serous
> s. cystadenoma of the pancreas
> s. tumor

Serpalan

serpentine receptor

SERPIN
> serine protease inhibitor

serpin protein

S

NOTES

Serratia marcescens
Ser/Thr
　serine/threonine
Ser/Thr-Tyr-Ser
Sertoli
　S. cell
　S. cell-only syndrome
　S. cell testicular tumor
Sertoli-Leydig
　S.-L. cell
　S.-L. cell tumor
sertraline
serum, pl. **sera, serums**
　s. acid phosphatase test
　s. alanine aminotransferase
　s. albumin
　s. albumin concentration
　s. aldosterone
　s. alkaline phosphatase
　s. antiinsulin antibody
　antilymphocytic s. (ALS)
　s. bicarbonate
　s. cholesterol concentration
　s. corticosterone
　s. C-peptide level
　s. creatine phosphokinase
　s. dehydroepiandrosterone sulfate
　　level
　s. endoprotease
　s. erythropoietin
　s. estradiol
　s. estrogen-receptor modulator
　s. estrone
　s. fibronectin
　s. fluoride
　s. free T_4
　s. free testosterone
　s. fructosamine level
　s. glutamic-oxaloacetic transaminase
　　(SGOT)
　s. glutamic-pyruvic transaminase
　　(SGPT)
　s. growth hormone level
　s. 18-hydroxycorticosterone
　　concentration
　s. IGFBP-3 concentration
　s. IGF-1 concentration
　s. inorganic phosphorus
　s. insulinlike growth factor-1
　s. insulinlike growth factor binding
　　protein-3 concentration
　s. insulinlike growth factor-1
　　concentration
　s. ionized calcium
　s. ionized calcium concentration
　s. leptin concentration
　s. microsomal antibody
　s. osmolality
　s. Osteocalcin

　s. parathyroid hormone level
　s. phosphorus goal
　s. prolactin
　s. response element
　s. response element binding protein
　　(SREBP)
　s. sodium
　s. tartrate-resistant acid phosphatase
　s. thrombomodulin
　s. thymic factor
　s. thyroglobulin
　s. thyroid hormone-binding protein
　thyrotropin s.
　s. thyroxine-binding globulin
　s. total T_4
　s. total testosterone
　triiodothyronine s.
　s. vasopressinase activity
serum-to-ascitic albumin gradient
SES
　socioeconomic status
sestamibi
　99m-technetium s.
　technetium-99m s.
sestamibi-pertechnetate subtraction
　scintigraphy
set
　s. point abnormality
　s. point for insulin secretion
SETTLE
　spindled and epithelial tumor with
　　thymus-like differentiation
sevalemer
sevenless
　son of s. (SOS)
seven-transmembrane-domain receptor
severe
　s. acute pancreatitis (SAP)
　s. combined immunodeficiency
　s. combined immunodeficiency
　　disease (SCID)
　s. insulin resistance
Sevier-Munger stain technique
sex
　s. chromatin
　s. chromosome aneuploidy
　s. cord stromal tumor
　s. cord tumor with annular tubule
　　(SCTAT)
　dosage-sensitive s. (DSS)
　s. hormone-binding globulin
　　(SHBG)
　S. Maturity Rating (SMR)
　s. steroid
　s. steroid-binding globulin (SSBG)
　s. steroid hormone
　s. steroid level
sex-binding globulin

sex-determining
  s.-d. region of the Y chromosome (SRY)
  s.-d. region Y gene (SRY)
  s.-d. region Y gene detection
sex-linked
  s.-l. adrenoleukodystrophy
  s.-l. inheritance
sexual
  s. differentiation
  s. differentiation disorders
  s. dimorphic physical change
  s. dimorphism
  s. dysfunction
  s. functioning
  s. infantilism
  s. infantility
  s. precocity
  s. sensation
sexually
  s. dimorphic
  s. dimorphic nucleus
  s. transmitted infection (STI)
SF-1
  steroidogenic factor-1
SFO
  subfornical organ
SGA
  small for gestational age
SGLT
  sodium-dependent glucose transporter family
  sodium glucose cotransporter
SGLT1
  sodium glucose cotransporter-1
SGLT2
  sodium glucose cotransporter-2
SGOT
  serum glutamic-oxaloacetic transaminase
SGP
  stress-generated potential
SGPT
  serum glutamic-pyruvic transaminase
SH
  sulfhydryl
  SH2
  SH compound
sharing
  United Network for Organ S. (UNOS)
SHBG
  sex hormone-binding globulin

Shc-dependent pathway
Sh2-containing inositol 5'-phosphatase 2
Sheehan syndrome
sheet
  arachnoidal s.
shell
  trophoblastic s.
SHH
  syndrome of hyporeninemic hypoaldosteronism
shin
  saber s.
  s. spot
shiner
  allergic s.
shivering thermogenesis
shock
  cardiogenic s.
  circulatory s.
  hypoglycemic s.
  hypovolemic s.
  insulin s.
  neuronal s.
  s. syndrome
  s. wave lithotripsy
Shohl solution
short
  s. bowel syndrome (SBS)
  s. chain acyl-CoA dehydrogenase deficiency (SCAD)
  s. luteal phase
  s. stature
  s. stature homeobox (SHOX)
  s. tandem repeat (STR)
  s. tandem repeat marker
  s. time inversion recovery sequence
  s. T1 inversion recovery (STIR)
short-acting insulin
shortened luteal phase
shortening
  acromelic s.
  fractional s.
  mesomelic s.
  rhizomelic s.
short-limbed dwarfism
short-loop
  s.-l. feedback
  s.-l. inhibition
short-stature homeobox-containing gene (SHOX)
shoulder-hand syndrome

NOTES

S

SHOX
>short stature homeobox
>short-stature homeobox-containing gene
>>SHOX gene

SHP
>small heterodimer partner

SHP-1
>Src homology containing phosphatase 1

SHP-2
>Src homology containing phosphatase 2

shunt
>Denver s.
>glandulocavernosal s.
>LeVeen s.
>peritoneovenous s.
>portacaval s.
>portasystemic s.
>transjugular intrahepatic
>>portosystemic stent s. (TIPS)
>ventriculoperitoneal s.

shuttle
>carnitine s.

Shwachman syndrome
Shy-Drager syndrome
SIADH
>syndrome of inappropriate secretion of
>antidiuretic hormone

sialadenitis
sialic
>s. acid
>s. acid content
>s. acid storage disease

sialidosis
sialoadenectomy
sialoadenitis
sialoglycolipid
sialography
>parotid s.

sialoprotein
>biglycan bone s.
>bone s. (BSP)

sialylated
>s. hCG
>s. human chorionic gonadotropin

sialylation
sialyl Lewis[a]
Sibley-Lehninger test
sibling
>haploidentical s.
>identical s.

sibship
sibutramine hydrochloride monohydrate
sick
>euthyroid s.
>s. euthyroid syndrome

sickle
>s. cell (SC)
>s. cell anemia
>s. cell disease

side
>s. chain cleavage (SCC)
>s. chain cleavage deficiency
>s. chain cleavage enzyme

side-chain composition
side-effect profile of use
sideroblastic anemia
side-to-side pancreaticojejunostomy
sign
>Chvostek s.
>Collier s.
>Cullen s.
>Dalrymple s.
>Darier s.
>double-duct s.
>Graefe s.
>Grey Turner s.
>infiltrative eye s.
>Joffroy s.
>Kussmaul s.
>mask s.
>Pemberton s.
>pyramidal tract s.
>Schultze s.
>Stellwag s.
>Thorn s.
>Trousseau s.
>Unschuld s.
>von Graefe s.

signal
>afferent s.
>autoimmune s.
>B-cell second s.
>gastrointestinal s.
>hormonal s.
>humoral s.
>long-loop feedback s.
>metabolic s.
>s. patch
>s. peptid
>s. peptidase
>s. peptide
>phosphatidylinositol s.
>s. processor
>radiofrequency s.
>s. recognition particle receptor
>stomach-derived paracrine s.
>SV40 polyadenylation s.
>s. transducer
>s. transducer and activator of
>>transcription (STAT)
>s. transducer and activator of
>>transcription-4 (Stat4)
>s. transducer and activator of
>>transcription-5 (Stat5)
>s. transducer and activator of
>>transcription-4 transcription factor
>s. transducer and activator of
>>transcription-5 transcription factor

signaling
activin s.
bone morphogenetic factor 7 s.
cell s.
intracellular s.
melanocortin s.
PDX-1 IRS-2 s.
s. pheromone
suppressor of cytokine s. (SOCS)
suppressor of cytokine s. 3
(SOCS-3)
signalosomes
signal-transduction pathway
signet-ring appearance
significance
monoclonal gammopathy of
unknown s. (MGUS)
Silain
Silapap
Silastic
S. ring
S. rod
sildenafil citrate
silencing
s. mediator of retinoic acid and
thyroid hormone receptor (SMRT)
transcriptional s.
silent
s. ACTH adenoma
s. autoimmune thyroiditis
s. corticotrope adenoma subtype I,
II, III
s. corticotroph cell adenoma
s. gonadotroph cell adenoma
s. microadenoma
s. somatotroph adenoma
silicon
Sillence
S. classification scheme
S. type I, II, III, IV
silver-impregnated semithin section
simethicone
aluminum hydroxide, magnesium
hydroxide, and s.
calcium carbonate and s.
magaldrate and s.
simian sarcoma virus genome
Simmonds disease
simple
s. carbohydrate
s. nonendemic goiter

s. tandem repeat polymorphism
(STRP)
s. virilizer
s. virilizing hydroxylase deficiency
variant
simplex
thyroiditis akuta s.
SimpleXx
Norditropin S.
Simron
Sims-Huhner test
Simulect
simultaneous
s. pancreas-kidney (SPK)
s. pancreas and kidney (SPK)
s. pancreas-kidney transplant
s. pancreas-kidney transplantation
simvastatin with fenofibrate
Sindh
dwarfism of S.
sine
s. qua non
s. qua nonsuppressed thyroid-
stimulating hormone
sinensis
Clonorchis s.
single
s. gateway hypothesis
s. hormone deficiency
s. nucleotide polymorphism (SNP)
s. thyroid nodule
single-bladed Kurze microscissors
single-chain polypeptide
single-pass transmembrane protein
single-photon
s.-p. absorptiometry (SPA)
s.-p. emission computed
tomography (SPECT)
**single-serum dehydroepiandrosterone
sulfate value**
**single-strand conformation polymorphism
(SSCP)**
**single-stranded conformation
polymorphism analysis**
singlet oxygen
single-transmembrane-domain receptor
sinonasal
s. complication
s. surgery
sinugram
sinus
basilar s.

S

NOTES

sinus *(continued)*
>   carotid s.
>   cavernous s.
>   conchal-type sphenoid s.
>   inferior petrosal s.
>   lactiferous s.
>   petrosal s.
>   sphenoid s.
>   superior petrosal s.
>   urogenital s.

sinusoid
sinusoidal pattern
Sipple syndrome
siRNA
>   small interference RNA

sirolimus
SIRS
>   systemic inflammatory response
>   syndrome

sister
>   s. chromatid
>   S. Mary Joseph node

Sistrunk
>   S. operation
>   S. procedure

site
>   extragonadal s.
>   extrahypothalamic s.
>   injection s.
>   Maillard s.
>   protease-sensitive s.
>   putative-binding s.
>   thyroid hormone-binding s.
>   tyrosine phosphorylation s.
>   zona pellucide recognition s.

site-directed mutagenesis
site-specific ovarian cancer syndrome
sitostanol
sitosterolemia
sitotherapy
situs
>   s. inversus
>   s. inversus viscerum totalis

sivelestat
size
>   age, metastases, extent and s.
>   (AMES)
>   phallic s.

Sjögren syndrome
skeletal
>   s. deformity
>   s. fluoride
>   s. homeostasis
>   s. mass
>   s. muscle
>   s. muscle glycogen storage
>   s. muscle ischemia
>   s. muscle spontaneous infarction
>   s. regeneration

>   s. resistance
>   s. scintigraphy
>   s. sclerosis

skeleton
>   appendicular s.
>   axial s.
>   computer tomographic methods of
>   axial s. (axial QCT)
>   computer tomographic methods of
>   peripheral s. (pQCT)

Skelid
Skene paraurethral gland
skin
>   Composite Cultured S.
>   diabetic thick s.
>   s. fold measurement
>   s. fold thickness
>   hyperpigmented s.
>   perforating disorder of the s.
>   s. thinning
>   waxy s.
>   yellow s.

skull
>   s. base
>   salt and pepper appearance of s.
>   scaphocephalic s.

S/L
>   A-Spas S.

SLC12A1 gene
SLC12A3 gene
SLE
>   systemic lupus erythematosus

sleep-associated penile tumescence
Sleep Sentry
sleep-wake
>   s.-w. cycle
>   s.-w. homeostasis

slice
>   coronal s.

sliding scale
Slo-bid
Slo-Niacin
Slo-Phyllin GG
sloppy pacemaker
slow
>   S. Fe
>   s. relaxation phase of deep tendon
>   reflex

slow-release
>   Bontril S.-r.
>   s.-r. lanreotide

slow-twitch oxidative fiber
slow-wave (SW)
SLS
>   scleroderma-like syndrome

sludge
>   biliary s.

Sly syndrome

SMA
  superior mesenteric artery
Sm-A
  somatomedin A
Smad
small
  s. bowel diabetes
  s. cell carcinoma
  s. cleaved lymphoma
  s. fiber polyneuropathy
  s. for gestational age (SGA)
  s. goiter
  s. heterodimer partner (SHP)
  s. interference RNA (siRNA)
  s. noncleaved lymphoma
  s. nuclear ribonucleic acid
    (snRNA)
small-fiber type of diabetic neuropathy
small-volume pituitary tumor
Sm-C
  somatomedin C
smear
  buccal s.
  Pap s.
  Papanicolaou s.
  vaginal s.
Smith-Lemli-Opitz syndrome
Smith-Magenis syndrome
**smooth endoplasmic reticulum (SER,
  sER)**
SM-PVC
  superior mesenteric-portal vein
    confluence
SMR
  Sex Maturity Rating
SMRT
  silencing mediator of retinoic acid and
    thyroid hormone receptor
SMS
  stiff man syndrome
SMV
  superior mesenteric vein
SNAP
  soluble *N*-ethylmaleimide-sensitive factor
    attachment protein
    SNAP receptor
Snaplets-FR Granule
SNARE
  soluble *N*-ethylmaleimide-sensitive factor
    attachment protein receptor
    SNARE hypothesis

SNP
  single nucleotide polymorphism
Snp5
  S. c/c
  S. t/c
  S. t/t
snRNA
  small nuclear ribonucleic acid
SNS
  sympathetic nervous system
society
    North American Menopause S.
      (NAMS)
socioeconomic status (SES)
socks
    Thorlo padded s.
SOCS
  suppressor of cytokine signaling
SOCS-3
  suppressor of cytokine signaling 3
sodium
  s. acetate
  alendronate s.
  s. antiport
  s. ascorbate
  s. azide
  s. bicarbonate
  s. bicarbonate therapy
  s. chloride tablet
  cromolyn s.
  s. excess
  s. fluoride
  s. glucose cotransporter (SGLT)
  s. glucose cotransporter-1 (SGLT1)
  s. glucose cotransporter-2 (SGLT2)
  s. glucose transporter
  s. homeostasis
  s. iopanoate
  s. ipodate
  s. lactate
  levothyroxine s.
  liothyronine s.
  s. nitrite
  phenytoin s.
  s. phosphate
  plasma s.
  PMS-Levothyroxine S.
  s. polystyrene sulfonate
  risedronate s.
  s. salicylate
  serum s.

NOTES

S

sodium *(continued)*
 thiopental s.
 s. wasting
sodium-dependent glucose transporter family (SGLT)
sodium-iodide symporter (NIS)
sodium/iodine cotransporter gene
sodium-lactate cotransporter
sodium-potassium
 s.-p.-2 chloride cotransporter (NKCC2)
 s.-p. adenosine triphosphatase
 s.-p. pump
sodium-potassium-2 chloride cotransporter (NKCC2)
SOF
 Study of Osteoporotic Fractures
SOFA
 stromal osteoclast-forming activity
soft
 s. tissue nodule
 s. tissue swelling
Sof-Tact
 S.-T. Diabetes glucose monitor
 S.-T. test strip
Softgels
 Vita-Plus E S.
soft-tissue
 s.-t. calcification
 s.-t. infection
software
 Accutility S.
 Gammaplan s.
solid
 s. cell nest
 s. cystic tumor (SCT)
 s. phase support
 s. pseudopapillary tumor
solid-phase
 s.-p. minisequencing
 s.-p. radioimmunoassay
solitarius
 nucleus of the tractus s. (NTS)
 nucleus tractus s. (NTS)
 tractus s.
solitary
 s. adenoma
 s. nontoxic nodule
 s. thyroid nodule
 s. unilateral macroadenoma
solium
 Taenia s.
soluble
 s. complement receptor (sCR1)
 s. fiber
 s. *N*-ethylmaleimide-sensitive factor attachment protein (SNAP)
 s. *N*-ethylmaleimide-sensitive factor attachment protein

 s. *N*-ethylmaleimide-sensitive factor attachment protein receptor (SNARE)
Solu-Cortef Injection
Solu-Medrol Injection
Soluspan
 Celestone S.
solute
 s. diuresis
 intracellular s.
solution
 albumin s.
 aqueous s.
 balanced electrolyte s. (BES)
 Dakin s.
 Euro-Ficoll s.
 Krebs-Ringer s.
 Los Angeles preservation s. 1 (LAP-1)
 Lugol s.
 modified University of Wisconsin s.
 mUW s.
 original University of Wisconsin s.
 oUW s.
 Resectisol irrigation s.
 Shohl s.
 University of Wisconsin s.
 UW s.
solvent drag
somatic
 s. amplification
 s. deletion
 s. phenotype
 s. PTEN mutation
 s. RET protooncogene mutation
somatocrinin
SomatoKine
somatoliberin
somatomammotropic hormone
somatomammotropin
 chorionic s. (CS)
 human chorionic s. (hCS)
somatomedin
 s. A (Sm-A)
 s. C (Sm-C)
 s. C level
 s. C protein
 hepatic s.
 s. hypothesis
somatomegaly
somatopause
somatosensory-evoked potential recovery period
somatostatin (SS, SST)
 s. analog
 s. analogue octreotide
 s. gene
 s. infusion

s. receptor
s. receptor scintigraphy (SRS)
somatostatin-14, -18, -25
somatostatinergic innervation
somatostatinoma
somatostatin-producing delta cell
somatotrope
somatotroph
s. acidophil
s. adenoma of pituitary gland
s. cell
s. cell adenoma
s. cell proliferative rate
s. hormone (STH)
s. hypoplasia
s. tumor
somatotrophinoma
somatotropic
s. axis
s. cell
s. hormone
somatotropin (hGH)
s. deficiency
s. release factor (SRF)
s. release-inhibiting factor (SRIF)
s. release-inhibiting hormone (SRIH)
somatotropinoma
isolated familial s.
pituitary s.
somatrem
somatropin of rDNA origin
Somavert
Somogyi
S. effect
S. hypothesis
S. phenomenon
Somogyi-Nelson method
somostatin
SON
supraoptic nucleus of the hypothalamus
sonographic halo
son of sevenless (SOS)
sorbent dialysis cartridge
Sorbinil Retinopathy Trial
sorbitol
SOS
son of sevenless
Soto syndrome
sound
Korotkoff s.
South American blastomycosis

southern
S. blot
S. blot analysis
SOX9 gene
soy
s. isoflavone
s. phytoestrogen extract (SPE)
s. protein
soybean protein
Soyselect
Sp1 motif
SPA
single-photon absorptiometry
space
anterior incisural s.
extradural s.
intertrabecular s.
intervillous s.
periosteocytic s.
perivitelline s.
subarachnoid s.
suprasellar s.
Virchow-Robin s.
spacing
interdental s.
Span-FF
spare receptor
sparse body fat
spasm
carpopedal s.
tonic s.
spasmodic dysphonia
Spasmolin
spasmus nutans
spastic paraplegia
SPE
soy phytoestrogen extract
specialist
insulin infusion s.
specialization
ectoplasmic s.
species
reactive oxygen s. (ROS)
specific gravity
specificity
s. test
tissue s.
SPECT
single-photon emission computed tomography
spectrometer

S

NOTES

spectrometry
  mass s.
spectrophotometry
  atomic absorption s.
spectroscopy
  affinity attenuated total
    reflectance s.
  affinity evanescent wave s.
  affinity fluorescence s.
  affinity surface plasmon s.
  fluorescence quencing s.
  magnetic resonance s. (MRS)
  potassium s.
SpectRx glucose monitor
speech dyspraxia
sperm
  artificial insemination with donor s.
  s. autoantibody
  female s.
  s. function test
  s. granuloma
  s. kinematics
  male s.
  s. transport disorder
  s. velocity
spermacrasia
spermarche
spermatic cord leiomyoma
spermatid
spermatocyte
  postmeiotic s.
  preleptotene primary s.
  primary s.
  secondary s.
spermatocytogenesis
spermatogenesis
spermatogonia
  type A s.
  type Ad s.
  type A dark s.
  type Ap s.
  type B s.
spermatogonium
  stem s.
spermatogram
spermatozoa
  capacitation of the s.
sperm-cervical mucus interaction
spermiation
spermicide
spermiogenesis
SpermMar test
SPGR pulse sequence
S-phase fraction
sphenoethmoidal encephalocele
sphenoid
  s. bone
  s. septum
  s. sinus

sphenoidale
  midline jugum s.
  planum s.
sphenoorbital encephalocele
spherocytosis
sphincter
  lower esophageal s. (LES)
  s. of Oddi dysfunction
  s. of Oddi manometry
  s. vesicae
sphincteroplasty
sphincterotomy
  endoscopic s.
sphingolipidosis
sphingomyelin
spike
  cholesterol s.
spilling point
spillover syndrome
spinal
  s. accessory nerve
  s. cord compression
  s. muscular atrophy types I, II, III
spindle
  s. cell
  s. cell carcinoma
**spindled and epithelial tumor with
  thymus-like differentiation (SETTLE)**
spindle-shaped fibroplastic morphology
spine
  ankylosing hyperostosis of s.
  flattened lumbar s.
  rugger-jersey s.
spin-echo magnetic resonance
spin-lattice relaxation time
spinnbarkeit
spinobulbar muscular atrophy
**spinocerebellar ataxia types I, II, III,
  VI, VII**
spinosum
  foramen s.
  stratum s.
spinothalamic tract
spin-spin relaxation time
spiral
  s. computed tomography
  s. CT
spirit
  aromatic ammonia s.
spirometry
  flow-volume loop s.
spironolactone
SPK
  simultaneous pancreas-kidney
  simultaneous pancreas and kidney
  SPK transplant
splanchine glucose uptake
splanchnic nerve

spleen
>   upper pole of s.
>   s. volume

Splenda

splenic
>   s. artery
>   s. involution
>   s. vein (SPV)

splenomegaly

splice motif

spliceosome

split mixed insulin program

spoiled
>   s. gradient-recalled
>   s. gradient-recalled acquisition pulse sequence

spondylitis

spondylodysplastic

spondyloepiphyseal dysplasia (SED)

spondylolisthesis

spondylometaphyseal dysplasia

sponge
>   Gelfoam s.
>   polyvinyl s.
>   Protectaid s.

spongiform encephalopathy

spongiosa
>   primary s.

spongiosum
>   corpus s.

spongy bone

spontaneous
>   s. autoimmune antiinsulin antibody syndrome
>   s. autoimmune thyroiditis (SAT)
>   s. bacterial peritonitis
>   s. diuresis
>   s. hypokalemia
>   s. pituitary necrosis
>   s. primary hypothyroidism
>   s. secretion

sporadic
>   s. carcinoid
>   s. congenital hypothyroidism
>   s. goiter
>   s. silent thyroiditis
>   s. testitoxicosis
>   s. thyroid tumor

Sporothrix schenckii

sporotrichosis
>   lymphocutaneous s.

spot
>   café au lait s.
>   cotton-wool s.
>   G s.
>   Graefenberg s.
>   hot s.
>   pituitary bright s.
>   shin s.

spotted bone

spotting
>   midcycle s.

SPPARM
>   selective PPAR-gamma modulator

sprinkle
>   Humibid S.

26S proteasome

20S proteasome

sprue
>   celiac s.
>   nontropic s.
>   nontropical s.

SP-1 transcription factor

spurious elevation

spuriously elevated hemoglobin A1$_c$

spurt
>   growth s.
>   pubertal growth s.

SPV
>   splenic vein

squamous
>   s. cell nest
>   s. cell rest
>   s. follicular epithelium

Src
>   S. homology containing phosphatase 1 (SHP-1)
>   S. homology containing phosphatase 2 (SHP-2)
>   S. homology 2 domain
>   S. protein

SRC-1 coactivator

SREBP
>   serum response element binding protein
>   sterol regulatory element binding protein

SRF
>   somatotropin release factor

SRIF
>   somatotropin release-inhibiting factor

SRIH
>   somatotropin release-inhibiting hormone

SR-NaF
>   sustained-release sodium fluoride

NOTES

SRS
somatostatin receptor scintigraphy
SRY
sex-determining region of the Y chromosome
sex-determining region Y gene
SRY chromosome
SRY detection
SRY gene
SRY transcription factor
SS
somatostatin
SSBG
sex steroid-binding globulin
SSCP
single-strand conformation polymorphism
SSKI
saturated solution of potassium iodide
supersaturated potassium iodide
SSP
sequence-specific primer
SSRI
selective serotonin reuptake inhibitor
SST
somatostatin
St.
S. Anthony fire
S. Louis encephalitis
stability
platelet s.
stack
Golgi s.
stadiometer
Harpenden s.
stage
colloid s.
follicular s.
PAHO s. 0, Ia, Ib, II, III
precolloid s.
Tanner s. (I–V)
Stagesic
staghorn stone
staging
Tanner s.
staining
immunocytochemical s.
immunogold s.
immunohistochemical s.
periumbilical s.
thyroglobulin s.
vital s.
stalk
hypophysial s.
infundibular s.
neural s.
neurohypophysial s.
pituitary s.
s. section effect
stalkitis

stalled puberty
standard
Greulich and Pyle growth measurement s.
stanolone
stanozolol
Staphylococcus
S. aureus
S. epidermidis
S. non-aureus
S. pneumoniae
S. pyogenes
staphylomata
peripapillary s.
StAR
steroid acute regulatory protein
steroid acute respiratory protein
steroidogenic acute regulatory protein
StAR deficiency
StAR protein
starburst artifact
stare
thyroid s.
Starling
S. curve of the pancreas
S. force
Starlix
starvation ketosis
stasis, pl. stases
urinary s.
STAT
signal transducer and activator of transcription
Janus kinase STAT
Stat4
signal transducer and activator of transcription-4
Stat4 transcription factor
Stat5
signal transducer and activator of transcription-5
Stat5 transcription factor
state
diabetic hyperosmolar s. (DHS)
enhanced oxidative s.
eumetabolic s.
euthyroid s.
hormone-resistant s.
hyperadrenal s.
hyperandrogen s.
hyperandrogenic s.
hypercalciuric hypophosphatemic s.
hypercontractile s.
hyperestrogenic s.
hypergonadotropic s.
hypertrophic s.
hypoadrenal s.
hypocorticotropic s.
induced hypermetabolic s.

insulin-resistant s.
lampbrush s.
nonketotic hyperosmolar s.
postabsorptive s.
postprandial s.
pseudo-Cushing s.
redox s.
resistance s.
statin catabolism
stature
excessive s.
idiopathic short s. (ISS)
nongrowth hormone-deficient
short s.
short s.
tall s.
status
s. epilepticus
socioeconomic s. (SES)
thyroid hormone s.
thyrometabolic s.
tumor receptor s.
Staub-Traugott effect
staurosporine
steady-state plasma glucose test
steal syndrome
stearic acid
stearoyl acyl-CoA desaturase
steatoma
steatorrhea
pancreatic s.
steatosis
diet-induced s.
hepatic s.
Stein-Leventhal syndrome
Stellwag sign
stem
s. cell
s. cell factor (SCF)
s. spermatogonium
Stemex
stenbolone
stenosis, pl. **stenoses**
papillary s.
stenting
step 2 diet
stercoralis
Strongyloides s.
stereochemistry
stereoisomer
stereotactic
s. hypophysectomy

s. radiosurgery
s. radiotherapy
stereotaxy
frameless s.
sterility
sterna (*pl. of* sternum)
sternocleidomastoid muscle
sternohyoid muscle
sternothyroid muscle
sternum, pl. **sterna**
tie s.
steroid
s. acne
s. acute regulatory protein (StAR)
s. acute regulatory protein
deficiency
s. acute respiratory protein (StAR)
s. acute respiratory protein
deficiency
alkylated androgenic s.
s. 5-alpha-reductase deficiency
anabolic s.
anabolic-androgenic s.
s. analog
s. biosynthesis
C-18 s.
C-19 s.
C-21 s.
circannual rhythmicity of s.
s. dose
estrogen C_{19} s.
gonadal s.
s. hormone
s. hormone receptor
s. hormone receptor activation
s. hormone receptor antihormone
s. hormone-receptor hormone-
response element
s. hormone receptor zinc finger
s. hormone resistance syndrome
hybrid s.
s. hydroxylase
intralesional fluorinated s.
ketogenic s.
17-ketogenic s.
s. prohormone
s. replacement therapy
sex s.
s. sulfatase
s. sulfatase deficiency
s. sulfotransferase

S

NOTES

steroid *(continued)*
    urine s.
    s. withdrawal syndrome
steroid-dependent tumor
steroid-induced
    s.-i. diabetes
    s.-i. osteoporosis
steroidogenesis
    adrenal s.
    gonadal s.
    ovarian s.
steroidogenic
    s. acute regulatory protein (StAR)
    s. acute regulatory protein deficiency
    s. cytoplasmic pool
    s. enzyme
    s. enzyme function
    s. factor-1 (SF-1)
    s. pathway
steroid-releasing intrauterine device
steroid/thyroid hormone receptor
sterol
    s. carrier protein-2 (SCP-2)
    s. hormone
    s. metabolism
    s. regulatory element binding protein (SREBP)
    s. response element
    s. secretion
    s. synthesis
    vitamin D s.
Stevia rebaudiana
steviol
stevioside
Stewart-Treves syndrome
STF-1
    sensitive transcription factor-1
STH
    somatotroph hormone
STI
    sexually transmitted infection
Stickler syndrome
sticky colloid
stiff
    s. hand syndrome
    s. man syndrome (SMS)
stigma, pl. **stigmata**
    stigmata of Cushing disease
    Turner s.
stilbestrol
Stilphostrol
Stimate
stimulant
    luteinization s.
stimulation
    blunt estrogenic s.
    breast s.
    bystander s.

    dexamethasone-suppressed corticotropin-releasing hormone s.
    dexamethasone-suppressed CRH s.
    gastric electrical s.
    ligand-independent s.
    osteoclastic s.
    plasminogen-activator s.
    s. test
    thyrotropin-releasing hormone s.
    vagal s.
stimulator
    adenylate cyclase s.
    allosteric s.
    long-acting thyroid s. (LATS)
    Triax metabolic s.
stimulator-protector
    long-acting thyroid s.-p. (LATS-P)
stimulatory
    s. G protein
    s. immunoglobulin
    s. receptor (R_s)
stimulus, pl. **stimuli**
    diabetogenic s.
    dipsogenic s.
    kaliuretic s.
    nonosmotic s.
    osmotic s.
    stimuli of thirst
stimulus-secretion coupling
stippled epiphysis
STIR
    short T1 inversion recovery
    STIR sequence
stochastic theory of aging
Stockholm
    S. Diabetes Intervention Study
    S. trial
stocking
    TheraPress DUO Lite s.
stocking-glove distribution
stomach
    thoracic s.
stomach-derived paracrine signal
stomatitis
stomodeal
    s. ectoderm
    s. hypophysial pouch
stomodeum
stone
    ampullary s.
    calcium oxalate renal s.
    cystine renal s.
    infection s.
    noncalcareous s.
    pancreatic s.
    staghorn s.
    uric acid renal s.
storage
    glycogen s.

intracellular insulin s.
skeletal muscle glycogen s.
store
    energy s.
    glycogen s.
    intracellular s.
storm
    thyroid s.
    thyrotoxic s.
STR
    short tandem repeat
    STR marker
strap muscle
strategy
    positional cloning s.
stratum
    s. basale
    s. functionale
    periventricular s.
    s. spinosum
strawberry lesion
streak
    fatty s.
    s. gonad
    s. ovary
    retinal angioid s.
strength
    Acutrim II, Maximum S.
    Excedrin, Extra S.
    hand grip s.
    ionic s.
Streptococcus
    group A *S.*
    S. hemolyticus
    S. mutans
    S. pneumoniae
    S. pyogenes
streptokinase
streptolysin O, S
streptozocin
streptozotocin (STZ)
stress
    catabolic s.
    end-systolic s.
    fluid shear s.
    s. fracture
    s. hormone
    oxidative s.
    s. response of Selye
stress-activated protein kinase 2 (SAPK2)
stress-generated potential (SGP)

stress-relevant amygdalar nucleus
Stresstabs 600 Advanced Formula Tablets
stretched penile length
stretch receptor
stria, pl. **striae**
    abdominal s.
    striae medullaris thalami
    purple s.
    purplish s.
    s. terminalis
    violaceous s.
striata
    osteopathia s.
striation
    radiodense s.
stridor
strip
    Accu-Chek Comfort Curve test s.
    Ascensia Autodisc test s.
    Ascensia Elite test s.
    Excel GE electrochemical glucose monitoring test s.
    fibrillar collagen s.
    Focus test s.
    FreeStyle test s.
    Hypoguard Advance test s.
    MediSense Q.I.D. test s.
    MediSense 2 test s.
    Microflo test s.
    OneTouch Ultra test s.
    Precision Xtra test s.
    Prestige Smart System test s.
    QuickTek test s.
    QuickVue UrinChek urine test s.
    reagent s.
    ReliOn test s.
    Sof-Tact test s.
    Supreme test s.
    SureStep test s.
stroke
    alcohol, epilepsy, insulin, overdose, uremia, trauma, infection, psychiatric, s. (AEIOU TIPS, AEIOU TIPS)
    coronary artery disease, hypertension, adult-onset diabetes, obesity, and s. (CHAOS)
stroma, pl. **stromata**
    bone marrow s.
    desmoplastic s.
    echogenic ovarian s.

NOTES

stroma *(continued)*
  endometrial s.
  hematopoiesis-supporting s.
  interfollicular s.
  thyroid s.
stromal
  s. cell
  s. enlargement
  s. hyperplasia
  s. hyperthecosis
  s. osteoclast-forming activity
    (SOFA)
stromelysin
stromelysin-1
strong
  S. Heart Study
  Thyroid S.
Strongyloides stercoralis
strongyloidosis
  disseminated s.
strontium
STRP
  simple tandem repeat polymorphism
structural gene defect
structure
  axonemal s.
  helix-loop-helix s.
  heterodimeric s.
  mediobasal brain s.
  müllerian duct derived s.
  pentalaminar tubular s.
  PPAR protein s.
  tennis racket-shaped pentalaminar
    tubular s.
  thyroglobulin regional s.
  widened cranial s.
Strudwick-type spondyloepimetaphyseal
  dysplasia
struma, pl. **strumae**
  s. granulomatosa
  s. lymphomatosa
  s. ovarii
  Riedel s.
  substernal s.
struvite
  s. crystal
Stuart
  S. factor
  S. Prenatal
Stuartnatal 1 + 1
study
  Canadian/European Cyclosporine S.
  CARE s.
  cell culture s.
  Cholesterol and Recurrent Events s.
  contrast dynamic s.
  coronal postgadolinium s.
  Da Qing s.

Deutsch Nicotinamide Diabetes
  Intervention S. (DENIS)
Diabetes Atherosclerosis
  Intervention S. (DAIS)
Diabetes in Early Pregnancy S.
Diabetes Epidemiology Collaborative
  Analysis of Diagnostic Criteria in
  Europe s. (DECODE)
Diabetes Mellitus Insulin-Glucose
  Infusion in Acute Myocardial
  Infection s.
Diabetes Prevention Trial
  research s.
Diabetic Retinopathy S. (DRS)
Diabetic Retinopathy Vitrectomy S.
  (DRVS)
DIAD s.
DIGAMI s.
DIPP S.
Dipyridamole Aspirin
  Microangiopathy of Diabetes S.
DPT-1 research s.
Early Treatment Diabetic
  Retinopathy S. (ETDRS)
EUCLID s.
euglycemic clamp s.
EURODIAB Controlled Trial of
  Lisinopril in Insulin Dependent
  Diabetes s.
EURODIAB Insulin-Dependent
  Diabetes Mellitus
  Complications S.
FDG-PET s.
^{18}F-fluorodeoxyglucose positron
  emission tomography s.
Finnish Diabetes Prevention S.
Finnish DIPP s.
Framingham Nutrition S.
German Multicenter BABY-
  DIAB s.
glucose clamp s.
Heart and Estrogen/Progestin
  Replacement S. (HERS)
histomorphometric s.
Honolulu Asia Aging S.
hormonal s.
Islet Cell Antibody Registry of
  Users S. (ICARUS)
Kabi International Growth S.
  (KIGS)
National Cooperative Growth S.
  (NCGS)
neurodiagnostic s.
neuroimaging s.
North American Pediatric Renal
  Transplant Cooperative S.
  (NAPRTCS)
Nurses' Health S.
S. of Osteoporotic Fractures (SOF)

O'Sullivan-Mahan s.
PAQUID s.
Personnes Agées Quid s.
Pima Indian s.
postgadolinium s.
pregadolinium s.
pressure-flow s.
psychophysiological s.
radioautographic s.
radionuclide gastric emptying s.
Randomized Aldactone
  Evaluation S. (RALES)
saline suppression s.
San Antonio Heart S.
Scandinavian Simvastatin
  Survival S. (4S)
selective arterial calcium
  stimulation s.
Stockholm Diabetes Intervention S.
Strong Heart S.
swallow s.
Third National Health and
  Nutrition Examination S.
thyrotropin-releasing hormone s.
Ticlopidine Microangiopathy of
  Diabetes S.
Toronto Renal Osteodystrophy S.
TRH s.
TRIPOD s.
twin s.
type 1 diabetes mellitus twin s.
Type 1 Diabetes Prediction and
  Prevention S. (DIPP)
United Kingdom Prospective
  Diabetes S. (UKPDS)
Whitehall S.
whole-body ^{131}I-MIBG s.
whole-genome association s.
xenon-133 washout s.

stunning
  thyroid s.
stuttering impotence
stylohyoid muscle
styrene
STZ
  streptozotocin
subacute
  s. granulomatous thyroiditis
  s. hyperthyroidism
  s. painful thyroiditis
subarachnoid
  s. fluid

s. space
s. space of Virchow-Robin
subcapsular follicular microcyst
subchondral cyst
subclavian pocket
subclinical
  s. hyperthyroidism
  s. hypothyroidism
  s. pheochromocytoma
  s. thyrotoxicosis
subcommissural organ (SCO)
subcutaneous
  s. fat necrosis
  s. insulin
subendothelium
subependymal plexus
subfornical organ (SFO)
subfrontal surgery
sublabial
  s. transseptal approach
  s. transseptal technique
Sublimaze Injection
subluxation
  globe s.
submicromolar
subsalicylate
  bismuth s.
subset
  T-cell s.
substance
  goitrogenic s.
  ground s.
  s. K
  müllerian-inhibiting s. (MIS)
  Nissl s.
  noncholecystokinin s.
  s. P
substantia nigra
substernal
  s. goiter
  s. struma
  s. thyroid
substitute
  DiabetiSweet sugar s.
  sugar s.
substitution
  amino acid s.
  ether bridge s.
substrate
  s. cycle
  insulin receptor s. (IRS)
  protein kinase B s.

S

NOTES

substrate-1
    insulin receptor s.-1 (IRS-1)
substrate-2
    insulin receptor s.-2 (IRS-2)
substrate-limited hypoglycemia
subthalamus
subtilisin
subtilisin-related endoprotease
subtotal
    s. parathyroidectomy
    s. thyroidectomy
subtraction thyroid scan
subtunical venous plexus
subunit
    acid-labile s. (ALS)
    alpha-thyroid stimulating
      hormone s.
    alpha-TSH s.
    glucose-6-phosphatase catalytic s.
    P85 s.
succinate
    hydrocortisone sodium s.
succinylacetone
succinyl-CoA
sucked-candy appearance
suckling reflex
Sucraid
sucralfate suspension
sucralose
sucrase
sucrose
sudanophilic leukodystrophy
Sudeck atrophy
sudomotor
    s. sympathetic function
    s. system
sugar
    s. alcohol
    blood s.
    capillary blood s. (CBS)
    s. diabetes
    s. diary
    fingerstick blood s.
    s. log
    s. substitute
    s. watch
sulcus, pl. **sulci**
    chiasmatic s.
    hypothalamic s.
    s. limitans
    pontomesencephalic s.
sulfadiazine
sulfaguanidine
sulfamethoxazole
    trimethoprim s. (TMP-SMX)
sulfasalazine
sulfatase
    steroid s.

sulfate
    cellulose s.
    chondroitin s.
    s. conjugate
    dehydroepiandrosterone s. (DHEAS, DHEA-S)
    dermatan s.
    DHEA s.
    estrone s.
    ferrous s.
    glucosamine s.
    heparan s.
    indoxyl s.
    keratan s.
    magnesium s.
    morphine s.
    piperazine estrone s.
    terbutaline s.
    zinc s.
sulfatide
sulfatidosis
    juvenile Austin-type s.
sulfation factor
sulfhydryl (SH)
    s. amino acid
    s. compound
sulfisoxazole
sulfoconjugation
sulfocysteine
sulfocysteinuria
sulfonamide
sulfonate
    sodium polystyrene s.
sulfonylurea
    s. agent
    bedtime insulin, daytime s. (BIDS)
    s. hypoglycemic drug
    plasma s.
    s. receptor (SUR)
    s. receptor 1 (SUR1)
    s. receptor 2 (SUR2)
    s. receptor gene
sulfotransferase
    s. enzyme
    phenol s.
    steroid s.
sulfur
sulindac
sulphate
    dihydroepiandrosterone s. (DHEA)
sum
    vectorial s.
Sumacal
sump syndrome
Sumycin Oral
supercoiled chromatin
superfamily
    adenosine triphosphate binding cassette s.

protein-tyrosine phosphatase
enzyme s.

superfecundation

superficial

s. dermal perivasculitis

s. fascia

s. perineal muscle

supergene

superior

s. colliculus

s. hypophyseal artery

s. laryngeal nerve

s. limbic keratoconjunctivitis

s. mesenteric artery (SMA)

s. mesenteric-portal vein confluence (SM-PVC)

s. mesenteric vein (SMV)

s. oblique palsy

s. ophthalmic vein obstruction

s. orbital fissure syndrome

s. orbital fossa

s. pancreaticoduodenal artery

s. parathyroid artery

s. parathyroid gland

s. petrosal sinus

s. vascular pedicle

superotemporal hemianoptic defect

superovulation

superoxide dismutase

supersaturated potassium iodide (SSKI)

supersaturation

superselective microcoil embolization

supersensitive

supplement

Alphabetic multivitamin s.

botanical dietary s. (BDS)

dehydroepiandrosterone s.

supplementation

cyclical s.

supply

anastomotic blood s.

support

solid phase s.

ventilatory s.

suppository

Dilaudid s.

progesterone s.

Supprelin

suppressant

appetite s.

Suppressant/Expectorant

Diabetic Tussin DM Maximum Strength Cough S.

suppressed plasma renin activity

suppression

gonadal s.

high-dose dexamethasone s. (HDDS)

HPA axis s.

hypothalamic-pituitary-adrenal axis s.

suppressive therapy

suppressor

autocrine s.

s. of cytokine signaling (SOCS)

s. of cytokine signaling 3 (SOCS-3)

growth s.

s. T cell

tumor s.

suppressor/cytotoxic T-lymphocyte

Supprettes

B&O S.

suppurative

s. hydradenitis

s. thyroiditis

suprachiasmatic

s. nucleus (SCN)

s. nucleus of the hypothalamus

s. region

suprachiasmic nucleus

supraclavicular

s. fat pad

s. fullness

supraclinoid

supradiaphragmatic extrusion

suprahyoid

Supranol

supranormal gonadal steroid level

supranumerous mammary glands and nipples

supraoptic

s. nucleus

s. nucleus of the hypothalamus (SON)

s. region

supraopticohypophysial

s. cell

s. tract

supraphysiologic dose

suprapineal recess

S

NOTES

suprasellar
- s. cistern
- s. compartment
- s. cystic lesion
- s. disease
- s. epidermoid cyst
- s. extension
- s. germ cell tumor
- s. germinoma
- s. region
- s. space
- s. vein

Supreme
- S. II blood glucose meter
- S. test strip

suprofen

Suprol

SUR
- sulfonylurea receptor

SUR1
- sulfonylurea receptor 1

SUR2
- sulfonylurea receptor 2

sural nerve

suramin

Surbex-T Filmtabs

Surbex With C Filmtabs

SureStep
- S. glucose monitor
- S. test strip

surface
- basal s.
- erosion surface per bone s. (ES/BS)
- hypocellular bone s.
- luminal s.
- osteoid s.

surfactant-associated protein

surfactant protein gene expression

surge
- blunting of nocturnal thyroid-stimulating hormone s.
- blunting of nocturnal TSH s.
- catecholamine s.
- nocturnal thyroid-stimulating hormone s.
- nocturnal TSH s.

surgery
- cytoreduction s.
- cytoreductive s.
- endonasal endoscopic pituitary s.
- palliative s.
- pituitary s.
- sinonasal s.
- subfrontal s.
- transsphenoidal s.
- tumor-reduction s.

surgical
- s. adenomectomy

- s. andropause
- s. extirpation
- s. menopause
- s. thyroidectomy

surrogate
- s. beta cell
- insulin s.

survey
- National Health Interview S. (NHIS)
- National Health and Nutrition Examination S. (NHANES)
- pharmacoepidemiologic s.
- Second National Health and Nutrition Examination S.
- Whickham s.

survival
- living segmental donor s.

suspension
- Nephrox S.
- sucralfate s.

suspensory ligaments of Cooper

sustained-release sodium fluoride (SR-NaF)

Sustanon 100, 250

suture
- lambdoidal s.

Suzuki duodenopancreatobiliary reconstruction

SV40
- S. large T antigen
- S. large T-antigen gene
- S. polyadenylation signal
- S. virus

SV40-transformed human fibroblast

SVR
- systemic vascular resistance

SW
- slow-wave

swallow
- barium s.
- s. study

sweating
- excessive s.
- gustatory s.

sweetener
- alternative s.

swelling
- periorbital s.
- soft tissue s.

Swiss cheese disease

Swyer syndrome

Sylvius
- aqueduct of S.

Symlin

symmastia

symmetrical
- s. distal polyneuropathy
- s. peripheral polyneuropathy

symmetric distal polyneuropathy
sympathectomy
sympathetic
    s. cell
    s. chain
    s. denervation
    s. ganglia
    s. nerve
    s. nervous system (SNS)
    s. plexus
    s. postganglionic
    s. preganglionic axon
sympathoadrenal neuroendocrine system
sympathogonia
sympatholytic drug
sympathomimetic
    s. amine
    s. drug
sympathoneural
symphony
    hormonal s.
symporter
    iodide s.
    sodium-iodide s. (NIS)
symptom
    acromegalic s.
    humoral s.
    local s.
    neuroglycopenic s.
    postprandial s.
    preprandial recurrent s.
    Prospective Record of the Impact and Severity of Menstrual S.'s
    systemic s.
symptomatic
    s. hyperglycemia
    s. hypocalcemia
    s. hyponatremia
    s. therapy
symptothermal rhythm method
Synacthen test
Synalgos-DC
synapse
    ganglionic s.
synaptic
    s. cleft
    s. transmission
    s. vesicle
synaptobrevin
synaptophysin
synaptosome
Synarel

syncytial trophoblast
syncytiotrophoblast
    s. cell
    s. mass
syndactyly
syndrome
    achalasia-addisonianism-alacrima s.
    ACL s.
    acquired immune deficiency s. (AIDS)
    acquired immunodeficiency s. (AIDS)
    acromegaly, cutis verticis, leukoma s.
    ACTH-dependent Cushing s.
    ACTH-independent Cushing s.
    acute phase response s.
    adiposogenital s.
    adrenocorticotropic hormone-dependent Cushing s.
    adrenogenital s.
    adult respiratory distress s.
    Alagille s.
    Albright hereditary osteodystrophy s.
    Allgrove s.
    Alstrom s.
    amenorrhea-galactorrhea s.
    androgen insensitivity s. (AIS)
    androgen resistance s.
    Angelman s.
    antenatal Bartter s.
    antiphospholipid s.
    Apert s.
    s. of apparent mineralocorticoid excess
    Arnold-Healy-Gordon s.
    Asherman s.
    autoimmune polyendocrine s. (APS)
    autoimmune polyendocrine s. 1 (APS-1)
    autoimmune polyendocrine s. 2 (APS-2)
    autoimmune polyendocrine s. 3 (APS-3)
    Bamforth-Lazarus s.
    Bannayan-Ruvalcaba-Riley s.
    Bannayan-Zonana s.
    Bardet-Biedl s.
    bare lymphocyte s.
    Bartter s.
    basal cell nevus s.

S

NOTES

syndrome *(continued)*

Bassen-Kornzweig s.
Beckwith-Wiedemann s.
Berardinelli-Seip s.
beta cell dysmaturation s.
s. of bioinactive growth hormone
Blackfan-Diamond s.
blepharophimosis, ptosis, epicanthus inversus s.
blind-loop s.
Bloom s.
blue-diaper s.
blue-toe s.
Borjeson-Forssman-Lehman s.
bowel-associated dermatosis-arthritis s.
breast/ovarian cancer s.
bronchial carcinoid variant s.
BRR s.
Buschke-Ollendorff s.
Caffey s.
candidiasis endocrinopathy s.
capillary leak s.
carbohydrate-deficient glycoprotein s.
carcinoid s.
cardiofaciocutaneous s.
cardiometabolic s.
cardiovascular dysmetabolic s.
Carney s.
Carpenter s.
CATCH 22 s.
caudal regression s.
cavernous sinus s.
Cayler cardiofacial s.
Chediak-Higashi s.
Chiari-Frommel s.
chiasmal s.
chiasmatic s.
childhood Cushing s.
chronic fatigue s.
chylomicronemia s.
Cockayne s.
Coffin-Lowry s.
Cohen s.
compensatory hyperinsulinemia insulin-resistance s.
complete androgen insensitivity s. (CAIS)
s. of complete androgen resistance
congenital GH resistance s.
congenital growth hormone resistance s.
congenital rubella s. (CRS)
Conn s.
contiguous gene s.
Cope s.
Cornelia de Lange s.
corticotropin-dependent Cushing s.

cortisol resistance s.
Cowden s.
cri du chat s.
Crouzon s.
Cushing s.
Dandy-Walker s.
de Lange s.
de Morsier s.
Denys-Drash s.
diabetes associated with certain s.
diabetes-deafness s.
diabetic foot s.
diabetic hand s.
diencephalic s.
diet-induced metabolic s.
DiGeorge s.
DIMOAD s.
Donohue leprechaun s.
Down s.
Drash s.
Dubovitz s.
dumping s.
Dunnigan s.
ectopic ACTH s.
ectopic adrenocorticotropic hormone s.
ectopic corticotropin-releasing hormone s.
ectopic CRH s.
ectopic Cushing s.
ectopic hormone s.
Ehlers-Danlos s. types I, II, III, IV, VII
elfin facies s.
Ellis-van Creveld s.
embryonic testicular regression s.
empty sella s.
endocrine tumor s.
entrapment s.
eosinophilia myalgia s.
euthyroid sick s. (ESS)
familial atypical multiple mole-melanoma s.
familial Down s.
FAMMM s.
Fanconi s.
feminizing adrenal s.
fertile eunuch s.
fetal alcohol s. (FAS)
fetal hydantoin s.
food-dependent Cushing s.
fragile X s.
fragile X-E s.
Fraser s.
FRAXE s.
Freeman-Sheldon s.
Fröhlich s.
galactorrhea-amenorrhea s.
Gardner s.

gastric carcinoid variant s.
s. of generalized thyroid hormone resistance
genetic hormone resistance s.
GH insensitivity s.
Gitelman s.
s. of globus hystericus
glucagonoma s.
goiter-deafness s.
Goltz s.
Goodpasture s.
Gordon s.
Gorlin s.
growth hormone resistance s.
Guillain-Barré s.
HAIRAN s.
hairless woman s.
Hartnup s.
HDL-C insulin resistance s.
HELLP s.
hemolysis, elevated liver enzymes, and low platelets s.
Hercules s.
s. of hereditary hypophosphatemic rickets with hypercalciuria (HHRH)
hereditary nonpolyposis colon cancer/ovarian cancer s.
Hermansky-Pudlak s.
Herrmann s.
Hirata s.
hirsutism-anovulation s.
HLA-DRB1 autoimmune polyendocrine s.
Hoffmann s.
Holmes-Adie s.
Horner s.
hungry bone s.
Hunter s.
Hurler s.
Hurler-Scheie s.
Hutchinson-Gilford s.
hyperchylomicronemic s.
hyperglycemic hyperosmolar s. (HHS)
hyperinsulinemic polycystic ovary s.
hyperprostaglandin E s.
hypertonic s.
hypoglycemia s.
hypoglycemia unawareness s.
hypoplastic left heart s.

s. of hyporeninemic hypoaldosteronism (SHH)
hypotonic s.
iatrogenic Cushing s.
idiopathic postprandial s.
immunodysregulation, polyendocrinopathy, enteropathy, X-linked s.
s. of inappropriate antidiuretic hormone secretion
s. of inappropriate secretion of antidiuretic hormone (SIADH)
s. of inappropriate somatotropin secretion
s. of inappropriate thyroid-stimulating hormone
s. of incomplete androgen resistance
infertile male s.
inherited hormone resistance s.
insulin-autoimmune s.
s. of insulin resistance
insulin-resistance s.
insulin-resistant s. X
IPEX s.
Jackson-Weiss s.
Jerusalem s.
Johanson-Blizzard s.
Kahn s.
Kallmann s.
Kartagener s.
Kearns-Sayre s.
Kennedy s.
Kenny Caffey s.
Kleine-Levin s.
Klinefelter s.
Klippel-Trenaunay-Weber s.
Klüver-Bucy s.
Kobberling-Dunnigan s.
Kocher-Debré-Sémélaigne s.
kwashiorkor s.
Laron s.
late dumping s. (LDS)
Laurence-Moon s.
Laurence-Moon-Biedl s.
Lawrence s.
Lemmel s.
lentiginosis s.
Lenz-Majewski s.
leprechaunism s.
Lesch-Nyhan s.
Liddle s.

S

NOTES

syndrome *(continued)*

Li-Fraumeni s.
linear nevus sebaceous s.
lipodystrophic s.
lipodystrophy s.
lipotoxicity metabolic s.
Louis-Bar and Nijmegen
 breakage s.
low bone turnover s.
low-density lipoprotein cholesterol
 and insulin-resistance s.
Lowe s.
low-T_3 s.
low-triiodothyronine s.
luteinized unruptured follicle s.
 (LUFS)
Lynch s.
malabsorption s.
male Turner s.
marasmus s.
Marfan s.
Marine-Lenhart s.
maternal deprivation s.
Mauriac s.
Mayer-Rokitansky-Küster-Hauser s.
McCardle s.
McCune-Albright s. (MAS)
s. of melancholia
MELAS s.
MEN s.
mendelian obesity s.
Mendenhall s.
metabolic s.
milk-alkali s.
Milkman s.
Miller s.
Miller-Dicker s.
Möbius s.
Modigliani s.
Morgagni s.
Morquio s.
Morris s.
müllerian duct s.
multiple hamartoma s.
Münchausen s.
musculoskeletal s.
Nager s.
nail-patella s.
Najjar s.
Nelson s.
nephrotic s.
neuroleptic malignant s.
nonthyroidal illness s.
Noonan s.
obesity/type 2 diabetes s.
orbital apex s.
osteomalacia s.
ovarian hyperstimulation s. (OHSS)
overlap s.

Pallister-Hall s.
paraneoplastic s.
parasellar s.
parathyroid hormone resistance s.
Parinaud s.
PCO s. (PCOS)
Pearson s.
Pendred s. (PDS)
penis at twelve s.
Perheentupa s.
perimenopausal s.
Perrault s.
persistent müllerian duct s.
Peutz-Jeghers s.
Pfeiffer s.
pickwickian s.
pituitary isolation s.
pituitary resistance to thyroid
 hormone s.
pituitary stalk interruption s.
plantar fascia s.
plasma cell dyscrasia with
 polyneuropathy, organomegaly,
 endocrinopathy, M protein in
 plasma, and skin changes s.
POEMS s.
polar T_3 s.
polar triiodothyronine s.
polycystic ovarian s. (PCOS)
polycystic ovary s. (PCOS)
s. of polycystic ovary
polyendocrine deficiency s.
polyendocrine failure type I s.
polyglandular autoimmune s.
polyglandular autoimmune s. type
 II (PGA-II)
polyuric s.
postprandial s.
postprandial lipemia insulin-
 resistance s.
PPAR-gamma resistance s.
Prader-Labhart-Willi s.
Prader-Willi s. (PWS)
premenstrual s. (PMS)
primary antiphospholipid s.
primary empty sella s.
s. of primary hyperaldosteronism
PRTH s.
pseudo-Cushing s.
pseudo-Turner s.
Rabson-Mendenhall s.
Reaven s.
Recklinghausen s.
Refetoff s.
Reifenstein s.
Reiter s.
renal Fanconi s.
resistant ovary s.
respiratory distress s. (RDS)

Reye s.
rheumatic s.
Richner-Hanhart s.
Rieger s.
Riley-Day s.
Riley-Smith s.
Rokitansky-Küster s.
Rokitansky-Kuster-Hauser s.
Roux stasis s.
rubella s.
Rubinstein-Taybi s.
Russell-Silver s.
Saethre-Chotzen s.
Sanfilippo s.
Savage s.
Scheie s.
Schmidt s.
Schwartz-Bartter s.
scleroderma-like s. (SLS)
Seckel s.
secondary empty sella s.
second hormone s.
sedentary death s. (SeDS)
Sedlackova s.
Seip-Berardinelli s.
serotonin s.
Sertoli cell-only s.
Sheehan s.
shock s.
short bowel s. (SBS)
shoulder-hand s.
Shwachman s.
Shy-Drager s.
sick euthyroid s.
Sipple s.
site-specific ovarian cancer s.
Sjögren s.
Sly s.
Smith-Lemli-Opitz s.
Smith-Magenis s.
Soto s.
spillover s.
spontaneous autoimmune antiinsulin
   antibody s.
steal s.
Stein-Leventhal s.
steroid hormone resistance s.
steroid withdrawal s.
Stewart-Treves s.
Stickler s.
stiff hand s.
stiff man s. (SMS)

sump s.
superior orbital fissure s.
Swyer s.
systemic inflammatory response s.
   (SIRS)
Takatsuki s.
testicular regression s.
thyroid hormone adaptation s.
thyroid hormone resistance s.
thyroid storm s.
Tolosa-Hunt s.
toxic shock s.
tumor-induced osteomalacia s.
tumor lysis s.
Turner s.
type A s.
type B extreme insulin
   resistance s.
type II autoimmune
   polyglandular s.
type 1 polyglandular s.
Ullrich s.
ulnar-mammary s.
undervirilized fertile male s.
vanishing testis s.
vascular steal s.
vasopressin resistance s.
velocardiofacial s.
Verner-Morrison s.
virilizing adrenal s.
von Hippel-Lindau s.
wasting s.
Waterhouse-Friderichsen s.
s. of water intoxication
watery diarrhea s.
s. of watery diarrhea, hypokalemia,
   and achlorhydria
WDHA s.
Werdnig-Hoffman s.
Werner s.
Wernicke-Korsakoff s.
Williams s.
Williams-Beuren s.
Wilms tumor-aniridia-genital
   anomalies-mental retardation s.
   (WAGR)
Wilson s.
Wilson-Turner s.
Wiskott-Aldrich s.
Wolcott-Rallison s.
Wolf-Hirschhorn s.
Wolfram s.

S

NOTES

syndrome *(continued)*
    s. X
    xeroderma pigmentosa/Cockayne s.
    X-linked immunodeficiency s.
    Young s.
    Young-Simpson s.
    Zellweger s.
    Zieve s.
    Zollinger-Ellison s.
synechia, pl. **synechiae**
    asymptomatic s.
synergism
synergistic necrotizing cellulitis
synexin
Synflex
SYNIP
    syntaxin 4-interacting protein
synkinesis
    bimanual s.
synostosis
syntaxin 4-interacting protein (SYNIP)
synteny
synthase
    carbamoyl phosphate s.
    citrate s.
    cystathionine s.
    endothelial nitric oxide s. (eNOS)
    estrogen s.
    fatty acid s.
    glycogen s.
    lactose s.
    nitric oxide s. (NOS)
    NO s. (NOS)
    phosphoribosylpyrophosphate s.
    porphobilinogen s.
    prostaglandin H s. (PGHS)
    PRPP s.
synthesis, pl. **syntheses**
    aldosterone s.
    calcium-binding protein s.
    collagen s.
    de novo s.
    eicosanoid s.
    endothelin-induced protein s.
    estrogen s.
    glycogen s.
    glycosaminoglycan s.
    growth hormone s.
    hepatic glycogen s.
    immunoglobulin s.
    pituitary s.
    prolactin s.
    protein s.
    sterol s.
    testosterone s.
    thrombospondin s.
    thyroglobulin s.
    thyroid hormone s.
    thyroid peroxidase s.
    thyroid-stimulating hormone s.
synthesis-secretion coupling
synthetase
    dihydrobiopterin s.
    fatty acid s. (FAS)
synthetic
    s. bCgA
    s. conjugated estrogen
    s. corticotropin-releasing hormone
    s. glucocorticoid
    s. human insulin
Synthroid
syntrophoblast
syphilitic gumma
Syp protein
Syprine
system
    Accu-Chek Advantage non-wipe blood glucose monitoring s.
    Accu-Chek Complete blood glucose monitoring s.
    Accu-Chek Complete glucose meter s.
    Accu-Chek Simplicity blood glucose monitoring s.
    actin scavenger s.
    Acusyst-Xcell monoclonal antibody culturing s.
    adenohypophysial s.
    adenylate cyclase s.
    ADICOL s.
    adrenergic nervous s.
    adrenomedullary hormonal s.
    AERx diabetes management s.
    afferent s.
    American Diabetes Association classification s.
    amphetamine-related transcript s.
    amplification refractory mutation s. (ARMS)
    Androderm Transdermal S.
    Appraise diabetes monitoring s.
    Ascensia Breeze blood glucose monitoring s.
    Ascensia DEX2 diabetes care s.
    Ascensia Elite XL diabetes care s.
    Assure blood glucose monitoring s.
    AtLast blood glucose monitoring s.
    autocrine s.
    autonomic nervous s.
    Behavioral Risk Factor Surveillance S. (BRFSS)
    blood glucose buffer s.
    cardiac endocrine aldosterone s.
    cardiac steroidogenic s.
    catecholaminergic s.
    central nervous s. (CNS)
    CFC BioScanner S.

closed-loop insulin delivery s.
COBE 2991 computerized
  centrifuge s.
continuous glucose monitoring s.
  (CGMS)
countertransport s.
CozMore insulin technology s.
diffuse endocrine s.
diffuse neuroendocrine s. (DNES)
dopaminergic s.
dynorphin s.
efferent s.
enkephalin s.
enteric nervous s. (ENS)
excurrent duct s.
extrahypothalamic nervous s.
extraneuronal amine transport s.
FastTake blood glucose
  monitoring s.
Focus glucose monitoring s.
GABA/BZD s.
gamma-aminobutyric
  acid/benzodiazepine s.
Genotropin s.
Glucometer DEX diabetes care s.
Glucometer II home glucose
  monitoring s.
GlucoWatch G2 Biographer
  diabetes monitoring s.
Greenberg retractor mounting s.
haversian s.
hematopoietic s.
HemoCue blood glucose s.
hormone-sensitive adenylate
  cyclase s.
hypophysial-hypothalamic portal s.
hypophysial portal s.
hypophysiotropic s.
hypothalamohypophysial portal s.
  (HHPS)
immune s.
In Charge Diabetes Control S.
insulin-IGF signaling s.
insulin-sensitive signaling s.
insuloacinar portal s.
insuloductular portal s.
kallikrein-kinin s.
lacrimal s.
LifeGuide S.
limbic s.
magnocellular neurosecretory s.
matrix transdermal s.

Medi-Ject needle-free insulin
  injection s.
Medi-Jector Choice needle-free
  insulin injection s.
melanocortin receptor s.
neuroendocrine s.
nonoral estradiol delivery s.
nucleolar channel s.
OneTouch II hospital blood
  glucose monitoring s.
osteocytic membrane s.
paracrine s.
parasympathetic nervous s.
peripheral nervous s. (PNS)
portable endocrine s.
portal s.
Precision Xtra Advanced Diabetes
  Management S.
primary central nervous s. (PCNS)
renin-angiotensin s.
renin-angiotensin-aldosterone s.
  (RAAS)
reservoir transdermal s.
reticuloendothelial s.
reverse hemolytic plaque assay s.
Santorini duct s.
Schwann cell s.
Select GT blood glucose s.
serotonergic s.
sudomotor s.
sympathetic nervous s. (SNS)
sympathoadrenal neuroendocrine s.
TD Glucose Monitoring s.
Testoderm testosterone
  transdermal s.
testosterone transdermal s.
tissular hormonal s.
TLX alloantigen s.
Toronto Clinical Scoring S.
transdermal testosterone delivery s.
transscrotal testosterone delivery s.
trophoblast-lymphocyte cross-reactive
  alloantigen s.
tuberoinfundibular s.
two-cell s.
ubiquitin/proteasome s.
urogenital s.
uterine-endocrine s.
vitamin D endocrine s.
WHO classification s.
wolffian s.

S

NOTES

system *(continued)*
World Health Organization Expert Committee on Diabetes classification s.

systemic
s. arterial hypertension
s. estrogen
s. inflammatory response syndrome (SIRS)
s. lupus erythematosus (SLE)
s. symptom
s. vascular resistance (SVR)
s. vasculitis
s. virilization

Sytobex

T

testosterone
T cell
T helper 1, 2 cell
T lymphocyte

^{201}T1

thallium-201

T_4

thyroxine
fetal T_4
free T_4
peripheral T_4
serum free T_4
serum total T_4
total T_4 (TT_4)

T_3

3,5,3'-triiodo-I-thyronine
triiodothyronine
free T_3
T_3 receptor (TR)
T_3 resin uptake (T_3RU)
T_3 resin uptake test
T_3 responsive element (T_3RE)
reverse T_3 (rT_3)
T_3 suppression test
total T_3 (TT_3)

T_m

tubular transport maximum

T1-weighted image
T2-weighted spin-echo image
T3 toxicosis
TAA

premature top codon

tab

Meda T.

Tabby gene
tabes dorsalis
table

Bailey-Pinneau t.

tablet

Amaryl glimepiride t.
Dostinex t.
Ergoset t.
K-Phos Neutral t.
sodium chloride t.
Stresstabs 600 Advanced
Formula T.'s

TACE

transcatheter arterial chemoembolization

Tace
tachyarrhythmia

atrial t.

tachycardia

ventricular t.

tachygastria

tachykinin
tachyphylaxis
tachysterol
Tac-3, -40 Injection
tacrolimus
TAD

thiazolidinedione
trans-activation domain

Taenia solium
TAF

transactivation factor

TAG

total available glucose

tag

expressed sequence t. (EST)

tagging

haplotype t.

tailing
Takatsuki syndrome
TAL

thick ascending limb

tall

t. cell
t. stature

5T allele
T alpha$_1$

thymosin alpha$_1$

Tamm-Horsfall protein
tamoxifen
tamsulosin
Tangier disease
tannate

pitressin t.

Tanner

T. stage (I–V)
T. staging

tanycyte
TAO

thyroid-associated ophthalmopathy

TAP

trypsinogen-activating peptide

Tapanol
Tapazole
tape

Deknatel t.

taper

prednisone t.

tapering dose
***Taq*I restriction enzyme**
tarda

porphyria cutanea t.

target

accommodative t.
t. cell
t. gland function

target *(continued)*
    t. height
    t. organ resistance
    t. of rapamycin (TOR)
    t. of rapamycin kinase
    t. tissue
targeting
    gene t.
Targretin
tarsorrhaphy
tartrate
    belladonna, phenobarbital, and
      ergotamine t.
    pentolinium t.
tartrate-resistant acid phosphatase (TR-ACP, TRAP)
taste receptor
TATA-binding protein (TBP)
TATA box
taurine
tautomycin
tax protein
Tay-Sachs disease
TB
    total bound
Tb$_4$
    thymosin b$_4$
    thymosin beta$_4$
TBBMC
    total body bone mineral content
TBBMD
    total body bone mineral density
TBG
    thyroid-binding globulin
    thyroxine-binding globulin
      TBG deficiency
      TBG excess
TBII
    thyrotropin-binding inhibitory
      immunoglobulin
    TSH-binding inhibitory immunoglobulin
      TBII assay
T-box gene family
TBP
    TATA-binding protein
TBPA
    thyroid-binding prealbumin
    thyronine-binding prealbumin
TBS
    total body scan
TC
    total cholesterol
TC-10
    T. cell
    T. cell activation
^{99m}Tc
    technetium-99m
      ^{99m}Tc sestamibi scintigraphy

t/c
    Snp5 t/c
TC-6 cell
TCA
    tricarboxylic acid
TCDD
    2,3,7,8-tetrachlorodibenzo-*p*-dioxin
^{99m}Tc-DMSA
    technetium-99m dimercaptosuccinic acid
T-cell
    T.-c. antigen
    T.-c. epitope
    T.-c. growth factor (TCGF)
    T.-c. lymphoma
    T.-c. mediated cytotoxicity
    T.-c. protein tyrosine phosphatase
      (TCPTP)
    T.-c. receptor (TCR)
    T.-c. repertoire
    T.-c. response
    T.-c. subset
    T.-c. tolerance
TCGF
    T-cell growth factor
TCL
    thyroid T-cell line
Tc-99m
    T. MIBI
    T. sestamibi scintigraphy
Tc-99m-TcO4
    pertechnetate
TCP
    tropical calcific pancreatitis
^{99m}Tc-pentavalent dimercaptosuccinate
TCPTP
    T-cell protein tyrosine phosphatase
TCR
    T-cell receptor
^{99m}Tc-sestamibi
^{99m}Tc-tetrafosmin
TD
    thyroid dysgenesis
      TD Glucose meter
      TD Glucose Monitoring system
TDA
    testis-determining antigen
T$_4$5′-deiodinase type 2 (D2)
TDF
    testis-determining factor
TDI
    therapeutic donor insemination
T2DM
    type 2 diabetes mellitus
TDP
    time-dependent potentiation
TDT
    transmission disequilibrium test
TdT
    terminal deoxynucleotide transferase

tear
retinal t.
Tebamide
TeBG
testosterone-binding globulin
T/EBP
thyroid-specific enhancer-binding protein
TechLite lancet
technetium
t. bone scan
t. pertechnetate
t. pertechnetate scan
t. pyrophosphate
t. sestamibi scintigraphy
triple-phase scan with t.
technetium-99m (^{99m}Tc)
t. dimercaptosuccinic acid (^{99m}Tc-DMSA)
t. tetraforsmin
technetium/thallium subtraction nuclear scanning
technique
aldehyde thionin staining t.
assisted reproduction t.
coital alignment t. (CAT)
coupled amplification and sequencing t.
deuterated water t.
double-labeling t.
dye-diluting t.
endonasal endoscopic t.
endoscopic pituitary surgery t.
euglycemic glucose clamp t.
fast spin-echo t.
Grimelius stain t.
histomorphometric t.
hyperinsulinemic-euglycemic clamp t.
imaging t.
immunogold-labeling t.
immunohistochemical staining t.
immunohistochemistry t.
immunoperoxidase t.
interstitial hyperthermic t.
Karydakis t.
neuroanatomic t.
nonisotropic t.
pause and squeeze t.
perimetric t.
recombinant DNA t.
regular spin-echo t.
septal pushover t.

Sevier-Munger stain t.
sublabial transseptal t.
tetracycline double-labeling t.
thermodilution t.
thyroglobulin t.
Uchida t.
technology
Affymetrix GeneChip t.
assisted reproductive t.
gene-transfer t.
Kumetrix microneedle t.
Tedral
TEF
thyrotroph embryonic factor
T-effector lymphocyte
Tega-Vert Oral
tegmentum
telachoroidea
telangiectasia
ataxia t.
hereditary hemorrhagic t.
t. macularis eruptiva perstans
venous t.
telencephalon
basal t.
Telepaque
television-watching obesity
telogen effluvium
telomerase enzyme
telopeptide
C-terminal type I collagen t.
type I collagen C-terminal t.
temperature
ambient t.
basal body t. (BBT)
thermoneutrality t.
temporal
t. balding
t. bone osteomyelitis
t. fiber
t. horn
temporary
t. delayed puberty
t. end-organ resistance
Tempra
Tenderlett
T. Jr. lancing device
T. Toddler lancing device
tendinous xanthoma
tendon xanthoma
tennis racket-shaped pentalaminar tubular structure

NOTES

T

tenosynovitis
tense tumor capsule
tensin homologue
tension
  decreased oxygen t.
  oxygen t.
tentorial incisura
Tenuate Dospan
teratocarcinoma
teratogenic
teratogenicity
teratoma
  atypical t.
  benign cystic t.
  mature t.
  ovarian t.
  thyroid t.
terazosin
terbinafine
terbutaline sulfate
terconazole
teriparatide
terminal
  autonomic postganglionic nerve t.
  t. deoxynucleotide transferase (TdT)
  t. hair
  t. nerve ending
  t. nerve fiber
  neurohypophysial nerve t.
  t. oxidase
  presynaptic nerve t.
terminalis
  lamina t.
  organum vasculosum of the
    lamina t. (OVLT)
  organum vasculosum laminae t.
    (OVLT)
  stria t.
terminus
  amino t.
ternary complex
terpin
  t. hydrate
  t. hydrate and codeine
Terry nail
tertiary
  t. adrenal insufficiency
  t. chorionic villus
  t. follicle
  t. hyperaldosteronism
  t. hyperparathyroidism
  t. hypogonadism
  t. hypothyroidism
  t. messenger
Tesamone Injection
TESE
  testicular sperm extraction
Teslac

test
  Access Ostase blood t.
  adrenocorticotrophin stimulation t.
  alkaline phosphatase antialkaline
    phosphatase antibody t.
  Allen t.
  alternate cover t.
  antibody-dependent cytotoxicity t.
  arginine infusion t.
  arginine tolerance t. (ATT)
  ascitic fluid t.
  Benedict t.
  [13C]-acetate t.
  calcium stimulation t.
  captopril t.
  chorionic gonadotropin
    stimulation t.
  Chvostek t.
  clomiphene citrate challenge t.
    (CCCT)
  clonidine suppression t.
  [13C]-octanoic acid t.
  corticotroph stimulation t.
  corticotropin-releasing hormone t.
  Cortrosyn stimulation t.
  cosyntropin stimulation t.
  C-peptide suppression t.
  CRH stimulation t.
  crossed t.
  Cytomel suppression t.
  deferoxamine t.
  dexamethasone suppression t.
  DFO t.
  2,4-dinitrophenylhydrazine t.
  duodenal intubation t.
  epinephrine provocation t.
  ether-stimulation t.
  fecal chymotrypsin t.
  ferric chloride t.
  fructosamine t.
  get up and go t.
  glucagon stimulation t.
  glucose challenge t.
  glucose oxidase t.
  glucose polymer challenge t.
  glucose tolerance t. (GTT)
  Glycosal diabetes t.
  gonadotropin-releasing hormone t.
  hCG pregnancy t.
  high-dose dexamethasone
    suppression t.
  human zona pellucide binding t.
  hydrogen breath t.
  insulin tolerance t. (ITT)
  intravenous glucose tolerance t.
    (IVGTT)
  iodine-perchlorate discharge t.
  KetoSite t.
  Kveim t.

late-night salivary cortisol t.
LDL direct t.
L-dopa t.
Liddle t.
low-dose dexamethasone t.
low-dose short synacthen t.
  (LDSST)
methasone-suppressed corticotropin-
  releasing hormone t.
metrapone stimulation t.
metyrapone t.
Michigan Neuropathy Screening T.
Micral urine dipstick t.
morning corticotropin-releasing
  hormone t.
morning CRH t.
nitroblue tetrazolium t.
oral glucose tolerance t. (OGTT)
osmolality dehydration t.
overnight high-dose dexamethasone
  suppression t. (ONDST)
overnight metyrapone t.
overnight 1-mg dexamethasone
  suppression t.
pancreatic functioning diagnostant t.
pancreolauryl t.
pancreozymin secretin t.
pentagastrin provocation t.
pentagastrin stimulation t.
perchlorate discharge t.
PFD t.
pituitary dynamic t.
pituitary target organ t.
postcoital t.
posture stimulation t.
predictive value t.
pregnancy thyroid function t.
progesterone challenge t.
protein truncation t. (PTT)
provocation t.
PS t.
Quantitative Autonomic Function T.
Quantitative Sensory T.
radioiodine uptake t.
radiolabeled breath t.
random glucose t.
RET oncogene t.
S t.
saline suppression t.
Schilling t.
Schirmer t.
secretin stimulation t.

semen fructose t.
sensitivity t.
serum acid phosphatase t.
Sibley-Lehninger t.
Sims-Huhner t.
specificity t.
sperm function t.
SpermMar t.
steady-state plasma glucose t.
stimulation t.
Synacthen t.
Thorn t.
Thyrogen serum thyroglobulin t.
thyroidal radioactive iodine
  uptake t. (RAIU)
thyroid function t.
thyroperoxidase antibody t.
thyrotropin-releasing hormone t.
thyroxine suppression t.
tolbutamide stimulation t.
transmission disequilibrium t. (TDT)
T_3 resin uptake t.
TRH stimulation t.
triiodothyronine resin uptake t.
triiodothyronine suppression t.
Trousseau t.
T_3RU t.
TSH stimulation t.
T_3 suppression t.
two-day high-dose dexamethasone
  suppression t.
van den Bergh t.
Wassermann t.
water deprivation t.
water restriction t.
zona-free hamster oocyte
  penetration t.

testicular
  t. atrophy
  t. choriocarcinoma
  t. enzyme defect
  t. feminization
  t. fluid
  t. Leydig cell tumor
  t. regression syndrome
  t. sperm extraction (TESE)
  t. volume

testing
  acute insulin response t.
  blood glucose t.
  Cortrosyn stimulation t.
  fludrocortisone suppression t. (FST)

NOTES

testing *(continued)*
  metyrapone t.
  Monojector fingerstick device for blood glucose t.
  nocturnal penile tumescence t.
  NPT t.
  provocative t.
  quantitative autonomic functioning t. (QAFT)
  quantitative sensory t. (QST)
  thyroid antibody t.
  urine t.
  vibration perception t.
  water deprivation t.
testis
  canalicular t.
  feminizing t.
  intraabdominal t.
  Leydig cells of the t.
  mediastinum t.
  rete t.
  varicocele t.
testis-determining
  t.-d. antigen (TDA)
  t.-d. factor (TDF)
testitoxicosis
  familial t.
  sporadic t.
Testoderm
  T. testosterone transdermal system
  T. TTS
testolactone
  aromatase inhibitor t.
Testopel Pellet
testosterone (T)
  buccal t.
  t. buciclate
  t. cyclodextrin
  t. cypionate
  t. enanthate
  endogenous t.
  t. ester
  estradiol and t.
  t. estradiol-binding globulin
  ethinyl t.
  free t.
  t. implant
  intramuscular t.
  plasma t.
  t. propionate
  serum free t.
  serum total t.
  t. skin patch
  t. synthesis
  total t.
  t. transdermal system
  t. undecenoate
testosterone-binding globulin (TeBG)
testosterone-deficient patient

Testoviron Depot 50, 100
testoxicosis
Testred
tetany
  cerebral t.
  hypocalcemic t.
  latent t.
  uterine t.
tethered
  t. cord
  t. cord release
  t. ligand thrombin receptor
Tetracap Oral
2,3,7,8-tetrachlorodibenzo-*p*-dioxin (TCDD)
tetracycline
  t. double-labeling technique
  t. labeling
tetradecapeptide
tetraforsmin
  technetium-99m t.
tetraglycine hydroperiodide
tetrahydroaldosterone
tetrahydrobiopterin
tetrahydrocortisol (THC)
tetrahydrocortisone (THC)
tetraiodoacetic acid
tetraiodo-L-thyronine
tetraiodothyroacetic acid
tetralogy of Fallot
tetramer
tetranitrate
  pentaerythritol t.
tetrapeptide
texture
  inhomogeneous t.
TF5
  thymosin fraction 5
TG
  thyroglobulin
  triacylglycerol
  turtle TG
Tg
  thyroglobulin
TgAb
  thyroglobulin antibody
TGBI
  thyroid growth-blocking immunoglobulin
T-Gen
T-Gesic
TGF
  transforming growth factor
  tubuloglomerular feedback
  TGF system
TGF-A
  transforming growth factor alpha
TGF-B
  transforming growth factor beta

TGI
thyroid growth immunoglobulin
TGN
trans-Golgi network
TH
thyroid hormone
TH beta-receptor deficiency
Th1 cell
Th2 cell
thalami
striae medullaris t.
thalamic nucleus
thalamus
nucleus ventralis anterior of t.
thalassemia major
thalidomide
Thalitone
thallium-201 (^{201}T1)
thallium chloride (TI-201)
thallium-pertechnetate subtraction scintigraphy
thallium-technetium dual isotope scintigraphy
THAM
tromethamine
THAM-E
tromethamine E
thanatophoric dysplasia type I, II
THBG
thyroid hormone-binding globulin
THBR
thyroid hormone-binding ratio
THC
tetrahydrocortisol
tetrahydrocortisone
THDA
tuberohypophyseal dopaminergic neuron
theca
t. cell androgen production
t. externa
t. externa cell
t. folliculi
t. interna
t. interna cell
t. interstitial cell
t. interstitial cell dysregulation
t. lutein cell
thecal
t. dysregulation
t. hyperplasia
theca-lutein cyst
thecoma

The Diabetes A1C Initiative
thelarche
premature t.
Theo-24
Theobid
theobromine
Theochron
Theoclear-80
Theo-Dur
Theolair
theophylline
t. intoxication
t. metabolism
t. toxicity
theophylline-induced hypercalcemia
theory
chronic autoimmune t.
second attack t.
Theo-Sav
Theostat-80
Theovent
Theo-X
Therabid
Thera-Combex H-P Kapseals
Theragran Hematinic
Theragran-M
therapeutic
t. donor insemination (TDI)
t. irrigation
TheraPress DUO Lite stocking
therapy
acarbose combination t.
aminoglutethimide t.
anabolic t.
androgen-lowering t.
androgen replacement t. (ART)
antigen-specific preventive t.
antihypertensive t.
antimicrobial t.
antiresorptive t.
antiretroviral t.
basal insulin t.
behavioral t.
bicarbonate t.
BIDS t.
blood purification t.
bolus t.
Bragg peak proton irradiation t.
bromocriptine t.
B vitamin t.
calcitriol t.
coherence t.

NOTES

355

therapy *(continued)*
    combination t.
    combined t.
    complementary and alternative t.
    continuous-combined estrogen-progestogen t. (CC-EPT)
    continuous-combined hormone replacement t. (ccHRT)
    continuous hormone replacement t.
    conventional t.
    corticosteroid t.
    cyclical hormone replacement t.
    deferoxamine t.
    desferrioxamine t.
    dexamethasone suppression t.
    dialytic t.
    diuretic t.
    D-Modem and insulin pump t.
    dopamine agonist t.
    electroconvulsive t.
    electrolyte t.
    endocrine t.
    Enterra t.
    estrogen t. (ET)
    estrogen/androgen t.
    estrogen-progesterone t. (EPT)
    estrogen replacement t. (ERT)
    exogenous glucocorticoid t.
    fludrocortisone replacement t.
    fluid t.
    foscarnet t.
    fractionated radiation t.
    gene t.
    glucocorticoid replacement t.
    gonadotropin-releasing hormone-agonist t.
    growth factor t.
    growth hormone t.
    hemodialysis t.
    hormonal add-back t.
    hormone replacement t. (HRT)
    hydrocortisone replacement t.
    ^{131}I t.
    insulin pump t.
    intensified conventional t.
    intensive t.
    interferon t.
    intracystic radiation t.
    iodine-131 t.
    levothyroxine suppression t.
    lipid-lowering t.
    medical nutrition t.
    metyrapone t.
    mineralocorticoid replacement t.
    multiport collimated cobalt-60 t.
    natural hormone t. (NHT)
    neurotrophic t.
    nutrition t.
    octreotide t.

    pathogenesis-specific t.
    pharmacologic t.
    phosphate t.
    postnatal t.
    PPAR-gamma t.
    pregnancy radioiodine t.
    preventive hormone t.
    primary t.
    proton beam t.
    pulsatile gonadotropin-releasing hormone t.
    pulsed progestin hormone replacement t.
    radiation t. (XRT)
    radioablation t.
    radioactive iodine t.
    radioiodine ablation t.
    recombinant enzyme replacement t.
    replacement t.
    salvage t.
    sequential hormone replacement t.
    serotonergic t.
    steroid replacement t.
    suppressive t.
    symptomatic t.
    thionamide drug t.
    thyroid hormone replacement t.
    thyrotropin suppressive t.
    thyroxine replacement t.
    tolerogenic t.
    vasodepressor drug t.
    vidarabine t.
    warfarin t.

Therasense
    T. FreeStyle
    T. subcutaneous glucose sensor

thermal
    t. cycler
    t. injury
    t. perception

thermic effect of food

thermocoagulation

thermodilution technique

thermogenesis
    basal t.
    facultative t.
    nonshivering t.
    obligatory t.
    shivering t.

thermogenic

thermography
    imaging t.

thermolabile receptor

thermolability

thermoneutrality temperature

thermoregulation

thermosensitive neuron

thermostatic hypothesis

thiabendazole

thiamine
thiazide
t. diuretic
t. diuretic agent
thiazolidinedione (TAD, TZD)
thick ascending limb (TAL)
thickened
t. acral part
t. adrenal limb
thickening
calvarial t.
t. of cortex
thickness
endometrial t.
intimal wall t. (IWT)
osteoid seam t.
skin fold t.
thick-walled hypha
thiethylperazine
Thigh Thing pump holder
thinning
t. fat pad
skin t.
trabecular t.
thin-walled simple cyst
thiocyanate
granidinium t.
thioglucoside
thioguanine
thiolase
acetoacetyl-CoA t.
thionamide
t. antithyroid drug
t. drug therapy
thionin
aldehyde t.
thiopental sodium
thiophorase
thioredoxin
thiouracil
thiourea
t. compound
t. drug
ethylene t.
thioureylene group
thioxanthine
third
t. complementarity determining region (CDR3)
T. National Health and Nutrition Examination Study
t. ventricle

third-generation assay
thirst
impaired t.
intense t.
t. mechanism
stimuli of t.
t. threshold
thoracic stomach
Thorazine
Thorlo padded socks
Thorn
T. sign
T. test
THOX
thyroid oxidase
Thr
threonine
Thr-410
Thra gene
Thrb gene
thread
mucus t.
three-compartment model
threonine (Thr)
threshold
glucose t.
kidney t.
osmotic t.
renal t.
thirst t.
vibration t.
thrift
metabolic t.
thrifty
t. gene
t. genotype
t. genotype hypothesis
thrive
failure to t. (FTT)
thrombin
t. generation
t. receptor-activating peptide 6 (TRAP-6)
thrombocytopenia
thromboembolic event
thromboembolism
venous t. (VTE)
thrombolytic therapy
thrombomodulin
serum t.
thrombophilia

NOTES

T

thrombophlebitis
    cavernous sinus t.
thrombopoietin (TPO)
thrombosis
    adrenal vein t.
    cerebral vein t.
    exuberant t.
    vascular t.
thrombospondin synthesis
thromboxane (TX)
    t. A2 (TXA2, TxA2)
    t. analog
    t. B2 (TXB2, TxB2)
thrombus
    t. formation
    nascent t.
thyamidine autoradiography
thymectomy
thymic
    t. branch
    t. carcinoid
    t. hyperplasia
    t. involution
    t. lymphocyte
thymicolymphaticus
thymidine autoradiography
thymocyte
thymoma
    ACTH-producing t.
thymosin
    t. alpha$_1$ (T alpha$_1$)
    t. b$_4$ (Tb$_4$)
    t. beta$_4$ (Tb$_4$)
    t. fraction 5 (TF5)
    t. peptide
thymoxamine
thymulin
thymus
    t. gland
    t. hypertrophy
Thypinone
Thyrar
thyroacetic acid
thyroarytenoid
Thyro-Block
thyrocalcitonin
thyrocardiac disease
thyrocervical trunk
thyrocyte
Thyrogen
    T. radioiodine scan
    T. serum thyroglobulin test
thyrogenic carcinoma
thyroglobin synthesis defect
thyroglobulin (TG, Tg)
    t. antibody (TgAb)
    t. antigen
    t. asparagine
    t. assay

    t. autoantibody
    t. binding
    t. biosynthesis
    t. cellular uptake
    t. expression
    t. gene
    t. glycosylation
    human t. (hTg)
    t. hydrolysis
    t. iodination
    t. level
    t. protein
    t. proteolytic
    t. regional structure
    t. secretion
    serum t.
    t. staining
    t. synthesis
    t. technique
thyroglobulin-producing tissue
thyroglossal
    t. duct
    t. duct carcinoma
    t. duct cyst
    t. duct remnant
    t. tract
thyroglucase
    gold t.
thyroid
    t. ablation with ^{131}I
    t. acropachy
    t. adenylate cyclase
    t. agenesis
    t. angiosarcoma
    t. anlage
    t. antibody testing
    t. antigen-antibody nephritis
    Armour T.
    t. axis
    t. biopsy
    black t.
    t. bud
    t. cancer
    t. capsule
    t. carcinosarcoma
    t. cartilage
    t. C cell
    t. chemodectoma
    t. colloid
    t. computed tomography
    t. cork phenomenon
    t. crisis
    t. deficiency cell
    t. dermopathy
    desiccated t.
    t. diverticulum
    t. dysfunction
    t. dysgenesis (TD)
    t. dyshormonogenesis

ectopic t.
t. enlargement
t. epithelial cell
t. extract
t. eye disease
t. follicle
t. follicular cell
t. function
t. function test
t. gland
t. gland ablation
t. gland adenoma
t. gland autonomy
t. gland carcinoma
t. gland development
t. growth-blocking immunoglobulin (TGBI)
t. growth immunoglobulin (TGI)
gummata of the t.
t. hemosiderosis
t. hormone (TH)
t. hormone action
t. hormone adaptation syndrome
t. hormone autoantibody
t. hormone-binding globulin (THBG)
t. hormone-binding ratio (THBR)
t. hormone-binding site
t. hormone metabolism
t. hormone nuclear receptor isoform
t. hormone production
t. hormone receptor auxiliary antibody protein
t. hormone receptor defect
t. hormone receptor homodimer
t. hormone receptor monomer
t. hormone receptor-retinoid X receptor (TR-RXR)
t. hormone replacement
t. hormone replacement therapy
t. hormone resistance
t. hormone resistance syndrome
t. hormone-response element (TRE)
t. hormone status
t. hormone synthesis
t. hormone target gene
t. hormone transport protein
t. hormonogenesis
t. hormonogenesis defect IIB
t. hyperplasia
t. ima artery

t. inflammatory disease
t. iodide transporter
t. iodide trap
t. iodine transport
t. isthmus
lateral aberrant t.
lingual t.
t. lymphoma
t. magnetic resonance imaging
medullary carcinoma of the t. (MCT)
t. microsomal antibody
t. migration
t. morphogenesis
t. mucoepidermoid carcinoma
t. necrosis
t. neuroendocrine tumor
t. nodule
t. ophthalmopathy
t. orbitopathy
t. organogenesis
t. overactivity
t. oxidase (THOX)
t. papillary carcinoma
t. parafollicular cell
t. paraganglioma
t. parenchyma
t. peroxidase (TPO)
t. peroxidase activity
t. peroxidase antibody
t. peroxidase antigen
t. peroxidase autoantibody
t. peroxidase synthesis
t. plasmacytoma
porcine t.
t. radioiodine uptake
t. remnant
t. reserve
t. response element (TRE)
t. scan
t. scintigraphy
t. scintiscan
t. screening
t. secretion
t. squamous cell carcinoma
t. stare
t. stimulation-blocking antibody (TSBAb)
t. storm
t. storm hyperthermia
t. storm syndrome
t. stroma

NOTES

359

thyroid *(continued)*
    T. Strong
    t. stunning
    substernal t.
    t. symptom checklist
    t. T-cell line (TCL)
    t. technetium pertechnetate uptake
    t. teratoma
    t. transcription factor (TTF)
    t. transcription factor 1 (TTF-1)
    t. transcription factor 2 (TTF-2)
    t. trapping activity
    t. tumorigenesis
    t. ultrasound
    t. uptake probe
    t. venous effluent
    t. volume

thyroidal
    t. ablation
    t. autoantibody secretion
    t. C cell
    t. hypothyroidism
    t. radioactive iodine uptake test
      (RAIU)

thyroid-associated ophthalmopathy (TAO)

thyroid-binding
    t.-b. globulin (TBG)
    t.-b. prealbumin (TBPA)

thyroidectomy
    t. cell
    near-total t.
    subtotal t.
    surgical t.

thyroiditis
    acute lymphocytic t.
    acute suppurative t.
    agoiterous autoimmune t.
    t. akuta simplex
    Aspergillus t.
    atrophic chronic autoimmune t.
    atrophic Hashimoto t.
    autoimmune t.
    bacterial t.
    chronic autoimmune t.
    chronic fibrous t.
    chronic lymphocytic t.
    Coccidioides immitis t.
    coccidioidomycosis-induced t.
    cytokine-induced t.
    de Quervain nonsuppurative t.
    destruction t.
    echinococcal t.
    experimental autoimmune t. (EAT)
    giant-cell t.
    goitrous chronic autoimmune t.
    goitrous Hashimoto t.
    granulomatous t.
    hamburger t.
    Hashimoto t.
    infectious t.
    interferon-alpha-induced t.
    invasive fibrous t.
    lymphocytic t.
    painful subacute t.
    painless postpartum t.
    palpation t.
    perineoplastic t.
    Pneumocystis carinii t.
    postpartum lymphocytic t.
    postpartum painless t.
    postpartum silent t.
    pseudogranulomatous t.
    pseudotuberculous t.
    pyogenic t.
    radiation t.
    radiation-induced t.
    Riedel t.
    silent autoimmune t.
    spontaneous autoimmune t. (SAT)
    sporadic silent t.
    subacute granulomatous t.
    subacute painful t.
    suppurative t.

thyroidologist

thyroidology

thyroid-releasing hormone-degrading ectoenzyme

thyroid-specific
    t.-s. enhancer-binding protein (T/EBP)
    t.-s. tracer

thyroid-stimulating
    t.-s. antibody (TSAb)
    t.-s. hormone abnormality
    t.-s. hormone-binding inhibitor antibody
    t.-s. hormone-binding inhibitor immunoglobulin assay
    t.-s. hormone deficiency
    t.-s. hormone receptor (TSH-R, TSHR)
    t.-s. hormone receptor antibody (TSH-RAb)
    t.-s. hormone receptor autoantibody (TSH-RAb)
    t.-s. hormone receptor expression
    t.-s. hormone receptor mutation
    t.-s. hormone-releasing hormone
    t.-s. hormone-secreting pituitary tumor
    t.-s. hormone synthesis
    t.-s. immunoglobulin (TSI)

thyroid-stimulating-blocking antibody (TSBAb)

Thyrolar

thyromegaly

thyrometabolic status

thyromimetic
t. action
t. compound
thyronine-binding prealbumin (TBPA)
thyroparathyroidectomy (TPTX)
thyroperoxidase (TPO)
t. antibody (TPO Ab)
t. antibody test
thyroperoxidase-iodide complex
thyropexin
thyrostatic
ThyroTest rapid assay
thyrotoxic
t. crisis
t. Graves disease
t. myopathy
t. osteodystrophy
t. periodic paralysis
t. phase
t. storm
thyrotoxicity
thyrotoxicosis
accelerated t.
amiodarone t.
amiodarone-associated t.
amiodarone-induced destructive t.
apathetic t.
autoimmune t.
destruction-induced t.
destructive t.
exogenous t.
extrathyroidal t.
t. factitia
gestational transient t. (GTT)
hamburger t.
hereditary t.
t. of hyperemesis gravidarum
iatrogenic t.
iodine-induced t.
lithium-associated t.
t. medicamentosa
mild overt t.
neonatal t.
pituitary-dependent t.
pregnancy t.
subclinical t.
T_3-predominant t.
transient t.
TSH-dependent t.
TSH-induced t.
thyrotoxicosis medicamentosa
thyrotrope adenoma

thyrotroph
t. carcinoma
t. cell
t. cell adenoma
t. cell hyperplasia
t. embryonic factor (TEF)
thyrotroph-derived adenoma
thyrotropic cell
thyrotropin
t. alfa
t. alpha
chorionic t.
human chorionic t.
nonpituitary t.
pituitary t.
t. receptor (TSH-R)
t. receptor antibody
t. receptor autoantibody (TRAb)
t. receptor-stimulating antibody (TSH-RAb)
t. release factor (TRF)
t. serum
t. suppressive therapy
thyrotropin-binding inhibitory immunoglobulin (TBII)
thyrotropinoma
thyrotropin-receptor activating mutation
thyrotropin-releasing
t.-r. hormone (TRH)
t.-r. hormone-induced refractoriness
t.-r. hormone receptor (TRH-R)
t.-r. hormone stimulation
t.-r. hormone study
t.-r. hormone test
thyrotropin-secreting
t.-s. pituitary adenoma
t.-s. pituitary tumor
thyrotropin-stimulating
t.-s. hormone (TSH)
t.-s. hormone-expressing cell
thyroxine, thyroxin (T_4)
basal t.
blood free t.
free t. (FT_4)
peripheral t.
t. radioisotope assay (T_4RIA)
t. replacement
t. replacement therapy
t. suppression test
thyroxine-binding
t.-b. globulin (TBG)
t.-b. globulin deficiency

T

NOTES

thyroxine-binding *(continued)*
    t.-b. globulin excess
    t.-b. prealbumin
Thytropar
TI-201
    thallium chloride
tibolone
Ticlopidine Microangiopathy of Diabetes Study
Ticon
TIDA
    tuberoinfundibular dopaminergic neuron
tie sternum
TIF2
    transcriptional intermediary factor 2
    TIF2 coactivator
tige pituitaire
tight junction
tiglic acid
tiludronate disodium
TIM
    T. gene
    T. protein
time
    ankle reflex t.
    longitudinal relaxation t.
    mineralization lag t.
    t. sense
    spin-lattice relaxation t.
    spin-spin relaxation t.
    transverse relaxation t.
    T1, T2 relaxation t.
Timecelles
time-dependent potentiation (TDP)
timing
    meal t.
timolol
TIMP
    tissue inhibitor of metalloproteinase
TIMP-1
    tissue inhibitor of metalloproteinase-1
tinctorial feature
tincture
    iodine t.
    opium t.
tinea versicolor
tiopronin
TIPS
    transjugular intrahepatic portosystemic stent shunt
      AEIOU TIPS
        alcohol, epilepsy, insulin, overdose, uremia, trauma, infection, psychiatric, stroke
tiratricol
tissue
    aberrant mediastinal thyroid t.
    adipose t.
    adrenal rest t.

t. aluminum
t. aluminum toxicity
brown adipose t. (BAT)
chromaffin t.
t. concentration
connective t.
ectopic thyroid t.
endomysial connective t.
erectile t.
excitable t.
fibroglandular t.
goitrous t.
granulation t.
gut-associated lymphoid t. (GALT)
hyperfunctioning t.
t. inhibitor of metalloproteinase (TIMP)
t. inhibitor of metalloproteinase-1 (TIMP-1)
insulin-producing t.
insulin target t.
juxtathyroidal t.
t. kallikrein
lateral aberrant thyroid t.
lean t.
marginal zone/mucosa-associated lymphoid t.
mucosa-associated lymphoid t. (MALT)
t. necrosis factor (TNF)
t. nonspecific alkaline phosphatase gene
orbital t.
pancreatic endocrine t.
parasellar t.
pathological endocrine t.
pericardial bioprosthetic t.
peripheral t.
t. regeneration
remnant hyperplastic t.
t. repair
retroocular t.
retroorbital adipose t.
retroorbital connective t.
t. senescence
t. specificity
target t.
thyroglobulin-producing t.
trophoblastic t.
white adipose t. (WAT)
tissue-type plasminogen activator
tissular hormonal system
Titanic phenomenon
titanium mesh
titer
    antibody t.
    antithyroid antibody t.
    microsomal antibody t.
^{201}Tl-thallous chloride

TLX
> trophoblast-lymphocyte cross-reactive
> TLX alloantigen system

T-lymphocyte
> beta-cell cytotoxic T.-l.
> helper/inducer T.-l.
> T.-l. insulin binding and
> degradation
> suppressor/cytotoxic T.-l.

TMG
> toxic multinodular goiter

TMP-SMX
> trimethoprim sulfamethoxazole

TNF
> tissue necrosis factor
> tumor necrosis factor

TNF-alpha
> tumor necrosis factor-alpha

TNF-beta
> tumor necrosis factor-beta

TNFR
> tumor necrosis factor receptor

TNF-related apoptosis inducing ligand (TRAIL)

TNF-weak homologue (TWEAK)

TNG
> toxic nodular goiter

TNM
> tumor/node/metastases
> TNM classification

TOBEC
> total body electrical conductivity

tocolysis
tocolytic agent
tocopherol
tocophersolan
toe
> t. box
> t. pressure

tolazamide
tolbutamide stimulation test
Tolectin
tolerance
> glucose t.
> impaired glucose t. (IGT)
> insulinopenic impaired glucose t.
> T-cell t.

tolerogenic
> t. protocol
> t. therapy

Tolinase
tolmetin

Tolosa-Hunt syndrome
tolrestat
tomography
> computed t. (CT)
> dual-phase spiral computed t.
> dynamic computed t.
> ^{18}F-fluorodeoxyglucose positron
> emission t. (FDG-PET)
> helical computed t.
> parathyroid computed t.
> positron emission t. (PET)
> quantified computed t. (QCT)
> single-photon emission computed t.
> (SPECT)
> spiral computed t.
> thyroid computed t.

tone
> dopaminergic t.
> hypothalamic opioidergic t.
> peroxide t.

Tongyi Tang Diabetes capsule
tonicity
tonic spasm
tonofilament
Top2
> DNA topoisomerase II

topical
> t. antimicrobial
> Aquacare T.
> Carmol T.
> Lanaphilic T.
> Nutraplus T.
> Rogaine T.
> Ultra Mide T.
> Ureacin-20 T.

Topiglan
topiramate
topoisomerase
> DNA t. II (Top2)

topotecan
TOR
> target of rapamycin

toremifene
Toronto
> T. Clinical Scoring System
> T. Renal Osteodystrophy Study

Torpedo californica
torsades de pointes
tortuous blood vessel
Tostrex
total
> t. alopecia

T

total (*continued*)
t. androgen binding
t. available glucose (TAG)
t. blood volume
t. body bone mineral content (TBBMC)
t. body bone mineral density (D_{beta}, TBBMD)
t. body electrical conductivity (TOBEC)
t. body iodide pool
t. body nitrogen
t. body potassium
t. body scan (TBS)
t. body water
t. bound (TB)
t. Ca^{2+}
t. cholesterol (TC)
t. deoxypyridinoline cross-link
t. hormone
t. intestinal calcium
t. Mg^{2+}
t. pancreatectomy
t. parathyroidectomy
t. parenteral nutrition (TPN)
t. peripheral resistance
t. renin
t. serum calcium concentration
t. T_3 (TT_3)
t. T_4 (TT_4)
t. testosterone
t. testosterone assay
t. thyroidectomy

totalis
situs inversus viscerum t.

totipotent
TouchTrak glucose sensor
toxemia of pregnancy
toxic
t. adenoma
t. calcinosis
t. delirium
t. diffuse goiter
t. epidermal necrolysis
t. multinodal goiter
t. multinodular goiter (TMG)
t. nodular goiter (TNG)
t. pemphigus foliaceus
t. porphyria
t. shock syndrome
t. solitary nodule
t. thyroid nodule (TTN)

toxicity
aluminum t.
cell-mediated t.
glucose t.
pancreatic islet beta-cell glucose t. in diabetes mellitus type 2
postprandial glucose-mediated t.

theophylline t.
tissue aluminum t.

toxicosis
T3 t.
triiodothyronine t. (T_3-toxicosis)

toxin
botulinum A t.
cholera t.
pertussis t.

toxin-induced diarrhea
toxin-sensitive
pertussis t.-s.

Toxoplasma gondii
toxoplasmosis
T-Phyl
TPN
total parenteral nutrition

TPO
thrombopoietin
thyroid peroxidase
thyroperoxidase
TPO Ab

T_3-predominant thyrotoxicosis
TPTX
thyroparathyroidectomy

TR
T_3 receptor
TR homodimer
TR monomer

TRAb
thyrotropin receptor autoantibody

trabecular
t. adenoma
t. bone
t. osteopenia
t. pattern
t. plate
t. thinning

trabecule
Trace-4
trace metal
tracer
T. Blood Glucose Micro-monitor
isotopic glucose t.
radioactive glucose t.
thyroid-specific t.
t. uptake

tracheomalacia
trachomatis
Chlamydia t.

TrackEASE glucose monitor
TR-ACP
tartrate-resistant acid phosphatase

tract
aerodigestive t.
geniculohypothalamic t. (GHT)
hypothalamohypophysial nerve t.
hypothalamoneurohypophysial t.
mammillothalamic t.

optic t.
pyramidal t.
retinohypothalamic t.
spinothalamic t.
supraopticohypophysial t.
thyroglossal t.
tuberohypophyseal t.
urinary t.
tractus solitarius
TRAF
    tumor necrosis factor receptor-associated
    factor
trafficking
    membrane t.
TRAIL
    TNF-related apoptosis inducing ligand
training
    biofeedback t.
    exertional t.
trait
    Fitzgerald t.
    Flaujeac t.
    Fujiwara t.
    monogenic Mendelian t.
    Williams t.
TRAM
    transverse rectus abdominis muscle
TRAM-1 coactivator
TRANCE
    tumor necrosis factor-related activation-
    induced cytokine
Trandate
tranexamic acid
tranexamine acid
tranquilizer
    major t.
    minor t.
trans
    t. clomiphene citrate
    t. mechanism
trans-acting factor
transactivation
    t. factor (TAF)
    t. function 1, 2
trans-activation domain (TAD)
transaminase
    alanine t.
    beta-alanine t.
    isoleucine t.
    ornithine t.
    ornithine-ketoacid t. (OKT3)

serum glutamic-oxaloacetic t.
  (SGOT)
serum glutamic-pyruvic t. (SGPT)
valine t.
transamination
transcallosal-transforaminal approach
transcaltachia
transcarbamylase
    ornithine t. (OTC)
transcatheter
    t. arterial chemoembolization
    (TACE)
    t. celiac artery embolization
transcellular
    t. fluid compartment
    t. water
transcortin
transcript
    agouti-related t.
    cocaine and amphetamine
      regulated t. (CART)
    cocaine and amphetamine-
      responsive t.
    CRH-mRNA t.
    GHRH-mRNA t.
    X-inactive specific t. (Xist)
transcriptase
    reverse t.
transcription
    gene t.
    insulin gene t.
    monoallelic t.
    parathyroid hormone gene t.
    prolactin t.
    signal transducer and activator
      of t. (STAT)
transcription-4
    signal transducer and activator
      of t.-4 (Stat4)
transcription-5
    signal transducer and activator
      of t.-4 (Stat5)
transcriptional
    t. activation
    t. cross-talk
    t. intermediary factor 2 (TIF2)
    t. silencing
transcriptome
transcutaneous oxygen pressure
transcytosis
transdermal
    Alora t.

T

NOTES

transdermal *(continued)*
    Climara t.
    Duragesic t.
    Esclim t.
    Estraderm t.
    t. estradiol
    t. estrogen
    t. hydroalcoholic gel
    t. scrotum testosterone patch
    t. testosterone delivery system
    t. torso testosterone patch
    Vivelle t.
Transderm Scop
transducer
    signal t.
transducin
transepithelial phosphate transport
transethmoidal basal encephalocele
transfect
transfection
    rearranged during t. (RET)
transfer
    embryo t. (ET)
    gamete intrafallopian t. (GIFT)
    gene t.
    insulin gene t.
    peritoneal oocyte and sperm t.
      (POST)
    placental t.
    t. ribonucleic acid (tRNA)
    in vivo insulin gene t.
    zygote intrafallopian t. (ZIFT)
transferase
    chloramphenicol acetyl t. (CAT)
    gamma glutaryl t.
    glutamyl t.
    3-oxoacid-CoA t.
    terminal deoxynucleotide t. (TdT)
    UDP-galactosyl t.
transferrin receptor
transforming
    t. growth factor (TGF)
    t. growth factor alpha (TGF-A)
    t. growth factor beta (TGF-B)
transfusion
    neonatal exchange t.
transgastric endoscopic ultrasound
transgene
    beta-cell t.
    CD4+ T-cell receptor t.
    CD8+ T-cell receptor t.
transgenic
    t. models for autoimmunity
    t. mouse model
trans-Golgi network (TGN)
transhepatic portal venous sampling
transhydrogenase
    glutathione-insulin t. (GIT)

transient
    t. amplifying cell
    t. diabetes insipidus
    t. hypoparathyroidism
    t. neonatal diabetes
    t. neonatal hypoglycemia
    t. neonatal hypothyroidism
    t. neonatal thyroid dysfunction
    t. postradioiodine hypothyroidism
    t. thyrotoxicosis
transition
    luteal-follicular t.
transjugular intrahepatic portosystemic stent shunt (TIPS)
transketolase (TRK)
translateral retroperitoneal approach
translation
translocase
    adenine nucleotide t.
    fatty acid t. (FAT)
translocation
    bacterial t.
    chromosome t.
    glucose transporter t.
    nuclear t.
    t. process
translocator
    AhR nuclear t. (ARNT)
transmembrane domain
transmeridian travel
transmission
    t. disequilibrium test (TDT)
    synaptic t.
    vertical t.
transmitter
    excitatory t.
    inhibitory t.
transmucosal
    Actiq Oral T.
    t. calcium flux
transnasal-transseptal approach
transplacental antibody
transplant
    beta cell t.
    encapsulated islet t.
    enterically drained simultaneous
      pancreas and kidney t.
    fetal pancreas t.
    islet cell t.
    renal t.
    segmental pancreas and kidney t.
    simultaneous pancreas-kidney t.
    SPK t.
transplantation
    bone-forming cell t.
    bone marrow t.
    cadaveric pancreas t.
    Center for Human Islet T.
    islet cell t.

living segmental donor pancreas t.
organ t.
orthotopic liver t.
PAK t.
pancreas after kidney t.
renal t.
segmental t.
simultaneous pancreas-kidney t.
whole-organ pancreatic t.

transport
active salt t.
beta-granule plasma membrane t.
calcium t.
cholesterol t.
glucose t.
insulin calcium t.
insulin-stimulated glucose t.
iodide t.
ionic t.
plasma membrane beta-granule t.
Pl3K-independent glucose t.
t. protein
reverse cholesterol t.
thyroid iodine t.
transepithelial phosphate t.

transporter
euthyroid brain glucose t.
facilitative glucose t.
glucose t. (GLUT)
glucose t. 1 (GLUT-1)
glucose t. 2 (GLUT-2)
glucose t. 3 (GLUT-3)
glucose t. 4 (GLUT-4)
glucose t. 5 (GLUT-5)
glucose t. 6 (GLUT-6)
glucose t. 7 (GLUT-7)
glucose t. 8 (GLUT-8)
glucose t. 9 (GLUT-9)
glucose t. 10 (GLUT-10)
glucose t. 11 (GLUT-11)
glucose t. 12 (GLUT-12)
norepinephrine t. (NET)
sodium glucose t.
thyroid iodide t.
uptake-1, -2 t.
urea t. (UT)
vesicular monoamine t. (VMAT)

transracial mapping
transrectal ultrasound measurement
trans-retinoic acid (RAR)
transscrotal testosterone delivery system

transsphenoidal
t. approach
t. bipolar forceps
t. debulking
t. encephalocele
t. hypophysectomy
t. microadenomectomy
t. microsurgical adenomectomy
t. pituitary adenomectomy
t. selective adenomectomy
t. surgery

transsulfuration
transthyretin (TTR)
t. thyroid hormone analogue complex

transthyretin-ligand complex
transudate
transurethral
t. incision of the prostate (TUIP)
t. resection of the prostate (TURP)
t. ultrasound (TRUS)
t. ureterolithotripsy (TUL)

transverse
t. arytenoid
t. rectus abdominis muscle (TRAM)
t. relaxation time
t. vaginal septum

transversus perinei superficialis muscle
TRAP
tartrate-resistant acid phosphatase

TRAP-6
thrombin receptor-activating peptide 6

trap
iodide t.
thyroid iodide t.

trapping
iodide t.
radioiodine t.

travel
transmeridian t.

TRE
negative T_3 response element
thyroid hormone-response element
thyroid response element

T_3RE
T_3 responsive element

treatment
gestagen t.
gonadal suppression t.
high-dose statin t.
Hypertensive Optimal T. (HOT)

NOTES

T

treatment *(continued)*
    multidose insulin t.
    neuraminidase t.
    pharmacologic t.
    primary adjuvant t.
    recombinant human growth
      hormone t.
    RHGH t.
tremor
    intention t.
tremulousness
trenbolone
trench
    resorption t.
Trendar
trended
TRF
    thyrotropin release factor
TRH
    thyrotropin-releasing hormone
      TRH mRNA
      Relefact TRH
      TRH stimulation test
      TRH study
TRH-DE
    TRH-degrading ectoenzyme
TRH-degrading ectoenzyme (TRH-DE)
TRH-induced refractoriness
TRH-R
    thyrotropin-releasing hormone receptor
T₄RIA
    thyroxine radioisotope assay
TRIAC
    3,5,3′-triiodothyroacetic acid
Triacin-C
triacylglycerol (TG)
triad
    Carney t.
    t. of Carney
    fragile histidine t. (FHIT)
    Whipple t.
trial
    Advicor Versus Other Cholesterol-
      Modulating Agents T.
      (ADVOCATE)
    Arterial Disease Multiple
      Intervention T.
    catch t.
    clinical t.
    Diabetes Control and
      Complications T. (DCCT)
    Diabetes Prevention T.
    EPILOG t.
    EPISTENT t.
    European Nicotinamide Diabetes
      Intervention T. (ENDIT)
    Fracture Intervention T. (FIT)
    HOPE t.
    HOT T.

    Hypertensive Optimal Treatment T.
      (HOT)
    Intranasal Insulin T. (INIT)
    Multiple Risk Factor
      Intervention T. (MRFIT)
    Postmenopausal Estrogen/Progestin
      Interventions T. (PEPI)
    Raloxifene Use for The Heart T.
    randomized control t. (RCT)
    randomized controlled t. (RCT)
    T. to Reduce Incidence of
      Diabetes in Genetically at Risk
      (TRIGR)
    RUTH T.
    Schwabing Insulin Prophylaxis T.
    Sorbinil Retinopathy T.
    Stockholm t.
    Veteran Affairs Cooperative Study
      on Glycemic Control and
      Complications in Type 2
      Diabetes T.
    Veteran Affairs HDL
      Intervention T. (VA-HIT)
    Veterans Administration Cooperative
      Study on Glycemic Control and
      Complications in Type 2
      Diabetes T.
    Women's Estrogen-Progestin Lipid-
      Lowering Hormone Atherosclerosis
      Regression T. (WELL-HART)
    Women's Estrogen for Stroke T.
    Women's Health, Osteoporosis,
      Progestin, Estrogen t.
Triam-A Injection
triamcinolone
Triam Forte Injection
Triamonide Injection
triamterene
triangle
    gastrinoma t.
    Ward t.
triangular facies
triantennary
Triax
    T. Metabolic Accelerator
    T. metabolic stimulator
tricarboxylic acid (TCA)
trichilemmoma
trichlormethiazide
Trichomonas
trichomoniasis
trichorrhexis nodosa
trichothiodystrophy
TriCor
tricuspid regurgitation
tricyanoaminopropene
Tri-Cyclen
    Ortho T.-C.
tricyclic dibenzodiazepine

tridihexethyl
trientine
trifluoroacetate salt
triflupromazine
triflutate
    corticorelin ovine t.
trifunctional pyridinium cross-link
trigeminal
    t. nerve
    t. schwannoma
trigger
    environmental t.
triglyceride
Trigonella foenum-graecum
TRIGR
    Trial to Reduce Incidence of Diabetes in
    Genetically at Risk
triiodothyronine
triiodoacetic acid
3,5,3′-triiodo-I-thyronine (T_3)
triiodo-L-thyronine
3,5,3′-triiodothyroacetic acid (**TRIAC**)
triiodothyroacetic acid
triiodothyronine (T_3)
    free t. (FT_3)
    t. monomer
    t. resin uptake (T_3RU)
    t. resin uptake test
    reverse t.
    t. serum
    t. suppression test
    t. toxicosis (T_3-toxicosis)
triiodothyronine/thyroxine ratio
Tri-Kort Injection
Trilafon
Tri-Levlen
Trilisate
Trilog Injection
Trilone Injection
trilostane
Trimazide
trimegestone
trimer
    G-protein t.
trimethadione
trimethaphan camsylate
trimethobenzamide
trimethoprim sulfamethoxazole (**TMP-SMX**)
Trimox
Tri-Norinyl

trinucleotide
triopathy
triose
    t. isomerase
    t. isomerase protein
Triostat Injection
tripeptide amide
triphasic
    t. diabetes insipidus
    t. response
Triphasil
triphenylethylene
triphosphatase
    adenosine t. (ATPase)
    guanosine t. (GTPase)
    hydrogen adenosine t. (H^+-ATPase)
    sodium-potassium adenosine t.
triphosphate
    adenosine 5′ t. (ATP)
    deoxyinosine t. (dITP)
    deoxynucleotide t. (dNTP)
    guanosine 5′ t. (GTP)
    inositol t. (IP3)
    nucleotide t.
1,4,5-triphosphate
4,5-triphosphate
    phosphatidylinositol 4,5-t. (PIP3)
triple
    t. oral combination therapy for
    type 2 diabetes mellitus
    t. response of Lewis
triple-phase scan with technetium
triploidy
TRIPOD
    Troglitazone in the Prevention of
    Diabetes
    TRIPOD study
tripyrrole
trisalicylate
    choline magnesium t.
trisilicate
    aluminum hydroxide and
    magnesium t.
Trisoject Injection
trisomy
    t. 21
    t. X mosaicism
Tri-Tannate Plus
triventricular dilation
Tri-Vi-Flor
Tri-Vi-Sol

T

NOTES

369

TRK
>transketolase
>>protooncogene TRK

TRK-A
>tyrosine receptor kinase A

TRK-B
>tyrosine receptor kinase B

tRNA
>transfer ribonucleic acid
>>tRNA mitochondrial myopathy

trochlear nerve

troglitazone
>t. monotherapy
>T. in Prevention of Diabetes (TRIPOD)

troleandomycin

tromethamine (THAM)
>ketorolac t.

tromethamine E (THAM-E)

trophectoderm
>mural t.

trophic
>t. factor
>t. hormone

trophoblast
>t. cell
>intermediate t.
>syncytial t.
>villous t.

trophoblastic
>t. cell column
>t. disease
>t. lesion
>t. neoplasm
>t. shell
>t. tissue

trophoblast-lymphocyte
>t.-l. cross-reactive (TLX)
>t.-l. cross-reactive alloantigen system

trophoblastoma

trophosphate
>guanosine t.

tropic
>t. anterior pituitary hormone
>chronic calcific pancreatitis of the t.'s (CCPT)

tropical
>t. calcific pancreatitis (TCP)
>t. diabetes mellitus

troponin C protein

Trousseau
>T. sign
>T. test

Trovert

Trovett pegvisomant

TR-RXR
>thyroid hormone receptor-retinoid X receptor
>>TR-RXR heterodimer

T₃RU

>T_3 resin uptake
>triiodothyronine resin uptake
>>T_3RU test

Tru-Cut needle

true
>t. hermaphroditism
>t. periodic biorhythm
>t. precocious puberty

truncal
>t. adiposity
>t. mononeuropathy
>t. obesity

trunk
>thyrocervical t.

TRUS
>transurethral ultrasound

Trypanosoma brucei

trypanosomiasis
>African t.

trypsin

trypsinization

trypsinogen-activating peptide (TAP)

tryptamine

tryptophan hydroxylase

TSA
>tumor-specific antigen

TSAb
>thyroid-stimulating antibody

TSBAb
>thyroid-stimulating-blocking antibody
>thyroid stimulation-blocking antibody
>TSH stimulation blocking antibody

TSC1
>tuberous sclerosis complex 1

TSC2
>tuberous sclerosis complex 2

TsF
>T-suppressor factor

TSG
>tumor-suppressor gene

TSH
>thyrotropin-stimulating hormone
>>TSH deficiency
>>inappropriate secretion of TSH
>>TSH receptor (TSH-R)
>>TSH receptor antibody measurement
>>TSH receptor autoantibody
>>TSH receptor-blocking antibody
>>TSH receptor expression
>>TSH receptor mutation
>>TSH receptor-stimulating antibody
>>recombinant human TSH (rhTSH)

TSH stimulation blocking antibody (TSBAb)

TSH stimulation test

TSH-binding

T.-b. inhibitory antibody

T.-b. inhibitory immunoglobulin (TBII)

TSH-dependent thyrotoxicosis

TSH-induced thyrotoxicosis

TSH-oma

TSH-secreting pituitary adenoma

TSH-R

thyroid-stimulating hormone receptor

thyrotropin receptor

TSH receptor

TSH-R antibody

TSH-R gene

TSHR

thyroid-stimulating hormone receptor

TSH-RAb

thyroid-stimulating hormone receptor antibody

thyroid-stimulating hormone receptor autoantibody

thyrotropin receptor-stimulating antibody

TSH-secreting

T.-s. pituitary adenoma (TSH-oma)

T.-s. pituitary tumor

TSH:T$_4$ ratio

TSI

thyroid-stimulating immunoglobulin

TSI assay

T-suppresser lymphocyte

T-suppressor factor (TsF)

TT$_3$

total T$_3$

TT$_4$

total T$_4$

t/t

Snp5 t.

TTF

thyroid transcription factor

TTF-1

thyroid transcription factor 1

TTF-2

thyroid transcription factor 2

TTN

toxic thyroid nodule

T$_3$-toxicosis

triiodothyronine toxicosis

TTR

transthyretin

T$_3$:T$_4$ ratio

T1, T2 relaxation time

TTR-ligand complex

TTR-thyroid hormone analogue complex

TTS

Estracomb TTS

Testoderm TTS

T-type calcium channel

tube

fallopian t.

gut t.

nasogastrojejunal t. (NGJT)

neural t.

uterine t.

tuber

t. cinereum

t. cinereum hamartoma

tuberalis

pars t.

tuberal region

tubercle bacillus

tuberculoma

intrasellar t.

tuberculosis

adrenal t.

miliary t.

Mycobacterium t.

pancreatic t.

V t.

tuberculous

t. endometritis

t. meningitis

t. orchitis

tuberohypophyseal

t. dopaminergic neuron (THDA)

t. tract

tuberoinfundibular

t. dopaminergic neuron (TIDA)

t. neuron

t. system

tuberous

t. sclerosis

t. sclerosis complex 1 (TSC1)

t. sclerosis complex 2 (TSC2)

t. xanthoma

tubular

t. bulbo complex

t. cristae

t. dialysis membrane

t. transport maximum (T$_m$)

t. ultrafiltrate

NOTES

T

tubule
> collecting t.
> dentinal t.
> distal convoluted t. (DCT)
> early collecting t.
> t. fluid
> late distal t.
> proximal convoluted t. (PCT)
> seminiferous t.
> sex cord tumor with annular t. (SCTAT)

tubulin
tubuli recti coalesce
tubuloalveolar salivary gland
tubuloglomerular feedback (TGF)
tubulointerstitial
> t. nephropathy
> t. renal disease

tubulovesicular mitochondria
tubulus rectus
TUIP
> transurethral incision of the prostate

TUL
> transurethral ureterolithotripsy

tumescence
> nocturnal penile t. (NPT)
> sleep-associated penile t.

tumor
> acidophilic t.
> activin-nonresponsive pituitary t.
> adenomatous t.
> alpha subunit-secreting t.
> androgen-producing t.
> brain t.
> breast t.
> Brenner t.
> brown t.
> carcinoid t.
> carcinoidlike t.
> carcinoma with thymus-like differentiation t.
> carotid body t.
> CASTLE t.
> t. cell
> chorionic gonadotropin-secreting t.
> chromophobe t.
> clinically silent t.
> corticotroph t.
> debulking of t.
> deoxycorticosterone-producing t.
> dumbbell-shaped t.
> ectopic ACTH-secreting t.
> ectopic neuroendocrine t.
> endocrine t.
> endodermal sinus t.
> endo-exocrine t.
> endometrioid t.
> enterohepatic t.
> estrogen-producing t.

> extragonadal germ cell t. (EGGCT)
> t. flare
> germ-cell t. (GCT)
> GHRH-secreting t.
> giant cell t.
> glial t.
> glioneural t.
> glomus jugulare t.
> glucagon-producing t.
> glucagon-secreting t.
> glycoprotein-secreting pituitary t.
> gonadotropin-secreting t.
> granular cell t.
> granulosa cell t.
> granulosa-theca cell t.
> growth hormone-producing t.
> growth hormone-releasing hormone-secreting t.
> growth hormone-secreting pituitary t.
> gsp-positive somatotroph t.
> Hardy classification of pituitary t.
> hepatic t.
> hepatocellular t.
> hormone receptor-negative t.
> hormone receptor-positive t.
> hormone-secreting adrenal t.
> hormone-secreting pituitary t.
> Hürthle cell t.
> hypothalamic t.
> hypothalamic-pituitary t.
> hypovascular islet cell t.
> islet cell t.
> lactotroph t.
> large cell calcifying Sertoli cell t.
> Leydig cell t.
> lipid t.
> lipid-containing t.
> lipoid cell t.
> luteinizing hormone-secreting t.
> t. lysis syndrome
> malignant islet cell t.
> malignant peripheral nerve sheath t. (MPNST)
> mesenchymal t.
> t. metastasis
> metastatic t.
> mixed phenotype t.
> Mostofi classification of testicular t.
> mucinous cystic t.
> t. necrosis factor (TNF)
> t. necrosis factor-alpha (TNF-alpha)
> t. necrosis factor-beta (TNF-beta)
> t. necrosis factor gene
> t. necrosis factor receptor (TNFR)
> t. necrosis factor receptor-associated factor (TRAF)

t. necrosis factor-related activation-
induced cytokine (TRANCE)
neural t.
neuroendocrine t.
nonaggressive t.
nonbeta cell t.
nonfunctioning pituitary t.
nongerminomatous germ cell t.
(NGGCT)
non-islet cell t.
nonsecreting pituitary t.
oncocytic t.
optic tract pituitary t.
osteoblastic t.
ovarian t.
pancreatic alpha-cell t.
pancreatic endocrine t.
pancreatic islet cell t.
pancreatic polypeptide-secreting t.
(PPoma)
paraneoplastic t.
parasellar t.
pineal t.
pituitary t.
prolactin-producing pituitary t.
prolactin-secreting pituitary t.
t. receptor status
recurrent pituitary t.
t. removal
residual pituitary t.
retinoblastoma t.
sellar t.
serous t.
Sertoli cell testicular t.
Sertoli-Leydig cell t.
sex cord stromal t.
small-volume pituitary t.
solid cystic t. (SCT)
solid pseudopapillary t.
somatotroph t.
sporadic thyroid t.
steroid-dependent t.
t. suppressor
suprasellar germ cell t.
testicular Leydig cell t.
thyroid neuroendocrine t.
thyroid-stimulating hormone-secreting
pituitary t.
thyrotropin-secreting pituitary t.
TSH-secreting pituitary t.
urothelial t.

vasoactive intestinal peptide-
secreting t. (VIPoma)
vasoactive intestinal polypeptide-
secreting t.
VIP-secreting t.
Wilms t.
Wilms t. 1 (WTI)
t. xenograft model
yolk sac t.
tumoral calcinosis
tumor-associated hypoglycemia
tumor-derived endothelium
tumor-forming pancreatitis
tumorigenesis
adrenocortical t.
colorectal t.
Knudson two-hit model of t.
pituitary t.
thyroid t.
tumorigenic
tumorigenicity
tumor-induced osteomalacia syndrome
tumorlet
tumor-like calcification
tumor/node/metastases (TNM)
tumor/node/metastases classification
tumor-reduction surgery
tumor-specific antigen (TSA)
tumor-suppressor gene (TSG)
tunica
t. media
t. vaginalis
turbid fluid
turcica
bridged sella t.
sella t.
Turkish saddle
Turner
T. mosaicism
T. stigma
T. syndrome
turnover
bone t.
iron t.
water t.
whole-body protein t.
TURP
transurethral resection of the prostate
turtle TG
Tussin
Diabetic T.

NOTES

TWEAK
TNF-weak homologue
twin study
two-cell system
two-day high-dose dexamethasone suppression test
two-site sandwich immunoassay
TX
thromboxane
TXA2, TxA2
thromboxane A2
TXB2, TxB2
thromboxane B2
Tyk-2
tyrosine kinase-2
Ty-Pap
type
t. A, B, C syndrome of insulin resistance
activin cell-surface receptor t. I, II
t. A dark spermatogonia
t. 1A diabetes mellitus autoimmunity
t. Ad spermatogonia
t. 1, 2 angioneurotic edema
apolipoprotein t. 3
t. Ap spermatogonia
t. A spermatogonia
t. A syndrome
t. 1 autosomal recessive vitamin D dependency (ARVDD-1)
11-beta-hydroxysteroid dehydrogenase t. 1 (11-beta-HSD1)
11-beta-hydroxysteroid dehydrogenase t. 2 (11-beta-HSD2)
t. B extreme insulin resistance syndrome
t. B spermatogonia
t. 1 deiodinase (D1)
t. 2 deiodinase (D2)
t. 3 deiodinase (D3)
t. 1, 2 diabetes
t. 1 diabetes mellitus
t. 2 diabetes mellitus (T2DM)
t. 1 diabetes mellitus autoantigen
t. 2 diabetes mellitus autoimmunity
t. 1 diabetes mellitus combination autoantibody assays
t. 2 diabetes mellitus lifestyle
t. 1 diabetes mellitus twin study
T. 1 Diabetes Prediction and Prevention Study (DIPP)
differentiated thyroid carcinoma, intermediate t.
distal renal tubular acidosis t. 4
dystonia t. 1
t. 2 energy pathway

familial multiple endocrine neoplasia t. 1
t. 1, 2 fiber
t. 1, 2, 3 gastric carcinoid
t. 2 helper T-cell cytokine
t. I collagen C-terminal telopeptide
t. I collagen heterotrimer
t. II autoimmune polyglandular syndrome
t. III hyperlipoproteinemia
t. I, II, IV, V congenital adrenal hyperplasia
t. I, II, IX, X collagen
t. III selenoenzyme
t. II multiple endocrine glandular failure
t. II muscle fiber
t. II muscle fiber atrophy
t. II vitamin D dependency rickets
insulin growth factor-binding protein t. 1–6
t. I procollagen
t. IV glycogen storage disease
t. IV hyperlipidemia
t. I von Willebrand disease
melanocortin receptor t. 4 (MCAR)
5′-monodeiodinase t. I
polyglandular autoimmune syndrome t. I (PGA-I)
t. 1 polyglandular syndrome
t. 1 procollagen peptide
t. pseudohypoaldosteronism
pseudohypoaldosteronism t. II (PHA II)
t. I regulatory dimer (RI)
t. II regulatory dimer (RII)
t. 4 RTA
Waardenburg syndrome t. I
typhi
Salmonella t.
typing
HLA allele molecular t.
tyramine
tyropanoate
tyrosinase
tyrosine
t. aminotransferase
t. aminotransferase enzyme
diiodinated t. (DIT)
t. hydroxylase
t. kinase
t. kinase-2 (Tyk-2)
t. kinase activity
t. kinase domain of insulin receptor
monoiodinated t. (MIT)
peptide tyrosine t.
t. phosphorylation
t. phosphorylation site

t. receptor kinase A (TRK-A)
t. receptor kinase B (TRK-B)
tyrosinemia
    t. I
    t. II

tyrosinosis
tyrosyl residue
TZD
    thiazolidinedione
T- and Z- scores of bone mass

NOTES

T

U
Humulin U

U-100
unit of insulin

U-500
Regular (Concentrated) Iletin II U.

UB
ultimobranchial body

ubiquinone

ubiquitin
u. fusion degradation 1 gene
u. mechanism

ubiquitin-proteasome pathway
ubiquitin/proteasome system
ubiquitinylated protein
Uchida
U. method
U. technique

UCP
uncoupling protein

UCP1
uncoupling protein 1

UDCA
ursodeoxycholic acid

UDP-galactosyl transferase
UFC
urine free cortisol

uFSH
urinary FSH

UGDP
University Group Diabetes Program

UGP
urinary gonadotropin peptide

UICC
Union Internationale Contre le Cancer

UKPDS
United Kingdom Prospective Diabetes
Study

ulcer
diabetic u.
foot u.
necrotic palatal u.
neuropathic u.
perforating u.

ulceration
corneal u.

Ulcogant
ulcus cruris
Ullrich syndrome
ulnar-mammary syndrome
ultimobranchial
u. body (UB)
u. gland
u. organ

ultra
LifeScan U.
U. Mide Topical

ultradian
u. oscillation
u. rhythm

ultrafiltrate
salivary u.
tubular u.

ultrafiltration
extracorporeal u.
u. rate

Ultralente insulin
Ultram
Ultrase MT
ultrasensitive
ultrashort-loop feedback
ultrasonography (US)
color Doppler u. (CDU)
color duplex u.

ultrasound
endoscopic u.
intraductal u. (IDUS)
intraoperative u. (IOUS)
u. mammography
parathyroid u.
pulsed Doppler u.
thyroid u.
transgastric endoscopic u.
transurethral u. (TRUS)

ultrastructural feature
ultrastructure
osteoclast u.

UltraSure DTU-one ultrasound scanner
ultrathin pancreatoscope
UltraTLC adjustable lancing device
ultraviolet (UV)
unawareness
hypoglycemia u.

unci (*pl. of* uncus)
uncompensated metabolic acidosis
uncoupling
u. protein (UCP)
u. protein 1 (UCP1)

uncus, pl. **unci**
undecenoate
testosterone u.

undercalcified bone
underfunction
pregnancy thyroid u.

underpneumatization
undervirilized
u. fertile male syndrome
u. male

underwater body weight

U

undifferentiated
>u. pattern
>u. sarcoma

UNE
>unopposed estrogen

unesterified arachidonic acid
unexplained microcytic anemia
unformed visual hallucination
Uni-Ace
Unicap
Unicelles
>Melfiat-105 U.

unilateral
>u. adrenal disease
>u. adrenalectomy
>u. aldosterone excess
>u. aldosterone-producing adenoma
>u. APA
>u. lobectomy
>u. renal agenesis
>u. salpingo-oophorectomy

uniloculate
uninodular goiter
union
>anomalous pancreaticobiliary u.
>U. Internationale Contre le Cancer (UICC)

uniparental disomy
Uniphyl
Uniplant contraceptive implant
Uni-Pro
unit
>basic multicellular u. (BMU)
>bone structural u.
>fetoplacental u.
>gamma u.
>granulocyte-macrophage colony-forming u. (GM-CFU)
>hormone response u. (HRU)
>u. of insulin (U-100)
>international u. (IU)

united
>U. Kingdom Prospective Diabetes Study (UKPDS)
>U. Network for Organ Sharing (UNOS)

Unithroid
Unitrol
universal
>u. gas constant
>u. pacemaker
>u. salt iodization (USI)
>u. screening

universalis
>calcinosis u.

university
>U. Group Diabetes Program (UGDP)

>U. of Wisconsin (UW)
>U. of Wisconsin solution

unliganded thyroid hormone receptor
unmineralized lamellar osteoid
unmutated receptor
unmyelinated nerve fiber
unopposed estrogen (UNE)
UNOS
>United Network for Organ Sharing

unresponsiveness
>hypoglycemia u.

unsaturated fatty acid
Unschuld sign
unstable
>u. Cushing disease
>u. diabetes

5′-untranslated region (UTR)
untranslated region (UTR)
upper
>u. clivus
>u. pole of spleen
>u. pretracheal node

upregulate
upregulation
upright plasma renin
Uprima
uptake
>bromodeoxyuridine u.
>calcium u.
>elevated radioactive iodine u.
>fluorodeoxyglucose u.
>glucose u.
>hepatic free fatty acid u.
>insulin-mediated glucose u.
>leg glucose u. (LGU)
>L-triiodothyronine u.
>net hepatic glucose u. (NHGU)
>radioactive iodine u. (RAIU)
>radiofluoride u.
>radioiodine u. (RAIU)
>radiostrontium u.
>resin u.
>splanchine glucose u.
>thyroglobulin cellular u.
>thyroid radioiodine u.
>thyroid technetium pertechnetate u.
>tracer u.
>T_3 resin u. (T_3RU)
>triiodothyronine resin u. (T_3RU)

uptake-1, -2 transporter
Urabeth
Uracel
uranium
urate
>amorphous u.
>u. nephropathy
>u. salt

urate-hydroxyl exchanger
urate-lactate exchanger

urea
  u. cycle
  u. cycle enzyme
  interstitial u.
  u. recycling
  u. transporter (UT)
Ureacin-20 Topical
ureagenesis
  inherited disorder of u.
urealyticum
  Ureaplasma u.
Ureaphil Injection
Ureaplasma urealyticum
urease
  enzyme u.
Urecholine
uremia
uremic
  u. diabetic patient
  u. metabolic acidosis
  u. osteodystrophy
  u. pruritus
  u. pseudodiabetes
ureter
ureterolithotomy
ureterolithotripsy
  transurethral u. (TUL)
ureteropelvic junction
ureterosigmoidoscopy
ureterovesical junction
urethra
  internal u.
  membranous u.
  penile u.
  prostatic u.
urethral gland
urethritis
urethrocystoscopy
uric
  u. acid
  u. acid crystal
  u. acid renal stone
uricase method
uricemia
uricosuric agent
uridine
  u. 5'-diphosphate
  u. diphosphate glucose
urinary
  u. calcium
  u. concentrating mechanism
  u. creatinine

  u. drainage
  u. follicle-stimulating hormone
  u. free cortisol
  u. FSH (uFSH)
  u. genistein excretion
  u. glucose
  u. gonadotropin peptide (UGP)
  u. 17-hydroxycorticosteroid
  u. hydroxyproline
  u. hydroxyproline excretion
  u. iodine/thiocyanate ratio
  u. 17-ketosteroid
  u. N-telopeptide collagen cross-link
  u. paraaminobutyric acid excretion
  rate
  u. phosphoethanolamine
  u. potassium wasting
  u. pyridinoline cross-link excretion
  u. retention
  u. stasis
  u. tract
  u. tract infection
urine
  u. aldosterone
  clean-catch u.
  u. collection
  u. concentration
  fractional u.
  u. free cortisol (UFC)
  u. glucose level
  u. hydroxyproline level
  hypotonic u.
  u. osmolality
  u. output
  u. pH
  u. phosphorus excretion
  u. steroid
  u. testing
urinometer
Urispas
urochrome
  pigment u.
urocortin fiber
urodilatin
uroerythrin
urofollitropin
urogenital
  u. diaphragm
  u. fold
  u. ridge
  u. sinus
  u. system

U

NOTES

urogenitogram
urography
> intravenous u.

urokinase plasminogen activator
urokinase-type plasminogen activator
Urolen blue
urolithiasis
uropontin
urotensin I–IV
urothelial tumor
ursodeoxycholic acid (UDCA)
urticaria pigmentosa
US
> ultrasonography

use
> side-effect profile of u.

USI
> universal salt iodization

USP
> uterine-stimulating potency

UT
> urea transporter

uteri (*pl. of* uterus)
uterine
> u. activity rhythm
> u. arcuate artery
> u. contractile activity
> u. contractile rhythm
> u. endometrium
> u. gland

> u. leiomyoma
> u. milk
> u. rhythmicity
> u. tetany
> u. tube

uterine-endocrine system
uterine-stimulating potency (USP)
utero
> in u.

uteroglobin antibody
uteroplacental blood flow
uterotonin
uterus, pl. **uteri**
> cervix u.
> corpus u.
> isthmus u.

utilization
> peripheral glucose u. (PGU)

UTR
> untranslated region
> 5′-untranslated region

utricle
> prostatic u.

UV
> ultraviolet

uveal coloboma
UW
> University of Wisconsin
> UW solution

V
- annexin V
- V tuberculosis

vaccine
- bacillus Calmette-Guérin v.
- BCG v.
- Heptavax-B v.
- pneumococcal v.
- 7-valent v.

vaccinia virus growth factor
vacor
Vaculance
- Microlet V.

vacuole
- secretory v.

vacuolization
- marrow cell v.

vacuum
- v. constrictive device
- v. tumescence device

vagal
- v. afferent
- v. neural crest
- v. nucleus
- v. stimulation

Vagifem 17B
vagina, pl. **vaginae**
vaginal
- v. candidiasis
- Cleocin V.
- v. fornix
- Ogen V.
- v. ring
- v. smear

vaginalis
- *Gardnerella v.*
- portio v.
- processus v.
- tunica v.

vaginitis
- atrophic v.
- candidal v.

vaginoplasty
vagotomy
vagus nerve
VA-HIT
- Veteran Affairs HDL Intervention Trial

Val-A3-Leu
valence
7-valent vaccine
valerate
- 17-beta-estradiol v.

Valertest No. 1
valgum
- genu v.

valgus
- cubitus v.

valine transaminase
valproic acid
value
- consciousness osmolarity v.
- insulin surrogate v.
- predictive v.
- single-serum dehydroepiandrosterone sulfate v.

Vamate Oral
VAMP
- vesicle-associated membrane protein

van
- v. Buchem disease
- v. den Bergh test
- v. Heuven anatomic classification of diabetic retinopathy

vanadate
- GLUT-4 v.

vanadium
Vancocin
- V. Injection
- V. Oral

Vancoled Injection
vancomycin
vanillylmandelic acid (VMA)
VANIQA cream
vanishing testis syndrome
Vaponefrin
vardenafil
variable
- v. number of tandem repeat (VNTR)
- v. number of tandem repeat markers

variant
- antenatal-hypercalciuric v.
- Burin v.
- fertile eunuch v.
- hypocalciuric-hypomagnesemic v.
- oncocytic v.
- salt-wasting hydroxylase deficiency v.
- simple virilizing hydroxylase deficiency v.

variation
- circadian v.

varicella zoster
varices (*pl. of* varix)
varicocele testis
varicosity
- neurophysin-positive v.

Varidase
varix, pl. **varices**

V

varum
>genu v.

vas, pl. **vasa**
>v. deferens
>vasa nervorum
>vasa recta

vascular
>v. calcification
>v. cell adhesion molecule-1 (VCAM-1)
>v. cell biology
>v. compliance
>v. element
>v. endocrine protein
>v. endothelial cell growth inhibitor (VEGI)
>v. endothelial growth factor (VEGF)
>v. inflammation
>v. injury
>v. permeability factor (VPF)
>v. remodeling
>v. resistance
>v. smooth muscle cell (VSMC)
>v. steal syndrome
>v. thrombosis

vasculitis
>systemic v.

vasculopathy
>aldosterone diabetic v.
>diabetic v.

vasculosum
>organum v.

vasculosyncytial membrane
vasectomy
vasoactive
>v. intestinal peptide (VIP)
>v. intestinal peptide receptor
>v. intestinal peptide-secreting tumor (VIPoma)
>v. intestinal polypeptide (VIP)
>v. intestinal polypeptide-secreting tumor

vasoconstricting factor
vasoconstriction
vasodepressor drug therapy
vasodilating factor
vasodilation
>beta-adrenergic v.
>cutaneous v.

vasodilator
>v. peptide
>v. prostaglandin

vasomotor flush
vasopressin
>arginine v. (AVP)
>desamino D-arginine v. (DDAVP)
>1-desamino-8-d arginine v.
>v. excess

>lysine v.
>v. neurophysin II
>v. receptor (V2R)
>v. resistance syndrome

vasopressinase
>placental v.

vasopressinergic fiber
vasopressor
vasospasm
>digital v.
>painless cold-sensitive digital v.

vasotocin
>arginine v. (AVT)

Vasoxyl
VCAM-1
>vascular cell adhesion molecule-1

VDAC
>voltage-dependent anion channel

VDCC
>voltage-dependent calcium channel

VDDR
>pseudovitamin D deficiency rickets

VDDR-II
>vitamin D-dependent rickets type II

VDR
>vitamin D receptor

VDRE
>vitamin D-response element

vector
>adeno-associated virus v.
>adenovirus v.
>baculovirus v.
>liposome v.
>nonviral v.
>oncoretrovirus v.
>retroviral v.
>viral v.

vectorial sum
vegetative
VEGF
>vascular endothelial growth factor

VEGI
>vascular endothelial cell growth inhibitor

vein
>adrenal v.
>emissary v.
>hepatic v.
>innominate v.
>internal jugular v. (IJV)
>percutaneous femoral v.
>portal v.
>splenic v. (SPV)
>superior mesenteric v. (SMV)
>suprasellar v.

vellus hair
velocardiofacial syndrome
velocimetry
>Doppler v.

velocity
    falling height v.
    growth v. (GV)
    nerve conduction v.
    sensory nerve conduction v.
    sperm v.
Velosulin
    V. BR
    V. BR insulin
velum interpositum
venlafaxine
venography
venous
    v. beading
    v. ovarian plasma progesterone
    v. sampling
    v. telangiectasia
    v. thromboembolic disease
    v. thromboembolism (VTE)
ventilatory
    v. control
    v. drive
    v. support
Ventolin Rotocaps
ventral adrenergic bundle
ventricle
    anteroventral 3rd v. (AV3V)
    third v.
ventricular
    v. fibrillation
    v. myxoma
    v. region
    v. septal defect (VSD)
    v. tachycardia
ventriculomegaly
ventriculoperitoneal shunt
ventrolateral medulla
ventromedial
    v. nucleus (VMN)
    v. nucleus of the hypothalamus
    (VMN)
vera
    polycythemia v.
veralipride
verapamil
v-*erb* A oncogene
vermis
    cerebellar v.
Verner-Morrison syndrome
vernix
verrucosity
verrucous vulgaris

Versaflow peristatic pump
versicolor
    tinea v.
vertebra, pl. **vertebrae**
    codfish v.
    rugger jersey appearance of v.
vertebral venous plexus
vertical
    v. banded gastroplasty
    v. ring gastroplasty
    v. transmission
verticis
    cutis v.
vertigo
very
    v. long chain acyl-CoA
    dehydrogenase (VLCAD)
    v. long chain acyl-CoA
    dehydrogenase deficiency
    v. low birth weight (VLBW)
    v. low calorie diet
    v. low density lipoprotein (VLDL)
    v. low density lipoprotein C
    (VLDL-C)
    v. low density lipoprotein fraction
vesica, pl. **vesicae**
    sphincter vesicae
vesicle
    acrosomal v.
    aldehyde-thionin-positive v.
    chromaffin v.
    clathrin-coated v.
    matrix v.
    phospholipid v.
    pinocytic v.
    secretory v.
    seminal v.
    sequestered v.
    synaptic v.
vesicle-associated membrane protein
(VAMP)
vesicular
    v. follicle
    v. monoamine transporter (VMAT)
Vesprin
vessel
    endoneurial blood v.
    epineurial blood v.
    extrahypophyseal portal v.
    hypothalamic-hypophyseal portal v.
    intrahypophyseal portal v.

V

NOTES

vessel *(continued)*
    neurosecretory v.
    tortuous blood v.
vestibule
vestibulum, pl. **vestibuli**
    bulbus vestibuli
veteran
    V. Affairs Cooperative Study on
    Glycemic Control and
    Complications in Type 2 Diabetes
    Trial
    V. Affairs HDL Intervention Trial
    (VA-HIT)
    V.'s Administration Cooperative
    Study on Glycemic Control and
    Complications in Type 2 Diabetes
    Trial
V-gene family
VHL
    von Hippel-Lindau
    VHL disease
    VHL tumor suppressor gene
Viagra
vibration
    v. perception testing
    v. threshold
vibratory sensation
Vibrio
    V. cholerae
    V. vulnificus
vibrios
    marine v.
Vicon-C
Vicon Plus
vidarabine therapy
vide infra
villous
    v. cytotrophoblast
    v. hypertrichosis
    v. trophoblast
villus, pl. **villi**
    chorionic v.
    primary v.
    secondary v.
    tertiary chorionic v.
Vim-Silverman needle
vinblastine
vincristine
vinculum, pl. **vincula**
vinpocetine
Viokase
violaceous stria
viosterol
Vioxx
VIP
    vasoactive intestinal peptide
    vasoactive intestinal polypeptide
    VIP receptor

VIPoma
    vasoactive intestinal peptide-secreting
    tumor
VIP-secreting tumor
viral
    v. infection
    v. oncogene
    v. orchitis
    v. vector
Virchow-Robin
    V.-R. space
    subarachnoid space of V.-R.
virilism
virilization
    systemic v.
virilized external genitalia
virilizer
    simple v.
virilizing adrenal syndrome
Virilon
virulence
virus
    adeno-associated v. (AAV)
    avian myeloblastosis v. (AMV)
    bovine viral diarrhea mucosal
    disease v.
    BVD-MD v.
    canine distemper v.
    EMC v.
    encephalomyocarditis v.
    Epstein-Barr v. (EBV)
    hepatitis A v.
    herpes simplex v. (HSV)
    human immunodeficiency v. (HIV)
    lymphadenopathy-associated v.
    (LAV)
    lymphocytic choriomeningitis v.
    (LCMV)
    mammary tumor v. (MTV)
    Mengo v.
    mumps v.
    myeloproliferative leukemia v.
    (MPLV)
    respiratory syncytial v.
    rubella v.
    SV40 v.
virus-induced diabetes
viscera *(pl. of* viscus*)*
visceral
    v. calcification
    v. fat accumulation
    v. obesity
visceromegaly
viscous
    v. colloid
    v. dietary fiber
viscus, pl. **viscera**
Visidex II

vision
    color v.
Vistacon-50 Injection
Vistaquel Injection
Vistaril
    V. Injection
    V. Oral
Vistazine Injection
visual
    v. acuity
    v. examination
    v. field assessment
    v. field defect
    v. field disturbance
    v. hallucination
    v. loss
    v. outcome
visual-evoked potential
visualization
    panoramic v.
visuotopic
Vita-C
vital
    v. capacity
    v. red
    v. staining
vitamin
    v. A
    v. A_2
    v. A_1
    v. A, D intoxication
    v. B_6
    v. B_x
    v. B_c
    v. B complex
    v. B complex with vitamin C
    v. B complex with vitamin C and folic acid
    v. C drops
    v. D
    v. D_1
    v. D_2
    v. D_3
    v. D analog
    v. D-binding globulin
    v. D-binding protein (DBP)
    v. D-binding protein macrophage-activating factor
    v. D-deficiency osteomalacia
    v. D-dependent rickets type II (VDDR-II)
    v. D effect

    v. D endocrine system
    v. D end-organ resistance
    v. D 24-hydroxylase (24-OHase)
    v. D metabolite
    v. D receptor (VDR)
    v. D receptor deficiency
    v. D-regulatory element
    v. D-replete child
    v. D-resistant rickets
    v. D-response element (VDRE)
    v. D sterol
    v. E
    v. F
    v. G
    v. H
    injectable multiple v.
    v. K_1
    v. K_2
    v. K_5
    v. K_6
    v. K_7
    v. L
    v. L_1
    v. L_2
    v. M
    oral multiple v.
    v. P
    pediatric multiple v.
    v. PP
    prenatal multiple v.
    v. T
    v. U
Vita-Plus E Softgels
Vitec
vitelline circulation
vitiligo
vitreal lysis
vitrectomy
    pars plana v.
vitreous hemorrhage
vitro
    in v.
vitronectin receptor
Vivelle transdermal
vivo
    in v.
VLBW
    very low birth weight
VLCAD
    very long chain acyl-CoA dehydrogenase
VLDL
    very low density lipoprotein

NOTES

VLDL *(continued)*
VLDL cholesterol/total triglyceride ratio
VLDL fraction
VLDL-C
very low density lipoprotein C
VMA
vanillylmandelic acid
VMAT
vesicular monoamine transporter
VMN
ventromedial nucleus
ventromedial nucleus of the hypothalamus
v-mpl protein
VNTR
variable number of tandem repeat
VNTR markers
vocal
v. cord disorder
v. cord paralysis
voglibose
Volkmann canal
Vollman cycle
voltage-dependent
v.-d. anion channel (VDAC)
v.-d. calcium channel (VDCC)
voltage-gated
v.-g. Ca^{2+} channel
v.-g. K^+ channel
v.-g. Na^+ channel
voltage gradient
voltammetric microelectrode
Voltaren Oral
Voltaren-XR Oral
volume
v. assessment
blood v.
v. depletion
effective circulating v.
end-systolic v.
extracellular fluid v. (EFV)
goiter v.
intravascular v.
liver v.
v. receptor
relative osteoid v.
sellar v.
spleen v.
testicular v.

thyroid v.
total blood v.
vomer
vomeronasal organ
vomerosphenoidal articulation
von
v. Basedow disease
v. Gierke disease
v. Graefe sign
v. Hippel-Lindau (VHL)
v. Hippel-Lindau disease
v. Hippel-Lindau syndrome
v. Hippel-Lindau tumor-suppressor gene
v. Recklinghausen disease
v. Recklinghausen disease of bone
v. Willebrand disease
v. Willebrand factor (vWF)
VP-16
VPF
vascular permeability factor
V2R
vasopressin receptor
V_1 receptor
V_{1b} receptor
V_{1a} receptor
V_2 receptor
VSD
ventricular septal defect
v-*sis* transforming gene
VSMC
vascular smooth muscle cell
VTE
venous thromboembolism
vulgaris
pemphigus v.
verrucous v.
vulnificus
Vibrio v.
vulva, pl. **vulvae**
hypoplastic v.
vulvitis
candidal v.
vulvodynia
vulvovaginal candidiasis
vulvovestibulitis
vWF
von Willebrand factor
Vytone

Waardenburg syndrome type I
waddling gait
WAGR
    Wilms tumor-aniridia-genital anomalies-mental retardation syndrome
WAI
    wheat amylase inhibitor
Waist It pump holder
waist-to-hip circumference ratio (WHR)
Wakayama
    insulin W.
walking
    repetitive stress of w.
wallerian degeneration
Warburg apparatus
Ward triangle
warfarin therapy
warm nodule
Warthin-like papillary carcinoma
Wassermann test
wasting
    cerebral salt w.
    w. disease
    nitrogen w.
    renal calcium w.
    renal phosphate w.
    renal sodium w.
    salt w.
    sodium w.
    w. syndrome
    urinary potassium w.
WAT
    white adipose tissue
watch
    sugar w.
water
    w. balance
    body w.
    w. composition
    w. deprivation
    w. deprivation test
    w. deprivation testing
    w. diuresis
    w. homeostasis
    w. intoxication
    w. metabolism
    w. restriction test
    total body w.
    transcellular w.
    w. turnover
Waterhouse-Friderichsen syndrome
water-soluble hormone

watery
    w. diarrhea, hypokalemia, achlorhydria (WDHA)
    w. diarrhea syndrome
waxy skin
WBC
    white blood cell
WBS
    whole-body scanning
w/C
    Aprodine w/C
w/Codeine
    Allerfrin w/C.
WDHA
    watery diarrhea, hypokalemia, achlorhydria
    WDHA syndrome
weakness
    muscular w.
    proximal muscle w.
web
    metabolic w.
webbed neck
wedge
    mucoid w.
Wegener granulomatosis
weight
    body w.
    desirable body w.
    F glucosidase inhibitor and body w.
    w. gain
    w. loss
    low birth w. (LBW)
    underwater body w.
    very low birth w. (VLBW)
weight-loss medicine
WELL-HART
    Women's Estrogen-Progestin Lipid-Lowering Hormone Atherosclerosis Regression Trial
Werdnig-Hoffman syndrome
Werner syndrome
Wernicke encephalopathy
Wernicke-Korsakoff syndrome
WESDR
    Wisconsin Epidemiologic Study of Diabetic Retinopathy
Western
    W. blot
    W. blot analysis
wet keratin
Wharton jelly
wheal and flare response
wheat amylase inhibitor (WAI)

W

Whickham survey
Whipple
    W. disease
    W. triad
    W. triad criteria
    W. trial of insulinoma
white
    w. adipose tissue (WAT)
    w. blood cell (WBC)
    W. classification
    W. classification of diabetes
    mellitus
    w. muscle
    w. ramus
Whitehall Study
WHO
    World Health Organization
    WHO class 1, 2, 3 anovulation
    WHO classification system
    WHO (type I, II, III)
whole-body
    w.-b. counter
    w.-b. ^{131}I-MIBG study
    w.-b. protein turnover
    w.-b. radioiodine scan
    w.-b. scanning (WBS)
    w.-b. scintigraphy
whole-cell K_{ATP} beta-cell
whole-genome association study
whole-organ pancreatic transplantation
WHR
    waist-to-hip circumference ratio
    WHR ratio
widened
    w. cranial structure
    w. palpebral fissure
    w. pulse pressure
wide osteoid seam
widespread xanthoma
width
    capillary basement membrane w.
    (CBMW)
wild-type
    w.-t. K-ras gene
    w.-t. receptor
Williams
    W. syndrome
    W. trait
Williams-Beuren syndrome
Wilms
    W. lung
    W. tumor
    W. tumor 1 (WTI)
    W. tumor-aniridia-genital anomalies-
    mental retardation syndrome
    (WAGR)
    W. tumor 1 gene
    W. tumor 1 transcription factor

Wilson
    W. disease
    W. syndrome
Wilson-Turner syndrome
winged
    w. helix family
    w. scapulae
Winpred
Winstrol
Wisconsin
    W. Epidemiologic Study of
    Diabetic Retinopathy (WESDR)
    modified University of W. (mUW)
    original University of W. (oUW)
    University of W. (UW)
Wiskott-Aldrich syndrome
Wnt protein
Wnt/Wingless signaling pathway
Wolcott-Rallison syndrome
Wolff-Chaikoff effect
wolffian
    w. duct
    w. system
Wolf-Hirschhorn syndrome
Wolfram syndrome
Wolman disease
woman
    eumenorrheic hirsute w.
    normoprolactinemic w.
Women
    Brief Index of Sexual Functioning
    for W.
Women's
    W. Estrogen-Progestin Lipid-
    Lowering Hormone Atherosclerosis
    Regression Trial (WELL-HART)
    W. Estrogen for Stroke Trial
    W. Health, Osteoporosis, Progestin,
    Estrogen trial
workup
    metabolic stone w.
world
    W. Health Organization (WHO)
    W. Health Organization Expert
    Committee on Diabetes
    classification system
    W. Health Organization (type I, II,
    III)
worm
    biliary w.
wormian bone
Wortmannin
wound
    w. dehiscence
    w. healing
woven
    w. bone
    w. osteoid

WTI
   Wilms tumor 1

WTI   gene
WTI   transcription factor

NOTES

X

    X body
    X chromatin
    X chromosome to autosome (X:A)
    X chromosome to autosome ratio
      (X:A ratio)
    X chromosome inactivation
    disseminated histiocytosis X
    histiocytosis X
    X inactivation center (Xic)
    X pacemaker
    X zone

X:A

    X chromosome to autosome
    X:A ratio

xanthelasma, pl. **xanthelasmata**
xanthine oxidase deficiency
xanthinuria
xanthochromic fluid
xanthoma, pl. **xanthomata**

    x. disseminatum
    eruptive x.
    x. homogenate
    palmar xanthomata
    planar x.
    tendinous x.
    tendon x.
    tuberous x.
    widespread x.

xanthomatosis

    aggressive x.
    cerebrotendinous x.

X-body
X-chromosome

    adhesion molecule-like from
      the X.-c. (ADMLX)
    X.-c. linkage

Xe

    xenon

¹³³Xe

    xenon-133

Xenical
XeniCare program
xenobiotic chemical
xenobiotic-response element (XRE)
xenogeneic
xenogenic
xenograft

    islet x.

xenografting
xenon (Xe)
xenon-133 (¹³³Xe)

    w. washout study

Xenopus

    X. laevis
    X. oocyte expression assay

xenorexia
xenotransplantation
xenotropic
xeroderma

    x. pigmentosa
    x. pigmentosa/Cockayne syndrome

xerophthalmia
xeroradiography
xerostomia
45,X gonadal dysgenesis
Xic

    X inactivation center

X-inactivation
X-inactive specific transcript (Xist)
xiphoid
Xist

    X-inactive specific transcript
    Xist gene

XL

    Glucotrol XL
    Lodine XL

XL-alpha protein
XL-alpha-s exon
XLH

    X-linked hypophosphatemia
    XLH rickets

X-linked

    X-l. diabetes insipidus
    X-l. dominant pedigree
    X-l. hydrocephalus
    X-l. hypohidrotic ectodermal
      dysplasia
    X-l. hypophosphatemia (XLH)
    X-l. ichthyosis
    X-l. immunodeficiency syndrome
    X-l. inheritance
    X-l. lymphoproliferative disease
    X-l. myotubular myopathy
    X-l. polyendocrinopathy immune
      dysfunction and diarrhea (XPID)
    X-l. recessive adrenoleukodystrophy
    X-l. recessive hypophosphatemic
      rickets
    X-l. severe combined immune
      deficiency (X-SCID)

XO/XY mosaicism
XPID

    X-linked polyendocrinopathy immune
      dysfunction and diarrhea

x-ray crystallography
XRE

    xenobiotic-response element

X

XRT
    radiation therapy
X-SCID
    X-linked severe combined immune
      deficiency
Xtra
    Medisense Precision X.

X-Trozine
46,XX gonadal dysgenesis
47,XXY mosaic
46,XY
    46,XY gonadal dysgenesis
    46,XY mosaic
xylitol

Y

Y body
Y chromatin
Y chromosome detection
Y chromosome microdeletion
Y chromosome mosaicism
Y chromosome RNA recognition motif (YRRM)
Y hormone
Y pacemaker

Yasmin

yellow

y. body
y. bone marrow
y. skin

Yersinia enterocolitica

yersiniosis

Yes protein

Yocon

Yodoxin

yohimbine

Yohimex

yolk sac tumor

young

Diabetes Autoimmunity Study in the Y. (DAISY)
mature-onset diabetes of the y. (MODY)
maturity-onset diabetes of the y. (MODY)
maturity-onset diabetes in the y. (MODY)
Y. syndrome

Young-Simpson syndrome

youth

maturity-onset diabetes of y. (MODY)

YRRM

Y chromosome RNA recognition motif

yttrium-90

y. radioactive isotope

yttrium-91

colloidal y.

YY

peptide YY (PYY)

Z

Z element
Z element insulin gene promoter
Z score
Zadine
Zanosar
zanoterone
Zartan
Z-disk
zearalanol
zein
zeism
Zeitgeber gene
Zellweger syndrome
Zemplar
ZFP

zinc finger protein
ZFP gene
Zhen Qi capsule
zidovudine
Ziehl-Neelsen method
Zieve syndrome
ZIFT

zygote intrafallopian transfer
zinc (Zn)

z. chloride
z. finger
z. finger protein (ZFP)
z. finger Y gene
z. metalloproteinase
z. sulfate
zinc-finger motif
Zinn annulus
zirconium-containing compound
zirconium oxide
Zn

zinc
ZNP Bar
ZOG

zona glomerulosa protein
ZOG protein
Zoladex Implant
zoledronate
zoledronic

z. acid
z. acid for injection
Zollinger-Ellison syndrome
Zoloft
zolpidem
Zometa
zona, pl. **zonae**

z. fasciculata
z. fasciculata cell
z. glomerulosa
z. glomerulosa cell

z. glomerulosa protein (ZOG)
z. incerta
z. pellucida
z. pellucida 1 (ZP1)
z. pellucida 2 (ZP2)
z. pellucida 3 (ZP3)
z. pellucida receptor for glycoprotein 3
z. pellucide recognition site
z. radiata
z. reaction
z. reticularis
zona-free hamster oocyte penetration test
zone

adult z.
clear z.
fetal z.
hole z.
hypothalamic z.
lateral z.
Looser z.
lucent z.
medial z.
midline z.
z. occludens
periventricular z.
z. of provisional calcification
z. reticularis
X z.
zonula, pl. **zonulae**

z. adherens
z. occludens
zonule
zoster

herpes z.
varicella z.
Zostrix
Zostrix-HP
Zovia
ZP1

zona pellucida 1
ZP2

zona pellucida 2
ZP3

zona pellucida 3
Z-score
Zuckerkandl

organ of Z.
Z. peduncle
Zuclomiphene citrate
zwitterion
zygoma

hypoplastic z.
zygomatic process

Z

zygomycosis
zygosity
zygote intrafallopian transfer (ZIFT)
zymogen
    z. granule

pancreatic digestive z.
proteolysis of pancreatic z.

Contents: The Appendices

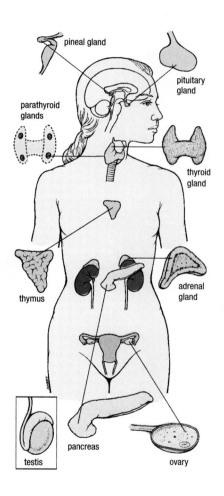

endocrine system, showing various endocrine glands

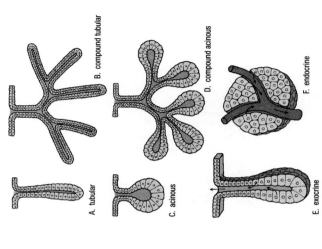

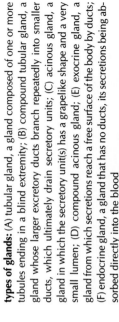

types of glands: (A) tubular gland, a gland composed of one or more tubules ending in a blind extremity; (B) compound tubular gland, a gland whose larger excretory ducts branch repeatedly into smaller ducts, which ultimately drain secretory units; (C) acinous gland, a gland in which the secretory unit(s) has a grapelike shape and a very small lumen; (D) compound acinous gland; (E) exocrine gland, a gland from which secretions reach a free surface of the body by ducts; (F) endocrine gland, a gland that has no ducts, its secretions being absorbed directly into the blood

A. tubular

B. compound tubular

C. acinous

D. compound acinous

E. exocrine

F. endocrine

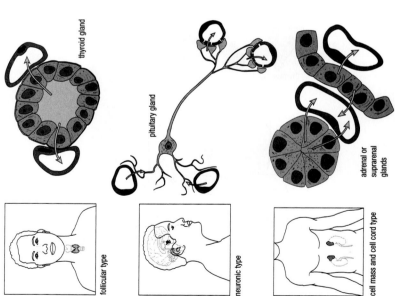

types of endocrine glands

thyroid gland

pituitary gland

adrenal or suprarenal glands

follicular type

neuronic type

cell mass and cell cord type

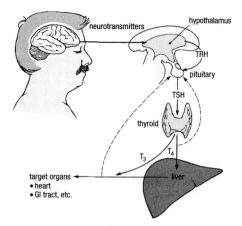

hypothalamic-pituitary-thyroid axis: thyrotropin-releasing hormone (TRH) from the hypothalamus stimulates the pituitary gland to secrete thyroid-stimulating hormone (TSH); TSH acts to produce thyroid hormone (T3 and T4); high circulating levels of T3 and T4 inhibit further TSH secretion and thyroid hormone production through a negative feedback mechanism (dashed lines)
This image was created by Mikki Senkarik for *Stedman's Medical Dictionary*, 27th Edition, Baltimore, Lippincott Williams & Wilkins, 2000, p. 865, and appears here with permission courtesy of Lippincott Williams & Wilkins.

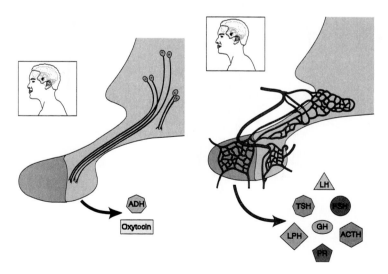

pituitary gland: consists of two major subdivisions, the neurohypophysis (left) and the adenohypophysis (right); ADH = antidiuretic hormone; LH = luteinizing hormone; TSH = thyroid-stimulating hormone; FSH = follicle-stimulating hormone; GH = growth hormone; LPH = lipotropic pituitary hormone; ACTH = adrenocorticotropic hormone; PR = prolactin

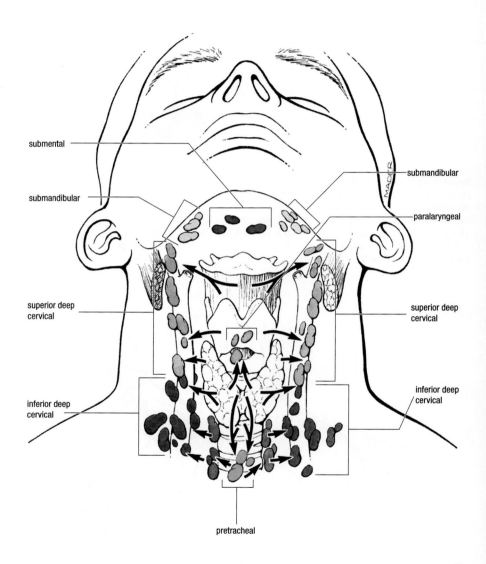

lymphatic drainage of the thyroid gland, larynx, and trachea

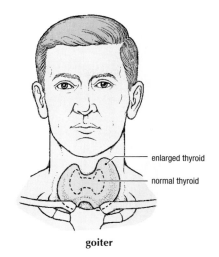

enlarged thyroid

normal thyroid

goiter

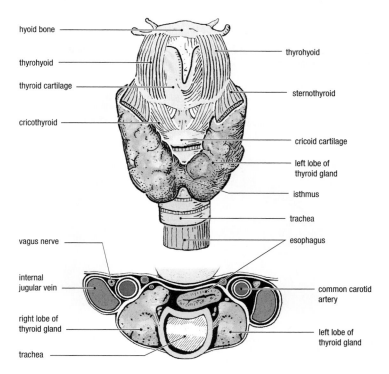

hyoid bone

thyrohyoid

thyrohyoid

thyroid cartilage

sternothyroid

cricothyroid

cricoid cartilage

left lobe of
thyroid gland

isthmus

trachea

vagus nerve

esophagus

internal
jugular vein

common carotid
artery

right lobe of
thyroid gland

left lobe of
thyroid gland

trachea

thyroid gland and its relations in anterior view (top) and transverse section (bottom)

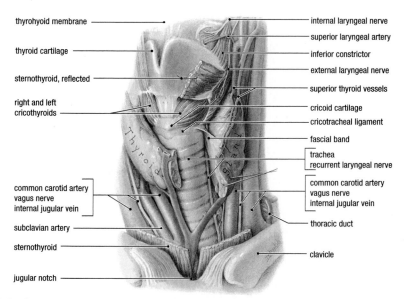

thyrohyoid membrane — internal laryngeal nerve
— superior laryngeal artery
thyroid cartilage — inferior constrictor
— external laryngeal nerve
sternothyroid, reflected — superior thyroid vessels
right and left cricothyroids — cricoid cartilage
— cricotracheal ligament
— fascial band
trachea
recurrent laryngeal nerve
common carotid artery
vagus nerve
internal jugular vein
common carotid artery
vagus nerve
internal jugular vein
subclavian artery — thoracic duct
sternothyroid — clavicle
jugular notch

thyroid gland retracted, anterolateral view of the neck; the isthmus of the thyroid gland is divided, and the left lobe is retracted

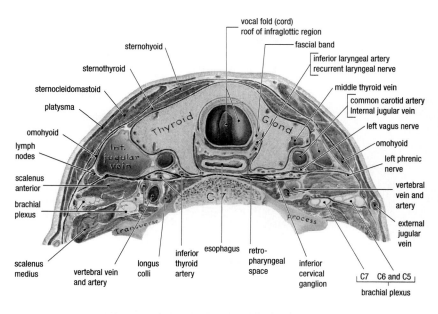

vocal fold (cord)
roof of infraglottic region
sternohyoid
fascial band
sternothyroid
inferior laryngeal artery
recurrent laryngeal nerve
sternocleidomastoid
middle thyroid vein
common carotid artery
platysma
Internal jugular vein
omohyoid
left vagus nerve
lymph nodes
omohyoid
scalenus anterior
left phrenic nerve
brachial plexus
vertebral vein and artery
external jugular vein
scalenus medius
vertebral vein and artery
longus colli
inferior thyroid artery
esophagus
retro-pharyngeal space
inferior cervical ganglion
C7 C6 and C5
brachial plexus

transverse section of neck through thyroid gland

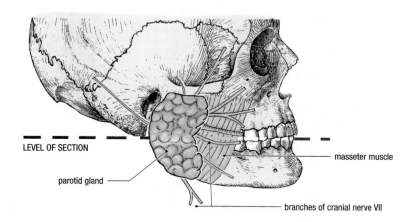

LEVEL OF SECTION

parotid gland

masseter muscle

branches of cranial nerve VII

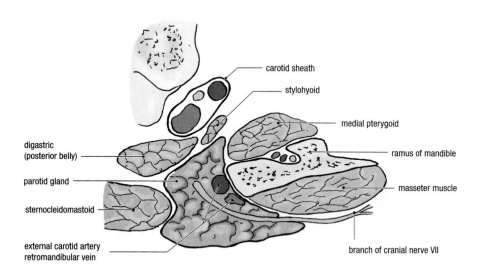

carotid sheath

stylohyoid

medial pterygoid

ramus of mandible

digastric
(posterior belly)

parotid gland

sternocleidomastoid

masseter muscle

external carotid artery
retromandibular vein

branch of cranial nerve VII

parotid gland and its topographic relations: orientation in lateral view and level section for the lower part of the illustration (top); transverse section demonstrates the relations of the gland to surrounding and traversing structures (bottom)

A7

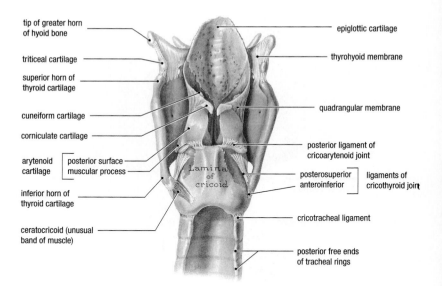

tip of greater horn of hyoid bone

triticeal cartilage

superior horn of thyroid cartilage

cuneiform cartilage

corniculate cartilage

arytenoid cartilage — posterior surface / muscular process

inferior horn of thyroid cartilage

ceratocricoid (unusual band of muscle)

epiglottic cartilage

thyrohyoid membrane

quadrangular membrane

posterior ligament of cricoarytenoid joint

posterosuperior / anteroinferior — ligaments of cricothyroid joint

cricotracheal ligament

posterior free ends of tracheal rings

Lamina of cricoid

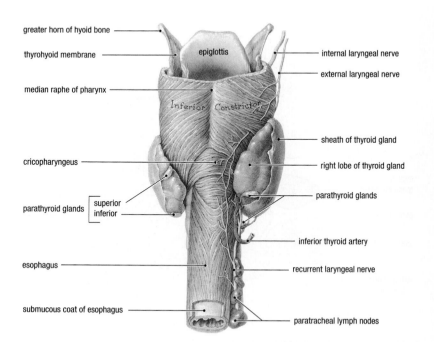

greater horn of hyoid bone

thyrohyoid membrane

median raphe of pharynx

cricopharyngeus

parathyroid glands — superior / inferior

esophagus

submucous coat of esophagus

epiglottis

Inferior Constrictor

internal laryngeal nerve

external laryngeal nerve

sheath of thyroid gland

right lobe of thyroid gland

parathyroid glands

inferior thyroid artery

recurrent laryngeal nerve

paratracheal lymph nodes

skeleton of larynx, posterior view (top); thyroid gland and laryngeal nerves, posterior view (bottom)

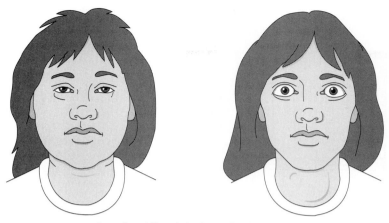

hypothyroidism (left); hyperthyroidism (right)

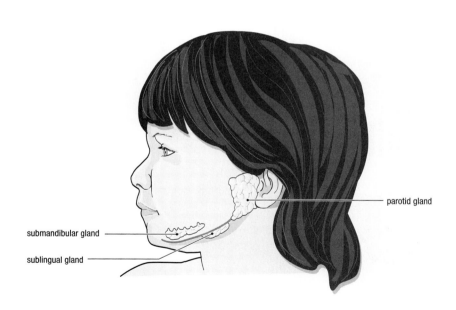

parotid gland

submandibular gland

sublingual gland

salivary glands: lateral view of child showing location

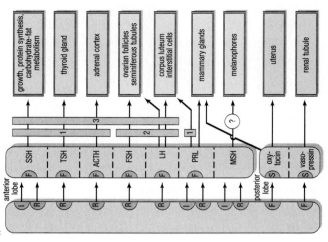

hypophyseal hormones: (I) inhibiting hormones; (R) releasing hormones; (F) formation; (S) storage; (1) metabolic hormones; (2) gonadotropins; (3) glandotropic hormones

This image was created by Mary Anna Barratt-Dimes for *Stedman's Medical Dictionary, 27th Edition*, Baltimore, Lippincott Williams & Wilkins, 2000, p. 831, and appears here with permission courtesy of Lippincott Williams & Wilkins.

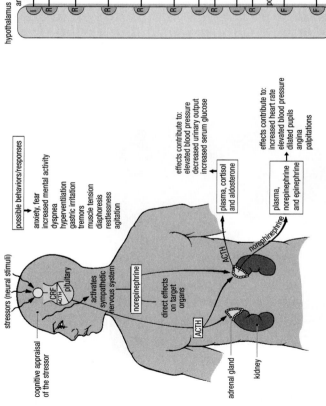

stress response: corticotropin releasing factor (CRF); adrenocorticotropic hormone (ACTH)

This image was created by Larry Ward for *Stedman's Medical Dictionary, 27th Edition*, Baltimore, Lippincott Williams & Wilkins, 2000, p. 1708, and appears here with permission courtesy of Lippincott Williams & Wilkins.

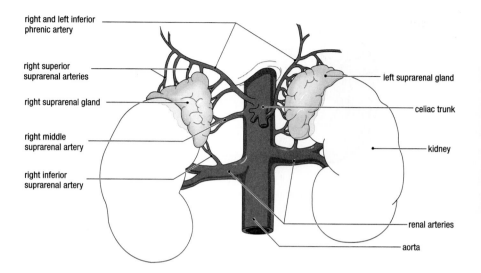

right and left inferior phrenic artery

right superior suprarenal arteries

right suprarenal gland

right middle suprarenal artery

right inferior suprarenal artery

left suprarenal gland

celiac trunk

kidney

renal arteries

aorta

arterial supply to adrenal glands and kidneys

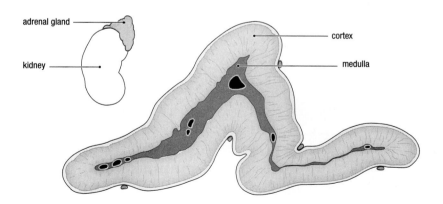

adrenal gland

kidney

cortex

medulla

cross-section of the adrenal gland with an orientation drawing indicating its location on the upper end of the kidney

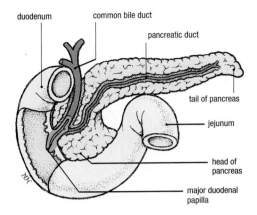

pancreas (and part of duodenum)

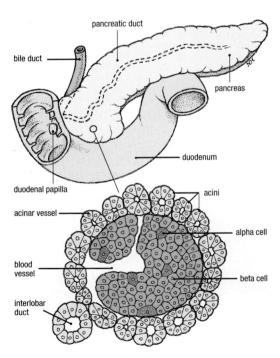

islets of Langerhans

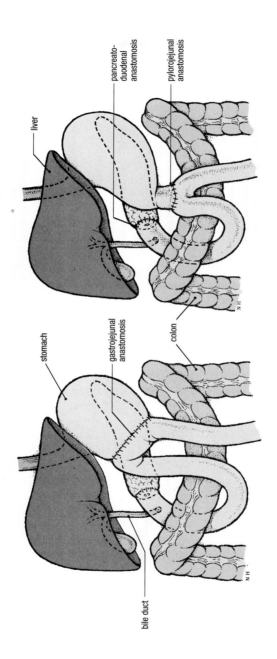

pancreatoduodenectomy: excision of all or part of the pancreas together with the duodenum and usually the distal stomach; the Whipple operation (left) removes the pylorus, while the pylorus-saving Whipple procedure (right) removes it

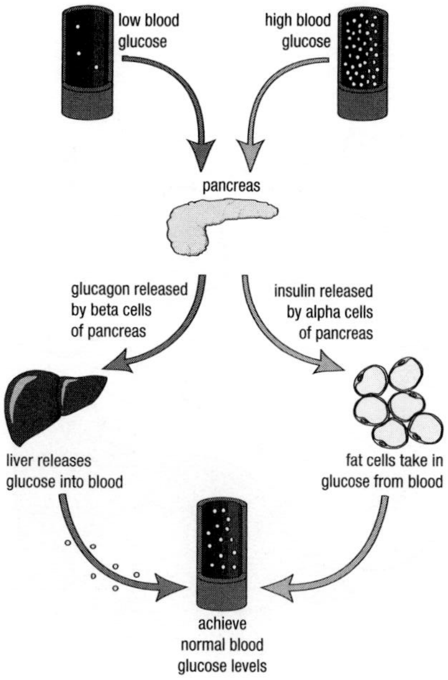

Insulin (metabolic effects)

Metabolic change	Effect	Mechanism	Main organ
1. Glucose transport	+	Unknown	Muscles, fatty tissue
2. Amino acid transport	+	Unknown	Muscles, fatty tissue
3. Potassium transport	+	Unknown; sometimes in connection with glucose transport	Liver, muscles
4. Glucose oxidation	+	Increased glucose transport into cells	Muscles, fatty tissue
5. Glycogen synthesis	+	Increased glucose transport into cells: activation of glycogen synthetase through dephosphorylation of the enzyme	Muscles, liver
6. Fatty acid synthesis	+	As in 4; plus reduction of acyl-CoA, incresed acetyl-CoA from glucose resulting from activation of pyruvate dehydrogenase, release of acetyl-CoA-carboxylase	Fatty tissue, liver
7. Lipid synthesis	+	As in 4; plus production of α-glycerophosphate from glucose	Fatty tissue, liver, muscles
8. Protein synthesis	+	Activation of ribosomes (translation of messenger RNA)	Muscles, fibroblasts
9. Lipolysis	–	Antagonistic to lipolytic hormones; inhibition of adenylate cyclase	Fatty tissue, liver
10. Ketogenesis	–	Inhibition of fatty acid production through anti-lipolysis (see 9)	Liver
11. Gluconeogenesis and glycogenolysis	–	Inhibition of glucagon-stimulated glucose release; inhibition of adenylate cyclase	Liver
12. Proteolysis	–	Unknown; inhibition of urea production in the liver, through reduced production of amino acids	Liver, muscle

insulin (metabolic effects)

This image was created by Susan Caldwell for *Stedman's Medical Dictionary, 27th Edition*, Baltimore, Lippincott Williams & Wilkins, 2000, p. 908, and appears here with permission courtesy of Lippincott Williams & Wilkins.

blood sugar regulation

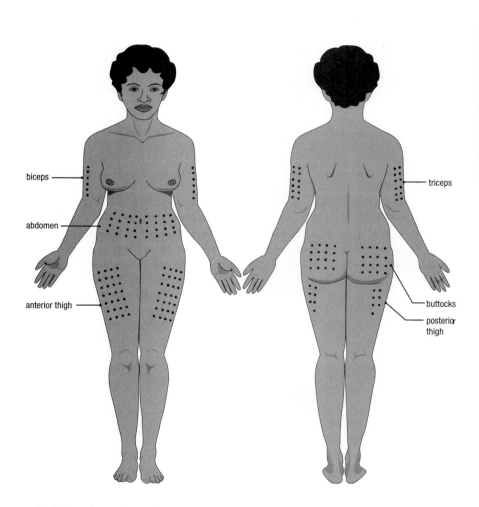

anterior (left) and posterior (right) views of adult female showing multiple sites for insulin injection

Diabetes mellitus (DM): Etiologic classification

I. Primary diabetes mellitus (types 1 and 2)

II. Secondary diabetes

A. Pancreatic diabetes
  - After total or partial pancreatectomy
  - With extensive destruction of pancreas
  - Through tumor or wound
  - Pancreatitis; hemochromatosis

B. Extrapancreatic/endocrine diabetes
  - With hypersomatotropism (acromegaly)
  - With hyperadrenalism (Cushing syndrome; Conn syndrome; pheochromocytoma)
  - With hyperthyroidism
  - With glucagonoma

C. Drug-induced diabetes
  - (Somatotropin; ACTH; adrenocorticoid [steroid diabetes]; thyroid hormone)
  - Thiazides

III. Rare, exceptional forms of diabetes
e.g., Lipoatrophic diabetes
(Lawrence); myatonic diabetes (Prader-Labhart-Willi); disturbance of insulin
receptors; DM with certain genetic syndromes

diabetes mellitus (DM): etiologic classification
This image was created by Susan Caldwell for *Stedman's Medical Dictionary, 27th Edition*, Baltimore, Lippincott Williams & Wilkins, 2000, p. 490, and appears here with permission courtesy of Lippincott Williams & Wilkins.

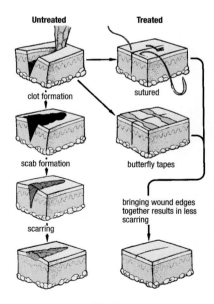

wound healing

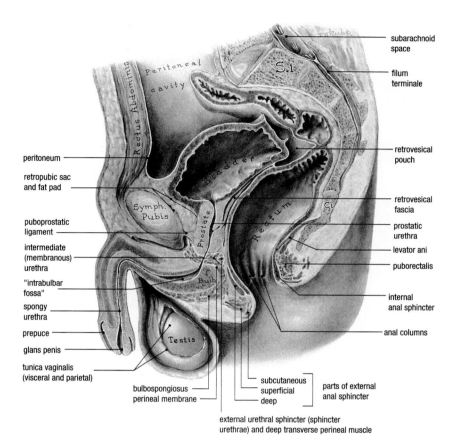

subarachnoid
space

filum
terminale

retrovesical
pouch

peritoneum

retropubic sac
and fat pad

retrovesical
fascia

puboprostatic
ligament

prostatic
urethra

intermediate
(membranous)
urethra

levator ani

puborectalis

"intrabulbar
fossa"

spongy
urethra

internal
anal sphincter

prepuce

anal columns

glans penis

tunica vaginalis
(visceral and parietal)

bulbospongiosus
perineal membrane

subcutaneous
superficial
deep

parts of external
anal sphincter

external urethral sphincter (sphincter
urethrae) and deep transverse perineal muscle

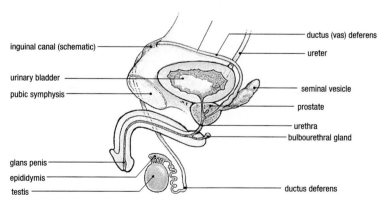

inguinal canal (schematic)

ductus (vas) deferens

ureter

urinary bladder

pubic symphysis

seminal vesicle

prostate

urethra
bulbourethral gland

glans penis

epididymis

testis

ductus deferens

male pelvis, median section (top); overview of urogenital system, median section (bottom)

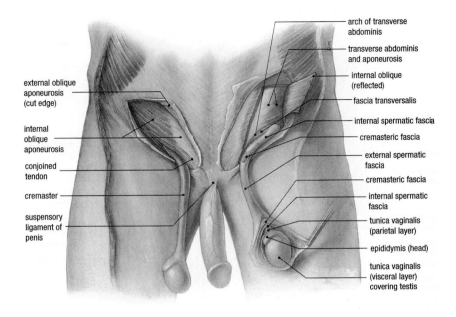

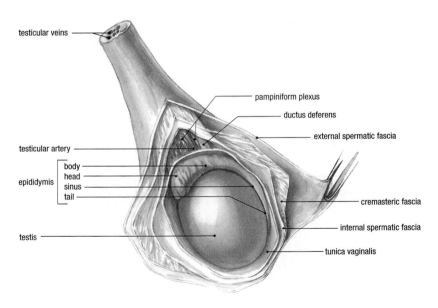

coverings of spermatic cord and testis, anterior view (top); sequential dissection of coverings of testis, anterior view (bottom)

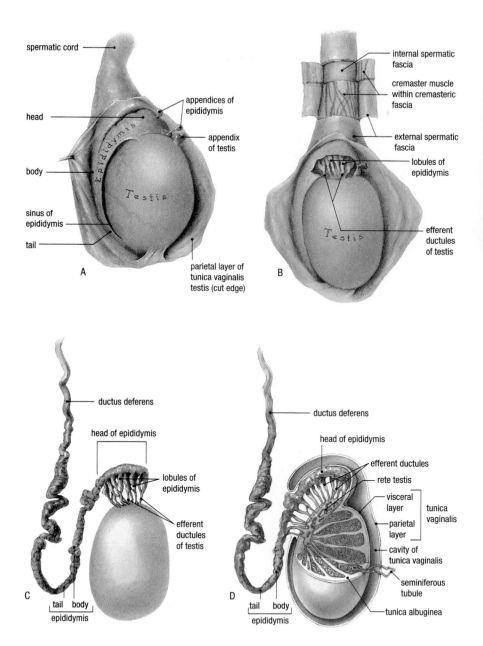

testis and spermatic cord: (A) testis, lateral view; (B) coverings of the spermatic cord, lateral view; (C) epididymis, lateral view; (D) structure of the epididymis and testis, schematic vertical section

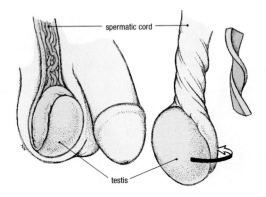

torsion of the spermatic cord

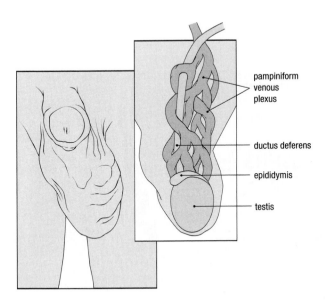

varicocele: image of male genitalia showing anatomical abnormality of left scrotum ("bag of worms" appearance); insert shows internal anatomy of scrotum with abnormal dilation of the cremaster and pampiniform venous plexuses surrounding the spermatic cord

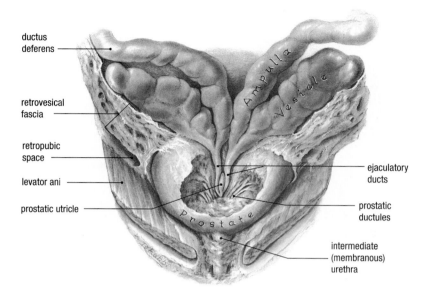

ductus deferens

retrovesical fascia

retropubic space

levator ani

prostatic utricle

Ampulla

Vesicle

prostate

ejaculatory ducts

prostatic ductules

intermediate (membranous) urethra

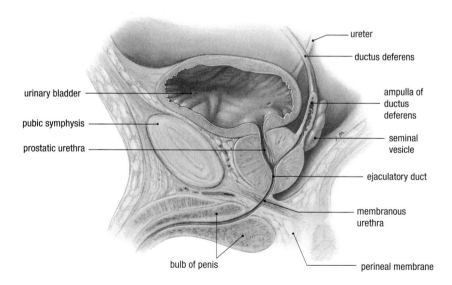

ureter

ductus deferens

urinary bladder

pubic symphysis

prostatic urethra

ampulla of ductus deferens

seminal vesicle

ejaculatory duct

membranous urethra

bulb of penis

perineal membrane

prostate, posterior view (top); bladder, prostate, and ductus deferens (bottom)

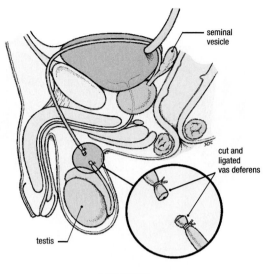

vasectomy

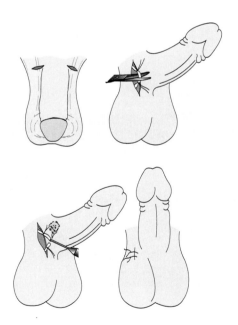

vasectomy: external view of male genitalia showing vasectomy procedure; site of incisions and location of vas deferens indicated (top left); vas deferens pulled outside of body and cut with surgical scissors (top right); cauterization of vas deferens (bottom left); skin suture (bottom right)

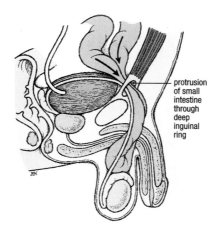

indirect inguinal hernia

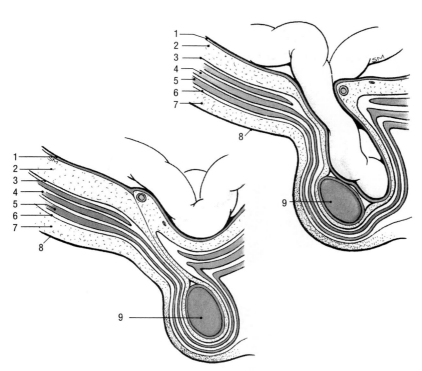

indirect inguinal hernia (right); direct inguinal hernia (left): (1) peritoneum; (2) extraperitoneal fat; (3) fascia transversalis; (4) transversus abdominis; (5) internal oblique; (6) external oblique aponeurosis; (7) subcutaneous fat; (8) skin; (9) testis descending

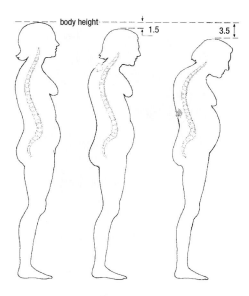

osteoporosis and aging: spinal column within outline of woman at 10 years post menopause (left); changes (loss of height) at 15 years post menopause (center); loss at 25 years post menopause (right)

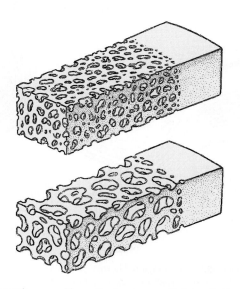

osteoporosis: normal bone (top); osteoporotic bone (bottom)

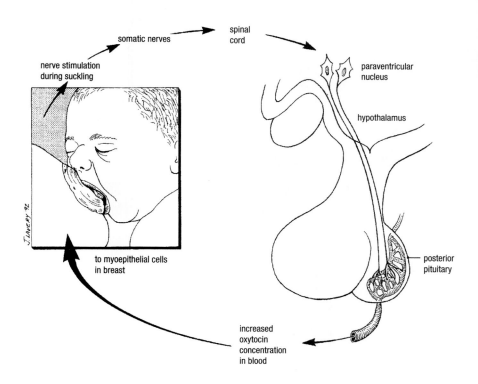

breast lactation: somatosensory pathways for the suckling-induced reduced reflex release of oxytocin

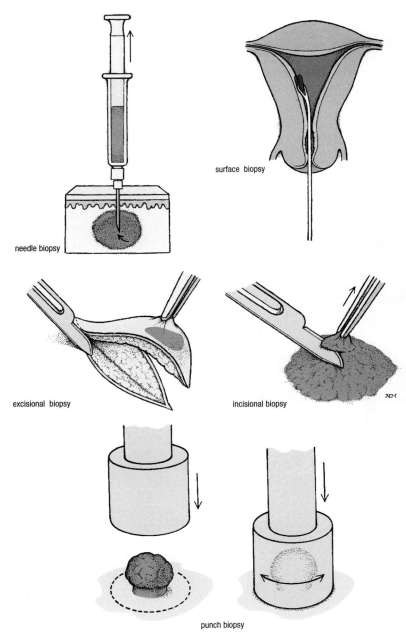

needle biopsy

surface biopsy

excisional biopsy

incisional biopsy

punch biopsy

biopsy techniques

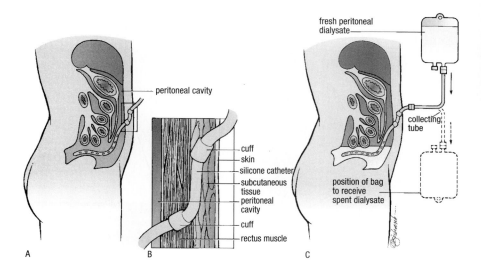

continuous ambulatory peritoneal dialysis: (A) the peritoneal catheter is implanted through the abdominal wall; (B) Dacron cuffs and a subcutaneous tunnel provide protection against bacterial infection; (C) dialysate flows by gravity into the peritoneal catheter and then into the peritoneal cavity; the fluid drains by gravity and is then discarded; additional solution is then infused into the peritoneal cavity until the next drainage period; dialysis thus continues on a 24-hour-a-day basis during which the patient is free to move around and engage in his or her usual activities

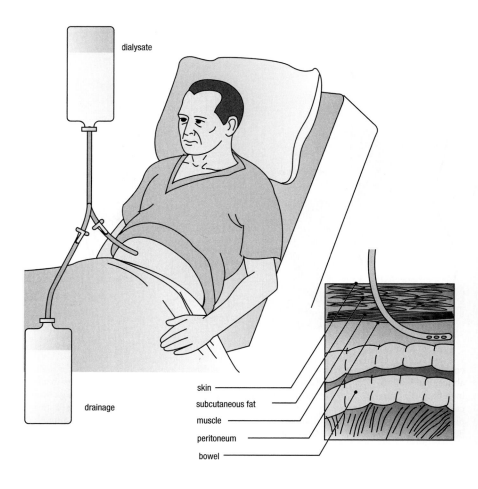

dialysate

drainage

skin

subcutaneous fat

muscle

peritoneum

bowel

peritoneal dialysis and acute intermittent peritoneal dialysis: dialysate is infused into the peritoneal cavity by gravity, after which the clamp on the infusion line is closed; after a dwell time (when the dialysate is in the peritoneal cavity), the drainage tube is unclamped and the fluid drains from the peritoneal cavity, again by gravity; a new container of dialysate is infused as soon as drainage is complete; the duration of the dwell time depends on the type of peritoneal dialysis

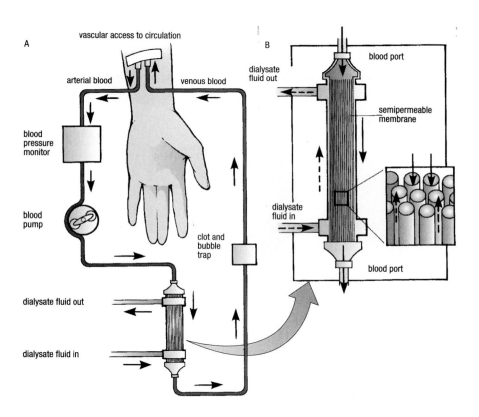

hemodialysis system: (A) blood from an artery is pumped into (B) a dialyzer where it flows through the cellophane tubes, which act as the semipermeable membrane (inset); the dialysate, which has the same chemical composition as the blood except for urea and waste products, flows in around the tubules; the waste products in the blood diffuse through the semipermeable membrane into the dialysate

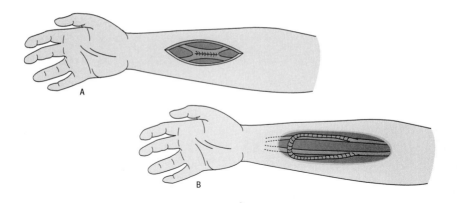

(A) internal arteriovenous fistula; (B) internal arteriovenous graft

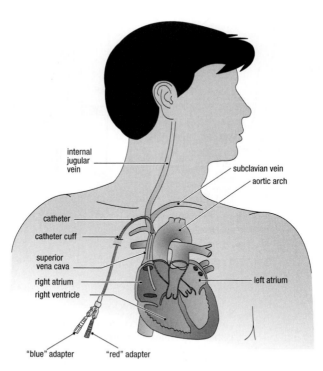

double-lumen, cuffed hemodialysis catheter used in acute hemodialysis: the red adapter (gray) is attached to a blood line through which blood is pumped from the patient; after the blood passes through the dialyzer (artificial kidney), it returns to the patient through the blue adapter (white)

Endocrine Glands: Locations and Functions

Endocrine glands release more than 20 major hormones directly into the
bloodstream so they can be transported to cells in other parts of the body.

Gland	Location and Function
adrenal	Two, one located on top of each kidney. Secrete hormones that influence the body's metabolism, blood chemicals, and body characteristics. Influence the part of the nervous system involved in response and defense against stress.
hypothalamus	Located in the lower central part of the brain. Main link between the endocrine and nervous systems. Controls the part of the nervous system regulating involuntary body functions, the hormonal system, and some body functions, such as regulating sleep and stimulating appetite.
ovary	Two, located in the pelvis. Produce eggs and secrete hormones that influence female characteristics.
pancreas	Located deep in the abdomen between the stomach and the spine. Secretes a hormone (insulin) that controls the use of glucose by the body.
parathyroid	Four small glands embedded in the posterior surface of the thyroid gland. Secretes a hormone that maintains the calcium level in the blood.
pineal	Located in the middle of the brain. Involved with regulating daily biological cycles.

pituitary Located at the base of the brain just beneath the hypothalamus. Often called the "master gland." Produces various hormones that influence other endocrine glands.

testis Two, located in the scrotum. Produce sperm and secrete hormones that influence male characteristics.

thymus Located in the upper center of the chest. Grows during childhood but gradually decreases in size after puberty. An integral part of the body's immune system.

thyroid Located in the front part of the lower neck. Produces hormones that control/regulate metabolism, stimulate body heat production, bone growth.

Endocrine Glands and Associated Products

Gland	Primary Products Secreted
adrenal	aldosterone, androstenedione, catecholamines, cortisol, dehydroepiandrosterone (DHEA), dehydroepiandrosterone sulfate (DHEAS), epinephrine (adrenaline), norepinephrine
hypothalamus	antidiuretic hormone (ADH), corticotropin-releasing hormone (CRH), dopamine, gonadotropin-releasing hormone (GnRH), growth hormone-releasing hormone (GHRH), somatostatin, thyrotropin-releasing hormone (TRH)
ovary	androstenedione, estradiol (E2), inhibin, testosterone, estrogen, progesterone
pancreas	glucagon, insulin, pancreatic polypeptide, somatostatin
parathyroid	parathyroid hormone (PTH)
pineal	melatonin
pituitary	adrenocorticotropic hormone (ACTH), antidiuretic hormone (ADH), corticotropin, endorphins, follicle-stimulating hormone (FSH), growth hormone (GH), luteinizing hormone (LH), melanocyte-stimulating hormone (MSH), oxytocin, prolactin (PRL), thyrotropin (thyroid-stimulating hormone/TSH)

testis   anti-müllerian hormone (AMH), estradiol,
                              inhibin, müllerian inhibitory hormone (MIH),
                              testosterone

thyroid   calcitonin, thyroxine (T4), triiodothyronine (T3)

Appendix 4
Common Disorders by Gland

Gland	Common Disorders
adrenal	Addison disease adrenal cortical hypofunction adrenal cortical hyperfunction Conn syndrome Cushing syndrome pheochromocytoma tumor
hypothalamus	hypothalamic neoplasm tumor
ovary	cancer cyst–functional, dermoid, cystadenoma, endometrioma polycystic ovary syndrome tumor
pancreas	cancer diabetes mellitus hyperglycemia hypoglycemia pancreatitis tumor
parathyroid	hyperparathyroidism osteoporosis tumor
pineal	cancer mood disorder seasonal affective disorder (SAD) sleep disorder
pituitary	acromegaly diabetes insipidus empty sella syndrome hypopituitarism tumor

A35

testis

cancer
hydrocele
hypogonadism
orchitis
priapism
prostatitis

thyroid

cancer–anaplastic, follicular, medullary, papillary
goiter
hyperthyroidism
hypothyroidism
nodules
thyroiditis–Hashimoto
tumor–Hürthle cell

Classification of Diabetes

Type	Characteristics
type 1 diabetes mellitus also called insulin-dependent diabetes mellitus (IDDM) or juvenile-onset diabetes	• Onset predominantly between 5 and 20 years of age but can occur at any age • Patient does not produce enough insulin and requires insulin to sustain life
type 1.5 diabetes mellitus also called slow onset type 1 or latent autoimmune diabetes	• Diagnosed as an adult • No immediate insulin requirement • Little or no insulin resistance • Generally not obese
type 2 diabetes mellitus also called non-insulin-dependent diabetes mellitus (NIDDM)	• Cause thought to be strongly genetic • Does not require insulin to sustain life • Has subgroups of obese and nonobese • Onset predominantly after age 40 but can occur at any age
gestational diabetes	• Glucose intolerance that frequently has onset or recognition during pregnancy
class A gestational diabetes	• Transient diabetes that reverts to normal after delivery
class B gestational diabetes	• Duration less than 10 years • Has been controlled by diet, but patient may become insulin-dependent during the pregnancy • May not need insulin after delivery • Onset after age 20
class C gestational diabetes	• Onset between ages of 10 and 19 • Patient has been insulin-dependent and will need increased doses during pregnancy, but will return to prepregnancy dose after delivery
class D gestational diabetes	• Duration more than 20 years • Hypertension, diabetic retinopathy, and peripheral vascular disease are present • Onset at less than age 10

class E gestational diabetes	• Calcification of pelvic vessels is present
class F gestational diabetes	• Diabetic nephropathy is present

Common Symptoms and Complications of Diabetes

Symptoms

blurred vision
excessive hunger
fatigue
frequent infections
frequent nausea
frequent urination
heartburn
high diastolic blood pressure
high systolic blood pressure
high triglycerides
irritability
low LDL levels
long menstrual cycles
low sex drive
numb/tingling/burning extremities
unusual thirst
unexplained weight gain
unexplained weight loss
slow wound healing

Complications

abscesses
aging
Alzheimer disease
birth/pregnancy complications
blindness
boils
carbuncles
cystic acne
diabetic retinopathy
foot complications
heart disease
kidney damage/failure
neuropathy/nerve damage
pancreatic cancer
respiratory problems/pneumonia
senile dementia
shortened lifespan
stroke
vascular dementia

Appendix 7
Wound Care Products

Bandages, Dressings (Including Foams and Gels)

ABD dressing
Absorptive Border
AcryDerm dressing
Adaptic gauze dressing
Allevyn foam dressing
Aquacel Hydrofiber wound dressing
Aquagel lubricating gel
Aquaphor gauze dressing
Aquasorb dressing
Bard Absorption Dressing
Bioclusive transparent dressing
Biolex
BioPatch foam dressing
BlisterFilm transparent film dressing
CarboFlex odor control dressing
CarraGauze
CarraSmart foam
CarraSorb gel
Carrasyn gel
ClearSite dressing
Coban bandage
CombiDERM
Curafoam hydrophilic foam wound
    dressing
Curagel hydrogel wound dressing
Curasol gel wound dressing
CURITY ABD
Cutinova foam dressing
DermaGauze
Derma-Gel
Dermagran hydrophilic dressing
Dermagran zinc-saline wet dressing
DermaMend foam dressing
DermAssist gauze
DermaSyn
DIAB GEL
DuoDERM hydrocolloid dressing

DuoDERM hydroactive gel
Elasto-Gel occlusive dressing
Elta Dermal
EXU-DRY wound dressing
Flexderm hydrogel dressing
FlexiGel
Flexzan foam dressing
Furacin dressing
Hyalofill dressing
Hydrogel sheet dressing
HyFil wound gel
Hypergel
Iamin wound gel
INTEGRA-GEL
IntraSite gel hydrogel wound dressing
LoProfile foam dressing
Lyofoam C odor control dressing
Lyofoam polyurethane foam dressing
Medipore dressing
Mepitel nonadhesive silicone dressing
Mepilex
Mepilex Border
Mepore
Microdon dressing
Mitraflex
Mitraflex Plus
MPM Conductive Gel Pad
MPM GelPad
MultiPad nonadherent wound dressing
Normlgel Impregnated Gauze
Nu Gauze dressing
Nu-Gel clear hydrogel wound dressing
NutraFill zinc hydrogel
Odob Absorbing Dressing
OpSite occlusive dressing
Owen gauze
Panogauze
PanoPlex
Polyderm foam dressing

Primapore dressing
ProCyte transparent film dressing
Purilon
Repair Hydrogel
Reston foam dressing
SAF-Gel
Silon Dual-Dress 04P Multi-Function
    Wound Dressing
Silon Dual-Dress 20F Multi-Function
    Wound Dressing
2nd Skin dressing
SkinTegrity
Sof-Kling conforming bandage
Sofsorb wound dressing
Soft Cloth adhesive wound dressing
SoloSite Gel
Tegaderm dressing
Tegapore dressing
Telfa dressing
Telfa Clear dressing
TELFAMAX
Tendersorb Wet-Pruf ABD pad
THINSite dressing
3M Foam Adhesive Dressing
3M Foam Dressing (nonadhesive)
Tielle hydropolymer dressing
Transorbent dressing
Ventex dressing
VigiFOAM
Vigilon gel dressing
Webril dressing
Xeroform dressing

Alginate Dressings

AlgiCell
AlgiDERM
Alginate dressing
AlgiSite
Algosteril
CarraSorb H
CURASORB
CURASORB Zinc
Dermacea

DermaGinate
FyBron
Gentell
Hyperion Advanced Alginate Dressing
KALGINATE
KALTOSTAT wound packing dressing
Maxorb
Melgisorb
PolyMem
Restore
Sorbalgon
SORBSAN wound dressing
SeaSorb
Tegagen HG
Tegagen HI

Antimicrobials

Acticoat
Acticoat 7
Arglase
Di-Dak-Sol
IODOFLEX gel pad dressing
IODOSORB gel
Kerlix AMD dressing
Silverlon

Cleansers

ALLCLENZ wound cleanser
Biolex wound cleanser
Cara-Klenz wound cleanser
Chloresium solution
Clean 'N Moist
ClinsWound wound cleanser
Constant-Clens
Curaklense wound cleanser
Debrisan wound cleaning paste
DermaKlenz
Dermagran wound cleanser
DermaMend
DiaB Klenz cleanser
DIAB KLENZ
Elta Dermal wound cleanser
Gentell foam cleanser

Gentell wound cleanser
Hyperion wound cleanser
Iamin wound cleanser
Lobana saline wound cleanser
MicroKlenz
MPM antimicrobial wound and skin
 cleanser
Optipore wound cleansing sponge
Puri-Clens wound deodorizer/cleanser
Repair Wound Cleanser
Restore wound cleanser
SAF-Clens wound cleanser
Sea-Clens wound cleanser
SeptiCare wound cleanser
Shur-Clens wound cleanser
Skintegrity wound cleanser
Techni-Care surgical scrub
UltraKlenz

Collagen Agents

BGC Matrix
FIBRACOL
hyCURE
hyCURE Smart Gel
Medifil
Skin Temp
WOUN'DRESS

Compression Dressings/Devices

Ace wrap
Aircast boot
Aircast EdemaFlow system
ArtAssist
Artiflex
CircAid Thera-Boot
CIRCULON
Coban elastic dressing
Comprilan
DuoDERM SCB
DYNA-FLEX
Elastikon tape
Elastoplast dressing
Foot Waffle air cushion

4-Layer Compression
Gelocast Unna Boot
PlexiPulse pneumatic compression
 device
Primer
Profore four-layer bandaging system
Profore LF
Profore Lite
Setopress high compression bandage
SurePress compression bandage
TENDERWRAP
Tricofix
Tubipad bandage
Unna boot
Unna-Pak
UnnaFlex bandage

Composite Dressings

AIRSTRIP
Alldress
Centurion SorbaView
COVADERM
Coverlet
CovRSite Plus
Cutifilm
MPM
OpSite Plus
OpSite Post-Op
Silon Dual-Dress 04P Multi-Function
 Wound Dressing
Silon Dual-Dress 20F Multi-Function
 Wound Dressing
StrataSorb
Tegaderm Transparent Dressing
 with Absorbent Pad
TELFA
VENTEX
Viasorb

Contact Layer Dressings

DERMANET
N-TERFACE
Mepitel

Profore Wound Contact Layer
Silon-TSR Temporary Skin
  Replacement
TELFA CLEAR
Tegapore

Debriding Agents
Accuzyme debriding ointment
Ethezyme 830 Papain Urea
  Debriding Ointment
Ethezyme Papain-Urea
  Debriding Ointment
Kovia Ointment
Panafil ointment
Pulsavac wound debridement system
Santyl debriding ointment
Ziox Ointment

Hydrocolloid Dressings
BGC Matrix
Comfeel
Cutinova Hydro
Cutinova Thin
DermaFilm HD
DermaFilm Thin
DuoDERM CGF
ExuDERM
Hydrocol
NU-DERM
RepliCare
SignaDRESS Sterile
Tegasorb
Tegasorb THIN
Ultec

Ointments, Creams, Lotions, Solutions
Amerigel ointment
Aquaphor ointment
Bactroban ointment
Baza cream
Betnovate

Biafine
Clinical Care solution
Cloderm cream
Dermagran ointment
Diabicream
Domeboro astringent
Eucerin cream
Lac-Hydrin cream
Lamisil cream
Meloderm ointment
Mitrazol cream
Mycolog cream
Neosporin ointment
Peri-Care Moisture Barrier Ointment
Panafil ointment
Polysporin ointment
Santyl ointment
Silvadene cream
Ureacin lotion
Vitamin A and D ointment

Powders (antibacterial, antifungal, adhesive)
Furacin powder
Mitrazol powder
Multidex powder
Nystatin powder
Stomahesive powder

Wound Fillers
AcryDerm Strands
BIAFINE
CURAFIL
Cutinova Cavity
DermAssist
Humatrix Microclysmic
Mesalt
MULTIDEX
PolyWic
Tegagel hydrogel filler

Normal Lab Values

Tests	Conventional Units	SI Units

Blood Values

acetone, serum
   qualitative — negative — negative
   quantitative — 0.3–2.0 mg/dL — 0.05–0.34 mmol/L

adrenocorticotropin
  (ACTH), plasma

   8 a.m. — <120 pg/mL — <26 pmol/L
    midnight (supine) — <10 pg/mL — <2.2 pmol/L

aldosterone, serum
   supine — 3–16 ng/dL — 0.08–0.44 nmol/L
   standing — 7–30 ng/dL — 0.19–0.83 nmol/L

androstenedione, serum
   male — 75–205 ng/dL — 2.6–7.2 nmol/L
   female — 85–275 ng/dL — 3.0–9.6 nmol/L

anion gap
  (Na – (Cl + HCO3)) — 7–16 mEq/L — 7–16 mmol/L
  ((Na + K) – (Cl + HCO3)) — 10–20 mEq/L — 10–20 mmol/L

calcium, serum — 8.6–10.0 mg/dL — 2.15–2.50 mmol/L
   (slightly higher in children) — (slightly higher in children)

calcium, ionized, serum — 4.64–5.28 mg/dL — 1.16–1.32 mmol/L

cortisol, serum
  plasma
   8 a.m. — 5–23 µg/dL — 138–635 nmol/L
   4 p.m. — 3–16 µg/dL — 83–441 nmol/L
   10 p.m. — <50% of 8 a.m. value — <0.5% of 8 a.m. value

creatine kinase (CK), serum
   male — 15–105 U/L (30°C) — 0.26–1.79 µkat/L (30°C)
   female — 10–80 U/L (30°C) — 0.17–1.36 µkat/L (30°C)
  Note: Strenuous exercise or intramuscular injections may cause transient elevation of CK.

cyclic AMP (cAMP)
  plasma
   male — 4.6–8.6 ng/mL — 14–26 nmol/L
   female — 4.3–7.6 ng/mL — 13–23 nmol/L

C-peptide, serum — 0.78–1.89 ng/mL — 0.26–0.62 nmol/L

dehydroepiandrosterone
  (DHEA), serum
   male — 180–1250 ng/dL — 6.2–43.3 nmol/L
   female — 130–980 ng/dL — 4.5–34.0 nmol/L

Tests	Conventional Units	SI Units
dehydroepiandrosterone sulfate, DHEAS, serum or plasma		
male	59–452 µg/dL	1.6–12.2 µmol/L
female		
premenopausal	12–379 µg/dL	0.8–10.2 µmol/L
postmenopausal	30–260 µg/dL	0.8–7.1 µmol/L
free thyroxine index (FTI), serum	4.2–13	4.2–13
glucose (fasting)		
blood	65–95 mg/dL	3.5–5.3 mmol/L
plasma or serum	74–106 mg/dL	4.1–5.9 mmol/L
glucose, 2 h postprandial, serum	<120 mg/dL	<6.7 mmol/L
glycated hemoglobin (hemoglobin A1C), whole blood	4.2%–5.9%	0.042–0.059
growth hormone, serum		
male	<5 ng/mL	<5 µg/L
female	<10 ng/mL	<10 µg/L
insulin, plasma (fasting)	2–25 µU/mL	13–174 pmol/L
L-lactate		
plasma		
venous	4.5–19.8 mg/dL	0.5–2.2 mmol/L
arterial	4.5–14.4 mg/dL	0.5–1.6 mmol/L
whole blood, at bed rest		
venous	8.1–15.3 mg/dL	0.9–1.7 mmol/L
arterial	<11.3 mg/dL	<1.3 mmol/L
lactate dehydrogenase (LDH) total (LrP), 37°C, serum		
newborn	290–775 U/L	4.9–13.2 µkat/L
neonate	545–2000 U/L	9.3–34 µkat/L
infant	180–430 U/L	3.1–7.3 µkat/L
child	110–295 U/L	1.9–5 µkat/L
adult	100–190 U/L	1.7–3.2 µkat/L
>60 y	110–210 U/L	1.9–3.6 µkat/L
magnesium, serum	1.3–2.1 mEq/L	0.65–1.07 mmol/L
	1.6–2.6 mg/dL	16–26 mg/L
osmolality, serum	275–295 mOsm/kg serum water	275–295 mmol/kg serum water
pH		
blood, arterial	7.35–7.45	7.35–7.45
phosphatase, alkaline (alkphos), total, serum	38–126 U/L (37°C)	0.65–2.14 µkat/L
phosphate, inorganic, serum		
adults	2.7–4.5 mg/dL	0.87–1.45 mmol/L
children	4.5–5.5 mg/dL	1.45–1.78 mmol/L

Tests	Conventional Units	SI Units
potassium (K), plasma		
male	3.5–4.5 mmol/L	3.5–4.5 mmol/L
female	3.4–4.4 mmol/L	3.4–4.4 mmol/L
potassium (K), serum		
premature		
cord	5.0–10.2 mmol/L	5.0–10.2 mmol/L
48 h	3.0–6.0 mmol/L	3.0–6.0 mmol/L
newborn cord	5.6–12.0 mmol/L	5.6–12.0 mmol/L
newborn	3.7–5.9 mmol/L	3.7–5.9 mmol/L
infant	4.1–5.3 mmol/L	4.1–5.3 mmol/L
child	3.4–4.7 mmol/L	3.4–4.7 mmol/L
adult	3.5–5.1 mmol/L	3.5–5.1 mmol/L
progesterone, serum		
adult		
male	13–97 ng/dL	0.4–3.1 nmol/L
female		
follicular phase	15–70 ng/dL	0.5–2.2 nmol/L
luteal phase	200–2500 ng/dL	6.4–79.5 nmol/L
pregnancy	varies with gestational week	
prolactin, serum		
male	2.5–15.0 ng/mL	2.5–15.0 µg/L
female	2.5–19.0 ng/mL	2.5–19.0 µg/L
protein, serum		
total	6.4–8.3 g/dL	64–83 g/L
albumin	3.9–5.1 g/dL	39–51 g/L
globulin		
alpha1	0.2–0.4 g/dL	2–4 g/L
alpha2	0.4–0.8 g/dL	4–8 g/L
beta	0.5–1.0 g/dL	5–10 g/L
gamma	0.6–1.3 g/dL	6–13 g/L
testosterone, serum		
male	280–1100 ng/dL	0.52–38.17 nmol/L
female	15–70 ng/dL	0.52–2.43 nmol/L
pregnancy	3–4 x normal	3–4 x normal
postmenopausal	8–35 ng/dL	0.28–1.22 nmol/L
thyroid-stimulating hormone (TSH), serum	0.4–4.2 µU/mL	0.4–4.2 mU/L
thyroxine (T4), serum	5–12 µg/dL (varies with age, higher in children and pregnant women)	65–155 nmol/L (varies with age, higher in children and pregnant women)
thyroxine, free, (free T4), serum	0.8–2.7 ng/dL	10.3–35 pmol/L

Tests	Conventional Units	SI Units
thyroxine binding globulin (TBG), serum	1.2–3.0 mg/dL	12–30 mg/L
triglycerides, serum, fasting		
desirable	<250 mg/dL	<2.83 mmol/L
borderline high	250–500 mg/dL	2.83–5.67 mmol/L
hypertriglyceridemia	>500 mg/dL	>5.65 mmol/L
triiodothyronine, total (T3), serum	100–200 ng/dL	1.54–3.8 nmol/L
urea nitrogen, serum	6–20 mg/dL	2.1–7.1 mmol Urea/L
urea nitrogen/creatinine ratio, serum	12:1 to 20:1	48-80 urea/creatinine mole ratio
zinc, serum	70–120 µg/dL	10.7–18.4 µmol/L

Urine Values

Tests	Conventional Units	SI Units
acetone, urine		
qualitative	negative	negative
aldosterone, urine	3–19 µg/24 h	8–51 nmol/24 h
calcium, urine		
low calcium diet	50–150 mg/24 h	1.25–3.75 mmol/24 h
usual diet, trough	100-300 mg/24 h	2.50-7.50 mmol/24 h
cortisol, free, urine	<50 µg/24 h	<138 mmol/24 h
cyclic AMP, urine, 24 h	0.3–3.6 mg/d or 0.29–2.1 mg/g creatinine	100–723 mmol/d or 100–723 mmol/mol creatinine
glucose, urine		
quantitative	<500 mg/24 h	<2.8 mmol/24 h
qualitative	negative	negative
17-hydroxycorticosteroids, urine		
male	3–10 mg/24 h	8.3–27.6 µmol/24 h (as cortisol)
female	2–8 mg/24 h	5.5–22 µmol/24 h (as cortisol)
17-ketosteroids, urine		
male	10–25 mg/24 h	38–87 µmol/24 h
female	6–14 mg/24 h (decreases with age)	21–52 µmol/24 h (decreases with age)
L-lactate, urine		
24 h	496–1982 mg/d	5.5–22 mmol/d
magnesium, urine	6.0–10.0 mEq/24 h	3.0–5.0 mmol/24 h

Tests	Conventional Units	SI Units
osmolality, urine	50–1200 mOsm/kg water	50–1200 mmol/kg water
ratio, urine:serum	1.0–3.0, 3.0–4.7 after 12 h fluid restriction	1.0–3.0, 3.0–4.7 after 12 h fluid restriction
pH, urine	4.6–8.0 (depends on diet)	4.6–8.0 (depends on diet)
phosphorus, urine	0.4–1.3 g/24 h	12.9–42 mmol/24 h
potassium, urine 24 h	25–125 mmol/d; varies with diet	25–125 mmol/d; varies with diet

Other Values

L-lactate, CSF	10–22 mg/dL	1.1–2.4 mmol/L
lactate dehydrogenase (LDH) CSF	10% of serum value	0.10 fraction of serum value
potassium, (CSF)	70% of plasma level or 2.5–3.2 mmol/L; rises with plasma hyperosmolality	0.70 of plasma level; rises with plasma hyperosmolality

Sample Reports

ADDISON DISEASE

PRIMARY DIAGNOSES: Hypocortisolism (addisonian).

SECONDARY DIAGNOSES
1. Previous Cushing syndrome (adrenocorticotropic hormone pituitary adenoma).
2. Chronic anxiety.
3. Chronic depression.

The patient is a 68-year-old married woman who was admitted to this hospital through the emergency department with complaints of generalized aches, pains, and weakness. She had been discharged from the hospital 5 days ago following a comprehensive investigation focused on endocrine workup. She was found to have normal thyroid function and normal a.m./p.m. cortisols; however, 24-hour cortisol excretion seemed very low.

The patient was noted to have a very cushingoid appearance in the summer of last year. Her investigation determined the presence of a tiny pituitary adenoma secreting excessive adrenocorticotropic hormone. She had a very long wait for neurosurgery and eventually was admitted for transsphenoidal hypophysectomy.

Further investigation during this admission showed that there had been further reduction in cortisol levels, specifically a.m. cortisol was only 59 on the day following admission.

The internal medicine specialist saw the patient in consultation, and he initially approved a trial of Florinef to treat postural hypotension. She was subsequently started on prednisone. Over the course of a very few days, her energy, vitality, and mood were significantly improved. The psychiatrist also saw her in consultation prior to discharge.

The patient was sent home in improved condition with arrangements to be seen in the office in 2 weeks.

COMPLETION THYROIDECTOMY

PREOPERATIVE DIAGNOSIS: Atypical left thyroid nodule.

POSTOPERATIVE DIAGNOSIS: Atypical left thyroid nodule.

PROCEDURE PERFORMED: Completion thyroidectomy with left thyroid lobectomy.

ANESTHESIA: General endotracheal anesthesia.

COMPLICATIONS: None.

FLUIDS GIVEN: 1200 mL.

DRAINS: One #7 Jackson-Pratt.

ESTIMATED BLOOD LOSS: Minimal.

SPECIMEN: Left thyroid lobe to pathology.

INDICATIONS FOR PROCEDURE: The patient is a 55-year-old woman who had previously undergone a right thyroid lobectomy with a partial left thyroid lobectomy. She was noted to have a left thyroid nodule and biopsy revealed atypia. The patient was advised to have surgery. The risks, benefits, and alternatives were discussed which included but were not limited to bleeding, infection, numbness, hoarseness, hypercalcemia, and need for further surgery. The patient accepted the risks and consented freely to the procedure.

PROCEDURE IN DETAIL: After patient was placed in the supine position and general anesthesia was induced, the patient was prepped and draped in the standard fashion. A transverse cervical incision was planned through her previous incision. The area was infiltrated with 0.5% Marcaine. Using a 15 blade, dissection was carried down to the subcutaneous tissue and platysma with electrocautery. Subplatysmal flaps were raised superiorly and inferiorly. Then the strap muscles were split in the midline and carefully carried down to the trachea anteriorly. The left strap muscles were attempted to be elevated off the left thyroid lobe. This was performed carefully due to the extensive scarring. As we approached laterally, the scar tissue became less prominent, and the superior pole was dissected. The blood supply was divided at the entrance to the thyroid capsule and controlled with 3-0 silk ties. Upon anterior and medial rotation of the superior pole, a superior parathyroid was identified. This was dissected off with its blood supply intact, and the trachea itself was entered where the recurrent laryngeal nerve was identified. This was followed to its entrance point to the larynx.

This allowed division of the inferior thyroid artery branches, which were controlled with 3-0 ties at each point, confirming the recurrent laryngeal nerve was well out of harm's way. Dissection was carried inferiorly, and the inferior parathyroid was also dissected off with its blood supply intact. The inferior pole vessels were dissected, divided, and ligated with 2-0 silk ties. Then the remaining venous ligaments and attachments to the anterior trachea were divided and controlled with 3-0 silk ties and divided. The avascular attachments to the anterior trachea were divided with bipolar cautery. The specimen, which was all remaining thyroid tissue, was removed and marked with a stitch in the superior pole. This was sent to pathology.

The wound was irrigated copiously, and hemostasis was confirmed. The recurrent laryngeal nerve was intact without evidence of injury. The parathyroids were intact and viable. The wound again was irrigated copiously. Hemostasis was confirmed. A #7 Jackson-Pratt drain was placed into the dissection and brought out through the incision. The wound was then closed with 3-0 Vicryl interrupted to reapproximate the strap muscles, 3-0 Vicryl interrupted to reapproximate the platysma, then 4-0 Monocryl subcuticular and 3-0 nylon was used to secure the drain to skin exit site. Counts were correct x2. Benzoin and Steri-Strips were applied. The patient was extubated and transferred to the recovery room in stable condition. As attending surgeon, I was present from the skin incision until the patient was transferred to the recovery room.

COMPLETION THYROID LOBECTOMY

PREOPERATIVE DIAGNOSIS: Papillary carcinoma of the thyroid.

POSTOPERATIVE DIAGNOSIS: Papillary carcinoma of the thyroid.

OPERATION: Left (completion) thyroid lobectomy.

ANESTHESIA: General anesthesia via endotracheal tube.

ESTIMATED BLOOD LOSS: 50 mL.

INDICATIONS: This is a patient who underwent a surgery for goiter. The goiter was on the right side. Frozen section demonstrated no evidence of malignancy. Final pathology actually demonstrated 2 different sites of papillary carcinoma, 1 measuring over 3 cm in diameter. Therefore the patient is returning for a completion thyroidectomy in anticipation of I-131 treatment.

PROCEDURE/FINDINGS: The patient was anesthetized with general anesthesia via endotracheal tube. The patient was put in a semi-sitting position. Her neck was hyperextended, a roll placed under her shoulder. The face, neck, and upper chest were prepped with DuraPrep and draped in a sterile fashion. We used evoked potential monitoring. We also used nerve stimulation.

The scar from her previous operation was excised and then the incision extended down through the platysma. Subplatysmal flaps were raised to the level of the thyroid cartilage and substernal notch. The strap muscles were divided in the midline and the left lobe identified. The left lobe overall appeared to be normal in size, perhaps even a little shrunken from before. There were no nodules. There were no signs of any lymphadenopathy. The gland was carefully dissected from surrounding tissues. There were minimal adhesions, less than anticipated. We were able to roll the gland medially and dissect it away from the surrounding muscle and other soft tissues. The upper pole was doubly ligated with 2-0 Vicryl, the lower pole was also ligated with 2-0 Vicryl, and the recurrent laryngeal nerve was identified. The inferior left parathyroid was also identified and preserved. The gland was dissected up off the trachea and removed.

The area was inspected. We did use nerve stimulation to confirm the presence of the recurrent laryngeal nerve and the fact that it was uninjured. There was no evidence from the evoked potential monitoring to indicate any neurologic injury. The area was inspected. Hemostasis was assured. Throughout the case hemostasis had been achieved either with 2-0 or 4-0 Vicryl, electrocautery where appropriate, and a rare Hemoclip.

To prevent injury to the recurrent laryngeal nerve, a trace of thyroid was left right at the area of insertion. This measured less than 2-3 mm in largest diameter.

When it was clear there was no bleeding, the strap muscles and platysma were closed with 2-0 Vicryl, and then the skin was closed with 4-0 Vicryl, benzoin, and Steri-Strips. Sponge and needle counts were correct. The patient tolerated the procedure well and returned to the recovery room awake and in stable condition.

DIABETES, COMPLICATION OF GANGRENE: DIGIT AMPUTATION

FINAL DIAGNOSES
1. Diabetes mellitus.
2. Gangrenous 4th toe, right foot.

SURGICAL PROCEDURE: Amputation, right 4th and 5th toes.

HISTORY: This 61-year-old diabetic with multiple complications from diabetes was brought to the hospital for amputation of his 4th and 5th toes for gangrene of his 4th toe, as this toe had been infected. We treated with antibiotics, and it seemed to have improved. We used a flap from the lateral 5th toe to fill in the defect.

Postoperatively, he was bothered with inflammation on the sole of his foot. He was continued on antibiotics for a long time, and he continued to have an elevated white count. We were able to manipulate his antibiotics.

Another complication of his diabetes is his chronic renal failure with creatinines in the 200-300 range. His foot was still tender. It was felt to be dangerous to do a CT scan angiogram. He has a pacemaker in place so we could not do an MR angiogram. We continued to observe him. We did a CT scan of his foot while in the hospital and repeated it a week later. There was swelling in the sole of the foot but no obvious abscess. He was followed by Orthopedics throughout his stay. Infectious Disease was also consulted and followed the patient during hospitalization. His foot seemed to improve a bit, and he was ultimately discharged to a rehab facility for ongoing care.

DIABETES CONTROL DISCHARGE SUMMARY

HISTORY: This is one of several admissions for this 32-year-old female who has had diabetes type 1 for several years. She was admitted due to poor diabetic control, having blood sugars in the 300 range prior to admission. In addition, she had hypertension and hypercalcemia. The patient currently is on a regimen of multiple daily injections of regular Humulin insulin and once-daily NPH at bedtime. With this schedule, she has been unable to maintain adequate blood sugar control. In addition the patient has hypothyroidism and takes Synthroid 100 mcg daily.

LABORATORY DATA: On admission the patient had a glucose level of 298. Her hemoglobin A1c was 11.1%, confirming the diagnosis of poorly controlled diabetes.

HOSPITAL COURSE: The patient was admitted to the medical service and placed on a 1200-calorie ADA diet. She was maintained on her Humulin regular insulin 6-12 units daily by sliding scale as well as 4 units of NPH at night. Initially blood sugars did not respond appropriately. She continued to have labile blood sugars with high fasting levels as well as high postprandial levels. However, after approximately 8 days in hospital, her blood sugars came under some control, and the patient was discharged home in somewhat improved condition.

MEDICATIONS ON DISCHARGE
1. Regular Humulin insulin 4 times daily according to sliding scale.
2. NPH 4 units daily at supper.
3. Synthroid 0.1 mg daily.
4. Captopril 25 mg b.i.d.

DISCHARGE DIAGNOSES
1. Diabetes type 1 with improved control.
2. Hypertension.
3. Hypothyroidism.

DIABETES MELLITUS HISTORY AND PHYSICAL

HISTORY OF PRESENT ILLNESS: This 63-year-old female patient was brought to the emergency room in the early morning hours with complaints of persistent vomiting over the last several hours. She reports she started vomiting shortly after supper the night previous and subsequently vomited at least 8 times. The patient is a known diabetic and had a fingerstick blood sugar reading of 427 at home.

REVIEW OF SYSTEMS: The patient complains of some chest pain, burning in nature, without radiation. She has no history of diarrhea. Otherwise review of systems was basically negative.

PAST SURGICAL HISTORY: Coronary artery bypass graft 3 years ago, cholecystectomy and appendectomy in the distant past.

SOCIAL HISTORY: The patient is married. She does not smoke and does not consume alcohol. She is a homemaker.

MEDICATIONS
1. Regular insulin 10 units every morning.
2. Lantus 12 units every evening.
3. Pentoxifylline 400 mg t.i.d. with meals.
4. Multivitamin daily.

PHYSICAL EXAMINATION
VITAL SIGNS: The patient's temperature was 98.7, pulse 62, respirations 22, and blood pressure was 112/60.

GENERAL APPEARANCE: The patient appeared pale and somewhat weak.

HEENT: Normocephalic, atraumatic. PERRLA and extraocular movements were intact. Her mucous membranes appeared dry.

HEART: Regular rate and rhythm without murmurs, rubs, or gallops.

LUNGS: Clear to auscultation bilaterally without wheezes or rales.

ABDOMEN: Soft with diffuse generalized tenderness; no masses detected.

EXTREMITIES: No clubbing, cyanosis, or edema.

ADMITTING LABORATORY DATA: The patient's serum glucose level was noted to be 503, serum sodium 132, and BUN was 30.

IMPRESSION
1. Diabetes mellitus, inadequate control.
2. Dehydration.
3. Electrolyte imbalance.

PLAN: The patient will be admitted to the medical service. An IV of normal saline was started, and she was also given Phenergan 25 mg IM for repeated episodes of vomiting. Further treatment will depend upon her clinical course.

DIABETES MELLITUS, NEWLY DIAGNOSED

This 12-year 9-month-old girl was referred by her family physician and admitted to the hospital with a diagnosis of newly diagnosed diabetes mellitus. She had been well until about 2 weeks previously when she had increased thirst, increased urine output, and she lost 10 pounds of weight. Her mouth felt dry, and she felt weak. On the day of admission, she had blurred vision of the left eye. In the past, she has had frequent tonsillitis and frequently enlarged cervical nodes. She is in grade 7 and progressing satisfactorily. She has had chickenpox. She has not had ear infections. Her immunizations are up-to-date. There are no known allergies. She had onset of menstrual periods at age 12, and these have been irregular. Her 2 brothers, ages 14 years and 22 years, are well, and 1 sister, age 19 years, is well. Her mother is working as a cook up north at a gas plant, and her father lives out of state. The patient lives with her sister and her sister's husband.

The patient appeared well. Her abdominal tissue elasticity was very slightly decreased, and she complained of dry mouth. General physical examination was normal. Height was 157 cm, weight 42.5 kg, blood pressure 121/72 mmHg, and other vital signs were normal.

Hemoglobin 16.0, WBC 10.9, and platelet count 582,000. Blood pH at the outside hospital was 7.22, and total CO_2 was 15. Blood glucose was 27.3. Sodium was 133, and other electrolytes were normal. Urea was slightly elevated at 8.7.

On the day of admission, her CO_2 was up to 20. Her urine glucose was 56 mmol/L and ketones 15 mmol/L. On the day after admission, the urine was clear of ketones. TSH was 2.60. Urine culture showed an insignificant growth of organisms.

The patient received an IV of saline with added KCl. Initially, she was given 4 units of Novolin insulin and NovoLog insulin prior to the 3 main meals of the day. By the time of discharge, she was on 16 units of Novolin NPH in the morning and 8 units of Novolin NPH in the evening and NovoLog 6 to 7 units prior to meals. Initially, she was on a 2200-calorie diabetic diet. She seemed to learn the principles of diabetes satisfactorily. Her weight was up to 45.3 kg at the time of discharge, and discharge physical examination was normal. She was seen in the office after discharge and at that time was doing well.

Because the patient lives away from her parents, it is necessary for her to take primary responsibility for her diabetes. She seems to be mature for her age and accepting of this responsibility.

MOST RESPONSIBLE DIAGNOSIS: Newly diagnosed diabetes mellitus with minimal ketoacidosis.

DIABETES MELLITUS TYPE 2 CONSULTATION

REASON FOR CONSULTATION: I was asked to see this 57-year-old female patient for evaluation of renal insufficiency.

HISTORY OF PRESENT ILLNESS: THe patient presented to the emergency room with diaphoresis, vomiting, and extreme weakness. Subsequently laboratory data revealed hypoglycemia. She had elevated potassium of 6.5 with evidence of renal insufficiency and was admitted to the medical floor.

I have seen this patient previously due to chronic renal failure and hyperkalemia.

Her medications on admission included DiaBeta 5 mg twice daily, Inderal 20 mg 3 times daily, ferrous sulfate and quinidine twice daily.

On examination, the patient was lying comfortably in bed. A detailed examination was not performed at this time although note was made that her mucous membranes were somewhat dry and she appeared somewhat lethargic.

DIAGNOSTIC IMPRESSIONS
1. Diabetes mellitus, type 2.
2. Hypoglycemia secondary to oral agents in the face of renal insufficiency.
3. Acute hyperkalemia, secondary to renal insufficiency and angiotensin-converting enzyme inhibitors.

TREATMENT RECOMMENDATIONS
1. Discontinue Inderal.
2. IV hydration with saline as I believe her renal failure is based on prerenal azotemia.
3. Administer sodium bicarbonate for treatment of metabolic acidosis.
4. Kayexalate to treat hyperkalemia.
5. Glucose infusion followed by regular insulin administration.

Thank you for asking me to see this pleasant woman. I will continue to follow her along with you.

DIABETIC FOOT INFECTION DEBRIDEMENT

DISCHARGE DIAGNOSIS: Diabetic foot infection.

PROCEDURE PERFORMED: Debridement of right foot.

HOSPITAL COURSE: This man was admitted through the outpatient clinic with an indolent infection of the right foot. I debrided his foot some months ago, and he had 2 open areas which seemed to be responding well to local treatment and also oral clindamycin. His wound was growing MRSA. He was admitted with cellulitis, low-grade fever, and increasing pain in the foot.

X-rays showed no significant evidence of osteomyelitis proximally. There was some destruction of the 2nd MTP joint, but this is probably due to neuropathic changes rather than osteomyelitis.

He was admitted, and after consultation with Internal Medicine, he was begun on intravenous vancomycin. After several days of vancomycin, his symptoms had resolved and the foot was looking better. I took him to the operating room and debrided both ulcers under the 2nd MTP joint, which showed solid bone and no sign of infection. We also debrided the more proximal wound from which I curetted some inflammatory material. I did a thorough curettage including removing some of the residual stump of the 1st metatarsal and this bone was quite solid and healthy. We continued with antibiotics for 48 hours and daily packings with Bactroban ointment and gauze.

Wound swabs came back MRSA negative. Plans were made to discharge him. He will return to see me in clinic in about 3 weeks.

PEDIATRIC DIABETIC KETOACIDOSIS

HISTORY: This is a 13-year-old female with known type 1 diabetes mellitus diagnosed in 2000 who presented to the ER with decreased p.o. intake, feeling dizzy all day, nausea, and a sore throat. Her blood sugar at home was 300, and she gave herself 30 units of NPH and 9 units of regular insulin. In the ER she was noted to have a blood sugar of 430. She was admitted to the pediatric ICU for DKA.

HOSPITAL COURSE: The patient did very well during her short stay in the pediatric ICU. Her blood sugars gradually decreased and normalized in the span of a day. Her bicarb was initially low but that normalized as well. Her urine had ketones and glucose that normalized as time went on. She was taking 30 units of NPH pre-breakfast and 14 units of NPH pre-dinner, and she was on a Humalog sliding scale. She had a Rapid Strep and throat culture that came back negative, and a urine culture that initially grew out greater than 100,000 strep B, and a repeat urine culture grew out greater than 100,000 colonies of mixed flora. All of her UAs had no leukocyte esterase and no nitrites. There was a third urine culture that was done before discharge, and that is still pending. She was also on an insulin drip, but that was discontinued after a day. Her hemoglobin A1c came back high at 13.4. Endocrine was following her on the case as well as Social Work due to her noncompliance. She was on a low-carb ADA diet and was sent home on insulin. She was to follow up with Endocrinology 2 days after discharge.

FINAL DIAGNOSIS: A 13-year-old female status post diabetic ketoacidosis.

FOLLICULAR ADENOMA OF THE THYROID SOAP NOTE

S: This 79-year-old female patient was noted to have an enlarging lesion in the left thyroid lobe. Nuclear medicine scans revealed this was a cold nodule. Her thyroid function studies remained in normal limits. Previous fine-needle aspiration suggested Hürthle cell adenoma.

O: The patient was a well-developed, well-nourished female in no apparent distress. Examination of the neck revealed a 2 x 1 x 1.5-cm mass in the left upper pole of the thyroid gland. No lymphadenopathy was present. The remainder of her physical examination was basically within normal limits.

A: Follicular adenoma, left thyroid lobe with Hürthle cell changes.

P: The patient will be booked for a right neck exploration and probable left thyroid lobectomy. All risks, benefits, and possible complications associated with surgery were discussed with the patient and she consented to the procedure.

GRAVES DISEASE SOAP NOTE

S: The patient is a 27-year-old female referred to me for Graves disease. Shortly after the patient became pregnant, she was found on lab work to be hyperthyroid. At this time she was placed on PTU 350 mg daily in divided doses until 1 week prior to delivery. The patient manifests all classical symptoms of hyperthyroidism including tremors, frequent soft stool, feeling flushed, insomnia, leg weakness, and exophthalmos.

O: Her extraocular eye movements were normal with the exception of convergence. On examination of her neck, the thyroid gland palpated at least twice normal size. The gland felt soft, compatible with hyperthyroidism. No distinct nodules were felt. The patient overall had normal hair distribution on her forearms but extension of hair on the dorsal aspect of the hands bilaterally. In addition, she is beginning to develop hair on the upper lip.

A/P: Graves disease. I had a lengthy discussion with the patient about her condition. After she has been euthyroid for a period of time, we will consider checking an androgen level. The patient was asked to discontinue her PTU for the time being and was sent to the lab for T3 and T4. She will be booked for a nuclear medicine uptake scan and subsequent therapy next week.

HYPOTHYROIDISM CONSULTATION

FINAL DIAGNOSES
1. Hypothyroidism.
2. Depression with panic features, likely secondary to hypothyroidism.

PRESENTATION AND COURSE: The patient is a very pleasant 21-year-old woman who is referred to me by her family physician after presenting to his office with recurrent palpitations, hyperventilation, and presyncope with numbness on her face transiently.

There is little past significant medical history in this young nonsmoker who denies alcohol or recreational drug use. She denies any heart disease history, and there is no family history of any early heart disease.

She described many social stressors over the last 6-12 months, including having a 5-year-old child with the father being her abusive former boyfriend, financial stressors, having grown apart from friends, mother with issues with alcohol use, and divorced parents. She did admit to having a supportive present boyfriend and siblings, as well as her family physician but, up to this point, has not felt that she could confide in them.

She described a 6-month history of fear of the dark, nightmares, poor sleep, decreased interest, decreased energy, weight gain with compulsive eating, guilt over not living up to others' expectations, mental and physical slowness, and decreased mood. Importantly, she denies any suicidal or harmful ideation, and I believe her with respect to this.

With respect to these symptoms, I asked Psychiatry to see her, and I know that that did occur, but I am not privy to the actual dictation at this time.

The incident of palpitations, hyperventilation, and presyncope was limited to a number of minutes on today's occasion but had lasted in the past up to hours at a time.

Physical exam revealed a tearful young woman with decreased affect. Pulse was 66 and regular, oxygen saturation 98% on room air, and blood pressure normal at 130/85 mmHg. Normal heart sounds, chest clear, and abdomen within normal limits. No focal neurologic signs.

Electrocardiogram revealed sinus arrhythmia. Chest x-ray was normal. CBC, D-dimer, and electrolytes were normal. Of peculiar note was a TSH which came back at greater than 100.

ASSESSMENT: The patient very likely has Hashimoto hypothyroidism. On review, she does have a mild-to-moderate goiter with no nodularity or tenderness. This likely, in whole or in part, explains her recent depression and panic state. Free T4 was ordered, but this is very likely just a technicality. I have started her on Synthroid at 112 mcg daily. Serum antithyroid antibodies are not necessary at this time. Given that Psychiatry has seen her and has arranged some type of followup, she is okay to be discharged, and that was done today. I have asked her to see her family physician in followup, and I would suggest having her TSH rechecked in about 3 months' time for further titration, either up or down, of her thyroid medicine.

LOBECTOMY, LEFT THYROID

PREOPERATIVE DIAGNOSIS: Left thyroid mass.

POSTOPERATIVE DIAGNOSIS: Left thyroid mass.

PROCEDURE PERFORMED: Left thyroid lobectomy.

INDICATIONS FOR PROCEDURE: This lady has had an ultrasound of her neck done. This demonstrated a 2-cm lesion in the left lobe of her thyroid. Aspiration biopsy demonstrated cells suspicious for papillary carcinoma. We decided to proceed with thyroid lobectomy.

PROCEDURE IN DETAIL: The patient was brought to the operating room, and a general anesthetic was administered. Airway was maintained with the use of an endotracheal tube. A nerve monitor tube was used. The neck was prepped and draped in an extended position. A skin crease incision was made above the sternal notch. Dissection was carried through the subcutaneous and platysmal layers. Flaps were elevated superiorly and inferiorly. The strap muscles were then split in the midline, and the face of the thyroid gland was isolated on each side. Dissection was carried around the left lobe of the gland. The upper pole vessels were skeletonized and doubly tied. Posteriorly, the gland was cleared. The recurrent laryngeal nerve was identified. This was confirmed with a nerve stimulator. The gland was gradually dissected inferior to the nerve. I felt that 2 definite parathyroid glands were identified and preserved in the neck. These had good blood supply. There was a relatively large vein entering the mid portion of the gland. This was tied with chromic and cut. The gland was then rotated forward off the upper trachea and larynx. It was cut across at the isthmus and sent for frozen section.

Frozen section suggested benign disease. Therefore it seemed apparent that nothing further should be done.

A Jackson-Pratt drain was brought out through a separate stab wound on the right side. The strap muscles and platysmal layer were closed with interrupted sutures of 3-0 chromic. The skin was closed with a running suture of 4-0 nylon, and the procedure was terminated.

The patient tolerated the procedure well and left the operating room in good condition.

LOBECTOMY, LEFT TOTAL THYROID

PREOPERATIVE DIAGNOSIS: Previous right thyroid cancer.

POSTOPERATIVE DIAGNOSIS: Pending pathology.

OPERATIVE PROCEDURE: Left total thyroid lobectomy.

INDICATIONS: This pleasant young lady had a right papillary carcinoma, which was resected a few months ago. She is back for completion thyroidectomy preparatory to consideration of radioactive iodine.

FINDINGS: The patient had a normal-looking, slightly cystic left lobe of the thyroid, which was normal size. There was no sign of any adenopathy or disease extension. The area of the previous cancer, which was just off to the right side of the isthmus, was carefully examined, and there was no sign of any recurrence.

DESCRIPTION OF PROCEDURE: With the patient under general endotracheal anesthesia and prepped and draped in the usual manner with the shoulders elevated on a sandbag, the previously used transverse incision was reopened, and the subplatysmal flaps were raised sharply with electrocautery. The superficial cervical fascia in the midline was picked up and incised, and the edges were retracted to the left, and then the thyroid was carefully mobilized in the usual fashion. The middle thyroid vein, superior and inferior thyroid arteries and veins were divided and taken down with 2-0, 3-0, and 4-0 Vicryl ligatures as appropriate. Other small feeding blood vessels were carefully controlled as encountered. The inferior parathyroid on the left and the recurrent laryngeal nerve were carefully preserved. The superior parathyroid was never identified.

The wound was hemostatic at the end of the case, and the superficial cervical fascia was closed using 3-0 PDS. The skin was closed with a running 5-0 Dexon after closing platysma with 3-0 Vicryl. A dry dressing was applied. The patient tolerated the procedure well, and there were no complications.

LOBECTOMY, RIGHT THYROID

PREOPERATIVE DIAGNOSIS: Right thyroid mass.

POSTOPERATIVE DIAGNOSIS: Right thyroid mass.

PROCEDURE PERFORMED: Right thyroid lobectomy.

INDICATIONS FOR PROCEDURE: This lady presents with a slowly advancing mass in the right lobe of the thyroid gland. Aspiration biopsy has demonstrated a follicular lesion. The mass is now over 3 cm in size, and due to its growth we decided to proceed with removal.

DETAILS OF PROCEDURE: The patient was brought to the operative room and a general anesthetic administered. Airway was maintained with the use of an endotracheal tube. Special monitoring tube was used to help monitor the recurrent laryngeal nerve. The neck was prepped and draped in an extended position. Electrodes were placed over the upper chest.

A skin crease incision was made above the sternal notch. Dissection was carried through the subcutaneous tissue and platysmal. Strap muscles were split in the midline. A relatively firm mass was present in the right lobe of the gland. The overlying strap muscles were somewhat attached. These were gradually cleared off the face of the gland. The left lobe appeared normal. Resection was carried around the right side posteriorly. The upper pole vessels were skeletonized and doubly tied. They were then cut. The inferior veins were gradually isolated and tied. The inferior thyroid artery was isolated and tied. The recurrent laryngeal nerve was identified where it entered the posterior larynx. There was a parathyroid gland apparent with this, which was preserved with good blood supply. There was a second gland inferiorly, which was also preserved. The recurrent laryngeal nerve was confirmed with the nerve monitor. The right thyroid lobe was then elevated off the larynx and upper trachea. It was cut across at the isthmus and removed totally. There was no significant bleeding encountered. Following the dissection, the nerve was again stimulated to confirm that it was intact. A Jackson-Pratt drain was brought out through a separate stab wound on the left. Strap muscles were reapproximated with 3-0 chromic. Platysmal layer also closed with 3-0 chromic. A running 4-0 nylon suture was used on the skin.

The patient tolerated the procedure well and left the operative room in good condition.

RIGHT THYROID LOBECTOMY DISCHARGE SUMMARY

This gentleman presented with a relatively large mass in the right lobe of his thyroid gland. This has been increasing in size. Aspiration and biopsy had suggested benign disease, but the lesion was vague and advancing in size. The patient was therefore admitted for thyroid lobectomy.

He does have a history of hypertension. He, however, had not continued with his therapy. He was mildly hypertensive when admitted.

He underwent his surgery on the day of admission. This was well tolerated. He remained hypertensive postoperatively. Internal Medicine reviewed him in this regard and recommended therapy with HCTZ 12.5 mg daily. The patient will be discharged on this. He does not have a general practitioner that he deals with regularly, and I will review him in the office next week for removal of sutures. At that time he will have decided on a general practitioner. The information about his hypertensive therapy will be forwarded.

We do not have a final pathology report back on the thyroid mass.

DISCHARGE DIAGNOSIS: Right thyroid nodule, final pathology report not yet available.

PRINCIPAL PROCEDURE: Right thyroid lobectomy.

Lymphoma Removal, Left Neck

Preoperative Diagnosis: Possible lymphoma, left neck.

Postoperative Diagnosis: Possible lymphoma, left neck.

Procedure Performed: Removal of lymph nodes, left neck.

Indications for Surgery: This lady presents with a mass in the left lower neck. She thinks this has been stable in size through the last month. Aspiration biopsy had been performed and suggested a diagnosis of lymphoma. She did have a previous history of a left parotid tumor being resected and treated with radiotherapy. This was about 40 years ago. She was admitted for open biopsy of this neck mass.

Operative Procedure: The patient was brought to the operative room, and a general anesthetic was administered. Airway was maintained with the use of an endotracheal tube. The left neck was prepped and draped in the usual manner. A skin crease incision was made, and this was carried down through the subcutaneous and platysmal layers. The mass was identified without difficulty. We approached it from the posterior aspect of the sternomastoid muscle where it was most apparent. Gradually dissection was carried out around the mass. This was obvious to be a group of lymph nodes. They did extend anteriorly to the carotid sheath. The mass of nodes, however, was resected completely. It was sent to the pathologist as fresh tissue so that cell studies could be completed.

The wound was drained with 1/4-inch Penrose. Deep layers were closed with interrupted sutures of 3-0 chromic. The skin was closed with a running suture of 4-0 nylon. The drain was sutured in place. The procedure was then terminated.

The patient tolerated the procedure well and left the operative room in good condition.

Parathyroidectomy

Preoperative Diagnosis: Hyperparathyroidism.

Postoperative Diagnosis: Hyperparathyroidism.

Operation: Parathyroidectomy.

Anesthesia: General anesthesia with endotracheal tube.

INDICATIONS: This is a female with hypercalcemia found to have hyperparathyroidism on endocrine workup. The risks and benefits of surgery were discussed with the patient including the possibility of missing the gland that may be involved. The patient understands and agrees to proceed.

PROCEDURE/FINDINGS: The patient was taken to the operating room and placed supine on the OR table. General anesthesia was induced, and she was intubated without difficulty. A slight sheet roll was placed underneath the shoulders, and the neck was placed in extension taking great care to make sure that the occiput was padded. The arms were tucked at her sides, and she was placed in somewhat of the reverse Trendelenburg position.

The neck and upper chest were then prepped and draped in sterile fashion. A transverse low-collar incision was then performed and deepened down through the platysma muscle layer which was very thin. Hemostasis was achieved with both electrocautery and with Vicryl ties along larger veins. A superior flap was made to the thyroid notch, inferiorly to the suprasternal notch. Subsequently the strap muscles were retracted laterally by dividing along the median raphe. We dissected down to the thyroid gland, and then the strap muscles were brought laterally. We first addressed the right side of the patient. The middle thyroid vein was tied off with silk ligatures. With careful dissection, peeling the thyroid gland medially, I identified a large parathyroid, what appeared to be an adenoma, measuring over 1.5 cm. Care was taken to assure good hemostasis by both clips and silk ligatures. In this fashion, the right inferior parathyroid gland was removed in toto. This was sent for frozen section which confirmed removal of parathyroid tissue.

Attention was directed over to the left side. The thyroid gland here appeared to be somewhat full but containing no nodules. Peeling this medially as well, a normal-appearing parathyroid gland was visualized. This was left intact and no dissection occurred in this area. No biopsy of this was performed.

The neck was irrigated with sterile fluid. Hemostasis was noted. The strap muscles were then brought back medially and together with a running suture of 2-0 Vicryl, the platysmal muscle layer was closed with running 3-0 Vicryl, and the skin was closed with a subcuticular suture of 4-0 Monocryl. Steri-Strips were applied. A sterile dressing was placed. The patient was then awakened and extubated and taken to the recovery room in stable and satisfactory condition. Sponge and needle counts were correct at the end of the case.

Of note, the clips will identify where the parathyroid enlarged gland was removed. It appeared to be just below the inferior thyroid artery.

Parathyroidectomy and Thyroid Lobectomy

Preoperative Diagnosis: Hyperparathyroidism.

Postoperative Diagnoses
1. Hyperparathyroidism.
2. Thyroiditis.

Operation
1. Neck exploration.
2. Parathyroidectomy.
3. Right thyroid lobectomy with frozen section.

Anesthesia: General anesthesia via endotracheal tube.

Estimated Blood Loss: Less than 100 mL.

Procedure/Findings: The patient was anesthetized with general anesthesia via endotracheal tube. A roll was placed under her shoulder and her neck hyperextended. The face, neck, and upper chest were prepped with DuraPrep and draped in a sterile fashion. The patient had received a sestamibi injection prior to the procedure, although preoperatively the findings on a sestamibi scan were ambiguous at best. We decided to optimize our chance of finding the abnormality since there was a slight asymmetry to her preoperative study. In addition, the patient received 500 mg of methylene blue intravenously after being induced. The patient tolerated these without any problems. The line of incision was marked using a marking pen, and examining the patient with the gamma probe demonstrated that on the right side the signal was considerably stronger than the left. On the right side in the midportion of the thyroid, the signal was approximately 2100-2500, whereas on the left side, it was approximately 1400-1700.

Initially we made an opening in the left side of the incision and extended it through the platysma. We retracted the strap muscles medially and went over the medial edge of the sternocleidomastoid to examine that area, since it appeared to be hot by the gamma probe; however, the thyroid lobe itself appeared grossly enlarged and perhaps had a nodule in it; therefore we abandoned that approach. The incision was extended to create a curved incision following the skin lines centered about the midline and extended through the platysma. The strap muscles were divided in the midline and retracted, and the thyroid gland exposed. We dissected the thyroid gland free. Ultimately we exposed the inferior pole vessels bilaterally, the recurrent laryngeal nerve bilaterally, and the upper pole. There was no obvious abnormality. Again, the strongest signal from the gamma probe was in the midportion of the thyroid, and this area was very hard.

Examining the usual locations for the parathyroids did not reveal any suspicious findings initially. There were some lymph nodes on the left side, and a tiny nodule immediately adjacent to the thyroid on the edge of the inferior thyroid artery, and again the indurated area within the right lobe of the thyroid. We examined along the space between the trachea and esophagus bilaterally and also along the carotid sheath bilaterally. No specific abnormality could be identified, either by the gamma probe or by dissection. Therefore, we decided to remove the right lobe of the thyroid with the slight possibility that there was a parathyroid within it. This was dissected free. Again, we had identified the recurrent laryngeal nerve. Vessels were ligated with either 4-0 or 2-0 Vicryl ties. The upper pole vessels were doubly ligated and the thyroid gland clamped at its isthmus and then the specimen excised.

The stump of the isthmus was suture ligated with 2-0 Vicryl, and the right lobe thyroid, the 2 lymph nodes from the left lower pole, the nodule near the right lower pole, and 1 other nodule slightly to the left of midline below the isthmus were all sent for frozen section. These ultimately revealed thyroiditis. The nodule on the right lower pole was just additional thyroid tissue. The lymph nodes were as suspected, and the sub-isthmus nodule, which measured about 8 mm in largest diameter, was parathyroid. It should be noted that it did not seem to be stained particularly darkly.

The area was reexamined with the gamma probe. The signal where there was still thyroid gland remained relatively constant. No other hot spot could be found. There was a nodular area in the lower pole of the left lobe of the thyroid just distal to the inferior thyroid vessels. A clamp was placed. This was excised. Frozen section demonstrated it was thyroid tissue. The amputation site was suture ligated with 2-0 Vicryl. The neck was re-explored again along the carotid sheath and the tracheoesophageal groove and all of the soft tissue below. Recurrent laryngeal nerves were seen. Again, they appeared to be unharmed, and no other abnormality could be identified. No other abnormality could be palpated within the thyroid lobe. Therefore we decided to close.

The wound was irrigated. We used some Gelfoam and topical thrombin to obtain hemostasis, and then the strap muscles and platysma were closed with 2-0 Vicryl. The skin was closed with 4-0 Vicryl, benzoin, and Steri-Strips. Sponge and needle counts were correct. The patient tolerated the procedure well and returned to the recovery room awake and in stable condition.

PAROTIDECTOMY, LEFT SUPERFICIAL WITH FACIAL NERVE DISSECTION

PREOPERATIVE DIAGNOSIS: Left parotid tumor.

POSTOPERATIVE DIAGNOSIS: Left parotid tumor.

OPERATION: Left superficial parotidectomy with facial nerve dissection.

FINDINGS: The patient is an 82-year-old female with an enlarging mass on the left parotid area, superficial lobe, lower pole. This measured approximately 2.5 cm. There was an enlarged lymph node attached to it. Identification of the main trunk and the different branches of the facial nerve on the left side was accomplished, and they were protected from injury. At the completion of the operation, the integrity of the branches was found to be preserved and also with good response to nerve stimulation. The patient tolerated the procedure well.

PROCEDURE IN DETAIL: The patient was brought to the operating room and placed under adequate general endotracheal anesthesia by the anesthetist who also monitored the patient throughout the procedure. The patient was placed in a semisitting position, slightly tilting her head to the right side. Appropriate exposure was then accomplished, and the skin edges were outlined, starting at the level of the zygomatic arch and following the skin fold on the preauricular area, and then going around the tragus and around a curve turn going down to the superior neck fold approximately 2 cm distal to the angle of the jaw. It extended anterior to the facial vessels. Appropriate prepping with Betadine solution was accomplished. Sterile cotton was placed in the ear canal and then removed at the completion of the operation and draping was accomplished.

Dissection was then carried through the subcutaneous tissues. Dissection was carried in order to elevate the flap anterior, and this was accomplished by identifying the anterior border of the sternocleidomastoid muscle on the most posterior aspect of the incision and then carried forward toward the anterior aspect of the parotid gland proper. This was done with cautery set at 25. Appropriate sutures were placed in order to expose the area, and then the dissection was carried to the preauricular area by following the cartilage, and this was done mostly bluntly and with the bipolar for cauterization after elevating and identification of tissues. The main trunk was eventually identified following the point as outlined by the preauricular cartilage of the area, and then once the main trunk had been identified, appropriate exposure was accomplished again by blunt dissection and elevating the tissue after visualization of the different branches of the nerve, and then using the bipolar and transecting. Branches of the posterior facial vein were identified and tied by means of 3-0 silk. The upper division of the nerve was then dissected free, including zygomatic and temporal, and then anterior aspect of the gland on the upper aspect was dissected free, separated, and dissection was carried toward the area of the mass proper which was as previously stated on the lower pole of the thyroid. Again following the lower division of the main trunk, the mandibular and cervical branches were also identified as a buckle, and again the dissection was carried separating from the mass proper, and total excision of the mass was accomplished after controlling the superior facial vessels and making sure that the mandibular branch was preserved and running anteriorly to them as normal.

Once the mass had been removed, irrigation was accomplished until returns were clear. Further stimulation was checked by means of the nerve stimulator with good response of peripheral branches, and integrity was found to be preserved, and then a round Silastic 10-French drain was left in place and brought out through a stab wound, secured in placed by 3-0 nylon. Approximation of the wound was then accomplished by means of 3-0 chromic to the subcutaneous and dermis area. The posterior lip of the anterior flap was then transected in order to increase its vascularity and then properly attached to the rest of the incision. The skin was then closed by means of running subcuticular suture of 4-0 Monocryl. There was good vacuum produced by the drain proper with collapsing of the flaps, and then Steri-Strips were applied, and the operation was considered terminated.

DISPOSITION: The patient tolerated the procedure without any apparent complications and was transferred to recovery in stable condition.

DRAINS: 10-French round Silastic through a stab wound.

ESTIMATED BLOOD LOSS: 150 mL.

SPECIMEN: Left parotidectomy with attached tumor.

PAROTID TUMOR DISCHARGE SUMMARY

DISCHARGE DIAGNOSES
1. Lymphoma, right cervical region.
2. Right hydronephrosis due to lymphatic enlargement and obstruction.
3. Anxiety state.
4. Previous uterine and breast cancer.

HISTORY: The patient is a 72-year-old woman admitted to the hospital because of an enlarging mass in her right parotid area. While in the hospital she was investigated with a CT scan of her neck and abdomen, which showed a mass in her right side of her neck in the parotid region, which turned out to be a malignant lymphoma. She also was found to have a right hydronephrosis probably due to an enlarging lymph gland in the area. Over the course in hospital, she was taken to the operating room for surgery on the parotid tumor, which turned out to be a lymphoma. She was followed in the hospital by Internal Medicine with plans for outpatient followup. Prior to discharge, she recovered quite remarkably. She was having a lot less pain and after discharge will be followed in the office.

THYROIDECTOMY, PAPILLARY CARCINOMA

PREOPERATIVE DIAGNOSIS: Papillary carcinoma, thyroid.

POSTOPERATIVE DIAGNOSIS: Papillary carcinoma, thyroid.

PROCEDURE PERFORMED: Excision, thyroid gland.

INDICATIONS FOR PROCEDURE: This young lady has presented with a 3-cm mass in the medial portion of the left lobe of her thyroid gland. This had been slowly enlarging. Aspiration biopsy had demonstrated papillary carcinoma. She was admitted for thyroid surgery and underwent her operation on the day of admission.

OPERATIVE DETAILS: General anesthetic was administered. The neck was prepped and draped in an extended position. A skin crease incision was made above the sternal notch. Dissection was carried through the subcutaneous and platysmal layers. Flaps were elevated superiorly and inferiorly. Strap muscles were split in the midline. The thyroid gland was exposed. The mass within the left lobe was readily apparent. The lobe was gradually dissected. The parathyroid glands were readily identified and preserved with good blood supply. The upper pole vessels were skeletonized and tied. The lobe was gradually mobilized and removed. This was sent for frozen section.

The report of frozen section was somewhat inconclusive. With the aspirate report, however, and the fact that the parathyroid tissue was easily identified, I thought the best approach was to complete the thyroidectomy. The right lobe of the gland was therefore also isolated. The upper pole vessels were tied. Again, the parathyroid tissue was well identified and preserved with good blood supply. The recurrent laryngeal nerve was also readily identified. Gradually this entire lobe was mobilized and removed. There was no lymphadenopathy apparent throughout the anterior compartment of the neck. A Jackson-Pratt drain was placed through a separate stab wound. Strap muscles and platysmal layer were closed with interrupted sutures of 3-0 chromic. The skin was closed with a running suture of 4-0 nylon, and the drain was also sutured in place. The procedure was then terminated. The patient tolerated this procedure well and left the operating room in good condition.

PAPILLARY CARCINOMA OF THE THYROID

PREOPERATIVE DIAGNOSIS: Papillary carcinoma of the thyroid gland.

POSTOPERATIVE DIAGNOSIS: Papillary carcinoma of the thyroid gland.

PROCEDURE PERFORMED: Left thyroidectomy.

INDICATIONS FOR PROCEDURE: This lady had a right thyroidectomy last fall, which demonstrated a papillary carcinoma of the thyroid, greater than 1 cm. Completion thyroidectomy is proposed, having discussed the options including risks of surgery.

DETAILS OF PROCEDURE AND FINDINGS: The patient was placed in the supine position under general anesthesia. The neck was somewhat extended, and she was suitably prepped and draped. A transverse incision was made through the old scar, and that was extended a little bit laterally to the left side for better exposure. Platysmal layer was divided, and the strap muscles were separated in the midline. The left thyroid lobe was exposed. The inferior thyroid artery was divided between clamps and ligated with 3-0 Vicryl. The middle thyroid vein was similarly isolated, clamped, and ligated before dividing it. Smaller vessels were cauterized or ligated with Vicryl. Attention was taken to stay right on the thyroid gland to avoid damaging the parathyroids. There was some fatty tissue toward the inferior pole, which could have contained the inferior parathyroid gland, although this was not certain. It was all preserved by staying on the thyroid. There was a little bit of yellowish tissue, which came out and was buried in the sternomastoid muscle on the left side in case it did represent some parathyroid tissue. The upper pole gland was divided within the substance of the gland between clamps, and 3-0 Vicryl ties were used on the upper pole vessels. The thyroid lobe was rotated off the trachea from medial to lateral using cautery, taking with it the isthmus, which had been left behind. The recurrent laryngeal nerve was identified and traced up to its point where it pierced the cricopharyngeus muscle. It was protected throughout this. The thyroid was separated off the trachea. The isthmus was tagged with a stitch, as was the upper pole, and these were labeled as per the pathology sheet. The superior parathyroid gland looked like it was left in the patient. It was a little bit bruised and was located just lateral to the recurrent laryngeal nerve superiorly.

Hemostasis was achieved with pressure and a small piece of Surgicel. The strap muscles were reapproximated in the midline with interrupted 3-0 Vicryl sutures. Platysma was closed with 3-0 Vicryl, and the skin was closed with 4-0 Vicryl subcuticular stitch and Steri-Strips. Marcaine with epinephrine was infiltrated for postoperative analgesia. She tolerated the procedure without complications and was transferred to the recovery room in satisfactory condition.

Common Terms by Procedure

Addison Disease
Addison disease
addisonian
adrenocorticotropic hormone pituitary
   adenoma
cortisol
Cushing syndrome
cushingoid appearance
Florinef
hypocortisolism
postural hypotension
prednisone
transsphenoidal hypophysectomy

Completion Thyroidectomy
15 blade
2-0 silk ties
3-0 silk ties
3-0 Vicryl interrupted
3-0 nylon
4-0 Monocryl
anterior trachea
avascular attachments
benzoin
bipolar cautery
dissection
electrocautery
endotracheal anesthesia
extubated
hemostasis
hypercalcemia
inferior thyroid artery branches
inferior parathyroid
inferior pole vessels
Jackson-Pratt drain
larynx
Marcaine
nodule
platysma

recurrent laryngeal nerve
skin exit site
Steri-Strips
strap muscles
subcutaneous tissue
subcuticular
subplatysmal flaps
superior pole
superior parathyroid
supine position
thyroid lobectomy
thyroid lobe
trachea
transverse cervical incision
venous ligaments

Completion Thyroid Lobectomy
2-0 Vicryl
4-0 Vicryl
adhesions
benzoin
completion thyroidectomy
doubly ligated
DuraPrep
electrocautery
endotracheal tube
evoked potential monitoring
Hemoclip
hemostasis
hyperextended
I-131 treatment
lower pole
lymphadenopathy
nerve stimulation
papillary carcinoma
parathyroid
platysma
recurrent laryngeal nerve
semi-sitting position

Steri-Strips
strap muscles
subplatysmal flaps
substernal notch
thyroid cartilage
trachea
upper pole

Diabetes, Complication of Gangrene: Digit Amputation

abscess
amputation
antibiotics
chronic renal failure
computed tomography (CT) angiogram
computed tomography (CT) scan
creatinine
diabetes mellitus
gangrene
gangrenous
inflammation
magnetic resonance (MR) angiogram
orthopedics
rehab facility

Diabetes Control Discharge Summary

American Diabetes Association (ADA)
   diet
blood sugar
diabetes type 1
glucose level
hemoglobin A1c
high fasting levels
high postprandial levels
Humulin insulin
hypercalcemia
hypertension
labile blood sugars
NPH (insulin)
sliding scale

Diabetes Mellitus History and Physical

blood urea nitrogen (BUN)
dehydration
electrolyte imbalance
fingerstick blood sugar reading
Lantus
normal saline
pentoxifylline
regular insulin
serum glucose level
serum sodium

Diabetes Mellitus, Newly Diagnosed

blood pH
blood glucose
blurred vision
carbon dioxide (CO2)
diabetic diet
dry mouth
electrolytes
enlarged cervical nodes
hemoglobin
increased thirst
increased urine output
ketoacidosis
ketones
Novolin NPH
NovoLog
platelet count
potassium chloride (KCl)
sodium
thyroid-stimulating hormone (TSH)
tonsillitis
urea
urine glucose
white blood cell (WBC)

Diabetes Mellitus Type 2 Consultation
angiotensin-converting enzyme inhibitors
chronic renal failure
DiaBeta
diaphoresis
elevated potassium
glucose infusion
hyperkalemia
hypoglycemia
Kayexalate
metabolic acidosis
prerenal azotemia
renal insufficiency
sodium bicarbonate
vomiting
weakness

Diabetic Foot Infection Debridement
Bactroban ointment
cellulitis
clindamycin
curettage
curetted
debridement
diabetic foot infection
first metatarsal
indolent infection
inflammatory material
metatarsophalangeal (MTP) joint
methicillin-resistant Staphylococcus aureus (MRSA)
neuropathic changes
osteomyelitis
residual stump
ulcers
vancomycin

Pediatric Diabetic Ketoacidosis
bicarb
diabetic ketoacidosis (DKA)
glucose
hemoglobin A1c
Humalog sliding scale
insulin drip
ketones
leukocyte esterase
low-carb American Diabetes Association (ADA) diet
mixed flora
nitrites
NPH (insulin)
pediatric intensive care unit (ICU)
rapid strep and throat culture
regular insulin
strep B
type 1 diabetes mellitus
urine culture

Follicular Adenoma of the Thyroid
cold nodule
fine-needle aspiration
Hürthle cell adenoma
nuclear medicine scan
thyroid function studies
thyroid lobectomy

Graves Disease
androgen level
euthyroid
exophthalmos
flushed
frequent soft stool
hyperthyroid
insomnia
nuclear medicine uptake scan
propylthiouracil (PTU)
T3
T4
tremors
weakness

Hypothyroidism Consultation
chest x-ray
complete blood count (CBC)
D-dimer
electrocardiogram
electrolytes
free T4
goiter
Hashimoto hypothyroidism
hyperventilation
numbness
palpitations
presyncope
serum antithyroid antibodies
sinus arrhythmia
Synthroid
thyroid-stimulating hormone (TSH)

Lobectomy, Left Thyroid
3-0 chromic
4-0 nylon
aspiration biopsy
benign disease
chromic
dissection
doubly tied
endotracheal tube
extended position
flaps
frozen section
interrupted sutures
isthmus
Jackson-Pratt drain
larynx
nerve monitor tube
parathyroid glands
platysmal layers
recurrent laryngeal nerve
running suture
skeletonized
stab wound
sternal notch

strap muscles
subcutaneous layers
trachea
ultrasound
upper pole vessels

Lobectomy, Left Total Thyroid
2-0 Vicryl ligatures
3-0 Vicryl ligatures
3-0 Polydioxanone Sutures (PDS)
4-0 Vicryl ligatures
adenopathy
completion thyroidectomy
cystic left lobe
electrocautery
feeding blood vessels
general endotracheal anesthesia
hemostatic
inferior parathyroid
isthmus
middle thyroid vein
papillary carcinoma
platysma
radioactive iodine
recurrent laryngeal nerve
running 5-0 Dexon
sandbag
subplatysmal flaps
superficial cervical fascia
superior parathyroid
thyroid lobectomy
transverse incision

Lobectomy, Right Thyroid
3-0 chromic
4-0 nylon suture
aspiration biopsy
dissection
doubly tied
electrodes
endotracheal tube
follicular lesion
inferior veins

A75

inferior thyroid artery
isthmus
Jackson-Pratt drain
larynx
left lobe
monitoring tube
nerve monitor
parathyroid gland
platysmal layer
posterior larynx
recurrent laryngeal nerve
resection upper pole vessels
right lobe
skeletonized
skin crease incision
stab wound
sternal notch
strap muscles
subcutaneous tissue
thyroid lobectomy
upper trachea

Right Thyroid Lobectomy Discharge Summary

aspiration biopsy
benign disease
hydrochlorothiazide (HCTZ)
hypertensive
thyroid lobectomy
thyroid nodule

Lymphoma Removal, Left Neck

1/4-inch Penrose
3-0 chromic
4-0 nylon
aspiration biopsy
carotid sheath
cell studies
endotracheal tube
fresh tissue
interrupted sutures
lymph nodes

lymphoma
open biopsy
parotid tumor
platysmal layer
radiotherapy
running suture
skin crease incision
sternomastoid muscle
subcutaneous layer

Parathyroidectomy

2-0 Vicryl
3-0 Vicryl
4-0 Monocryl
adenoma
biopsy
electrocautery
endotracheal tube
frozen section
hemostasis
hypercalcemia
hyperparathyroidism
inferior parathyroid gland
inferior thyroid artery
median raphe
occiput
parathyroid
parathyroidectomy
platysmal muscle layer
reverse Trendelenburg position
silk ligatures
slight sheet roll
sterile fluid
Steri-Strips
strap muscles
subcuticular suture
superior flap
suprasternal notch
thyroid notch
transverse low-collar incision
Vicryl ties

Parathyroidectomy and Thyroid Lobectomy

2-0 Vicryl ties
4-0 Vicryl ties
amputation site
benzoin
carotid sheath
curved incision
DuraPrep
endotracheal tube
esophagus
frozen section
gamma probe
Gelfoam
hemostasis
hot spot
hyperparathyroidism
indurated area
inferior pole vessels
inferior thyroid artery
inferior thyroid vessels
isthmus
methylene blue
nodule
parathyroidectomy
parathyroids
platysma
recurrent laryngeal nerve
sestamibi injection
sestamibi scan
Steri-Strips
sternocleidomastoid
strap muscles
sub-isthmus nodule
thyroid lobectomy
thyroid lobe
thyroiditis
topical thrombin
trachea
tracheoesophageal groove
upper pole

Parathyroidectomy, Left Superficial with Facial Nerve Dissection

3-0 silk
3-0 nylon
3-0 chromic
4-0 Monocryl
Betadine solution
bipolar
buckle
cautery
cervical branch
dermis area
dissection
ear canal
endotracheal anesthesia
facial nerve dissection
facial vessels
lower pole
main trunk
mandibular branch
nerve stimulator
parotid tumor
parotid gland proper
peripheral branches
preauricular area
preauricular cartilage
round Silastic 10-French drain
semisitting position
stab wound
sterile cotton
Steri-Strips
sternocleidomastoid muscle
subcutaneous tissues
subcuticular suture
superficial parotidectomy
superficial lobe
temporal
tragus
zygomatic arch

Parotid Tumor Discharge Summary

computed tomography (CT) scan
hydronephrosis
lymphatic enlargement
lymphatic obstruction
lymphoma
malignant lymphoma

Thyroidectomy, Papillary Carcinoma

3-0 chromic
4-0 nylon
anterior compartment of the neck
aspirate report
aspiration biopsy
dissection
drain
extended position
flaps
frozen section
interrupted sutures
Jackson-Pratt drain
papillary carcinoma
parathyroid glands
parathyroid tissue
platysmal layers
recurrent laryngeal nerve
running suture
skeletonized
stab wound
sternal notch
strap muscles
subcutaneous
upper pole vessels

Papillary Carcinoma of the Thyroid

3-0 Vicryl ties
4-0 Vicryl subcuticular stitch
cautery
completion thyroidectomy
cricopharyngeus muscle
epinephrine
fatty tissue
hemostasis
inferior thyroid artery
inferior parathyroid gland
inferior pole
interrupted 3-0 Vicryl sutures
isthmus
Marcaine
middle thyroid vein
papillary carcinoma
platysmal layer
postoperative analgesia
recurrent laryngeal nerve
Steri-Strips
sternomastoid muscle
strap muscles
superior parathyroid gland
supine position
Surgicel
thyroid lobe
thyroidectomy
trachea
transverse incision
upper pole gland
upper pole vessels

Drugs by Indication

ACIDOSIS (METABOLIC)
Alkalinizing Agent
  Cytra-K (US)
  Neut® (US)
  Polycitra®-K (US)
  potassium citrate and citric acid
  sodium acetate
  sodium bicarbonate
  sodium lactate
  THAM® (US)
  tromethamine
Electrolyte Supplement, Oral
  Fleet® Phospho®-Soda Accu-Prep™
    (US-OTC)
  Fleet® Phospho®-Soda Oral
    Laxative (Can)
  Fleet® Phospho®-Soda (US-OTC)
  sodium phosphates
  Visicol™ (US)

ACROMEGALY
Ergot Alkaloid and Derivative
  Apo-Bromocriptine® (Can)
  bromocriptine
  Parlodel (US/Can)
  pergolide
  Permax® (US/Can)
  PMS-Bromocriptine (Can)
Growth Hormone Receptor Antagonist
  pegvisomant
  Somavert® (US)
Somatostatin Analog
  octreotide
  Sandostatin LAR® (US/Can)
  Sandostatin® (US/Can)

ADDISON DISEASE
Adrenal Corticosteroid
  A-HydroCort® (US)

betamethasone (systemic)
Celestone® Soluspan® (US/Can)
Celestone® (US)
Cortef® Tablet (US/Can)
cortisone acetate
Cortone® (Can)
hydrocortisone (systemic)
Hydrocortone® Phosphate (US)
Solu-Cortef® (US/Can)
Adrenal Corticosteroid
    (Mineralocorticoid)
  Florinef® (US/Can)
  fludrocortisone
Diagnostic Agent
  Cortrosyn® (US/Can)
  cosyntropin

ADENOSINE DEAMINASE DEFICIENCY
Enzyme
  Adagen™ (US/Can)
  pegademase (bovine)

ADRENOCORTICAL FUNCTION ABNORMALITIES
Adrenal Corticosteroid
  A-HydroCort® (US)
  A-methapred® (US)
  Apo-Prednisone® (Can)
  Aristocort® Forte Injection (US)
  Aristocort® Intralesional Injection (US)
  Aristocort® Tablet (US/Can)
  Aristospan® Intraarticular Injection
    (US/Can)
  Aristospan® Intralesional Injection
    (US/Can)
  betamethasone (systemic)
  Celestone® Soluspan® (US/Can)

Celestone® (US)
Cortef® Tablet (US/Can)
corticotropin
cortisone acetate
Cortone® (Can)
Decadron® (US/Can)
Deltasone® (US)
Depo-Medrol® (US/Can)
Dexamethasone Intensol® (US)
dexamethasone (systemic)
DexPak® TaperPak® (US)
Diodex® (Can)
H.P. Acthar® Gel (US)
hydrocortisone (systemic)
Hydrocortone® Phosphate (US)
Kenalog® Injection (US/Can)
Medrol® (US/Can)
methylprednisolone
Orapred™ (US)
Pediapred® (US/Can)
PMS-Dexamethasone (Can)
Prednicot® (US)
prednisolone (systemic)
Prednisol® TBA (US)
prednisone
Prednisone Intensol™ (US)
Prelone® (US)
Solu-Cortef® (US/Can)
Solu-Medrol® (US/Can)
Sterapred® DS (US)
Sterapred® (US)
triamcinolone (systemic)
Winpred™ (Can)
Adrenal Corticosteroid
(Mineralocorticoid)
Florinef® (US/Can)
fludrocortisone

ALDOSTERONISM
Diuretic, Potassium Sparing
Aldactone® (US/Can)
Novo-Spiroton (Can)
Spironolactone

ALOPECIA
Antiandrogen
finasteride
Propecia® (US/Can)
Progestin
hydroxyprogesterone caproate
Topical Skin Product
Apo-Gain® (Can)
Minox (Can)
minoxidil
Rogaine® (Can)
Rogaine® Extra Strength for Men
(US-OTC)
Rogaine® for Men (US-OTC)
Rogaine® for Women (US-OTC)

AMENORRHEA
Ergot Alkaloid and Derivative
Apo-Bromocriptine® (Can)
bromocriptine
Parlodel® (US/Can)
PMS-Bromocriptine (Can)
Gonadotropin
Factrel® (US)
gonadorelin
Lutrepulse™ (Can)
Progestin
Alti-MPA (Can)
Apo-Medroxy® (Can)
Aygestin® (US)
Camila™ (US)
Crinone® (US/Can)
Depo-Provera® Contraceptive (US)
Depo-Provera® (US/Can)
Errin™ (US)
Gen-Medroxy (Can)
hydroxyprogesterone caproate
Jolivette™ (US)
medroxyprogesterone acetate
Micronor® (US/Can)
Nora-BE™ (US)
norethindrone
Norlutate® (Can)

Nor-QD® (US)
Novo-Medrone (Can)
Prochieve™ (US)
Progestasert® (US)
progesterone
Prometrium® (US/Can)
Provera® (US/Can)

ANGIOEDEMA (HEREDITARY)
Anabolic Steroid
    stanozolol
    Winstrol® (US)
Androgen
    Cyclomen® (Can)
    danazol
    Danocrine® (US/Can)

BARTTER SYNDROME
Nonsteroidal Antiinflammatory Drug
    (NSAID)
    Advil® Children's (US-OTC)
    Advil® Infants' (US-OTC)
    Advil® Junior (US-OTC)
    Advil® Migraine (US-OTC)
    Advil® (US-OTC/Can)
    Apo-Ibuprofen® (Can)
    Apo-Indomethacin® (Can)
    Genpril® (US-OTC)
    Ibu-200 (US-OTC)
    ibuprofen
    Indocid® (Can)
    Indocid® P.D.A. (Can)
    Indocin® I.V. (US)
    Indocin® SR (US)
    Indocin® (US/Can)
    Indo-Lemmon (Can)
    indomethacin
    Indotec (Can)
    I-Prin (US-OTC)
    Menadol® (US-OTC)
    Midol® Maximum Strength Cramp
      Formula (US-OTC)

Motrin® Children's (US-OTC/Can)
Motrinv IB (US-OTC/Can)
Motrin® Infants' (US-OTC)
Motrin® Junior Strength (US-OTC)
Motrin® Migraine Pain (US-OTC)
Motrin® (US/Can)
Novo-Methacin (Can)
Novo-Profen® (Can)
Nu-Ibuprofen (Can)
Nu-Indo (Can)
Rhodacine® (Can)
Ultraprin (US-OTC)

BREAST ENGORGEMENT (POSTPARTUM)
Estrogen Derivative
    Alora® (US)
    Cenestin® (US/Can)
    C.E.S.® (Can)
    Climara® (US/Can)
    Congest (Can)
    Delestrogen® (US/Can)
    Depo®-Estradiol (US/Can)
    Esclim® (US)
    Estrace® (US/Can)
    Estraderm® (US/Can)
    estradiol
    Estradot® (Can)
    Estrasorb™ (US)
    Estring® (US/Can)
    EstroGel® (US/Can)
    estrogens (conjugated A/synthetic)
    estrogens (conjugated/equine)
    Femring™ (US)
    Gynodiol® (US)
    Menostar™ (US)
    Oesclim® (Can)
    Premarin® (US/Can)
    Vagifem® (US/Can)
    Vivelle-Dot® (US)
    Vivelle® (US/Can)

CACHEXIA
Progestin
Apo-Megestrol® (Can)
Lin-Megestrol (Can)
Megace® OS (US)
Megace® (US/Can)
megestrol acetate
Nu-Megestrol (Can)

CARCINOMA
Androgen
Andriol® (Can)
Androderm® (US/Can)
AndroGel® (US/Can)
Android® (US)
Andropository (Can)
bicalutamide
Casodex® (US/Can)
Deca-Durabolin® (Can)
Delatestryl® (US/Can)
Depotest® 100 (Can)
Depo®-Testosterone (US)
Durabolin® (Can)
Everone® 200 (Can)
Methitest® (US)
methyltestosterone
nandrolone
Striant™ (US)
Teslac® (US/Can)
Testim™ (US)
Testoderm® (Can)
testolactone
Testopel® (US)
testosterone
Testred® (US)
Virilon® (US)
Antiandrogen
Alti-CPA (Can)
Androcur® (Can)
Androcur® Depot (Can)
Apo-Flutamide® (Can)
cyproterone (Can)

Euflex® (Can)
Eulexin® (US/Can)
flutamide
Gen-Cyproterone (Can)
Novo-Flutamide (Can)
PMS-Flutamide (Can)
Antineoplastic Agent, Estrogen
Receptor Antagonist
Faslodex® (US)
fulvestrant
Antineoplastic Agent, Hormone
(Antiestrogen)
Femara® (US/Can)
letrozole
Estrogen and Androgen Combination
Estratest® H.S. (US)
Estratest® (US/Can)
estrogens (esterified) and
methyltestosterone
Estrogen Derivative
Alora® (US)
C.E.S.® (Can)
Climara® (US/Can)
Congest (Can)
Delestrogen® (US/Can)
Depo®-Estradiol (US/Can)
Esclim® (US)
Estrace® (US/Can)
Estraderm® (US/Can)
estradiol
Estradot® (Can)
Estrasorb™ (US)
Estring® (US/Can)
EstroGel® (US/Can)
estrogens (conjugated/equine)
estrone
Femring™ (US)
Gynodiol® (US)
Menostar™ (US)
Oesclim® (Can)
Premarin® (US/Can)
Vagifem® (US/Can)
Vivelle-Dot® (US)

Vivelle® (US/Can)
Gonadotropin-Releasing Hormone
    Analog
    goserelin
    Zoladex® LA (Can)
    Zoladex® (US/Can)
Progestin
    Alti-CPA (Can)
    Alti-MPA (Can)
    Androcur® (Can)
    Androcur® Depot (Can)
    Apo-Medroxy® (Can)
    Crinone® (US/Can)
    cyproterone (Can)
    Depo-Provera® Contraceptive (US)
    Depo-Provera® (US/Can)
    Gen-Cyproterone (Can)
    Gen-Medroxy (Can)
    hydroxyprogesterone caproate
    medroxyprogesterone acetate
    Novo-Medrone (Can)
    Prochieve™ (US)
    Progestasert® (US)
    progesterone
    Prometrium® (US/Can)
    Provera® (US/Can)
Somatostatin Analog
    octreotide
    Sandostatin LAR® (US/Can)
    Sandostatin® (US/Can)
Thyroid Product
    Armour® Thyroid (US)
    Cytomel® (US/Can)
    Eltroxin® (Can)
    Levothroid® (US)
    levothyroxine
    Levoxyl® (US)
    liothyronine
    liotrix
    Nature-Throid® NT (US)
    Novothyrox (US)
    Synthroid® (US/Can)
    thyroid
    Thyrolar® (US/Can)

Triostat® (US)
Unithroid® (US)
Westhroid® (US)

CONGENITAL SUCRASE-ISOMALTASE DEFICIENCY
Enzyme
    sacrosidase
    Sucraid™ (US/Can)

CRYPTORCHIDISM
Gonadotropin
    chorionic gonadotropin (human)

CUSHING SYNDROME
Antineoplastic Agent
    aminoglutethimide
    Cytadren® (US)

CUSHING SYNDROME (DIAGNOSTIC)
Diagnostic Agent
    Metopirone® (US)
    metyrapone

CYSTIC FIBROSIS
Enzyme
    dornase alfa
    Pulmozyme® (US/Can)

DIABETES INSIPIDUS
Hormone, Posterior Pituitary
    Pitressin® (US)
    Pressyn® AR (Can)
    Pressyn® (Can)
    vasopressin
Vasopressin Analog, Synthetic
    Apo-Desmopressin® (Can)
    DDAVP® (US/Can)
    desmopressin acetate
    Minirin® (Can)
    Octostim® (Can)
    Stimate™ (US)

DIABETES MELLITUS, INSULIN-DEPENDENT (IDDM)

Antidiabetic Agent, Parenteral
  Apidra™ (US)
  Humalog® Mix 25™ (Can)
  Humalog® Mix 75/25™ (US)
  Humalog® (US/Can)
  Humulin® 50/50 (US)
  Humulin® 70/30 (US)
  Humulin® (Can)
  Humulin® L (US)
  Humulin® N (US)
  Humulin® R (Concentrated) U-500
    (US)
  Humulin® R (US)
  Humulin® U (US)
  Iletin® II Pork (Can)
  insulin preparations
  Lantus® (US)
  Novolin® 70/30 (US)
  Novolin® ge (Can)
  Novolin® N (US)
  Novolin® R (US)
  NovoLog® Mix 70/30 (US)
  NovoLog® (US)
  NovoRapid® (Can)
  NPH Iletin® II (US)
  Regular Iletin® II (US)

DIABETES MELLITUS, NONINSULIN-DEPENDENT (NIDDM)

Antidiabetic Agent
  Actos® (US/Can)
  Apo-Gliclazide® (Can)
  Diamicron® (Can)
  Diamicron® MR (Can)
  gliclazide (Can)
  nateglinide
  Novo-Gliclazide (Can)
  pioglitazone

  Starlix® (US/Can)
Antidiabetic Agent (Biguanide)
  Avandamet™ (US/Can)
  glipizide and metformin
  Metaglip™ (US)
  rosiglitazone and metformin
Antidiabetic Agent, Oral
  acarbose
  acetohexamide
  Albert® Glyburide (Can)
  Alti-Metformin (Can)
  Amaryl® (US/Can)
  Apo-Chlorpropamide® (Can)
  Apo-Glyburide® (Can)
  Apo-Metformin® (Can)
  Apo-Tolbutamide® (Can)
  chlorpropamide
  DiabBeta® (US/Can)
  Diabinese® (US)
  Euglucon® (Can)
  Fortamet™ (US)
  Gen-Glybe (Can)
  Gen-Metformin (Can)
  glimepiride
  glipizide
  Glucophage® (US/Can)
  Glucophage® XR (US)
  Glucotrol® (US)
  Glucotrol® XL (US)
  Glucovance™ (US)
  glyburide
  glyburide and metformin
  Glycon (Can)
  Glynase® PresTab™ (US)
  Glyset® (US/Can)
  metformin
  Micronase® (US)
  miglitol
  Novo-Glyburide (Can)
  Novo-Metformin (Can)
  Novo-Propamide (Can)
  Nu-Glyburide (Can)
  Nu-Metformin (Can)

PMS-Glyburide (Can)
PMS-Metformin (Can)
Prandase® (Can)
Precose® (US)
ratio-Glyburide (Can)
Rho®-Metformin (Can)
Rhoxal-metformin FC (Can)
tolazamide
tolbutamide
Tolinase® (US/Can)
Tol-Tab® (US)
Antidiabetic Agent, Parenteral
Apidra™ (US)
Humalog® Mix 25™ (Can)
Humalog® Mix 75/25™ (US)
Humalog® (US/Can)
Humulin® 50/50 (US)
Humulin® 70/30 (US)
Humulin® (Can)
Humulin® L (US)
Humulin® N (US)
Humulin® R (Concentrated) U-500
    (US)
Humulin® R (US)
Humulin® U (US)
Iletin® II Pork (Can)
insulin preparations
Lantus® (US)
Novolin® 70/30 (US)
Novolin® ge (Can)
Novolin® N (US)
Novolin® R (US)
NovoLog® Mix 70/30 (US)
NovoLog® (US)
NovoRapid® (Can)
NPH Iletin® II (US)
Regular Iletin® II (US)
Antidiabetic Agent (Sulfonylurea)
glipizide and metformin
Glucovance™ (US)
glyburide and metformin
Metaglip™ (US)

Antidiabetic Agent (Thiazolidinedione)
Avandamet™ (US/Can)
rosiglitazone and metformin
Hypoglycemic Agent, Oral
Apo-Gliclazide® (Can)
Avandia® (US/Can)
Diamicron® (Can)
Diamicron® MR (Can)
gliclazide (Can)
GlucoNorm® (Can)
Novo-Gliclazide (Can)
Prandin® (US/Can)
repaglinide
rosiglitazone
Sulfonylurea Agent
Apo-Gliclazide® (Can)
Diamicron® (Can)
Diamicron® MR (Can)
gliclazide (Can)
Novo-Gliclazide (Can)
Thiazolidinedione Derivative
Actos® (US/Can)
Avandia® (US/Can)
pioglitazone
rosiglitazone

DWARFISM
Growth Hormone
Genotropin Miniquick® (US)
Genotropin® (US)
human growth hormone
Humatrope® (US/Can)
Norditropin® Cartridges (US)
Norditropin® (US/Can)
Nutropin AQ® (US/Can)
Nutropine® (Can)
Nutropin® (US)
Protropine® (Can)
Protropin® (US/Can)
Saizen® (US/Can)
Serostim® (US/Can)
Zorbtive™ (US)

DYSMENORRHEA

Nonsteroidal Antiinflammatory Drug
  (NSAID)
  Advil® (US-OTC/Can)
  Aleve®(US-OTC)
  Alti-Flurbiprofen (Can)
  Anaprox® DS (US/Can)
  Anaprox® (US/Can)
  Ansaid® (US/Can)
  Apo-Diclo® (Can)
  Apo-Diclo Rapide® (Can)
  Apo-Diclo SR® (Can)
  Apo-Diflunisal® (Can)
  Apo-Flurbiprofen® (Can)
  Apo-Ibuprofen® (Can)
  Apo-Keto® (Can)
  Apo-Keto-E® (Can)
  Apo-Keto SR® (Can)
  Apo-Mefenamic® (Can)
  Apo-Napro-Na® (Can)
  Apo-Napro-Na DS® (Can)
  Apo-Naproxen® (Can)
  Apo-Naproxen SR® (Can)
  Apo-Piroxicam® (Can)
  Cataflam® (US/Can)
  diclofenac
  Diclotec (Can)
  diflunisal
  Dolobid® (US)
  EC-Naprosyn® (US)
  Feldene® (US/Can)
  flurbiprofen
  Froben® (Can)
  Froben-SR® (Can)
  Gen-Naproxen EC (Can)
  Gen-Piroxicam (Can)
  Genpril® (US-OTC)
  Ibu-200 (US-OTC)
  ibuprofen
  I-Prin (US-OTC)
  ketoprofen
  mefenamic acid

Menadol® (US-OTC)
Midol® Maximum Strength Cramp
  Formula (US-OTC)
Motrin® IB (US-OTC/Can)
Motrin® (US/Can)
Naprelan® (US)
Naprosyn® (US/Can)
naproxen
Naxen® (Can)
Novo-Difenac® (Can)
Novo-Difenac-K (Can)
Novo-Difenac® SR (Can)
Novo-Diflunisal (Can)
Novo-Flurprofen (Can)
Novo-Keto (Can)
Novo-Keto-EC (Can)
Novo-Naproc EC (Can)
Novo-Naprox (Can)
Novo-Naprox Sodium (Can)
Novo-Naprox Sodium DS (Can)
Novo-Naprox SR (Can)
Novo-Pirocam® (Can)
Novo-Profen® (Can)
Nu-Diclo (Can)
Nu-Diclo-SR (Can)
Nu-Diflunisal (Can)
Nu-Flurprofen (Can)
Nu-Ibuprofen (Can)
Nu-Ketoprofen (Can)
Nu-Ketoprofen-E (Can)
Nu-Mefenamic (Can)
Nu-Naprox (Can)
Nu-Pirox (Can)
Orudis® KT (US-OTC)
Orudis® SR (Can)
Oruvail® (US/Can)
Pamprin® Maximum Strength All
  Day Relief (US-OTC)
Pennsaid® (Can)
Pexicam®- (Can)
piroxicam
PMS-Diclofenac (Can)
PMS-Diclofenac SR (Can)

PMS-Mefenamic Acid (Can)
Ponstan® (Can)
Ponstel® (US/Can)
Rhodis™ (Can)
Rhodis-EC™ (Can)
Rhodis SR™ (Can)
Riva-Diclofenac (Can)
Riva-Diclofenac-K (Can)
Riva-Naproxen (Can)
Solaraze™ (US)
Ultraprin (US-OTC)
Voltaren® (US/Can)
Voltaren®-XR (US)

GALACTORRHEA
Ergot Alkaloid and Derivative
  Apo-Bromocriptine® (Can)
  bromocriptine
  Parlodel® (US/Can)
  PMS-Bromocriptine (Can)

GOITER
Thyroid Product
  Armour® Thyroid (US)
  Cytomel® (US/Can)
  Eltroxin® (Can)
  Levothroid® (US)
  levothyroxine
  Levoxyl® (US)
  liothyronine
  liotrix
  Nature-Throid® NT (US)
  Novothyrox (US)
  Synthroid® (US/Can)
  thyroid
  Thyrolar® (US/Can)
  Triostat® (US)
  Unithroid® (US)
  Westhroid® (US)

GROWTH HORMONE DEFICIENCY
Growth Hormone
  Genotropin Miniquick® (US)
  Genotropin® (US)
  human growth hormone
  Humatrope® (US/Can)
  Norditropin® Cartridges (US)
  Norditropin® (US/Can)
  Nutropin AQ® (US/Can)
  Nutropine® (Can)
  Nutropin® (US)
  Protropine® (Can)
  Protropin® (US/Can)
  Saizen® (US/Can)
  Serostim® (US/Can)
  Zorbtive™ (US)

GROWTH HORMONE (DIAGNOSTIC)
Diagnostic Agent
  Geref® Diagnostic (US)
  sermorelin acetate

HARTNUP DISEASE
Vitamin, Water Soluble
  Niacinamide

HORMONAL IMBALANCE (FEMALE)
Progestin
  Alti-MPA (Can)
  Apo-Medroxy® (Can)
  Aygestin® (US)
  Camila™ (US)
  Crinone® (US/Can)
  Depo-Provera® Contraceptive (US)
  Depo-Provera® (US/Can)
  Errin™ (US)
  Gen-Medroxy (Can)
  hydroxyprogesterone caproate
  Jolivette™ (US)

medroxyprogesterone acetate
Micronor® (US/Can)
Nora-BE™ (US)
norethindrone
Norlutate® (Can)
Nor-QD® (US)
Novo-Medrone (Can)
Prochieve™ (US)
Progestasert® (US)
progesterone
Prometrium® (US/Can)
Provera® (US/Can)

HYPERMENORRHEA (TREATMENT)
Contraceptive, Oral
Alesse® (US/Can)
Apri® (US)
Aviane™ (US)
Brevicon® 0.5/35 (Can)
Brevicon® 1/35 (Can)
Brevicon® (US)
Cryselle™ (US)
Cyclen® (Can)
Cyclessa® (US)
Demulen® 30 (Can)
Demulen® (US)
Desogen® (US)
Enpresse™ (US)
Estrostep® Fe (US)
ethinyl estradiol and desogestrel
ethinyl estradiol and ethynodiol
   diacetate
ethinyl estradiol and levonorgestrel
ethinyl estradiol and norethindrone
ethinyl estradiol and norgestimate
ethinyl estradiol and norgestrel
femhrt® (US/Can)
Junel™ (US)
Kariva™ (US)
Lessina™ (US)
Levlen® (US)
Levlite™ (US)

Levora® (US)
Loestrin® 1.5.30 (Can)
Loestrin® Fe (US)
Loestrin® (US/Can)
Lo/Ovral® (US)
Low-Ogestrel® (US)
Marvelon® (Can)
mestranol and norethindrone
Microgestin™ Fe (US)
Minestrin™ 1/20 (Can)
Min-Ovral® (Can)
Mircette® (US)
Modicon® (US)
MonoNessa™ (US)
Necon® 0.5/35 (US)
Necon® 1/35 (US)
Necon® 1/50 (US)
Necon® 7/7/7 (US)
Necon® 10/11 (US)
Nordette® (US)
Norinyl® 1+35 (US)
Norinyl® 1+50 (US)
Nortrel™ 7/7/7 (US)
Nortrel™ (US)
Ogestrel®
Ortho® 0.5/35 (Can)
Ortho® 1/35 (Can)
Ortho® 7/7/7 (Can)
Ortho-Cept® (US/Can)
Ortho-Cyclen® (US)
Ortho-Novum® 1/50 (US/Can)
Ortho-Novum® (US)
Ortho-Tri-Cyclen® Lo (US)
Ortho Tri-Cyclen® (US)
Ovcon® (US)
Ovral® (Can)
Portia™ (US)
PREVEN® (US)
Previfem™ (US)
Seasonale® (US)
Select™ 1/35 (Can)
Solia™ (US)
Sprintec™ (US)

Synphasic® (Can)
Tri-Cyclen® (Can)
Tri-Levlen® (US)
TriNessa™ (US)
Tri-Norinyl® (US)
Triphasil® (US/Can)
Tri-Previfem™ (US)
Triquilar® (Can)
Tri-Sprintec™ (US)
Trivora® (US)
Velivet™ (US)
Zovia™ (US)
Contraceptive, Progestin Only
norgestrel
Ovrette® (US/Can)

HYPERPARATHYROIDISM
Calcimimetic
cinacalcet
Sensipar™ (US)
Vitamin D Analog
doxercalciferol
Hectorol® (US/Can)
paricalcitol
Zemplar™ (US/Can)

HYPERTHYROIDISM
Antithyroid Agent
Iosat™ (US-OTC)
methimazole
Pima® (US)
potassium iodide
propylthiouracil
Propyl-Thyracil® (Can)
SSKI® (US)
Tapazole® (US/Can)
Beta-Adrenergic Blocker
Apo-Propranolol® (Can)
Inderal® LA (US/Can)
Inderal® (US/Can)
InnoPran XL™ (US)
Nu-Propranolol (Can)
propranolol
Propranolol Intensol™ (US)

HYPOALDOSTERONISM
Diuretic, Potassium Sparing
amiloride
Midamor® (Can)

HYPOGLYCEMIA
Antihypoglycemic Agent
B-D™ Glucose (US-OTC)
Dex4 Glucose (US-OTC)
diazoxide
GlucaGen® Diagnostic Kit (US)
GlucaGen® (US)
glucagon
Glucagon Diagnostic Kit (US)
Glucagon Emergency Kit (US)
glucose (instant)
Glutol™ (US-OTC)
Glutose™ (US-OTC)
Hyperstat® I.V. (Can)
Hyperstat® (US)
Insta-Glucose® (US-OTC)
Proglycem® (US/Can)

HYPOGONADISM
Androgen
Andriol® (Can)
Androderm® (US/Can)
AndroGel® (US/Can)
Android® (US)
Andropository (Can)
Delatestryl® (US/Can)
Depotest® 100 (Can)
Depo®-Testosterone (US)
Everone® 200 (Can)
Methitest® (US)
methyltestosterone
Striant™ (US)
Testim™ (US)
Testoderm® (Can)
Testopel® (US)
testosterone
Testred® (US)
Virilon® (US)
Diagnostic Agent

Factrel® (US)
gonadorelin
Lutrepulse™ (Can)
Estrogen Derivative
Alora® (US)
Cenestin® (US/Can)
C.E.S.® (Can)
Climara® (US/Can)
Congest (Can)
Delestrogen® (US/Can)
Depo®-Estradiol (US/Can)
Esclim® (US)
Estrace® (US/Can)
Estraderm® (US/Can)
estradiol
Estradot® (Can)
Estrasorb™ (US)
Estratab® (Can)
Estring® (US/Can)
EstroGel® (US/Can)
estrogens (conjugated A/synthetic)
estrogens (conjugated/equine)
estrogens (esterified)
estrone
estropipate
ethinyl estradiol
Femring™ (US)
Gynodiol® (US)
Menest® (US/Can)
Menostar™ (US)
Oesclim® (Can)
Ogen® (US/Can)
Ortho-Est® (US)
Premarin® (US/Can)
Vagifem® (US/Can)
Vivelle-Dot® (US)
Vivelle® (US/Can)

HYPOPARATHYROIDISM

Diagnostic Agent
Forteo™ (US)
teriparatide
Vitamin D Analog

Calciferol™ (US)
Calcijex® (US)
calcitriol
DHT™ Intensol™ (US)
DHT™ (US)
dihydrotachysterol
Drisdol® (US/Can)
ergocalciferol
Hytakerol® (US/Can)
Ostoforte® (Can)
Rocaltrol® (US/Can)

HYPOTHYROIDISM

Thyroid Product
Armour® Thyroid (US)
Cytomel® (US/Can)
Eltroxin® (Can)
Levothroid® (US)
levothyroxine
Levoxyl® (US)
liothyronine
liotrix
Nature-Throid® NT (US)
Novothyrox (US)
Synthroid® (US/Can)
thyroid
Thyrolar® (US/Can)
Triostat® (US)
Unithroid® (US)
Westhroid® (US)

IMPOTENCY

Androgen
Android® (US)
Methitest® (US)
methyltestosterone
Testred® (US)
Virilon® (US)
Phosphodiesterase (Type 5) Enzyme
Inhibitor
Cialis® (US)
Levitra® (US)
sildenafil

tadalafil
vardenafil
Viagra® (US/Can)
Vasodilator
ethaverine

INFERTILITY
Antigonadotropic Agent
Antagon® (US/Can)
ganirelix
Orgalutran® (Can)
Ovulation Stimulator
Follistim® (US)
follitropin alfa
follitropin beta

INFERTILITY (FEMALE)
Ergot Alkaloid and Derivative
Apo-Bromocriptine® (Can)
bromocriptine
Parlodel® (US/Can)
PMS-Bromocriptine (Can)
Gonadotropin
chorionic gonadotropin (human)
menotropins
Pergonal® (US/Can)
Repronex® (US/Can)
Ovulation Stimulator
Clomid® (US/Can)
clomiphene
Milophene® (Can)
Serophene® (US/Can)
Progestin
Crinone® (US/Can)
Prochieve™ (US)
Progestasert® (US)
progesterone
Prometrium® (US/Can)

INFERTILITY (MALE)
Gonadotropin
chorionic gonadotropin (human)
menotropins
Pergonal® (US/Can)
Repronex® (US/Can)

LACTATION (SUPPRESSION)
Ergot Alkaloid and Derivative
Apo-Bromocriptine® (Can)
bromocriptine
Parlodel® (US/Can)
PMS-Bromocriptine (Can)

MALNUTRITION
Electrolyte Supplement, Oral
Anuzinc (Can)
Orazinc® (US-OTC)
Rivasol (Can)
Zincate® (US)
zinc sulfate
Nutritional Supplement
cysteine
glucose polymers
Moducal® (US-OTC)
Polycose® (US-OTC)
Trace Element
Iodopen® (US)
Molypen® (US)
M.T.E.-4® (US)
M.T.E.-5® (US)
M.T.E.-6® (US)
M.T.E.-7® (US)
Multitrace™-4 Neonatal (US)
Multitrace™-4 Pediatric (US)
Multitrace™-4 (US)
Multitrace™-5 (US)
Neotrace-4® (US)
Pedtrace-4® (US)
P.T.E.-4® (US)
P.T.E.-5® (US)

Selepen® (US)
trace metals
zinc chloride
Vitamin
ADEKs (US-OTC)
Advanced NatalCare® (US)
A-Free Prenatal (US)
Aminate Fe-90 (US)
Anemagen™ OB (US)
Cal-Nate™ (US)
CareNate™ 600 (US)
Centrum® Kids Rugrats™ Complete
(US-OTC)
Centrum® Kids Rugrats™ Extra
Calcium (US-OTC)
Centrum® Kids Rugrats™ Extra C
(US-OTC)
Centrumv Performance™ (US-
OTC)
Centrum® Silver® (US-OTC)
Centrum® (US-OTC)
Chromagen® OB (US)
Citracal® Prenatal Rx (US)
Duet® DHA (US)
Duet® (US)
Flintstones® Complete (US-OTC)
Flintstones® Original (US-OTC)
Flintstones® Plus Calcium (US-
OTC)
Flintstones® Plus Extra C (US-
OTC)
Flintstones® Plus Iron (US-OTC)
Folbee (US)
Folgard RX 2.2® (US)
Folgard® (US-OTC)
folic acid, cyanocobalamin, and
pyridoxine
Foltx® (US)
Geritol® Tonic (US-OTC)
Iberet®-500 (US-OTC)
Iberet-Folic-500® (US)
Iberet® (US-OTC)
Infuvite® Adult (US)

Infuvite® Pediatric (US)
KPN Prenatal (US)
M.V.I.®-12 (US)
M.V.I.-Adult® (US)
M.V.I.-Pediatric® (US)
My First Flintstones® (US-OTC)
NataChew™ (US)
NataFort® (US)
NatalCare® CFe 60 (US)
NatalCare® GlossTabs™ (US)
NatalCare® PIC Forte (US)
NatalCare® PIC (US)
NatalCare® Plus (US)
NatalCare® Rx (US)
NatalCare® Three (US)
NataTab™ CFe (US)
NataTab™ FA (US)
NataTab™ Rx (US)
Nestabs® CBF (US)
Nestabs® FA (US)
Nestabs® RX (US)
Niferex®-PN Forte (US)
Niferex®-PN (US)
NutriNate® (US)
OB-20 (US)
Obegyn™ (US)
One-A-Day® 50 Plus Formula (US-
OTC)
One-A-Day® Active Formula (US-
OTC)
One-A -Day® Essential Formula
(US-OTC)
One-A-Day® Kids Bugs Bunny and
Friends Complete (US-OTC)
One-A-Day® Kids Bugs Bunny and
Friends Plus Extra C (US-OTC)
One-A-Day® Kids Extreme Sports
(US-OTC)
One-A-Day® Kids Scooby-Doo!
Complete (US-OTC)
One-A-Day® Kids Scooby Doo!
Plus Calcium (US-OTC)

One-A-Day® Maximum Formula (US-OTC)
One-A-Day® Men's Formula (US-OTC)
One-A-Day® Today (US-OTC)
One-A-Day® Women's Formula (US-OTC)
Poly-Vi-Flor® (US)
Poly-Vi-Flor® with Iron (US)
Poly-Vi-Sol® (US-OTC)
Poly-Vi-Sol® with Iron (US-OTC)
PreCare® (US)
Prenatal 1-A-Day (US)
Prenatal AD (US)
Prenatal H (US)
Prenatal MR 90 Fe™ (US)
Prenatal MTR with Selenium (US)
Prenatal Plus (US)
Prenatal Rx 1 (US)
Prenatal U (US)
Prenatal Z (US)
Prenate Elite™ (US)
Prenate GT™ (US)
Soluvite-F (US)
StrongStart™ (US)
Stuartnatal® Plus 3™ (US-OTC)
Stuart Prenatal® (US-OTC)
Theragran® Heart Right™ (US-OTC)
Theragran-M® Advanced Formula (US-OTC)
Tricardio B (Can)
Trinate (US)
Tri-Vi-Flor® (US)
Tri-Vi-Flor® with Iron (US)
Tri-Vi-Sol® (US-OTC)
Tri-Vi-Sol® with Iron (US-OTC)
Ultra NatalCare® (US)
Vicon Forte® (US)
Vicon Plus® (US-OTC)
Vi-Daylin® ADC + Iron (US-OTC)
Vi-Daylin® ADC (US-OTC)
Vi-Daylin® Drops (US-OTC)

Vi-Daylin®/F ADC + Iron (US)
Vi-Daylin®/F ADC (US)
Vi-Daylin®/F + Iron (US)
Vi-Daylin®/F (US)
Vi-Daylin® + Iron Drops (US-OTC)
Vi-Daylin® + Iron Liquid (US-OTC)
Vi-Daylin® Liquid (US-OTC)
Vitaball® (US-OTC)
Vitacon Forte (US)
vitamins (multiple/injectable)
vitamins (multiple/oral)
vitamins (multiple/pediatric)
vitamins (multiple/prenatal)
Vitamin, Fat Soluble
Aqua Gem E® (US-OTC)
Aquasol A® (US)
Aquasol E® (US-OTC)
E-Gems® (US-OTC)
Key-E® Kaps (US-OTC)
Key-E® (US-OTC)
Palmitate-A® (US-OTC)
vitamin A
vitamin E
Vitamin, Water Soluble
Allbee® C-800 + Iron (US-OTC)
Allbee® C-800 (US-OTC)
Allbee® with C (US-OTC)
Aminoxin® (US-OTC)
Apatate® (US-OTC)
Betaxin® (Can)
DiatxFe™ (US)
Diatx™ (US)
Gevrabon® (US-OTC)
NephPlex® Rx (US)
Nephrocaps® (US)
Nephron FA® (US)
Nephro-Vite® Rx (US)
Nephro-Vite® (US)
pyridoxine
Stresstabs® B-Complex + Iron (US-OTC)
Stresstabs® B-Complex (US-OTC)

Stresstabs® B-Complex + Zinc (US-OTC)
Surbex-T® (US-OTC)
Thiamilate® (US-OTC)
thiamine
Trinsicon® (US)
vitamin B complex combinations
Z-Bec® (US-OTC)

MARFAN SYNDROME
Rauwolfia Alkaloid
  reserpine

MENOPAUSE
Ergot Alkaloid and Derivative
  belladonna, phenobarbital, and
    ergotamine tartrate
  Bellamine S (US)
  Bellergal® Spacetabs® (Can)
  Bel-Tabs (US)
Estrogen and Progestin Combination
  Activella™ (US)
  ClimaraPro™ (US)
  CombiPatch® (US)
  Estalis® (Can)
  Estalis-Sequi® (Can)
  estradiol and levonorgestrel
  estradiol and norethindrone
  estradiol and norgestimate
  estrogens (conjugated/equine) and
    medroxyprogesterone
  Prefest™ (US)
  Premphase® (US/Can)
  Premplus® (Can)
  Prempro™ (US/Can)
Estrogen Derivative
  Alora® (US)
  Cenestin® (US/Can)
  C.E.S.® (Can)
  Climara® (US/Can)
  Congest (Can)
  Delestrogen® (US/Can)
  Depo®-Estradiol (US/Can)

Esclim® (US)
Estrace® (US/Can)
Estraderm® (US/Can)
estradiol
Estradot® (Can)
Estrasorb™ (US)
Estratab® (Can)
Estring® (US/Can)
EstroGel® (US/Can)
estrogens (conjugated A/synthetic)
estrogens (conjugated/equine)
estrogens (esterified)
ethinyl estradiol
Femring™ (US)
Gynodiol® (US)
Menest® (US/Can)
Menostar™ (US)
Oesclim® (Can)
Premarin® (US/Can)
Vagifem® (US/Can)
Vivelle-Dot® (US)
Vivelle® (US/Can)

MENORRHAGIA
Androgen
  Cyclomen® (Can)
  danazol
  Danocrine® (US/Can)

OBESITY
Amphetamine
  Desoxyn® (US/Can)
  Dexedrine® (US/Can)
  dextroamphetamine
  Dextrostat® (US)
  methamphetamine
Anorexiant
  Adipex-P® (US)
  benzphetamine
  Bontril® (Can)
  Bontril PDM® (US)
  Bontril® Slow-Release (US)
  Didrex® (US/Can)

diethylpropion
Ionamin® (US/Can)
Melfiat® (US)
Meridia® (US/Can)
Obezine® (US)
phendimetrazine
phentermine
Plegine® (Can)
Prelu-2® (US)
sibutramine
Statobex® (Can)
Tenuate® Dospan® (US/Can)
Tenuate® (US/Can)
Lipase Inhibitor
orlistat
Xenical® (US/Can)

OSTEOPOROSIS
Bisphosphonate Derivative
alendronate
Aredia® (US/Can)
Didronel® (US/Can)
etidronate disodium
Fosamax® (US/Can)
Gen-Etidronate (Can)
Novo-Alendronate (Can)
pamidronate
Electrolyte Supplement, Oral
calcium glubionate
calcium lactate
calcium phosphate (tribasic)
Posture® (US-OTC)
Estrogen and Progestin Combination
estrogens (conjugated/equine) and
medroxyprogesterone
Premphase® (US/Can)
Premplus® (Can)
Prempro™ (US/Can)
Estrogen Derivative
Alora® (US)
Cenestin® (US/Can)
C.E.S.® (Can)
Climara® (US/Can)

Congest (Can)
Delestrogen® (US/Can)
Depo®-Estradiol (US/Can)
Esclim® (US)
Estrace® (US/Can)
Estraderm® (US/Can)
estradiol
Estradot® (Can)
Estrasorb™ (US)
Estratab® (Can)
Estring® (US/Can)
EstroGel® (US/Can)
estrogens (conjugated A/synthetic)
estrogens (conjugated/equine)
estrogens (esterified)
ethinyl estradiol
Femring™ (US)
Gynodiol® (US)
Menest® (US/Can)
Menostar™ (US)
Oesclim® (Can)
Premarin® (US/Can)
Vagifem® (US/Can)
Vivelle-Dot® (US)
Vivelle® (US/Can)
Mineral, Oral
ACT® (US-OTC)
Fluor-A-Day (US-OTC/Can)
fluoride
Fluorigard® (US-OTC)
Fluorinse® (US)
Fluotic® (Can)
Flura-Drops® (US)
Flura-Loz® (US)
Gel-Kam® Rinse (US)
Gel-Kam® (US-OTC)
Lozi-Flur™ (US)
Luride® Lozi-Tab® (US)
Luride® (US)
NeutraCare® (US)
NeutraGard® (US-OTC)
Pediaflor® (US)
Pharmaflur® 1.1 (US)

Pharmaflur® (US)
Phos-Flur® Rinse (US-OTC)
Phos-Flur® (US)
PreviDent® 5000 Plus™ (US)
PreviDent® (US)
Stan-Gard® (US)
Stop® (US)
Thera-Flur-N® (US)
Polypeptide Hormone
Calcimar® (Can)
calcitonin
Caltine® (Can)
Miacalcin® NS (Can)
Miacalcin® (US)
Selective Estrogen Receptor Modulator
(SERM)
Evista® (US/Can)
raloxifene

OVARIAN FAILURE

Estrogen and Progestin Combination
estrogens (conjugated/equine) and
medroxyprogesterone
Premphase® (US/Can)
Premplus® (Can)
Prempro™ (US/Can)
Estrogen Derivative
Alora® (US)
Cenestin® (US/Can)
C.E.S.® (Can)
Climara® (US/Can)
Congest (Can)
Delestrogen® (US/Can)
Depo®-Estradiol (US/Can)
Esclim® (US)
Estrace® (US/Can)
Estraderm® (US/Can)
estradiol
Estradot® (Can)
Estrasorb™ (US)
Estratab® (Can)
Estring® (US/Can)
EstroGel® (US/Can)

estrogens (conjugated A/synthetic)
estrogens (conjugated/equine)
estrogens (esterified)
estrone
estropipate
Femring™ (US)
Gynodiol® (US)
Menest® (US/Can)
Menostar™ (US)
Oesclim® (Can)
Ogen® (US/Can)
Ortho-Est® (US)
Premarin® (US/Can)
Vagifem® (US/Can)
Vivelle-Dot® (US)
Vivelle® (US/Can)

OVULATION INDUCTION

Gonadotropin
chorionic gonadotropin (human)
chorionic gonadotropin
(recombinant)
menotropins
Ovidrel® (US)
Pergonal® (US/Can)
Repronex® (US/Can)
Ovulation Stimulator
chorionic gonadotropin
(recombinant)
Clomid® (US/Can)
clomiphene
Milophene® (Can)
Ovidrel® (US)
Serophene® (US/Can)
urofollitropin

PAIN (DIABETIC NEUROPATHY NEURALGIA)
Analgesic, Topical
Antiphlogistine Rub A-535
Capsaicin (Can)
ArthriCare® for Women Extra
Moisturizing (US-OTC)
ArthriCare® for Women Multi-
Action (US-OTC)
ArthriCare® for Women Silky Dry
(US-OTC)
ArthriCare® for Women Ultra
Strength (US-OTC)
Capsagel® (US-OTC)
capsaicin
Capzasin-HP® (US-OTC)
Zostrix®-HP (US-OTC/Can)
Zostrix® (US-OTC/Can)

PANCREATIC EXOCRINE INSUFFICIENCY
Enzyme
Cotazym® (Can)
Creon® 5 (Can)
Creon® 10 (Can)
Creon® 20 (Can)
Creon® 25 (Can)
Creon® (US)
Ku-Zyme® HP (US)
Lipram 4500 (US)
Lipram-CR (US)
Lipram-PN (US)
Lipram-UL (US)
Pancrease® MT (US/Can)
Pancrease® (US/Can)
Pancrecarb MS® (US)
pancrelipase
Pangestyme™ CN
Pangestyme™ EC
Pangestyme™ MT
Pangestyme™ UL

Ultrase® MT (US/Can)
Viokase® (US/Can)

PANCREATIC EXOCRINE INSUFFICIENCY (DIAGNOSTIC)
Diagnostic Agent
SecreFlo™ (US)
secretin

PITUITARY FUNCTION TEST (GROWTH HORMONE)
Diagnostic Agent
arginine
R-Gene® (US)

PSEUDOHYPO-PARATHYROIDISM
Vitamin D Analog
Calciferol™ (US)
Calcijex® (US)
calcitriol
DHT™ Intensol™ (US)
DHT™ (US)
dihydrotachysterol
Drisdol® (US/Can)
ergocalciferol
Hytakerol® (US/Can)
Ostoforte® (Can)
Rocaltrol® (US/Can)

PUBERTY (DELAYED)
Androgen
Andriol® (Can)
Androderm® (US/Can)
AndroGel® (US/Can)
Android® (US)
Andropository (Can)
Delatestryl® (US/Can)
Depotest® 100 (Can)
Depo®-Testosterone (US)

Everone® 200 (Can)
Methitest® (US)
methyltestosterone
Striant™ (US)
Testim™ (US)
Testoderm® (Can)
Testopel® (US)
testosterone
Testred® (US)
Virilon® (US)
Diagnostic Agent
Factrel® (US)
gonadorelin
Lutrepulse™ (Can)

PUBERTY (PRECOCIOUS)

Hormone, Posterior Pituitary
nafarelin
Synarel® (US/Can)
Luteinizing Hormone-Releasing
Hormone Analog
Eligard® (US)
leuprolide acetate
Lupron Depot-Ped® (US)
Lupron Depot® (US/Can)
Lupron® (US/Can)
Viadur® (US/Can)

SALIVATION (EXCESSIVE)

Anticholinergic Agent
Anaspaz® (US)
AtroPen® (US)
atropine
Atropine-Care® (US)
Buscopan® (Can)
Cantil® (US/Can)
Cystospaz-M® (US)
Cystospaz® (US/Can)
Dioptic's Atropine Solution (Can)
glycopyrrolate
hyoscyamine
Hyosine (US)

Isopto® Atropine (US/Can)
Isopto® Hyoscine (US)
Levbid® (US)
Levsinex® (US)
Levsin/SL® (US)
Levsin® (US/Can)
mepenzolate
Minim's Atropine Solution (Can)
NuLev™ (US)
Robinul® Forte (US)
Robinul® (US)
Sal-Tropine™ (US)
Scopace™ (US)
scopolamine
Spacol T/S (US)
Spacol (US)
Symax SL (US)
Symax SR (US)
Transderm Scop® (US)
Transderm-V® (Can)

SERUM THYROGLOBULIN (TG) TESTING

Diagnostic Agent
Thyrogen® (US/Can)
thyrotropin alpha

SWEATING

Alpha-Adrenergic Blocking Agent
Dibenzyline® (US/Can)
phenoxybenzamine

SYNCOPE

Adrenergic Agonist Agent
Adrenalin® (US/Can)
epinephrine
isoproterenol
Isuprel® (US)
Respiratory Stimulant
ammonia spirit (aromatic)

SYNDROME OF INAPPROPRIATE SECRETION OF ANTIDIURETIC HORMONE (SIADH)
Tetracycline Derivative
   Declomycin® (US/Can)
   demeclocycline

THYROID FUNCTION (DIAGNOSTIC)
Diagnostic Agent
  protirelin
  Relefact® TRH (Can)

THYROIDITIS
Thyroid Product
  Armour® Thyroid (US)
  Cytomel® (US/Can)
  Eltroxin® (Can)
  Levothroid® (US)
  levothyroxine
  Levoxyl® (US)
  liothyronine
  liotrix
  Nature-Throid® NT (US)
  Novothyrox (US)
  Synthroid® (US/Can)
  thyroid
  Thyrolar® (US/Can)
  Triostat® (US)
  Unithroid® (US)
  Westhroid® (US)

THYROTOXIC CRISIS
Antithyroid Agent
  Iosat™ (US-OTC)
  methimazole
  Pima® (US)
  potassium iodide
  propylthiouracil
  Propyl-Thyracil® (Can)

  SSKI® (US)
  Tapazole® (US/Can)

TURNER SYNDROME
Androgen
  Oxandrin® (US)
  oxandrolone

ULCER, DIABETIC FOOT OR LEG
Topical Skin Product
  becaplermin
  Regranex® (US/Can)

VASOACTIVE INTESTINAL PEPTIDE-SECRETING TUMOR (VIP)
Somatostatin Analog
  octreotide
  Sandostatin LAR® (US/Can)
  Sandostatin® (US/Can)

WILSON DISEASE
Chelating Agent
  Syprine® (US/Can)
  trientine

ZOLLINGER-ELLISON SYNDROME
Antacid
  calcium carbonate and simethicone
  Dulcolax® Milk of Magnesia (US-OTC)
  magaldrate and simethicone
  magnesium hydroxide
  magnesium oxide
  Mag-Ox® 400 (US-OTC)
  Phillips'® Milk of Magnesia (US-OTC)
  Titralac™ Plus (US-OTC)
  Uro-Mag® (US-OTC)
Antineoplastic Agent

streptozocin
  Zanosar® (US/Can)
Gastric Acid Secretion Inhibitor
  Aciphex® (US/Can)
  lansoprazole
  Losec® (Can)
  omeprazole
  Pariet® (Can)
  Prevacid® SoluTab™ (US)
  Prevacid® (US/Can)
  Prilosec OTC™ (US-OTC)
  Prilosec® (US)
  rabeprazole
  Zegerid™ (US)
Histamine H₂ Antagonist
  Alti-Ranitidine (Can)
  Apo-Cimetidine® (Can)
  Apo-Famotidine® (Can)
  Apo-Ranitidine® (Can)
  cimetidine
  famotidine
  Gen-Cimetidine (Can)
  Gen-Famotidine (Can)
  Gen-Ranitidine (Can)
  Novo-Cimetidine (Can)
  Novo-Famotidine (Can)
  Novo-Ranidine (Can)
  Nu-Cimet (Can)

Nu-Famotidine (Can)
Nu-Ranit (Can)
Pepcid® AC (US-OTC/Can)
Pepcid® I.V. (Can)
Pepcid® (US/Can)
PMS-Cimetidine (Can)
PMS-Ranitidine (Can)
ranitidine hydrochloride
ratio-Famotidine (Can)
Rhoxal-famotidine (Can)
Rhoxal-ranitidine (Can)
Riva-Famotidine (Can)
Tagamet® HB 200 (US-OTC/Can)
Tagamet® (US)
Zantac® 75 (US-OTC/Can)
Zantac® (US/Can)
Prostaglandin
  Apo-Misoprostil® (Can)
  Cytotec® (US/Can)
  misoprostol
  Novo-Misoprostol (Can)

ZOLLINGER-ELLISON SYNDROME (DIAGNOSTIC)
Diagnostic Agent
  SecreFlo™ (US)
  secretin